PENNSYLVANIA COLLEGE OF TECHNOLOGY LIBR
5 0608 01067523 8

D0085378

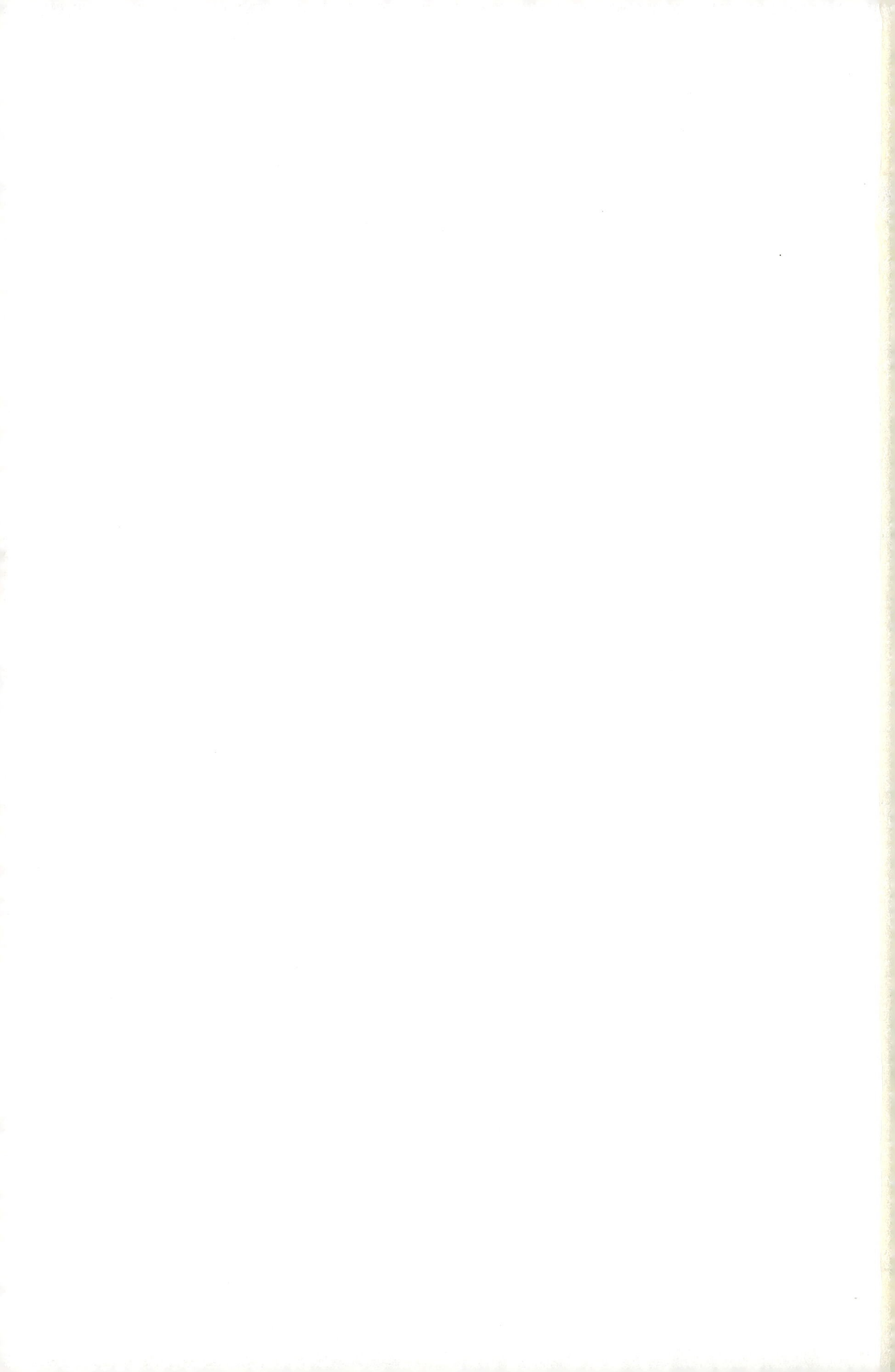

Health Care Ethics

Critical Issues for the 21st Century

John F. Monagle, MA, PhD, DASHRM
President
American Institute of Medical Ethics
Davis, California
Diplomate of the American Society for Healthcare Risk Management
of the American Hospital Association

David C. Thomasma, PhD
Professor and Director
Medical Humanities Program
Stritch School of Medicine
Loyola University Chicago
Maywood, Illinois

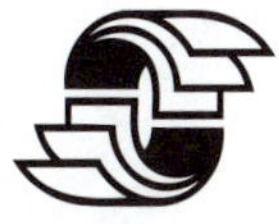

AN ASPEN PUBLICATION®
Aspen Publishers, Inc.
Gaithersburg, Maryland
1998

This publication is designed to provide accurate and authoritative information in regard to the Subject Matter covered. It is sold with the understanding that the publisher is not engaged in rendering legal, accounting, or other professional service. If legal advice or other expert assistance is required, the service of a competent professional person should be sought. (From a Declaration of Principles jointly adopted by a Committee of the American Bar Association and a Committee of Publishers and Associations.)

Library of Congress Cataloging-in-Publication Data

Monagle, John F.
Health care ethics: critical issues for the 21st century/John F. Monagle, David C. Thomasma.
p. cm.
Includes bibliographical references and index.
ISBN 0-8342-0911-X
1. Medical ethics. I. Thomasma, David C. II. Title.
R724.M66 1997
174'2.—dc21
97-23734
CIP

Orders: (800) 638-8437
Customer Service: (800) 234-1660

About Aspen Publishers • For more than 35 years, Aspen has been a leading professional publisher in a variety of disciplines. Aspen's vast information resources are available in both print and electronic formats. We are committed to providing the highest quality information available in the most appropriate format for our customers. Visit Aspen's Internet site for more information resources, directories, articles, and a searchable version of Aspen's full catalog, including the most recent publications: **http://www.aspenpub.com**

Aspen Publishers, Inc. • The hallmark of quality in publishing
Member of the worldwide Wolters Kluwer group.

Editorial Resources: Brian MacDonald
Library of Congress Catalog Card Number: 97-23734
ISBN: 0-8342-0911-X

Printed in the United States of America

2 3 4 5

This book is dedicated to the parents of John F. Monagle:
James and Margaret Mary Monagle; and the siblings of
David C. Thomasma: Robert Paul, Kathleen Rose, Elizabeth Ann,
Thomas Jonathan, Michael Joseph, and Teresa Mary Thomasma.

Table of Contents

Contributors .... **xv**

Preface .... **xxi**

Acknowledgments .... **xxiii**

PART I—REPRODUCTIVE ISSUES **1**

Chapter 1— Proposals for Human Cloning: A Review and Ethical Evaluation **3**
Kevin T. FitzGerald

Preventing Disease 5
Solving Reproductive Problems 5
Supplying Tissues or Organs for Transplantation 6
Replacing a Loved One 7
Conclusion 7

Chapter 2— The Moral Status of Gametes and Embryos: Storage and Surrogacy **8**
Glenn C. Graber

Chapter 3— Prenatal Diagnosis and the Ethics of Uncertainty **15**
Eric T. Juengst

Risk, Benefits, and Eligibility Criteria 16
Selective Abortion and the Therapeutic Imperative 18
Uncertainty and the Ethics of Reproductive Counseling 20
Prenatal Diagnosis for Sex Selection 22
Prenatal Diagnosis for a Treatable Defect 23
Public Health Uses of Prenatal Testing 25
Conclusions 26

Chapter 4— Prenatal Diagnosis of Fetal Disorders: Ethical, Legal, and Social Issues **29**
Diane Beeson and Patricia Jennings

Introduction 29
Testing and Screening Techniques 29

Support for Prenatal Screening and Testing 31
Critical Views on Prenatal Testing and Selective Abortion 33
Conclusion 41

Chapter 5— The Ethical Challenge of the New Reproductive Technology 45
Sidney Callahan

Two Inadequate Approaches to Alternative Reproductive Technology 45
The Basis for Developing an Ethical Position 46
A Proposed Ethical Standard 47
The Family 49
Donors and the Cultural Ethos 52
Conclusion 53

Chapter 6— Ethical Considerations of Preimplantation Genetic Diagnosis and Embryo Selection 56
Frank L. Barnes

Technology 56
Ethical Considerations 57

Chapter 7— Abortion: The Unexplored Middle Ground 60
Richard A. McCormick

Elements of a Middle Ground 61

Chapter 8— Women, Fetuses, Physicians, and the State: Pregnancy and Medical Ethics in the 21st Century 67
Michelle Oberman

Introduction 67
Pregnancy and the Advent of the Maternal–Doctor Relationship 68
High Technology and the Emergence of the Fetus as "Patient" 68
The Emerging Relationship between the State and the Fetus: Turning Doctors into Pregnancy Police 72
Conclusion 75

PART II—ADULT MEDICINE 79

Chapter 9— The Family in Medical Decision Making 81
Jeffrey Blustein

Family Decision Making and Competent Patients 82
The Communitarian Defense of Family Decision Making 84
How the Communitarian Challenge Fails 86
Family Involvement in the Process of Decision Making 88

Chapter 10—The Patient Self-Determination Act 92
David B. Clarke

Background 93
Statement of State Law 96
"On Admission..." 97
Ensuring Compliance 98
Objection on the Basis of Conscience 99
Nondiscrimination 99

Emergency Admissions ... 100
Psychiatric Admissions ... 101
Staff Education ... 102
Public Education ... 103
Five-Year Implementation Update ... 105

Chapter 11—Competency: What It Is, What It Isn't, and Why It Matters ... 117
Byron Chell

What Competency Is and Is Not ... 117
The Search for the Definition of *Competency* ... 118
The Essence of Competency ... 119
Competency is Compatible with "Irrationality"—Religious Refusals ... 120
Conclusions Relating to Competency ... 123
Why It Matters ... 124
Summary and Conclusion ... 125

Chapter 12—Domestic Violence: Changing Theory, Changing Practice ... 128
Carole Warshaw

Personal and Social Barriers ... 129
Systemic Barriers ... 129
Impact of Theory on Clinical Practice ... 130
Structural Constraints ... 132
Implications for Training and Practice ... 133
Conclusion ... 134

Chapter 13—Bioethical Dilemmas in Emergency Medicine and Prehospital Care ... 138
Kenneth V. Iserson

Safety Net ... 138
Emergency Medicine and Managed Care ... 139
Paternalism ... 140
Assisted Suicides and Emergency Department Resuscitations ... 140
Prehospital Advance Directives vs. Prehospital DNR Orders ... 141
Provider Safety and Security ... 142
Practicing and Teaching on the Newly Dead ... 142
Research under Unusual Circumstances ... 143
Other Troublesome Areas ... 144

Chapter 14—High-Technology Home Care: Critical Issues and Ethical Choices ... 146
Allen I. Goldberg, Eveline A. M. Faure, and John J. O'Callaghan

Introduction and Background ... 146
Understanding the Past ... 148
Analyzing the Present ... 152
Approaching the Future ... 155
Conclusion ... 161

Chapter 15—The Plight of the Deinstitutionalized Chronic Schizophrenics: Ethical Considerations ... 164
George B. Palermo

Historical Sketch ... 166
Life, Liberty, and the Pursuit of Happiness ... 168

Socioethical Considerations 169
Statistical Data 170
In Defense of Providing a New Type of Asylum 173
Conclusion 174

Chapter 16—Older People and Long-Term Care: Issues of Access 177
Robert H. Binstock

The Growing Population Needing Care 178
Issues of Access 180
Forces for Improving Access 183
What Prospects for Improved Access? 184

Chapter 17—Treating Senility and Dementia: Ethical Challenges and Quality-of-Life Judgements 189
Stephen G. Post

Diagnostic Disclosure 189
Autonomy 190
Quality of Life and Just Treatment Limitations 191
Long-Term Care 193
Behavior Control 196
Other Issues 198

Chapter 18—Respecting the Autonomy of Elders in Nursing Homes 200
George J. Agich

Independence, Rights, and the Paradox of Autonomous Life in a Nursing Home 200
Actual Autonomy and Identity 202
Nursing Homes 204
Safety Versus Autonomy 205
Identity and the Sense of Home 207
Conclusion 209

Chapter 19—The Ethics of Prediction: Genetic Risk and the Physician–Patient Relationship 212
Eric T. Juengst

Weather Watching, Fortunetelling, and Genetic Testing 213
The Challenges in Genetic Prediction 213
Public Policy Issues 218
Is Genetics Special? The Ideologic Archeology of Clinical Genetics 221
Conclusion: A New Lexicon for Genetic Diagnostics 223

Chapter 20—Human Experimentation and Clinical Consent 228
George J. Agich

The Definitional Problem 228
Practical Aspects 232

Chapter 21—The Ethics of Research on the Mentally Disabled **239**
Adil E. Shamoo and Joan L. O'Sullivan

History of the Medical Abuse of the Mentally Disabled 239
Current Practices 241
IRBs 242
Abuses of the Mentally Disabled 242
Informed Consent and the Mentally Disabled 244
Guidelines for Future Research Using the Mentally Disabled 245
Conclusions 247

Chapter 22—AIDS Activists and Their Legacy for Research Policy **251**
Loretta M. Kopelman

Traditional Methods under Attack 252
Critics of Research as a Cooperative Venture 255
Understanding or Control? 257
Moral and Value Judgments in Research 259
The Case for Research as a Cooperative Venture 261

Chapter 23—The IRB: Current and Future Challenges **265**
Kenneth C. Micetich

Clinical Research—The Protocol 266
Clinical Research Informed Consent 270
Summary 275

PART III—CRITICALLY ILL AND DYING PATIENTS **277**

Chapter 24—Ethical Issues in the Use of Fluids and Nutrition: When Can They Be Withdrawn? **279**
T. Patrick Hill

Chapter 25—Death, Medicine, and the Moral Significance of Family Decision Making **288**
James Lindemann Nelson

The Standard Approach: Romanticizing Death, Demonizing Families 289
A Revised Account: Dying in Intimacy 290
Conclusion: An Objection and a Reply 293

Chapter 26—Care of the Hopelessly Ill: Proposed Clinical Criteria for Physician-Assisted Suicide **295**
Timothy E. Quill, Christine K. Cassel, and Diane E. Meier

Physician-Assisted Suicide 296
A Policy Proposal 296
Proposed Clinical Criteria for Physician-Assisted Suicide 297
The Method 298
Balancing Risks and Benefits 299
Conclusion 300

Chapter 27—Ethical Issues Concerning Physician-Assisted Death **302**
Barbara Supanich and Howard Brody

Introduction and Key Definitions 302
Ethical Arguments 303
Clinical Management of Requests for Assisted Death 306
Placing the Debate in Context 308

Chapter 28—Euthanasia: The Way We Do It, the Way They Do It **311**
Margaret P. Battin

Introduction 311
Dealing with Dying in the United States 311
Dealing with Dying in the Netherlands 312
Facing Death in Germany 315
Objections to the Three Models of Dying 316
The Problem: A Choice of Cultures 318

Chapter 29—The Problem with Futility **323**
Robert D. Truog, Joel E. Frader, and Allan S. Brett

Paradigms of Futility 323
Futility and Values 324
Futility and Statistical Uncertainty 325
Futility and Resource Allocation 326
Moving Beyond Futility 326
Conclusion 328

Chapter 30—Is It Time To Abandon Brain Death? **330**
Robert D. Truog

Definitions, Concepts, and Tests 330
Critique of the Current Formulation of Brain Death 331
Alternative Approaches to the Whole-Brain Formulation 334
Turning Back 339

Chapter 31—Waste Not, Want Not: Communities and Presumed Consent **342**
Erich H. Loewy

The Problem Today 342
Community, Justice, and Mutual Obligation 344
Scarce Resources and Organ Donations 345
Objections to Customary Salvage 346
A Possible Resolution 347

PART IV—JUSTICE AND ECONOMICS IN HEALTH CARE **351**

Chapter 32—Intergenerational Justice: Is It Possible? **353**
Myles N. Sheehan

The Complexity of Justice 353
A Roman Catholic Perspective 356
Some Practical Suggestions on Policy 364

Chapter 33—Gender and Health Insurance **366**
Steven Miles and Kara Parker

Introduction 366
Nonelderly Adults and Private Insurance 366
Elderly Adults and Insurance 367
Medicaid: Old and Young Women Compete 368
Discussion 368

Chapter 34—Is Rationing of Health Care Ethically Defensible? **371**
Chris Hackler

Introduction 371
What is Rationing? 371
Is Rationing Ethically Justifiable? 373
Justifying Rationing in the Real World 374
Who Makes Rationing Decisions? 375
Summary 377

Chapter 35—The Social Obligations of Health Care Practitioners **378**
David T. Ozar

General Social Obligations 378
The Social Obligations of Health Care Practitioners 383
Managed Care 386
Conflict of Obligations 388

Chapter 36—Social Systems and Professional Responsibility **392**
Arlene Gruber

A New Model of Autonomy? 392
The Social Work Perspective 393
A New Bioethics 395
The Moral Universe of Professions 396
The Social Work Perspective 396
Conclusion 397

Chapter 37—Equality and Inequality in American Health Care **399**
Charles J. Dougherty

Inequalities, Born and Made 399
Building Equality 400
Justice, Prudence, and Equality 404

Part V—Institutional Issues **411**

Chapter 38—Rationing Health Care: The Ethics of Medical Gatekeeping **413**
Edmund D. Pellegrino

The De Facto Conflict of Interest 413
Three Forms of Gatekeeping 414
The Ethical Issues in Medical Gatekeeping 416
Some Social-Ethical Concomitants of Rationing 418
Is Rationing Inevitable? 419

Chapter 39—Multiculturalism, Bioethics, and End-of-Life Care: Case Narratives of Latino Cancer Patients **421**
Patricia A. Marshall, Barbara A. Koenig, Donelle M. Barnes, and Anne J. Davis

Cultural Diversity and Decisions at the End of Life: A Review of Empirical Studies 422
Disclosure of a Diagnosis of Terminal Illness 422
Advance Directives for End-of-Life Care 423
Case Narratives 425
Discussion 428

Chapter 40—Technology, Older Persons, and the Doctor-Patient Relationship **432**
Myles N. Sheehan

Technology and Human Relationships 433
Technology, Relationships, and Caring for the Elderly 437
Conclusion 440

Chapter 41—Ethically Important Distinctions among Managed Care Organizations **442**
Kate T. Christensen

Key Distinctions among MCOs 442
Consequences of Managed Care Financial Incentives 446
The Ethical HMO 447
Conclusion 448

Chapter 42—Outcomes Research: The Answer to All Our Health Care Questions or the Question to All Our Health Care Answers? **452**
Cory Franklin

Chapter 43—Hospital Ethics Committees: Roles, Membership, Structure, and Difficulties **460**
David C. Thomasma and John F. Monagle

Basic Roles of the Ethics Committee 460
Structures: Three Models 466
Difficulties and Needs: Ethics Committees and Ethicists 467
Conclusion 469

Chapter 44—Clinical Ethics Consultants: Survey and Practice **471**
Martha Jurchak

Introduction 471
Methodology 471
Establishment of Reliability and Validity 472
Demographic Description of the Sample 473
Findings on Ethics Case Consultation Process 477
Summary 481

Chapter 45—Can There Be Educational and Training Standards for Those Conducting Health Care Ethics Consultation? **484**
Mark P. Aulisio, Robert M. Arnold, and Stuart J. Youngner

Introduction: Motivating the Question 484
Background Questions 486

Central Questions 487
Conclusion 493

Chapter 46—Health Care Institutional Ethics: Broader Than Clinical Ethics 497
Dennis Brodeur

Clinical Concerns 498
Human Resources 498
Work and Human Resources 499
Organizational Identity and Strategic Direction 500
The Public Nature of the Corporation 502
Conclusion 504

Chapter 47—The Ethics of Health Care as a Business 505
Patricia H. Werhane

PART VI—METHODOLOGY 513

Chapter 48—Basic Theories in Medical Ethics 515
Glenn C. Graber

Moral Decisions 515
Ethical Judgements 515
Theories of Moral Obligation 517
Theories of Character 524
Narrative Approaches 524
Conclusion 525

Chapter 49—A Method of Ethical Decision Making 527
Edmund L. Erde

Some Key Concepts and Their Bearings on Dilemmas 527
Moral Theories 531
The Method 535
Conclusion 537

Chapter 50—Getting Down to Cases: The Revival of Casuistry in Bioethics 541
John D. Arras

The Revival of Casuistry 541
A "Case-Driven" Method 542
The Role of Principles in the New Casuistry 543
Problems with the Casuistical Method 546
Conclusion 551

Chapter 51—Literature and Medicine: Contributions to Clinical Practice 554
Rita Charon, Joanne Trautmann Banks, Julia Connelly, Anne Hunsaker Hawkins, Kathryn Montgomery Hunter, Anne Hudson Jones, Martha Montello, and Suzanne Poirier

The Patient's Life 555
The Physician's Work 556
Narrative Knowledge 557
Narrative Ethics 559

Literary Theory and Medicine 560
Discussion 561
Conclusions 561

Chapter 52—Ethically Responsibly Creativity—Friendship of an Understanding Heart: A Cognitively Affective Model for Bioethics Decision Making 566
John F. Monagle

Descriptive Definition of Ethically Responsible Creativity 567
The Cases of Nancy Beth Cruzan and Helga Wanglie 568
The ERC Model 570
Conclusion 575

Chapter 53—Bioethics as Social Problem Solving 578
Paul T. Durbin

Bioethics Philosophically Construed 578
Bioethics More Broadly Construed 582
Pragmatic Reflections on Philosophical Bioethics 583
Some Lessons 584

Chapter 54—Intercultural Reasoning: The Challenge for International Bioethics 587
Patricia A. Marshall, David C. Thomasma, and Jurrit Bergsma

Intercultural Experiences in Bioethical Reasoning 587
Concepts, Meaning, and Medical Morality in Transnational Context 589
Conclusion 591

Index 594

Contributors

George J. Agich, Ph.D.
F.J. O'Neill Chairman
Department of Bioethics
Cleveland Clinic Foundation
Cleveland, Ohio

Robert M. Arnold, M.D.
Associate Professor of Medicine
Division of General Internal Medicine
Center for Medical Ethics
Montefiore University Hospital
Pittsburgh, Pennsylvania

John D. Arras, Ph.D.
Division of Bioethics
Department of Epidemiology and Social Medicine
Albert Einstein College of Medicine
Montefiore Medical Center
Bronx, New York

Mark P. Aulisio, Ph.D.
Research Associate
School of Medicine
University of Pittsburgh
Associate, Center of Medical Ethics
University of Pittsburgh Medical Center
Pittsburgh, Pennsylvania

Joanne Trautmann Banks, Ph.D.
Adjunct Professor of Humanities
Department of Humanities
The Pennsylvania State University College of Medicine
Hershey, Pennsylvania

Donelle M. Barnes, Ph.D., R.N.
Assistant Clinical Professor
Department of Community Health Systems
School of Nursing
University of Texas
Austin, Texas

Frank L. Barnes, Ph.D.
Executive Laboratory Director
Pacific Fertility Medical Centers
Los Angeles, California

Margaret P. Battin, Ph.D.
Department of Philosophy
University of Utah
Salt Lake City, Utah

Diane Beeson, Ph.D.
Professor of Sociology
Department of Sociology and Social Services
School of Arts, Letters and Social Sciences
California State University, Hayward
Hayward, California

Jurrit Bergsma, Ph.D.
Medical Psychologist and Registered Psychotherapist
Institute for Medical and Psychological Consultations
The Netherlands
Permanent Visiting Professor
Loyola University Chicago Medical Center
Maywood, Illinois

Robert H. Binstock, Ph.D.
Professor of Aging, Health & Society
Department of Epidemiology & Biostatistics
School of Medicine
Case Western Reserve University
Cleveland, Ohio

Jeffrey Blustein, Ph.D.
Associate Professor of Bioethics
Albert Einstein College of Medicine
Adjunct Associate Professor of Philosophy
Barnard College
Columbia University
New York, New York

Allan S. Brett, M.D.
Director
Department of General Internal Medicine
Associate Professor
School of Medicine
University of South Carolina
Columbia, South Carolina

Rev. Dennis Brodeur, Ph.D.
Senior Vice President—Stewardship
SSM Health Care System
Adjunct
St. Louis University
School of Public Health
St. Louis, Missouri

Howard Brody, M.D., Ph.D.
Professor, Family Practice and Philosophy
Director, Center for Humanities in the Life Sciences
Michigan State University
East Lansing, Michigan

Sidney Callahan, Ph.D.
Professor of Psychology
Consultant to Hastings Center
Mercy College
Dobbs Ferry, New York

Christine K. Cassel, M.D.
Professor and Chair
The Henry L. Schwartz Department of Geriatrics and Adult Development
Mount Sinai Medical Center
New York, New York

Rita Charon, M.D.
Associate Professor of Clinical Medicine
Department of Medicine
Columbia University
New York, New York

Byron Chell, J.D.
General Counsel
California Medical Assistant Commission
Sacramento, California

Kate T. Christensen, M.D., F.A.C.P.
Internist; Regional Ethic Coordinator
Regional Health Education
Department of Ethics
The Permanente Medical Group, Inc.
Antioch, California

David B. Clarke, D.Min., J.D., M.P.H.
Director
Massachusetts Health Decisions
Sharon, Massachusetts

Julia Connelly, M.D.
Professor of Medicine
University of Virginia Health Sciences Center
Charlottesville, Virginia

Anne J. Davis, R.N., Ph.D.
Professor Emeritus
School of Nursing
University of California, San Francisco
San Francisco, California

Charles J. Dougherty, Ph.D.
Vice President
Academic Affairs
Creighton University
Omaha, Nebraska

Paul T. Durbin, Ph.D.
Professor of Philosophy
University of Delaware
Newark, Delaware

Edmund L. Erde, Ph.D.
Professor, Department of Family Practice
School of Osteopathic Medicine
University of Medicine & Dentistry of New Jersey
Stratford, New Jersey

Eveline A.M. Faure, M.D.
Associate Professor of Clinical Anesthesia
Department of Anesthesia and Critical Care
University of Chicago
Chicago, Illinois

Kevin T. FitzGerald, S.J., Ph.D.
Research Associate
Division of Hematology/Oncology
Department of Medicine
Medical Humanities Program
Loyola University Chicago
Maywood, Illinois

Joel E. Frader, M.D.
Associate Professor of Pediatrics
Associate Professor of Anesthesiology/Critical Care Medicine
Associate Director, Center for Medical Ethics
University of Pittsburgh
Children's Hospital of Pittsburgh
Pittsburgh, Pennsylvania

Cory Franklin, M.D.
Associate Professor
Medicine and Medical Ethics
University of Health Sciences
Chicago Medical School
Director, MICU
Cook County Hospital
Chicago, Illinois

Allen I. Goldberg, M.D., M.M., F.A.C.P.E.
Director, Pediatric Home Health
Professor of Pediatrics
Loyola University Chicago Medical Center
Maywood, Illinois

Glenn C. Graber, Ph.D.
Professor
Department of Philosophy
University of Tennessee
Knoxville, Tennessee

Arlene Gruber, M.S.W., M.A.
Rainbow Hospice
Park Ridge, Illinois
Teaching Associate
Stritch School of Medicine
Loyola University Chicago
Maywood, Illinois

Chris Hackler, Ph.D.
Director
Division of Medical Humanities
University of Arkansas for Medical Science
Little Rock, Arkansas

Anne Hunsaker Hawkins, Ph.D.
Associate Professor
Department of Humanities
Hershey Medical Center
The Pennsylvania State University College of Medicine
Hershey, Pennsylvania

T. Patrick Hill, M.A.
Research Scholar, Ethicist
Research Department
The Park Ridge Center for the Study of Health, Faith and Ethics
Chicago, Illinois

Kathryn Montgomery Hunter, Ph.D.
Director, The Medical Ethics and Humanities Program
Northwestern University Medical School
Chicago, Illinois

Kenneth V. Iserson, M.D., M.B.A., F.A.C.E.P.
Director, Arizona Bioethics Program
Professor of Surgery
Section of Emergency Medicine
University of Arizona College of Medicine
Tucson, Arizona

Patricia Jennings, B.A., M.A., Ph.D. Candidate
Department of Sociology
College of Arts and Sciences
University of Kentucky
Lexington, Kentucky

Anne Hudson Jones, Ph.D.
Professor of Literature & Medicine
Institute for the Medical Humanities
University of Texas, Medical Branch
Galveston, Texas

Eric T. Juengst, Ph.D.
Center for Biomedical Ethics
School of Medicine
Case Western Reserve University
Cleveland, Ohio

Martha Jurchak, R.N., C.S., Ph.D.
Chairman of Ethics
Psychiatric Liaison, Clinical Specialist
Faulkner Hospital
Boston, Massachusetts

Barbara A. Koenig, R.N., Ph.D.
Senior Research Scholar
Center for Biomedical Ethics
Stanford University
Stanford, California

Loretta M. Kopelman, Ph.D.
Professor and Chair
Department of Medical Humanities
School of Medicine
East Carolina University
Greenville, North Carolina

Erich H. Loewy, M.D.
Professor and Endowed Alumni Associate Chair of Bioethics Medical Center
Associate, Department of Philosophy
University of California, Davis
Sacramento, California

Patricia A. Marshall, Ph.D.
Associate Professor and Associate Director
Medical Humanities Program
Stritch School of Medicine
Loyola University Chicago
Maywood, Illinois

Richard A. McCormick, S.J., S.T.D.
John A. O'Brien Professor Emeritus
Department of Theology
University of Notre Dame
Notre Dame, Indiana

Diane E. Meier, M.D.
Department of Geriatrics and Adult Development
Mount Sinai Medical Center
New York, New York

Kenneth C. Micetich, M.D.
Professor of Medicine, Oncology
Chairman: Institutional Review Board for the Protection of Human Subjects
Loyola University Chicago
Maywood, Illinois

Steven Miles, M.D.
Associate Professor of Medicine
Soros Faculty Scholar
Project on Death in America
Department of Geriatric Medicine
St. Paul Ramsey Medical Center
St. Paul, Minnesota
Center for Biomedical Ethics
Department of Medicine and Department for Advanced Feminist Studies
University of Minnesota
Minneapolis, Minnesota

John F. Monagle, M.A., Ph.D., D.A.S.H.R.M.
President, American Institute of Medical Ethics
Davis, California
Diplomate of the American Society for Healthcare Risk Mangement of the American Hospital Association (D.A.S.H.R.M.)

Martha Montello, Ph.D.
Assistant Professor, Medical Humanities
Department of History and Philosophy of Medicine
University of Kansas Medical Center
Kansas City, Kansas

James Lindemann Nelson, Ph.D.
Professor of Philosophy
Department of Philosophy
University of Tennessee
Knoxville, Tennessee

Michelle Oberman, J.D., M.P.H.
Associate Professor of Law
College of Law
DePaul University
Chicago, Illinois

John J. O'Callaghan, S.J., M.A., S.T.D.
Adjunct Assistant Professor
Department of Medicine
Stritch School of Medicine
Loyola University Chicago
Maywood, Illinois

Joan L. O'Sullivan, J.D.
Visiting Assistant Professor
School of Law
University of Maryland at Baltimore
Baltimore, Maryland

David T. Ozar, Ph.D.
Director, Center for Ethics
Professor of Philosophy
Loyola University Chicago
Chicago, Illinois

George B. Palermo, M.D.
Clinical Professor of Psychiatry and Neurology
Medical College of Wisconsin
Milwaukee, Wisconsin
Adjunct Professor of Criminology
Marquette University
Milwaukee, Wisconsin
Lecturer in Ethics and Psychiatry
Stritch School of Medicine
Loyola University Chicago
Maywood, Illinois

Kara Parker, B.A.
Center for Biomedical Ethics
University of Minnesota
Minneapolis, Minnesota

Edmund D. Pellegrino, M.D.
John Carroll Professor of Medicine and Medical Ethics
Center for Clinical Bioethics
Georgetown University Medical Center
Washington, D.C.

Suzanne Poirier, Ph.D.
Associate Professor
Literature and Medical Education
Department of Medical Education
University of Illinois at Chicago
Chicago, Illinois

Stephen G. Post, Ph.D.
Center for Biomedical Ethics
School of Medicine
Case Western Reserve University
Cleveland, Ohio

Timothy E. Quill, M.D.
Professor of Medicine and Psychiatry
University of Rochester
Associate Chief of Medicine
The Genesee Hospital
Rochester, New York

Adil E. Shamoo, Ph.D.
Professor
Department of Biochemistry and Molecular Biology
School of Medicine
University of Maryland
Baltimore, Maryland

Myles N. Sheehan, S.J., M.D.
Assistant Professor of Medicine
Loyola University Medical Center
Maywood, Illinois

Barbara Supanich, R.S.M., M.D.
Associate Chair for Clinical Services
Assistant Professor
Department of Family Practice
College of Human Medicine
Michigan State University
Lansing, Michigan

David C. Thomasma, Ph.D.
Professor and Director
Medical Humanities Program
Stritch School of Medicine
Loyola University Chicago
Maywood, Illinois

Robert D. Truog, M.D.
Director, MICU
Boston Children's Hospital
Associate Professor of Anaesthesia (Pediatrics)
Harvard Medical School
Boston, Massachusetts

Carole Warshaw, M.D.
Director
Behavioral Science
Primary Care Internal Medicine
Director
Hospital Crisis Intervention Project
Cook County Hospital
Adjunct Assistant Professor of Psychiatry
University of Illinois
Chicago, Illinois

Patricia H. Werhane, Ph.D.
Peter and Adeline Ruffin Professor of Business Ethics
Darden School of Business Administration
University of Virginia
Charlottesville, Virginia

Stuart J. Youngner, M.D.
Professor of Medicine, Psychiatry and Biomedical Ethics
Case Western Reserve University
Cleveland, Ohio

Preface

This book is the third in our series of texts on biomedical ethics published by Aspen. The first, *Medical Ethics: A Guide for Health Professionals,* was published in 1988. The second, *Health Care Ethics: Critical Issues,* appeared in 1994. To both of those volumes we have added many new topics and dropped others, such that this work should not be seen as a revision or new edition, but rather as a brand new book. Of previously published chapters only a few appear here without substantial revision and updating.

Much has changed in biomedical ethics in the past four years. New issues are emerging or becoming more prominent. Accordingly we now include many new chapters. In keeping with our aim to include topics of interest to all health professionals, these new chapters include cloning; explorations of the rights of women and reproductive freedom; the role of the state in monitoring pregnancies of troubled women; the role of the family in medical decision making about children; prenatal diagnosis and the ethical challenges that are created for families; domestic violence; high-technology home care; the ethics of prediction about genetics; research on the mentally disabled; preimplantation embryo selection; challenges for Institutional Review Boards; new challenges for ethics committees; possible standards for ethics consultants; family decisions about the dying loved one; ethics of physician-assisted death and euthanasia; as well as intriguing ethical issues in intergenerational justice, rationing health care, gender and health insurance, managed care, outcomes research, literature and medicine, and multicultural and international challenges to medical ethics.

Near the end of editing this new volume, both of us, independently and in our own parts of the country, managed to fall and crack our ribs. We wonder if the closeness we have developed over the years both as colleagues and as friends, has now led to the requirement that to edit yet another volume together means that we must suffer the same medical fates!

We hope you enjoy this new book and find it helpful in your study and your work. If you have any suggestions or comments, please send them to us.

Acknowledgments

We are deeply grateful to our contributing authors for their willingness to labor under difficult deadlines to get their work to us. We wish to thank especially Robbin Hiller, research assistant and senior secretary in the Medical Humanities Program, for her exceptionally cooperative spirit and attention to detail that helped us put this book together. Robbin was the contact person for all correspondence and submissions. She assembled the book while corresponding with authors. Remarkably, Robbin did all this during her pregnancy and after the birth of her second child, so we owe her an even greater debt of gratitude than is normally the case. We also wish to thank Doris Thomasma, senior secretary, and Karin Dean, administrative secretary in the Medical Humanities Program, for their assistance with correspondence, telephoning, tracking submissions, getting permissions, and in some cases, typing and retyping manuscripts. We also wish to thank Jim Monagle for his help with editing and review. We also thank our editor at Aspen, Sandy Cannon, and the able assistance of the staff there in publishing and marketing the book; our freelance copyeditor, Jan Ortiz; and our freelance project editor, Sarah Andrus Kyle. Finally, and as always, we appreciate the support and love of our wives, Marjorie and Doris, for their constant and essential support.

John F. Monagle, Ph.D.
Davis, California

David C. Thomasma, Ph.D.
Maywood, Illinois

PART I

Reproductive Issues

Chapter 1

Proposals for Human Cloning: A Review and Ethical Evaluation

Kevin T. FitzGerald

In August of 1975, Dr. John Gurdon, a British scientist, reported the first successful cloning of frogs using nuclei from adult frogs transplanted into enucleated eggs.[1] This success generated great enthusiasm among scientists for developing techniques for cloning animals. Over the next two decades the initial enthusiasm greatly declined because not only did the cloned frogs never develop into adult frogs, but further experiments seemed to indicate that cloning a mammal from either adult or fetal tissue might never be possible. As scientific interest in cloning waned, so did the apparent need for extensive ethical discussion concerning the possibilities of human cloning. At times it seemed as though only Hollywood was still interested in human cloning with movies such as "The Boys from Brazil" and the more recent "Multiplicity."

On February 22, 1997, Dr. Ian Wilmut and his team of researchers from the Roslin Institute in Scotland regenerated scientific enthusiasm for animal cloning with their announcement of the successful cloning of a sheep. Concurrently, the media and the public reignited speculation about human cloning and its moral implications. In the wake of this renewed interest in human cloning came various proposals concerning what could, might, and should be done with regard to applying this new cloning technique to human beings. It is the intent of this article to review some of these proposals, and to evaluate them as to their scientific probability and ethical justification. Having evaluated these proposals, it will become clear that pursuit of human cloning at this time has neither scientific merit nor adequate ethical justification.

This article will begin the review at the most extreme end of the spectrum of proposals put forth. The journal *Nature Genetics* recently reported a statement made by Dr. Brigitte Boisselier declaring the rights of parents to clone themselves.[2] Dr. Boisselier is the scientific director of Clonaid—a Bahamas-based company that plans to offer human cloning for $200,000. How should one begin to respond to this offer and to Dr. Boisselier's claim for its ethical justification?

Before evaluating this particular news item, the wise course is to clarify the facts about mammalian cloning—at least inasmuch as they are presently known. Then the merits of the Clonaid offer, and other suggestions for the application of this new biotechnology to humans, can be considered.

Why the renewed excitement about mammalian cloning? The reasons for pursuing mammalian cloning have been enumerated in a variety of recent articles and reports. They include such diverse potential benefits as cloning mammals from endangered species, providing clones of genetically engineered animals that produce valuable medicines or tissues, creating mammalian animal models for research into diseases of human development, and furthering research into the aberrations in gene regulation that result in cancers.

The remarkable scientific article published by Wilmut et al., in the February 27 issue of the journal *Nature,* demonstrated that it was now possible to use cells from the differentiated tissue of an adult mammal to produce a clone of apparently normal characteristics.[3] Differentiated tissue is primarily composed of cells that have taken on specialized functions and, consequently, have turned off all the other genes not needed to perform these specialized functions. Many researchers had feared that it would never be possible to turn these genes back on so that cells from an adult mammal, or even a fetal mammal, might be used to produce a viable clone.

Though the cloning of Dolly has been rightly heralded as a major breakthrough in science, there still remain many obstacles to the application of this technology in other mammalian species, and even to its efficient use in sheep. In fact, there are characteristics of sheep embryological development that may account for the success of cloning an adult sheep while similar attempts in cattle, pigs, and mice have so far been unsuccessful.

One particular obstacle, which the Roslin researchers were able to circumvent in Dolly's case, is a natural incompatibility between the cellular activities of a differentiated cell and those of an egg cell.[4] In past experiments in mammals, this incompatibility has resulted in genetic abnormalities occurring within the developing cloned embryo that prove fatal to the clone. The Roslin researchers overcame this problem by starving the adult sheep cells until they became quiescent. Then when the adult cell was fused with the enucleated egg cell, the genetic material of the adult cell was presumably remodeled by the cellular components of the egg so that normal embryological development could ensue.

An advantageous aspect of sheep development is that the genes in the nucleus are not all turned on until after the fertilized egg has divided into 8 or 16 cells. This delay may allow enough gene remodeling to take place so that the embryos develop normally. Mouse experiments, on the other hand, may not work with this protocol because the mouse genes are activated during the two-cell stage. Extensive human gene activation occurs at the 4–8 cell stage, and this slightly earlier activation may affect the possibilities of applying the Roslin cloning technique to humans.

How, then, to evaluate Clonaid's bold offer? Since Clonaid made its announcement after Dolly arrived on the scene, it can be presumed that they intend to use the Roslin procedure in their attempt to clone human beings. If the question of the timing between gene modeling and gene activation raised above is taken into consideration, as well as the many other obstacles involved in cloning that can be discerned from the fact that so far there is only one Dolly, then Clonaid's offer may not just be another example of irresponsible advertising but also of irresponsible medicine.

Moving inward from this extreme end of the spectrum, more measured and reasonable proposals have been made concerning possible uses for human cloning in the future. All of them, of course, assume that animal research will indicate a strong possibility for success. Still, even these suggestions would eventually require attempting the refined cloning techniques on human beings who, it is hoped, will develop normally through birth to adulthood, and who then may desire to have children of their own. In the world medical community, research on human subjects requires that the research promise significant benefit to the human community and minimal risk to the subject before it can proceed.[5] Research into human cloning was considered unacceptable for federal funding when it was reviewed by the National Institutes of Health Human Embryo Research Panel (NIHHERP).[6] In light of this, then, any reasons put forward for attempting such cloning should decidedly outweigh the risks and costs to the clone, and to society.

These more moderate proposals for pursuing human cloning also spread out along a bit of a spectrum. They extend from responses to psychological grief at the loss of a loved one to possible medical interventions intended to prevent the passage of disease from one generation to the next. If the focus is first on the cases that represent the more traditional types of medical interventions, it will allow the presentation of scientific information that will also apply to the cases introduced later.

PREVENTING DISEASE

Not all genetic diseases are caused by mutations or abnormalities found within the genes located in the nucleus of a cell. Human cells contain many small structures outside the nucleus, called mitochondria, that are crucial to cell function, and that contain their own genes. Egg cells have many mitochondria, and even though sperm also have them, sperm mitochondria generally do not get into the egg when fertilization occurs. Therefore, only the mother has to be concerned about passing on a mitochondrial disease to her children.

One proposal that seeks to justify human cloning is the removal of a nucleus from an embryo that has inherited diseased mitochondria from the mother, and the implantation of that nucleus in an enucleated egg cell from healthy mitochondria. Hence the genetic characteristics inherited from both parents' chromosomes would remain and the diseased mitochondria would be eliminated. Since this procedure would be done directly to treat a disease that could be severely detrimental to the health of the offspring, it is proposed as conforming to the accepted medical ethos mentioned above of risking the health of the individual in order to achieve an even greater benefit.

The most direct ethical response to this proposal is to call attention to the fact that there is research presently being done on an alternative therapy that appears to have much less risk to the offspring and that can achieve the same medical benefit.[7] In this therapy the nucleus of the mother's egg is transferred to an enucleated egg cell with healthy mitochondria. If the transfer works, the new egg can be returned to its proper environment and hopefully be fertilized. The significant ethical difference here is that the human cloning procedure requires research on and manipulation of human embryos, while the nuclear transfer done just with eggs does not. Regardless of their final evaluation of the moral and legal status of human embryos, the vast majority of people involved with the topic of reproductive technology do not consider human eggs to have the same status as human embryos since the gametes themselves do not have the potential to develop and grow into individual human beings.

SOLVING REPRODUCTIVE PROBLEMS

What of parents who face both genetic and reproductive obstacles to having their own children? Some have proposed that human cloning could be another alternative in the array of assisted reproductive technologies (ART) offered to such couples. Again, one direct response would be to review all the options already available, or already being researched, for couples to combat genetic and infertility problems. Why risk the life and health of one's offspring by employing an experimental procedure of unknown, or at least lesser known, safety and predictability than the procedures already available? One could propose the possibility that no other alternatives are available to the couple except attempting to clone one of them. If cloning is the only option, should it be pursued? It is at this point in the ethical evaluation of the some of the proposals for human cloning that the impact of the more social aspects of medical technology becomes clear.

Proposing human cloning to solve reproduction problems, for example, depends heavily on the argument that people have the right to have genetically related offspring. When discussing such rights, it is important to distinguish between negative (liberty) rights and positive (welfare) rights. In 1994, the Ethics Committee of The American Fertility Society (now The American Society of Reproductive Medicine) stated that in the context of procreation, "A liberty right would encompass the moral freedom to reproduce or to assist others in reproducing without violating any countervailing moral obligations. A welfare right to reproduce would morally entitle one to be assisted by another party (or other parties) in achieving the goal of reproduction."[8]

Since the legal liberty right to reproduce is virtually unlimited in the United States, the Committee considered the possibilities of moral limitations on reproductive liberty rights.[9] They concluded that concerns about harm, specifically harm to the child but also harm to the public good, could limit reproductive liberty rights. As mentioned above, there is a significant chance of harm to the child even if the efficiency of the process can be improved in other species. This possible harm in itself could justify a prohibition on using human cloning to treat reproductive difficulties. Additional harm to the common good would tip the scales decidedly against human cloning.

Another part of this argument for using human cloning as a reproductive technology is the emphasis on having genetically related children. When pushed to an extreme such as the support for human cloning, it becomes evident that a genetic reductionism underlies this perspective. Are genes the only possible basis for the parent–child relationship? Is human identity and personality merely genetic? If all people are is contained within their genes, then genetic makeup is who human beings are and how human beings are related. But then what of adopted children who call their parents "mom and dad", or those who look to teachers or mentors as the ones who have been most instrumental in forming their identities?

A consistent response from scientists during this furor about the possibility of human cloning has been to remind people that we are more than our genes, even on a physiological level. One's environment plays a significant role in shaping one's identity and characteristics. For instance, whence comes the strong desire to have genetically related children? Is it a desire rooted in one's genes, or is it a social construct derived from a desire within a culture to search for technical solutions to all our difficulties? If indeed there is a social element, then it becomes crucial to investigate carefully how much of the individual and social environment people are willing to sacrifice in order to pursue the opportunity for anyone and everyone to have genetically related children. As soon as there is a good understanding of what this cloning technology can do, what is done with it will say a great deal about how people and communities see themselves and how they wish to relate to one another. Examining still another proposed use for human cloning will help elucidate this point.

SUPPLYING TISSUES OR ORGANS FOR TRANSPLANTATION

One of the first proposals for the use of human cloning was to supply needed tissues or organs for transplantation. In its most heartrending form, this proposal seeks to address the situation where a child or infant requires a transplantation in order to live. The parents, it is proposed, could clone the child to produce a genetically identical sibling. Presuming that the older child's disease does not have a genetic basis, the clone could then donate an organ or tissue to save the life of the older sibling. Again, it is helpful to check and see what the present state of medical research is, because in this case, buoyed by the Roslin progress, researchers are hoping to develop genetically engineered animals that could be sources of organs and tissue compatible for transplantation into humans.

This potential medical advance using animals is not the only reason, though, to refrain from using human cloning for transplantation purposes. Contemporary society holds that no adult should be forced to donate an organ or tissue against his or her will, not even to save the life of an innocent child. In an extension of this position, parents can speak for their child in volunteering to donate tissue if it will not threaten or impair the child's life.[10] But on what ethical grounds could one choose, in the name of an individual who does not, as yet, exist, to take the risks of applying cloning techniques to produce that individual when a central purpose of his or her existence will be to donate tissues or organs to someone else? (Ethics aside, what are the legal possibilities of a "wrongful life" suit?)

Some argue in defense of this proposal that the cloned child would be loved and cared for every bit as much as any child. In a society that places a value on providing love and care for all children, that is not the issue. The issue is that the cloned child was specifically created to donate part of his or her body to another. The tissue or organ donation is part of the reason for the clone's being. What sense of autonomy or equality or dignity does a child begin to possess when the realization dawns that he or she was produced/created/made/born principally to provide a biological part for another? In light of this potential for psychological and emotional harm to all who are cloned for such a purpose, as well as the potential for societal harm with the creation of an "underclass" of human donors, the balance of arguments is clearly against applying cloning techniques to humans.

REPLACING A LOVED ONE

Moving back toward the extreme end of the spectrum, it has been proposed that human cloning might be employed so that a couple could "replace" a dying child, or a person could replace a dying spouse. As in the previous case, there is a dangerous biological reductionism inherent in this proposal. No human being is replaceable—not even physiologically. We are all unique. The desire to clone a loved child or spouse to "replace" the lost loved one, therefore, may well indicate a retreat to a biological solution from the age-old problem of dealing with the grief and trauma of death. Even if the psychological struggle with the loss of a loved one is eventually dealt with successfully, the cloned child or spouse will always have to live with the reality of having been cloned to replace another.

Aside from suggesting that cloning technology be applied to human beings in order to achieve a particular benefit, might one argue that research into human cloning be done simply in the interest of discovering whatever knowledge could accrue from such research? Even to entertain such an argument it would have to be demonstrated that crucial scientific knowledge could not be obtained without the use of human subjects, as mentioned above (see note 5).

CONCLUSION

We have considered several proposals regarding the possibility of human cloning. These range from possible medical interventions for directly treating disease to meeting perceived psychological or societal needs. In the final analysis, there is presently no ethically justifiable reason to apply the recent advances in cloning techniques to human beings.

NOTES

1. J.B. Gurdon, R.A. Laskey, O.R. Reeves, "The developmental capacity of nuclei transplanted from keratinized skin cells of adult frogs," *Journal of Embryology and Experimental Morphology* 34 (1975): 93–112.
2. "News and views," *Nature Genetics* 15 (1997): 336.
3. I. Wilmut, A.E. Schnieke, J. McWhir, A.J. Kind, K.H.S. Campbell, "Viable offspring derived from fetal and adult mammalian cells," *Nature* 385 (1997): 810–13.
4. C. Stewart, "An udder way of making lambs," *Nature* 385 (1997): 770.
5. This ethos has been codified in many documents including *The Nuremberg Code* and the World Medical Association's *Declaration of Helsinki.*
6. U.S. National Institutes of Health, Human Embryo Research Panel (Ad Hoc Group of Consultants to the Advisory Committee to the Director, NIH), Report, Vol. 1, September 1994.
7. D.S. Rubenstein, D.C. Thomasma, E.A. Schon, M.J. Zinaman, "Germ-line Therapy to Cure Mitochondrial Disease: Protocol and Ethics of *In Vitro* Ovum Nuclear Transplantation." *Cambridge Quarterly of Healthcare Ethics* 4 (1995): 316–39.
8. The Ethics Committee of the American Fertility Society, *Fertility and Sterility* 62 (1994): Supp. 1, 18S.
9. Ibid., 19S.
10. G. Raanan, "Transplantation and ethics," in DC Thomasma and T Kushner, eds. *Birth to Death: Science and Bioethics* (Cambridge: Cambridge University Press, 1996), 106–118.

Chapter 2

The Moral Status of Gametes and Embryos: Storage and Surrogacy

Glenn C. Graber

Technology complicates issues about human reproduction by increasing the number of choices available to us. The chart in Table 2–1 that I have whimsically entitled "39 Ways to Make a Baby" illustrates this.

Technology has made possible a separation of the roles of genetic mother (who contributes germ cells, perhaps for in vitro fertilization) from that of gestational mother (in whose uterus the fetus develops); and the social mother (who cares for the child after its birth) may be different from either of these. The ultimate possibility is expressed in line 31 of the chart where the baby has five parents—or perhaps six if you count the technician who delivers the sperm to the ovum as a sort-of father.

Who among these five or six are *really* the parents of the resulting baby? Who should be given authority to make decisions about whether to continue the pregnancy if complications should develop? Who should have a say in decisions about terminating treatment after birth if the newborn is seriously compromised?

And, not only are these relationships complex, but the decision points are multiplied greatly beyond the traditional possibilities. Until the advent of the birth-control pill, there was no safe way to stop the process between fertilization and implantation, since these took place in the inaccessible regions of the woman's reproductive tract. Now many of the early steps in the reproductive process can be carried out in the laboratory, and we may have to decide at each stage whether to move forward to the next stage as well as with whom to consult about the decisions.

These are possibilities with which we are not conceptually, emotionally, or ethically prepared to deal. We must sort out myriad questions about the status of the entity at each stage and the relationship of the other parties to this entity.

I am convinced that the thorny question of the moral status of the materials of human reproduction will be settled, if at all, by decision rather than by discovery. It is less an ontological question than a political one (in the broadest sense of the term *political,* referring to the conventions and agreements among the members of a community or a society). Information about the entities in question may, of course, be relevant to the outcome—but not in anything like the way that further analysis of the molecular structure of a meteorite from Mars may furnish evidence for or against the question of whether there is life on that planet.

The issue here is to establish the boundaries of the moral community—who counts, morally; who stands, to us (those of us in the acknowledged moral community), in a way that requires us to take them into account in a central way in our decisions and actions. These boundaries are ones that the community *draws for itself,* not lines that we discover embedded in the ontological landscape.

This issue transcends the usual divide in ethical theory between teleological and deontological theories. Before teleologists begin to calculate the

Table 2–1 Thirty-Nine Ways To Make a Baby

		Source of Germ Cells		*Delivery of Sperm*	*Site of Fertilization*	*Site of Gestation*	*Social Parents*	
		♂	♀				♂	♀
1	traditional	S♂	S♀	S♂	S♀	S♀	S♂	S♀
2	AIH	S♂	S♀	technician	S♀	S♀	S♂	S♀
3	IVF	S♂	S♀	→	in vitro	S♀	S♂	S♀
4	DSI	S♂	S♀	direct sperm injection	in vitro	S♀	S♂	S♀
5	rent-a-womb	S♂	S♀	→	in vitro	surrogate	S♂	S♀
6	artificial womb	S♂	S♀	→	in vitro	artif. womb	S♂	S♀
7	adultery-a	G♂	S♀	G♂	S♀	S♀	?	S♀
8	AID	G♂	S♀	technician	S♀	S♀	S♂	S♀
9	AID + IVF	G♂	S♀	→	in vitro	S♀	S♂	S♀
10	AID + rent-a-womb	G♂	S♀	→	in vitro	surrogate	S♂	S♀
11	AID + artif. womb	G♂	S♀	→	in vitro	artif. womb	S♂	S♀
12	adultery-b	S♂	G♀	S♂	G♀	G♀	S♂	?
13	surrogate (AID)	S♂	G♀	technician	G♀	G♀	S♂	S♀
14	ovum donor	S♂	G♀	→	in vitro	S♀	S♂	S♀
15	surrogate (IVF)	S♂	G♀	→	in vitro	surrogate	S♂	S♀
16	#14 + artif. womb	S♂	G♀	→	in vitro	artif. womb	S♂	S♀
17	fornication	G♂	G♀	G♂	G♀	G♀	?	?
18	bachelor motherhood	G♂	S♀	G♂	S♀	S♀	—	S♀
19	#17 + AID	G♂	S♀	technician	S♀	S♀	—	S♀
20	#18 + IVF	G♂	S♀	→	in vitro	S♀	—	S♀
21	#19 + rent-a-womb	G♂	S♀	→	in vitro	surrogate	—	S♀
22	#19 + artif. womb	G♂	S♀	→	in vitro	artif. womb	—	S♀
23	bachelor fatherhood	S♂	G♀	S♂	G♀	G♀	S♂	—
24	#22 + AID	S♂	G♀	technician	G♀	G♀	S♂	—
25	#23 + IVF	S♂	G♀	→	in vitro	G♀	S♂	—
26	#24 + rent-a-womb	S♂	G♀	→	in vitro	surrogate	S♂	—
27	#24 + artif. womb	S♂	G♀	→	in vitro	artif. womb	S♂	—
28	adoption	G♂	G♀	G♂	G♀	G♀	S♂	S♀
29	#27 + AID	G♂	G♀	technician	G♀	G♀	S♂	S♀
30	#28 + IVF	G♂	G♀	→	in vitro	G♀	S♂	S♀
31	five parents (or is it six?)	G♂	G♀	→	in vitro	surrogate	S♂	S♀
32	#29 + artif. womb	G♂	G♀	→	in vitro	artif. womb	S♂	S♀
33	clone—male	S♂	—	→	in vitro	?	S♂	?
34	clone—female	—	S♀	→	in vitro	?	?	S♀
35	twin fission	?	?	?	twin fission	?	?	?
36	embryo transfer	G♂	G♀	G♂	embryo transfer	?	S♂	S♀
37	GIFT/POST/DIPI	S♂	S♀	technician	S♀	S♀	S♂	S♀
38	cryopreservation	?	?	?	?	?	?	?
39	genetic therapy	?	?	?	gene therapy	?	?	?

Note: S♂ = social father; S♀ = social mother; ? = unknown—indicates multiple possibilities; AID = artificial insemination by donor; DIPI = Direct Intraperitoneal Insemination; GIFT = Gamete Intrafallopian Transfer; POST = Peritoneal Ovum and Sperm Transfer; G♂ = genetic father (merely); G♀ = genetic mother (merely); — = none; AIH = artificial insemination by husband; DSI = Direct Sperm Injection; IVF = in vitro fertilization and embryo transfer.

Source: Reprinted with permission from G. Graber, Ethics and Reproduction, in *Bioethics,* R.B. Edwards and G. Graber, eds., p. 635, © 1988, Harcourt, Brace, and Jovanovich.

consequences of their actions, they must determine *whose* welfare is to count; only then can they begin the process of calculating which action is optimal. I have elsewhere[1] distinguished between several characterizations of what I there called the moral reference group (Table 2–2):

Two teleologists with identical theories of value may come up with very different assessments of a given course of action if they approach their welfare calculations from the perspective of different moral reference groups. For example, a thoroughgoing sexist, who refuses to take into account the interests of one gender, would come to a very different conclusion about the optimal division of household tasks in a typical family than one who took the interests of *all* members of the household into account.

Determination of the moral reference group is also a metatheoretical issue for deontologism. Kant's categorical imperative, for example, glosses together the moral reference group of personalism with that of humanism when it is phrased to read: "Act so that you treat humanity, whether in your own person or in that of another, always as an end and never as a means only."[2] It might be unclear whether this definition applies to persons only or to all humans, but it is clear that it does *not* countenance sexism, racism, or nationalism and that it does not include the lower animals in the moral community. Kant was no animal-rights advocate.

The debate about animal rights is instructive in illuminating the issues here. Animal-rights advocates point out the features of (lower) animals that are similar to human attributes (especially, the capacity to suffer pain) and accuse us of inconsistency if we uphold moral rules against certain sorts of treatment of humans at the same time that we allow similar treatment of animals. I contend that, even if successful, this argument is not enough to establish so-called rights in any full-blooded sense or to establish genuine moral standing for animals. Even if we are persuaded by these arguments that we have been needlessly cruel in our treatment of animals in food production, research, and so forth and resolve to treat them in less cruel and more humane ways in the future, we are still a long way from granting them genuine moral standing or membership in the moral community.

Moral standing entails going beyond describing actions as cruel or inhumane. For members of the moral community, there is possibly another, more serious category of wrong that goes beyond these—the wrong of moral affront, indignity, or disrespect. One can show disrespect without being cruel (through diffidence, for example); and one can cause pain (and perhaps even be cruel in a sense) without showing disrespect (as when a father refrains from rescuing his son from a painful experience in the interest of allowing him to experience the natural consequences of a mistake that he has made so that he will learn the wrongness of it). The common element in instances of disrespect or affronts to dignity has to do with the breakdown in an

Table 2–2 Moral Reference Groups

Label	*Scope of Moral Reference Group*
Personalism	Persons and only persons
Humanism	Humans and only humans
Vitalism	All and only living entities
Racism	All and only members of one race
Nationalism	All and only citizens of a nation
Sexism	All and only those of one gender
Universalism	All and only sentient creatures

established system of cooperative mutual interaction. Instead of treating you as a colleague engaged in a joint enterprise, I fail to acknowledge your interests or concerns and "use" you to further goals of my own. This notion of indignity or disrespect is the core notion in moral standing. If nothing we do qualifies as an indignity, they lack full moral standing.[3]

Individually, some of us may form such a bond with our pets that they are virtually admitted to our moral circle and thus we regard a slight to them as an indignity; but we are a long way as a society from having this regard for lower animals generally. The day might come when we do; and we might then look back on our treatment of animals nowadays with the same disdain as we hold for the institution of slavery in our nation's past. But, unless and until we reach this sort of general understanding of their status, it cannot be said that animals are admitted into the moral community.

It is difficult to say precisely when (if ever) the status of moral standing will have been established for animals. It is not enough for one or two visionaries to treat them in this way and to urge us to follow their example. It is also probably not necessary for every member of the moral community to acknowledge their standing. There is some (ill-defined) threshold of acceptance that would lead a moral anthropologist to say that this entity has become a full-fledged member of our moral community.

Questions can be raised, in this regard, as to whether children are fully established members of our moral community. Child-abuse statutes are on the books throughout our society, but they are not always seriously enforced. Gross abuse of children by their parents is all too often condoned by the authorities as acceptable discipline or as within the domain of the privacy of the family and therefore none of the community's business. If we are still at this stage with regard to children more than a century after humane societies were established to campaign against cruelty to children and animals, it is not surprising that we are uncertain about the moral standing of reproductive materials or of the embryo at various stages of its development.

Technological developments in the reproductive area not only increase the points at which we may (and perhaps must) make decisions, but they also have an ambiguous impact on our attitude toward the developing embryo. On the one hand, the use of ultrasound gives the expectant parent(s) prenatal contact with and experience of the embryo. I have heard more than one couple describe the ultrasound images of their fetus in utero as "our first baby pictures." On the other hand, the greater awareness of the uncertainties of pregnancy that have come through our diagnostic technologies have led to what one commentator has called "the tentative pregnancy,"[4] in which women do not fully acknowledge that they are pregnant (especially to their friends but also attitudinally to themselves) until early ultrasounds and/or amniocentesis have established that the fetus is free from the sort of significant problems that might lead to miscarriage or to a decision to have an elective abortion.

How does the separation of roles within the reproductive process affect the stake of the various parties in the decisions to be made? It is far from clear. Parents whom I know who have both one or more children who are genetically theirs and one or more who are adopted would insist that there is no fundamental difference in their commitment, emotional attachment, or sense of parenthood toward these children. Indeed, after a while, they may have to stop to remember which children are genetically theirs and which are not. Similarly, when the case was first in the news a few years ago about a child who had been switched at birth with another baby some dozen or so years earlier, I asked many of my friends who have children how they would feel if they were to learn after many years that the child they had been caring for was not genetically their child. I could not find any people who would begin to countenance the possibility of returning the child they now have to his or her genetic parents and taking on responsibility for the child that was genetically theirs. They uniformly and emphatically said that they considered the child now in their household as *their* child, and the other child, although having genetic links to them, would be a stranger to them.

And yet people expend enormous resources and effort in attempts to have a child who is genetically theirs—whereas many adoptable children languish in institutions or foster homes. To these people at this stage of the career of parenthood, genetics matters a great deal; to most people at a later stage of the career, it seems to matter a great deal less. The child that I have cared for and established a relationship with is clearly mine, no matter whether he or she is genetically mine; the child that I propose to care for is less obviously mine merely because I am entrusted with her or his care. I suggest that identification comes with extended contact with the child and getting to know that child as a person. Until that point has been reached, the child is, in a way, an abstraction—but the abstraction may be more nearly identified with myself if I am aware of our genetic linkage. All this suggests that genetics is far from fundamental to the long-range bond between child and parent.

The interest of adopted children in learning about their genetic parents raises similar ambiguities. Most (but not all) adopted children report a strong interest in learning about their genetic parentage; but most also insist that this interest does not interfere with or diminish their emotional ties to the parents who cared for them since birth.

There is one more complication introduced by new technologies: Even if the notion of the zygote and/or fetus as a potential person could be given sense in traditional reproduction—perhaps in terms of the course of development that would occur naturally if nature were left without interference to follow its course—this makes little or no sense nowadays. The natural course of events for a frozen preembryo is inertial—it will remain in suspended animation until some intervention occurs to change its status. There is little practical difference between the potential for personhood of a frozen preembryo and that for an individual germ cell that has not yet been joined with another. Only one additional laboratory step is required to move the individual sperm or ovum onto the path toward becoming a person. Only one additional step is required to move the frozen preembryo onto the same path. Without technical intervention, the potential is nil in both cases.

These several ambiguities cannot help but be reflected in our valuation of the entity in question and our decision making about it. A preembryo is not the same as a child; there is a vast gap between the ways we experience and think of this stage of the reproductive process and the ways we think of a child.

It is argued that the preembryo is already genetically individuated and thus that it should be accorded the respect due to any human being; but this overlooks at least two respects in which a preembryo falls short of human status. For one thing, twinning could occur after this stage, so we may have here the proto stage of *two* persons (i.e., identical twins) instead of one individual. Second, the cells at this stage are not yet differentiated in terms of which cell will become one organ and which another—and, indeed, some of the cells that form part of the unified organism at this point of development will differentiate into placental material and thus will ultimately be discarded. Thus, it flies in the face of genetic fact to insist at this stage that the person who will (perhaps) come into being is present in some inchoate form. Furthermore, the probabilities of carrying the preembryo to term are only in the neighborhood of 5 percent even if it is implanted, so the odds are decisively against having a child develop from this clump of cells.

These sorts of considerations led the Ethics Committee of the American Fertility Society to conclude:

> We find a widespread consensus that the preembryo is not a person but is to be treated with special respect because it is a genetically unique, living human entity that might become a person. In cases in which transfer to a uterus is possible, special respect is necessary to protect the welfare of the potential offspring. In that case, the

> preembryo deserves respect because it might come into existence as a person. This viewpoint imposes the traditional duty of reasonable prenatal care when actions risk harm to prospective offspring. Research on or intervention with a preembryo, followed by transfer, thus creates obligations not to hurt or injure the offspring who might be born after transfer.[5]

Applying this reasoning to the multitude of decisions that might arise leads to a sensitive and morally serious approach. The various parties affected by choices ought to have some significant voice in decisions, and all parties should take into account the special respect owed to these entities at every stage as well as the special precautions to be taken if the entities are to be implanted and allowed to develop.

Surrogate contracts ought not to be regarded as indistinguishable from, for example, a contract that a woman might enter into to keep some piece of property in trust for a period of time. In addition to fiduciary duties to the contracting parties, the surrogate mother has special obligations of due care to protect the life that is hoped to result. However, if her life or health became threatened from continuing the pregnancy, it would be unreasonable to expect her to jeopardize her future in order to continue the process—so she would retain her right to abortion. The legal right to elective abortion might remain even if her reasons for ending the pregnancy were less weighty (e.g., the notorious case of the threatened deposit on a scheduled cruise or pique over a late expense payment by the contracting parties); but ethically we would surely criticize her for failure to show the special respect that is due to the fetus.

Surrogacy arrangements ought to be developed with caution, recognizing that we are not dealing with a mere material possession here but with an entity that merits special respect and that may well generate intense emotions in the gestational mother, thus making it difficult for her to carry through agreements to give the child up and sever all ties.

It may be too much to expect the law to be responsive to all these ambiguities—at least immediately; but our ethical thinking in this area needs to take them into account. We are dealing here with issues in which our thinking must be stretched to provide nuanced, sensitive ethical guidance. It would be too heavy-handed to prohibit development of this technology because we do not have a ready set of rules for dealing with its ethical dimensions. It is simplistic to thrust these decisions into the procrustean bed of our moral rules for dealing with already-born children. Instead, we must undertake the task of sorting through the complexities and ambiguities of these unprecedented human dilemmas and attempt to come to consensus on the courses of action that maximize all the values involved. Casuistry (in the best sense) is called for, since we have a moral landscape before us that has been heretofore uncharted and that must be filled in through the most careful and sensitive analysis of all its features.

NOTES

1. G.C. Graber, A.D. Beasley, and J.A. Eaddy, *Ethical Analysis of Clinical Medicine: A Guide to Self-Evaluation* (Baltimore: Urban & Schwarzenberg, 1985), 256–258.
2. I. Kant, *Foundations of the Metaphysics of Morals,* translated by Lewis White Beck (Indianapolis, Ind.: Bobbs-Merrill, 1959), 47.
3. For a fuller account of this argument, see R.B. Edwards and G.C. Graber, *Bioethics* (New York: Harcourt, Brace, Jovanovich, 1988), 16–18.
4. B. Katz Rothman, *The Tentative Pregnancy: Prenatal Diagnosis and the Future of Motherhood* (New York: Viking/Penguin, 1986).
5. "Ethical Considerations of the New Reproductive Technologies" by the Ethics Committee of the American Fertility Society, *Fertility and Sterility,* Supplement 2, 53:6 (1990): 35S.

FURTHER READING

Glover, Jonathan. *Ethics of New Reproductive Technologies: The Glover Report to the European Commission.* DeKalb, Ill.: Northern Illinois University Press, 1989.

Grobstein, Clifford. "FETUS: I. Human Development from Fertilization to Birth." In *Encyclopedia of Bioethics.* Rev. ed., edited by Warren T. Reich. New York: Macmillan Library Reference, 1995.

Humber, James M., and Robert F. Almeder, eds. *Bioethics and the Fetus: Medical, Moral and Legal Issues.* Totowa, N.J.: Humana Press, 1991.

Mahowald, Mary B. "FETUS: II. Philosophical and Ethical Issues." In *Encyclopedia of Bioethics.* Rev. ed., edited by Warren T. Reich. New York: Macmillan Library Reference, 1995.

Walters, William, and Peter Singer. *Test-Tube Babies: A Guide to Moral Questions, Present Techniques, and Future Possibilities.* New York: Oxford University Press, 1982.

Chapter 3

Prenatal Diagnosis and the Ethics of Uncertainty

Eric T. Juengst

With the thirtieth anniversary of the first chromosomal analysis of human amniocytes, medicine celebrates three decades of experience with the practice of prenatal diagnosis.[1] The discussion of the moral problems that the practice can pose is almost as old.[2] This chapter reviews that discussion with an eye toward the issues that are particularly important for the practitioner. Many of the ethical issues that were raised during the infancy of prenatal diagnosis still influence clinical policies about its use. Some of these issues have been resolved with the accumulation of experience. The first part of the chapter surveys the points on which consensus has been reached. The second part examines the new questions that practitioners should prepare for as the practice of prenatal diagnosis matures.

There are now a number of techniques relevant to the diagnosis of diseases and defects in utero.[3] Some, like fetal biopsy techniques, are informative but relatively invasive.[4] Others, like maternal serum screening for fetal proteins, are less risky, but also less revealing.[5] This chapter concentrates on two techniques that occupy the middle ground: amniocentesis and chorionic villi sampling. In amniocentesis, a needle is inserted through the mother's abdominal and uterine walls into the amniotic sac to withdraw fluid containing fetal amniocytes.[6] Chorionic villi sampling involves passing a catheter vaginally into the uterus to aspirate a sample of fetal tissue from the developing placenta.[7] Both kinds of fetal tissue are then available for analysis by a growing number of cytological, biochemical, and molecular tests.[8] The next generation of prenatal diagnostic tools follows this model, either by isolating circulating fetal cells from maternal blood[9] or, in the context of in vitro fertilization, performing biopsies on totipotent preimplantation embryos.[10]

Amniocentesis is the oldest of the prenatal diagnostic techniques and has received the most ethical attention. The discussion has focused on four sets of questions, more or less in succession: (1) questions about how amniocentesis should be introduced into practice given the initial uncertainties that surrounded it; (2) questions about the purpose of amniocentesis and the appropriate indications for its use; (3) questions about the moral dynamics of the practitioner–patient relationship in light of the problems in identifying patients whom amniocentesis would benefit; and (4) questions about the future of prenatal diagnosis as a medical practice, and the consequences of such diagnosis for our cultural and professional values.

This chapter surveys the debate on these questions about amniocentesis and uses the review to highlight some issues raised by the newer

Note: The research and writing of this chapter was supported in part by a Multi-disciplinary Research Award from the Ethics and Values Studies program of the National Science Foundation. (RII-B511073), with cofunding from the National Institute of Child Health and Human Development.

techniques of chorionic villi sampling (CVS), circulating fetal blood-cell sampling, and preimplantation embryo biopsy. The latter two are still experimental procedures, but their promise as clinical alternatives to amniocentesis and CVS is great. Their potential to rapidly expand the scope of prenatal diagnostics suggests that the ethical issues that they raise will be the most prominent ones regarding prenatal diagnosis during its maturity.

Notice that all four sets of questions about amniocentesis involve forms of uncertainty: empirical uncertainty about the utility and safety of the technique, moral uncertainty about the justifications for its use, conceptual uncertainty about the "patient" it serves, and social uncertainty about its long-term effects. The ethics of uncertainty has provided a constant background to the discussion of amniocentesis. This background is emphasized in what follows to suggest some of its more important implications for the clinical practice of prenatal diagnosis.

RISK, BENEFITS, AND ELIGIBILITY CRITERIA

Two kinds of ethical questions almost always accompany the introduction of a new biomedical technology: questions about its unknown hazards and questions about its distribution. A novel technology, by definition, lacks the clinical record that usually supports medical assessments of risk. This raises concerns about how best to compile that record without placing patients in undue danger. A new technology is also usually scarce if only because there are few clinicians experienced in its use. This raises concerns about how best to allocate the new resource among the patients whom it might benefit.

Amniocentesis was no exception on either score. The earliest discussions focused on the procedure's unmeasured potential for infection, hemorrhage, spontaneous abortion, and developmental damages to the fetus.[11] The uncertainty that provoked these discussions was empirical: It was simply not known how safe the new technique might be. At the same time, there were only about 10 centers in the United States capable of offering amniocentesis to patients.[12] In this situation, the question of who should be eligible to undergo this uncertain procedure was an important one.

This initial concern remains important for practitioners because of the ways it has been addressed in the intervening years. The responses reflected a strategy for dealing with empirical uncertainty that is rooted in the traditional medical obligation to prevent harm in the process of providing benefit. The first step was to circumscribe the potential dangers of the technique until the relevant uncertainties could be substantially diminished. This had two implications for the clinical introduction of the technique. First, it suggested that the first patients undergoing the procedure should be known to have a risk of carrying a fetus affected with a diagnosable condition. For these patients, the relative burden of the procedure's unknown dangers would be minimized and the relative benefits of its uncertain efficacy enhanced. Second, it suggested that, within this class of potential patients, the procedure should be used in cases that could help generate the missing knowledge.

The second step was to undertake the systematic clinical assessments of amniocentesis that these preliminary risk-buffered eligibility criteria made possible. Those assessments yielded the relatively low-risk figures—less than 1 percent morbidity and mortality—that have come to be associated with the procedure.[13]

One might say that these preliminary access policies served as the apron strings of the technique's youth. They protected it from its own unpredictability by keeping it within the cautious research setting that gave it birth. There comes a time, however, when apron strings should be cut. Eligibility criteria based on the original uncertainties continue to influence the use of amniocentesis. Now that the safety and efficacy of the technique has been established, the ethical justification of some of those policies is being reassessed.

For example, some early commentators argued that only parents who were willing to undergo an abortion in the case of a positive diagnosis should be considered candidates for amniocentesis. On this view, running the unknown risks of the procedure could only be justified if all the benefits it could offer were actually going to be realized. In the face of the gravity of the potential hazards, being unwilling to carry through with an abortion when the procedure provided an opportunity to prevent harm was thought to tip its risk-benefit balance enough to make rejecting the intervention the only reasonable choice.[14]

Today, there is a broad consensus that parental commitment to abortion is an ethically inappropriate criterion for selecting candidates for amniocentesis.[15] As we shall see, there are powerful arguments against it that stem from the nature of the prenatal diagnostician's professional role and the place of abortion among the "benefits" of amniocentesis. The main point here is that, as the procedure's risk potential has now been determined, the argument in favor of the policy has lost its foundation. Not only do we know the risks (so that reasonable risk comparisons are possible), we also know them to be relatively low. Now that the dangers they would protect against have been dispelled, the paternalistic constraints of this particular apron string are no longer justifiable, even on their own terms.

Another eligibility policy that has roots in the initial uncertainties is the more common one of restricting amniocentesis—among candidates with no known family histories of diagnosable conditions—to women over the age of 35. Early studies indicated that the incidence of Down's syndrome increased dramatically in children born to mothers older than 35.[16] This meant that tests performed on those patients were likely to yield more positive diagnoses of the disease than tests performed on younger women. Thus, in the absence of known genetic risks, restricting amniocentesis to candidates over 35 would increase the procedure's effectiveness in preventing the disease and decrease the chances that a normal pregnancy would be endangered by its risks. Since the birthrate also declined steeply after age 35, using maternal age as a selection criterion also produced a set of candidates that the extant resources could accommodate.[17]

This policy was a justifiable way to introduce the technique, given the uncertainties that surrounded it. However, as the risks of amniocentesis have become established, and our knowledge of the incidence of Down's syndrome has improved, the rationale for this policy is beginning to be reexamined. Studies have shown that the incidence of Down's syndrome increases more gradually with maternal age than the earlier work indicated.[18] Meanwhile, the number of other age-independent disorders diagnosable through amniocentesis, many of which are far more devastating than Down's syndrome, continues to increase. As a result, providing amniocentesis to younger mothers now appears less risky and more likely to benefit than it did early on.

This new information raises questions about the fairness of access policies that still use age 35 as a cutoff for candidates who are not known to be at genetic risk for specific diagnosable conditions. Questions of fairness arise in considering the relevancy of the interpersonal differences we use to distribute our resources. Here, the concern is whether being 35 or younger is still a relevant difference for the purposes of allocating access to amniocentesis now that the original justification has been undermined.[19]

The maternal age criterion illustrates a general point about the risk-limiting strategy for dealing with empirical uncertainty. The logic of the strategy suggests that initial criteria for the use of innovative techniques will remain justifiable only if the worst-case risk scenarios are actually borne out by experience. In most situations, the strategy will include eventually loosening the apron strings and allowing the technology to benefit a broader range of patients.

Finally, it is important to note that eligibility criteria for newer prenatal diagnostic techniques may still be drawn cautiously. The systematic clinical assessments of the safety and efficacy of chorionic villi sampling are still unfolding.[20] Thus, experts advise that "meanwhile, it is judicious to exercise every caution in view of potential hazards to both mother and child."[21] For the moment, as we shall see, the apron strings that provide protections against such hazards also protect practitioners of CVS from having to deal with ethical issues quite unrelated to risk. As that technique matures, it will be important to make sure that outmoded constraints on the technique's use are not maintained simply to avoid dealing with those other issues.

Of course, even after the apron strings of a new technology have been cut, its use must still be governed by some criteria. If the initial criteria are now less defensible, how *should* the service of amniocentesis be delivered? Questions about how to deploy biomedical technologies are intimately connected with questions about the goals they help to achieve. In principle, the best way to use a technology is the way that best meets the needs that the technology was designed to address. For any specific technology, like amniocentesis, there will be issues about the proportion of our general medical resources that should go into alleviating the scarcity of the technology in order to meet such needs.[22] However, there are also issues at the clinical level having do with the definition of the needs that amniocentesis is intended to meet. These are the issues discussed in the next two sections.

SELECTIVE ABORTION AND THE THERAPEUTIC IMPERATIVE

In most discussions about allocating a medical technology, the purpose of the technology is unproblematic. Most technologies provide some preventive or therapeutic benefit for patients with particular needs, and the problem is deciding how to distribute that benefit. One of the interesting features of the discussion of amniocentesis, however, has been the persistence of the question as to its purpose. Given that the risks of the procedure are low, what are the benefits it offers and are they legitimate ones for health care professionals to provide?

Implicit in the early use of amniocentesis prior to abortion seemed to be a belief that the prevention of harm by the selective abortion of diseased fetuses was the primary benefit to be gained from amniocentesis. Much of the ethical discussion has centered on the merits of this view and its implications for the appropriateness of amniocentesis as a medical practice.

Concern over the legitimacy of the practice is usually based in the recognition that, in the absence of more effective uses for the knowledge it produces, selective abortion is the primary practical intention behind performing an amniocentesis.[23] Critics find the practice unacceptable because they claim that selective abortion is an ethically inappropriate medical response to the diagnosis of fetal disease. Many of the arguments for this position reflect particular philosophical and theological views on the status of the fetus as a person and the moral rights to life and equal protection that it might possess.[24] As such, they are arguments against selective abortion as a general social practice and, to the extent that they are persuasive, indict amniocentesis indirectly.

However, there are also concerns about selective abortion as a *medical* practice, quite aside from the question of its social acceptability. Some argue that for health care professionals, it is irrelevant whether the fetal subject of an amniocentesis is a person or possesses rights. As long as the fetus is a legitimate *patient,* it falls within the scope of the practitioners' professional obligations and enjoys the benefits of their protection.[25]

One of the practices that the professional ethics of medicine has traditionally prohibited is the killing of patients, either for their own benefit or for the benefit of others.[26] Commentators point out that if the fetus is the patient in prenatal diagnosis, it is misleading to call the sequelae of positive diagnoses "therapeutic abortions" or to justify them in terms of the "prevention of harm." Fetal patients are selectively aborted precisely because they have been diagnosed as already suffering from incurable harms. Selective abortion on these grounds is neither therapeutic nor preventive; they say: It is simply a form of euthanasia.[27] As a result, some wonder whether amniocentesis might be an unacceptable practice for health care practitioners simply by the internal moral standards for their profession.

These concerns have been addressed in several ways. Some agree that selective abortion is not an ethically attractive response to the diagnosis of fetal disease, but they assert that it is also not the only possible response. They claim that in fact the intended purpose of amniocentesis is "the treatment and eventual cure of disease in the fetus or infant."[28] It is only because prenatal treatment has not yet caught up to diagnosis that selective abortion is a "sad, negative alternative."[29] A National Institutes of Health (NIH) consensus conference task force on antenatal diagnosis summarized this approach when it wrote,

> Thus, the techniques of prenatal diagnosis are not, except in very few instances, associated with any medical therapies for the alleviation of the diagnosed disorder. Many leaders in the development of this technology recognize this is unsatisfactory. They affirm that studies of the etiology of genetic and hereditary disorders are of the greatest importance and that, based on knowledge of etiology, therapeutic measures must be developed. Thus, prenatal diagnosis, while presently most often associated with the choice of abortion, is not inextricably linked to abortion: it may provide information leading to the planning for the birth of a defective infant and it has the potential for the better understanding of, and therapeutic interventions in, the disease state.[30]

In trying to establish an appropriate therapeutic purpose for amniocentesis, this argument looks both toward the past and the future. It points to the rationale behind the technology's development and to the promise of its eventual uses. These appeals are persuasive as far as they go. But even if the original intentions were laudably therapeutic, the proponents recognize that "realistically, for generations to come, the power to diagnose fetal disease will outstrip the power to treat with effective therapies."[31] While the prospects of future treatments might justify the use of prenatal diagnosis in *research* efforts designed to shorten that lag, how do they help in addressing the critics' concerns about turning to the "sad, negative alternative" as a regular practice in the clinical setting?

A second response to these concerns is to agree that (for the time being) selective abortion is the principal clinical option after amniocentesis but then to argue that abortion is sometimes morally justified. Again, the consensus of the NIH task force:

> In addition, there is something profoundly troubling about allowing the birth of an infant who is known in advance to suffer from some serious disease or defect. While the prevention of that suffering is attained in this case by eliminating the potential sufferer rather than the cause of the suffering, many would consider it an act of mercy. Because the fetus holds so uncertain a place in the moral community, many (among them many who are deeply devoted to fetal well-being) consider that "act of mercy" to fall in quite a different moral category than a similar act performed on an already born human being of whatever age.[32]

As this quotation indicates, those who argue this way must distinguish the merciful killing of fetal patients, which they support, from active euthanasia in the clinical setting, which they condemn.

Again, an array of philosophical views about the ontological status of the fetus and its membership in "the moral community," can be drawn upon to make this distinction.[33] But the hallmark of those views, as of their counterparts among critics of abortion, is the extent and intensity of scholarly disagreement over their merits. By contrast, the resources of traditional professional medical ethics are fairly sparse on these matters and cannot provide much guidance on the relevant distinction without appealing to one or another of these background views.

For the practitioner trying to decide how best to use amniocentesis, this dispute over the purpose of prenatal diagnosis creates a genuine problem of moral uncertainty. Is selective abortion, on the one hand, an ethically appropriate response to fetal disease or not? Our cultural resources on the question are almost too rich, offering a perplexing variety of moral guidance, all of it equally controversial. The specific ethical resources of the profession, on the other hand, do not seem to provide enough guidance to definitively respond to the concerns. There are approaches to dealing with moral uncertainty, however, and in the next section one is outlined that allows practitioners to get beyond the moral quandary of selective abortion to the clinical business of prenatal diagnosis.

Before turning to that approach, there are two points about the moral quandary that are important to make. First, note that one of the primary clinical advantages of the newer prenatal diagnostic techniques is their capacity for circumventing some of that uncertainty. Unlike amniocentesis, CVS is performed during the first trimester of pregnancy, and the tissue samples it yields are immediately ready for laboratory analysis.[34] By allowing a diagnosis to be made much earlier in gestation, this technique allows the question of abortion to arise during a period in which the spontaneous abortion rate for defective fetuses is high and the philosophical status of the fetus, both as person and patient, is more tenuous than it is later. Screening maternal blood for circulating fetal cells also allows for earlier detection than amniocentesis and does so without the degree of invasiveness of CVS. And of course, preimplantation biopsy of an in vitro embryo represents the ultimate extension of that strategy, since it avoids the prospect of an abortion altogether. On that strategy, affected embryos would simply be "passed over" in the search for embryo transfer candidates.[35]

It is also important to notice the source of the uncertainty over prenatal diagnosis as a medical practice. Both the concerns and their responses were framed against the basic clinical imperative to treat and cure disease. All the arguments so far have assumed that, for a diagnostic tool to have a legitimate medical purpose, it should be used to help benefit the victim of the diseases it uncovers. When prenatal diagnosis is understood in terms of this therapeutic imperative, the discussion naturally focuses on how the information it yields can help alleviate the suffering of the afflicted fetus. This perspective makes the asymmetry between our abilities to diagnose and treat the fetus morally troubling and prompts the discussion of whether selective abortion (or embryo discard) is an acceptable way to balance the therapeutic scales. Our uncertainty on that score is what creates most of the moral tension that accompanies the practice of prenatal diagnosis.

As strong as that tension is, however, it has not paralyzed the conscientious medical use of prenatal diagnosis. That is largely because the practice of prenatal diagnosis is also informed by another moral point of view, one that *does* provide the practitioner with a way to address this problem of uncertainty.

UNCERTAINTY AND THE ETHICS OF REPRODUCTIVE COUNSELING

There is an important argument in defense of amniocentesis that was not mentioned with the others above, even though all are usually raised together. Proponents almost always stress that, in addition to its therapeutic goals, "we regard the provision of information as an important and legitimate purpose of prenatal diagnosis" independent of whether that information is used on behalf of the fetus.[36] One statement of this position is as follows:

> The desired and intended result of prenatal diagnosis is information about the presence or absence of a possible disease or defect in the fetus. In practice, the test results are negative in more than 96 percent of amniocentesis cases, providing these families with many months of relief from anxiety. . . .When diagnosis of the presence of disease or defect is

> made, parents and physicians use that information to make choices about subsequent action. . . . Ethical considerations make it imperative to separate the fact of a positive diagnosis from the choice about subsequent action. What parents and physicians decide to do is not automatically dictated by the diagnosis but ought to be shaped by their ethical and social views. . . . These guidelines were developed in a moral framework favoring the protection of individual choice and the autonomy of parents, even when we disagree with their course of action.[37]

Notice that this approach defines the aim of performing an amniocentesis in terms of the parents' problems, not the fetus's. Prenatal diagnosis is, in essence, an adjunct to a form of psychological counseling: It provides information the practitioners can use to alleviate the parents' anxieties during pregnancy and to help them work through difficult reproductive decisions.[38]

This obviously reflects an important shift in the orientation of the discussion. Again, the discussion thus far has been informed, and limited, by the traditional ethics of clinical medicine. This shift reflects the influence of another professional tradition relevant to the practice of prenatal diagnosis: that of the genetic counselor. As the last lines of the passage above suggest, the ethical resources that this tradition can contribute to the discussion have some important implications for the practitioner's response to the moral uncertainties of the practice.

The first important feature of this tradition is its relocation of the practitioner's primary professional obligations. As the purpose of amniocentesis shifts from helping the fetus to helping its parents, the latter become the practitioner's primary focus. The ethics of genetic counseling has traditionally been clear about the implications of this therapeutic shift for a counselor's professional commitments: "Counselors may find themselves pulled by an allegiance to the unborn child—whose well-being is, after all, the ultimate object of their concern as well as the motivating interest of the parents. As understandable as this concern may be, in the end it must give way to the duty owed to the counselee—the parents."[39]

The second important feature of this tradition is its substantive vision of the duties that the practitioner owes to the counselee. Along with duties to benefit and protect their patients, the ethics of clinical medicine commits physicians to the ideal of a physician-patient relationship marked by shared decision making.[40] In genetic counseling, the key to that relationship has been taken to be the practitioner's duty to respect patients' reproductive choices. Modern genetic counselors are especially careful not to impose their own values on their clients in the decision-making process. The goal of their practice is to improve their patients' abilities to cope with their reproductive experiences in their own terms. Thus, while counselors provide information, facilitate decision making, and make recommendations, they fully accept the obligation not to interfere with the reproductive decisions that their clients make after counseling.[41]

In part, this ethical orientation has historical roots in the reaction of postwar clinical geneticists to the excesses of their eugenic predecessors. However, it also reflects an important strategy for dealing with the moral uncertainties of the reproductive decisions that genetic counselors help their clients make.[42] This strategy assumes that where moral uncertainty is high—either because of a paucity of ethical guidance or a variety of equally defensible views—practitioners may accept conscientious decisions favoring either side of an issue. Moreover, since reproductive issues in general and abortion issues in particular are among the most highly controversial and culturally colored moral issues, professionals engaged in helping people make reproductive decisions have a special obligation to respect their patients' considered judgments about these issues.[43]

This strategy seems to stand behind defenses of prenatal diagnosis like the one mounted in the last passage quoted above. References to the "ethical considerations" that allow practitioners to divorce the propriety of their diagnostic interventions from what happens as a result and to the "moral framework" favoring parental autonomy "even when we disagree with their course of action" allude to the view that, in the face of a plurality of moral positions on abortion, practitioners should bracket their own uncertainties and focus on enhancing the parents' ability to make autonomous and conscientious reproductive decisions. Prenatal diagnosis is an acceptable medical practice, then, as a tool for helping parents to make those choices.

In the practice of prenatal diagnosis, this counseling model usually operates simultaneously with a therapeutic concern for the fetus. This is an effective combination in most cases, since the practitioner's respect for parental choice coincides with his or her obligations to the fetus. However, some of the more vivid ethical problems that the practitioner faces are created in the rare cases in which these points of view diverge. Then questions arise again about which patients should be eligible for prenatal diagnosis. Once the apron strings of the practice have been cut and its purposes have been clarified, how should it be used? In particular, what is the range of reproductive choices the practitioner may facilitate through prenatal diagnosis when those choices conflict with his or her therapeutic obligations to the fetus?

Two kinds of cases that are especially important for today's practitioner are requests for prenatal diagnosis for sex selection and curable diseases. These kinds of cases pose limited, though real, problems for the practice of amniocentesis. The ease and efficacy of techniques like CVS, however, suggest that they will become increasingly common in the future. This same convenience will also raise a third set of issues that amniocentesis does not: the prospect of the widespread use of prenatal testing for public health purposes.

PRENATAL DIAGNOSIS FOR SEX SELECTION

Is prenatal diagnosis that is performed in order to determine the gender of the fetus an acceptable practice in the absence of sex-linked genetic risks? Although this question has been faced by practitioners of amniocentesis, the maternal risks of late abortions and the experience of pregnancy past quickening have often been enough to dissuade candidates from the practice without having to deny them access to amniocentesis.[44] The main clinical promise of CVS, fetal cell sampling, and preimplantation embryo biopsies, however, is precisely that they avoid those barriers to selective abortion by allowing diagnosis early in gestation.[45] The newer techniques make it progressively easier, physically and emotionally, for the mother to stop a pregnancy, and there is also greater uncertainty about the moral status of the fetus early in gestation, making an abortion (or embryo discard) easier to justify. At present, the practitioners of CVS are depending on the apron strings of the technique's youth to convince people that using it for sex selection is an inappropriate way to allocate a scarce and experimental resource.[46] As time passes, however, and the even less invasive new approaches become available, practitioners will have to face the issue squarely—and when there is likely to be an increased demand.

Most commentators have been critical of sex selection, even if they would not ban it. For example, in an important report on social issues in genetic screening, the President's Commission for the Study of Ethical Problems in Medicine and Biomedical and Behavioral Research states,

> Despite the strong reasons for not precluding individuals from having access to genetic services on the basis of what they may do with the information, society may sometimes be warranted in discouraging certain uses. A striking example would be the use of prenatal diagnosis solely to determine the sex of the fetus and to abort a fetus of the unwanted sex.[47]

The commission summarized the four most prominent arguments why, beyond the question of scarce resources, prenatal diagnosis for sex selection is an inappropriate use of the technology. The first three arguments impugn the motives of parents who would make such a request.

First, such a request is often likely to be based on sexist thinking. Unlike selective abortion for defective fetuses, discrimination based on sheer prejudice against one gender is something that can be fairly confidently condemned as immoral. Second, the fact that parents are concerned enough to abort a child of the "wrong" sex raises questions about whether they are approaching the enterprise of having children responsibly or whether they are laboring under expectations that will end up working to the detriment of their children. Finally, the commission noted that "taken to an extreme, this attitude treats a child as an artifact and the reproductive process as a chance to design and produce human beings according to parental standards of excellence."[48]

Of course, these arguments rest on factual claims that may not be true for all parents who request prenatal diagnosis for sex selection. Thus, we cannot be sure, from the outset, that every request is a case of irrational sexism, nor can we determine how successfully prospective parents will raise their children or even what the final consequences of the practice would be on our cultural attitudes toward reproduction.[49] A 30-year-old mother of three boys who would like a girl may have quite good reasons for her choice. In the face of uncertainty about the parents' motives, some argue, the practitioner should not deny them the benefit of the doubt.

These uncertainties do suggest that blanket policies against releasing sex information on request might be unjustified. But the commission also presented a fourth argument that is based less on uncertain empirical facts. The commission argued that

> although every reproductive decision based on information gained from genetic screening involves the conscious acceptance of certain characteristics and the rejection of others, a distinction can be made between seeking genetic information in order to correct or avoid unambiguous disabilities, or to improve the well-being of the fetus, and seeking such information merely to satisfy parental preferences that are not only idiosyncratic but also unrelated to the good of the fetus. Although in some cases it will be difficult to draw a clear line between these two types of interventions, sex selection appears to fall in the latter class.[50]

This argument returns to the issue of using the prenatal diagnosis for guidance, and in the process it integrates the two moral contexts of the practice—the genetic counselor's and the fetal therapist's—in an interesting way. In essence, it says that the purpose of the practice is to provide information relevant to making a *special subset* of reproductive decisions: decisions that revolve around the health of the fetus. Although the counselor's stress on the importance of parental autonomy would keep those decisions in the parents' hands, the therapist's focus on the medical problems of the fetus tends to limit the range of decisions that the practice can serve to ones made in response to those problems. Since gender is not a pathological problem, requests for assistance in making gender-based reproductive decisions can be appropriately denied.

This response goes beyond simply combining the two ethical frameworks for prenatal diagnosis and using one or the other as the need arises. Its effect is to integrate the perspectives, so that prenatal diagnosis remains recognizably a medical practice (addressing the health problems of the fetus), but a practice that focuses primarily on helping parents make reproductive decisions in the light of those problems. This integrated framework allows practitioners to show why women at risk for fetal defects are appropriate candidates for prenatal diagnosis even in the absence of effective treatment and women at risk for carrying a fetus of a certain gender are not.

PRENATAL DIAGNOSIS FOR A TREATABLE DEFECT

The second kind of access question raises problems even within the context of the integrated approach of the President's Commission. The clinical advantages of CVS, fetal cell sampling, and preimplantation biopsy, together with the expanding ability to diagnosis genetic disorders at the molecular level, will mean increasing numbers of genetic diseases will be detectable in utero. Geneticists already promise that with chorionic villi sampling, "prodigious opportunities exist for the first-trimester diagnosis of many different genetic disorders as long as the safety and accuracy are first assured. It is expected that all chromosomal abnormalities, biochemical genetic disorders whose enzymatic deficiencies have been characterized in cell culture, and all disorders in which the gene defect has been delineated will be detectable.''[51] Of course, this will increase the *range* of detectable health-related fetal conditions as well as the number. As this happens, questions will become more frequent about the diagnosis of relatively minor conditions or of conditions like Huntington's disease or Alzheimer's disease that will not affect the fetus until much later in life.[52] Similarly, as more correlations are drawn between specific genetic markers and dispositions toward psychiatric conditions like depression, practitioners may face requests for testing for these markers. All of these questions will create tension between the practitioner's commitment to parental autonomy and his or her concern for fetal welfare. Perhaps most difficult will be requests for prenatal diagnosis for diseases for which there is effective therapy. Once the appropriate techniques are available, how should the practitioner respond to requests for prenatal diagnosis for a disease (e.g., phenylketonuria [PKU]) that is eminently treatable after birth?[53]

Here the two moral traditions that guide the practitioner seem at loggerheads. On one hand, the practitioner is committed to using prenatal testing to provide the parents with the information they need in order to make reproductive decisions that concern fetal health. On the other hand, from the purely therapeutic point of view, the important benefits that the practitioner can provide to the fetus make the obligation to do so in this case seem very strong. The conflict between the two perspectives generates conceptual uncertainty over who should be understood to be the primary patient. Usually, it is enough simply to accept, or reject, both parties as one's patients. Cases of treatable fetal problems, however, raise the necessity of arriving at some conclusion about the relative priority of the patients, even within the context of an integrated moral perspective that identifies them.[54]

A case can be made for placing the parents first, even in these hard cases. The argument starts with the merits of the genetic counselor's approach to the cultural and ethical complexities of reproductive decision making. Fetuses are patients only within the context of their parents' reproductive plans. These plans will be the starting point in all the cases that a practitioner faces, as long as the presenting parents are not brain dead, comatose, or otherwise incapable of making reproductive choices. And parents' reproductive choices, as genetic counselors recognize, will be influenced by serious considerations that go well beyond the practitioner's ability to assess. Moreover, there are also significant risks in giving priority to the welfare of the fetus when it can be enhanced. These are primarily social risks, concerned with the consequences of such a move for the "right of privacy" by which reproductive choices have been traditionally protected.

To give priority to the therapeutic imperative in these cases would be to assume that it is an unacceptable medical practice to selectively abort a fetus that can be successfully treated for its condition. On this view, for example, requests for prenatal diagnosis for PKU may be legitimately denied if they are made with the intent to abort affected fetuses. However, to subordinate parental autonomy to fetal welfare in the way required to deny prenatal diagnosis for PKU would also provide justification for an unacceptably large range of other limitations on parental decision making.

For example, practitioners might withhold the information that a fetus had PKU if they knew the parents would use that information to abort the fetus. Agreeing to treatment of the disease could be made a condition for the prenatal diagnosis. Moreover, if it is the fetal PKU victim's status as a *treatable patient* that justifies the restriction on parental access to prenatal diagnosis, would not a fetus who is prenatally treatable for other diseases merit similar protections? That is, might not clinics be justified in giving access only to parents committed to proceeding with prenatal therapies where they are available? In effect, limiting access to prenatal diagnosis would be a mirror image of the required-abortion policy. As the number of fetal treatments increased, the range of disorders for which selective abortion would no longer be held appropriate would grow, effectively limiting parental reproductive choice.[55]

Whether these developments would actually occur, of course, is uncertain. The point of the argument is not that giving priority to the therapeutic imperative would place us on some inevitable "slippery slope." The point is that doing so would by itself place us at the bottom of the slope—by providing the justification for all these coercive practices. Giving priority to the parents' autonomy, however, respects the context of the diagnostic intervention in the parents' reproductive decision making and protects the traditional moral privacy of those decisions. As the President's Commission stated,

> nowhere is the need for freedom to pursue divergent conceptions of the good more deeply felt than in decisions concerning reproduction. It would be a cruel irony if technological advances undertaken in the name of providing information to expand the range of individual choices resulted in unanticipated social pressures to pursue a particular course of action.[56]

PUBLIC HEALTH USES OF PRENATAL TESTING

For clinicians, one source of the "unanticipated social pressures" that the President's Commission warns of is the increasing use of prenatal diagnostic tools in the service of public health goals. To date, maternal serum alpha fetoprotein screening has been the only prenatal test inexpensive and noninvasive enough to be considered justifiable as a public health screening tool. However, fetal cell sampling from circulating maternal blood, which also requires only a simple blood drawing, will make the whole suite of DNA-based diagnostics available to public health officials without additional clinical effort. As the apron strings of this new technique are cut, its routinization as a public health tool to reduce the incidence of genetic disease will be an appealing prospect to states and institutions staggering under their populations' health care costs. However, to the extent that such testing programs are evaluated in terms of their success in reducing the incidence of particular diseases, practitioners in the programs will face pressure to ensure that their clients make the "right" reproductive decisions: that is, decisions not to bear children at risk for genetic disease.

This is a pressure that is already creating tensions within medical genetics, as the field attempts to accommodate itself to health care delivery systems that are managed with societal health costs in mind. For example, there has been a lively debate in the British medical literature about how genetic services should interpret the societal expectation that they will "pay their own way" within the national health budget. In that context, the prevailing clinical view is that:

> An unacceptable measure of outcome audit would be utilization of population-based data (e.g., numbers of terminations for a specified condition or a trend in birth incidence). If a department's work is to be measured in such terms, there will be subtle, and possibly less than subtle, pressure upon clinicians to maximize the rate of terminations of pregnancy for "costly" disorders: a completely unacceptable outcome which we must strive to prevent.[57]

Applying reproductive genetic tests to public health problems, in other words, imports a goal that challenges the prenatal diagnostician's ethos entirely by distracting the practitioner from both of its traditional injunctions: fetal therapists' concern for fetal welfare and genetic counselors' respect for the reproductive autonomy of those they serve.

CONCLUSIONS

The moral framework that will guide the practice of prenatal diagnosis as a mature medical technology is still emerging. Its foundations are in the ethical traditions of clinical medicine and genetic counseling, with their complementary imperatives to enhance fetal welfare and facilitate parental choice. During the discussions of the safety and purpose of amniocentesis that shaped the youth of prenatal diagnosis, these two traditions could often be used interchangeably in establishing the legitimate boundaries of the practice. As the next generation of diagnostic techniques raises new moral, conceptual, and social uncertainties, the relationship between these two traditions will become increasingly crucial to the moral stability of the practice. Different approaches to integrating the professional obligations that each tradition stresses will produce divergent responses to the hard questions of access and eligibility that practitioners of prenatal diagnosis will increasingly face. One approach, designed with the new uncertainties in view, would try to improve the fit between these traditions in two steps. First, it would rely on medicine's therapeutic imperative to limit the range of appropriately diagnosed conditions to those relevant to the medical welfare of the fetus. But within that clinical sphere, it would reaffirm the commitment of the practitioner, as counselor, to enhance the parent's autonomy to make reproductive and therapeutic decisions in light of the information that prenatal diagnosis can provide.

NOTES

1. M. Steele and W. Breg, "Chromosome Analysis of Human Amniotic Fluid Cells," *The Lancet* 1 (1966): 383.
2. M. Harris, ed., *Early Diagnosis of Human Genetic Defects: Scientific and Ethical Considerations,* NIH Publication no. 72–25 (Bethesda, Md.: National Institutes of Health, 1971).
3. M. Harrison, M. Golbus, and R. Filly, eds., *The Unborn Patient: Prenatal Diagnosis and Treatment* (New York: Grune & Stratton, 1984); National Institute of Child Health and Human Development, *Antenatal Diagnosis: Report of a Consensus Development Conference,* NIH Publication no. 79–1973 (Bethesda, Md.: National Institutes of Health, 1979).
4. Harrison, Golbus, and Filly, *The Unborn Patient,* 125–39.
5. National Institute of Child Health and Human Development, *Antenatal Diagnosis,* 118–28.
6. Ibid., 33.
7. G. Simoni et al., "Diagnostic Application of First Trimester Trophoblast Sampling in 100 Pregnancies," *Human Genetics* 66 (1984): 252–59; C.H. Rodeck and J.M. Morsman, "First Trimester Chorion Biopsy," *British Medical Bulletin* 39 (1983): 338.
8. F. Chervenak, G. Isaacson, and M. Mahoney, "Advances in the Diagnosis of Fetal Defects," *NEJM* 315 (1986): 305–7.
9. C. Camaschella, A. Alfarno, and E. Gattardi, "Prenatal Diagnosis of Fetal Hemoglobin Lepore-Boston Disease on Maternal Peripheral Blood," *Blood* 75 (1990): 2101.
10. J. J. Tarin and A.H. Handyside, "Embryo Biopsy Strategies for Preimplantation Diagnosis," *Fertility & Sterility* 59 (1993): 943–53.
11. H. Nadler, "Prenatal Detection of Hereditary Disorders," *Pediatrics* 42 (1968): 912; John Littlefield, "The Pregnancy at Risk for a Genetic Disorder," *New England Journal of Medicine* 282 (1970): 627–28.
12. National Institute of Child Health and Human Development, *Antenatal Diagnosis,* I-61.
13. Ibid., I-60–I-67.
14. Littlefield, "The Pregnancy at Risk," 627–28.
15. National Institute of Child Health and Human Development, *Antenatal Diagnosis,* I-185; Tabitha Powledge and John Fletcher, "Guidelines for the Ethical, Social, and Legal Issues in Prenatal Diagnosis," *New England Journal of Medicine* 300 (1979): 170–71.
16. The President's Commission for the Study of Ethical Problems in Medicine and Biomedical and Behavioral Research, *Screening and Counseling for Genetic Conditions* (Washington, D.C.: GPO, 1982), 77.
17. Ibid., 78.

18. L. Holmes, "Genetic Counseling for the Older Pregnant Woman: New Data and Questions," *New England Journal of Medicine* 298 (1978): 419.
19. E. W. Hook, "Genetic Triage and Genetic Counseling," *American Journal of Medical Genetics* 17 (1984): 531; M. Vekemans and A. Lippman, "Eligibility Criteria for Amniocentesis," *American Journal of Medical Genetics* 17 (1984): 531.
20. G. G. Rhoads, L. G. Jackson, and S. E. Schlesselman, et al., "The Safety and Efficacy of Chorionic Villus Sampling for Early Prenatal Diagnosis of Cytogenic Abnormalities," *New England Journal of Medicine* 320 (1989): 609–17.
21. A. Milunsky, "Prenatal Diagnosis: New Tools, New Problems," in *Genetics and Law III,* ed. A. Milunsky and G. Annas (New York: Plenum Press, 1985).
22. G. Omenn, "Prenatal Diagnosis and Public Policy," in *Genetic Disorders and the Fetus,* 2d ed., ed. A. Milunsky (New York: Plenum Press, 1986), 869–77.
23. J. Lejeune, "On the Nature of Man," *American Journal of Human Genetics* 22 (1970): 121–28.
24. L. Kass, "Implications of Prenatal Diagnosis for the Human Right to Life," in *Ethical Issues in Human Genetics,* ed. Bruce Hilton et al. (New York: Plenum Press, 1973), 185–99; Karen Lebacqz, "Prenatal Diagnosis and Selective Abortion," *Linacre Quarterly* 40 (1973): 109–27; Carol Tauer, "Personhood and Human Embryos and Fetuses," *Journal of Medicine and Philosophy* 10 (1985): 253–66.
25. Cf. Harrison, Golbus, and Filly, *The Unborn Patient,* 1–9; Roger Shinn, "The Fetus as Patient," in *Genetics and the Law III.*
26. G. Gruman, S. Bok, and R. Veatch, "Death, Dying and Euthanasia," in *The Encyclopedia of Bioethics,* ed. Warren Reich (New York: Macmillan, 1978).
27. P. Ramsey, "Reference Points in Deciding about Abortion," in *The Morality of Abortion,* ed. John Noonan (Cambridge, Mass.: Harvard University Press, 1970).
28. Powledge and Fletcher, "Guidelines," 170.
29. J. Fletcher and A. Jonsen, "Ethical Considerations," in *The Unborn Patient.*
30. National Institute of Child Health and Human Development, *Antenatal Diagnosis,* I-182, 183.
31. Fletcher and Jonsen, "Ethical Considerations," 166.
32. National Institute of Child Health and Human Development, *Antenatal Diagnosis,* I-192.
33. Cf. W. Bondeson et al., eds., *Abortion and the Status of the Fetus* (Boston: D. Reidel, 1983).
34. Milunsky, "Prenatal Diagnosis," 336–37.
35. A. McLaren, "Can we diagnose genetic disease in pre-embryos?" *New Scientist* 42 (Dec. 10, 1987): 42–3, 46–7.
36. Powledge and Fletcher, "Guidelines," 171.
37. Ibid., 170.
38. Thus, genetic counselors write that, far from simply "diagnosing" medical problems, "When the genetic counselor attempts to help the counselees reach appropriate health and reproductive decisions, he/she will probably use the same techniques that many psychotherapists would use under similar circumstances—clarification of motivations and beliefs, an examination of alternatives, with their pros and cons, a presentation of options not considered in the counselee's thinking, an identification and labeling of facts and fantasies, challenges to unrealistic beliefs and so on. In other words, assisting counselees to make realistic personal decisions, a major goal of genetic counseling, perhaps more than any other function, requires that the counselor employ the skills of the psychotherapist" (S. Kessler, "The Psychological Paradigm Shift in Genetic Counseling," *Social Biology* 27 [1980]: 167–85).
39. A. Capron, "Autonomy, Confidentiality and Quality Care in Genetic Counseling," in *Genetic Counseling: Facts, Values, and Norms,* Birth Defects: Original Article Series, vol. 15, no. 2, ed. Alexander Capron et al. (New York: Alan R. Liss, 1979), 334.
40. Cf. President's Commission for the Study of Ethics in Medicine and Biomedical and Behavioral Research, *Making Health Care Decisions: The Ethical and Legal Implications of Informed Consent in the Patient-Practitioner Relationship* (Washington, D.C.: GPO, 1982), 36.
41. Cf. A. Capron et al., eds. *Genetic Counseling: Facts, Values, and Norms,* Birth Defects Original Article Series, vol. 15, no. 2, ed. Alexander Capron et al. (New York: Alan R. Liss, 1979).
42. J. R. Sorenson, "Biomedical Innovation, Uncertainty, and Doctor–Patient Interaction," *Journal of Health and Social Behavior* 15 (1974): 366–74.
43. Thus, writers sensitive to the moral nuances of language have begun saying "intrauterine" instead of "prenatal" diagnosis to accommodate the focus of the parent and the possibility that the intervention may not precede a birth at all. Cf. L. Walters, "Ethical Issues in Intrauterine Diagnosis and Therapy," *Fetal Therapy* 1 (1986): 32–37.
44. H. Kazazian, "Prenatal Diagnosis for Sex Choice: A Medical View," *Hastings Center Report* 10 (1980): 17–18.
45. Milunsky, "Prenatal Diagnosis," 337.
46. K. Copeland, cited in "Gender Tests Leading to Abortions," *San Jose Mercury News* 11 February 1987.
47. President's Commission, *Screening and Counseling,* 56.
48. Ibid., 57.

49. J. Fletcher, "Ethics and Amniocentesis for Fetal Sex Identification," *New England Journal of Medicine* 301 (1979): 550–53; M. A. Warren, "The Ethics of Sex Preselection," in *Biomedical Ethics Reviews,* ed. J. Humbar and R. Almeder (Clifton, N.J.: Humana Press, 1985), 73–93.
50. President's Commission, *Screening and Counseling,* 58.
51. Milunsky, "Prenatal Diagnosis," 338.
52. J. Fletcher, "Ethical Issues in Genetic Screening and Antenatal Diagnosis," *Clinical Obstetrics and Gynecology* 24 (1981): 1156.
53. N. Holtzman, "Ethical Issues in the Prenatal Diagnosis of Phenylketonuria," *Pediatrics* 74 (1984): 424–27.
54. F. Schauer, "Slippery Slopes," *Harvard Law Review* 50 (1985): 361–83.
55. As is currently happening in other places: Cf. L. J. Nelson, B. Buggy, and C. Weil, "Forced Medical Treatment of Pregnant Women," *Hastings Law Journal* 37 (1986): 703–65; R. Hull, J. Nelson, and L. A. Gartner, "Ethical Issues in Prenatal Therapies," in *Biomedical Ethics Reviews: 1984,* ed. J. Humbar and R. Almeder (Clifton, N.J.: Humana Press, 1984).
56. President's Commission, *Screening and Counseling,* 56.
57. A. Clarke, "Genetics, Ethics and Audit," *The Lancet* 335 (1990): 1145–47.

CHAPTER 4

Prenatal Diagnosis of Fetal Disorders: Ethical, Legal, and Social Issues

Diane Beeson and Patricia Jennings

INTRODUCTION

Increased use of prenatal testing to detect fetal disorders creates the impression that it is a welcomed and unproblematic step toward better prenatal care. Many view the capacity to detect fetal anomalies prior to birth as enhancing reproductive choice and contributing to the reduction of human suffering. At the same time, more cautious and critical perspectives can be noted among some scholars, health care providers, social activists, and individuals with firsthand knowledge of this practice.

In this chapter we briefly describe the current state of prenatal screening and testing technology and then provide a broad overview of the major ethical, legal, and social implications of these practices and their impact on women, medical practice, and society. We first discuss the views of those who support and encourage the use of these technologies, and then we present some of the main concerns of those who are more critical of these developments. We will emphasize the concerns of critics in the hope that doing so is the most effective way to prevent abuses of these new technologies. In taking this approach, we hope to make clear the range of perspectives on prenatal testing and the complex interactions between clinical practice, social context, and individual choice.

TESTING AND SCREENING TECHNIQUES

Several diagnostic techniques provide information about the developing fetus. Amniocentesis was the first procedure to become well-established as a method of detecting fetal disorders in high-risk pregnancies. In the 1970s, the possibility of removing amniotic fluid during the second trimester gained utility with the discovery that the fetal cells it contained could be cultured and karyotyped.[1] This allowed for the detection of chromosomal and genetic as well as metabolic disorders. U.S. Supreme Court decisions in 1973, loosening restrictions on abortion, coincided with technical developments to bring second-trimester amniocentesis into widespread use.[2]

Amniocentesis is usually done between 15 and 20 weeks of gestation by inserting a long, thin needle through the pregnant woman's abdomen and extracting a small amount of the amniotic fluid that surrounds the developing fetus. This fluid contains fetal cells that can be examined for chromosomal abnormalities, such as Down's syndrome and other trisomies, and certain genetic disorders such as sickle cell disease, cystic fibrosis, and muscular dystrophy. The fluid can also be tested for neural tube defects (NTDs). Amniocentesis can now be done as early as 12 to 14 weeks, but at this stage it may not be as accurate in detecting neural tube defects. With most of these conditions, but particularly with NTDs, it is usually not possible to predict severity.

Ultrasound guidance has made amniocentesis safer and easier. This technology is also used independently to determine fetal age and to detect sex and certain malformations such as hydrocephaly. Perceptions of ultrasound as noninvasive, and the absence of evidence of fetal harm, have led to its increasing importance as a diagnostic tool. Routine ultrasound for every pregnant patient, regardless of age, is becoming increasingly common.[3]

A third technique, chorionic villi sampling (CVS), came into use in the 1980s. This procedure permits first-trimester prenatal diagnosis of fetal cells extracted by catheter from the villi of the placental chorion. The earlier diagnosis made possible through CVS has been regarded as preferable to amniocentesis because it permits earlier abortion when disorders are detected. In addition to more favorable timing for the procedure itself, CVS enables more rapid completion of most biochemical molecular diagnoses than the 10 to 30 days usually required after amniocentesis. This potential for producing earlier results has contributed to the diffusion of CVS, while at the same time other factors, including prohibitions on the use of federal funds for fetal research, have inhibited its development and proliferation.[4] CVS at its current stage of development still has a slightly higher risk of procedural failure and fetal loss than amniocentesis (1–3 percent instead of less than 1 percent) and usually costs more.[5] By 1992, however, more than 100,000 such procedures had been conducted as part of continuing efforts to assess safety and accuracy.[6]

The least invasive and most promising approach to prenatal diagnosis is maternal serum screening. With this procedure, information about the fetus is obtained simply by studying components of maternal blood. One widely studied component is alpha-fetoprotein (AFP), which is present at elevated levels when the fetus has a neural tube defect (anencephaly or spina bifida). A maternal serum AFP (MSAFP) test can be given as a screening device to identify high-risk pregnancies that can then be diagnosed more precisely using ultrasound and amniocentesis. By 1993, estimates were that half of the pregnancies in the United States were being screened for MSAFP.[7] More recently two additional markers in maternal serum have been found to be reliable indicators of certain aspects of the health of the fetus. As a result, today this test is often described as an "expanded," "triple marker," or "multiple marker" test because it now also measures HCG (human chorionic gonadotropin and UE [unconjugated estriol]). This means that it also provides information about the risk of abdominal wall defects and trisomies 18 and 21.[8] In California, for example, physicians are required to offer all pregnant women an "expanded AFP blood test" between their fifteenth and twentieth weeks of pregnancy.[9] Women who choose not to have their fetus screened, as well as those who do, must sign a consent form indicating this.

Ideally, prenatal diagnosis would permit treatment of fetuses identified as having disorders. However, in spite of promising developments, in the vast majority of cases of fetal anomalies, the only significant medical intervention to date is abortion. One way to receive the benefits of genetic testing without selective abortion is to have a preconception diagnosis prior to in vitro fertilization.[10] However, this is a complicated, stressful, and difficult procedure. Considering the high cost of in vitro fertilization and the relatively low rate of success, this option has limited feasibility.[11] More likely than finding a way around selective abortion, we can expect prenatal diagnosis to raise the question of abortion more and more frequently as utilization of prenatal diagnostic techniques and knowledge of the human genome expand.[12] Yet social, legal, and ethical questions regarding the type of genetic traits for which we should be testing, and those conditions for which abortion should be permitted, are generating increasingly intense debate. It is this close relationship of prenatal diagnosis to selective abortion and the implications of the former for the expanding use of the latter, that is the central focus of this chapter.

SUPPORT FOR PRENATAL SCREENING AND TESTING

Prenatal screening, testing, and the accompanying use of selective abortion appear to be broadly supported by the public. For instance, a recent national survey in the United States indicates that two-thirds of respondents would want to undergo prenatal diagnostic tests for themselves or partners and believe such tests will do more good than harm. This positive attitude toward prenatal testing is strongest among whites who are young and educated and who follow news about science and health.[13]

In general, those who favor prenatal diagnosis view such testing as a contribution to reproductive liberty and enhancement of choice. They view its utilization as an important expression of individual rights. Some assert that parents have a responsibility not to burden society with the health care of a disabled child or to bring into the world a child who would suffer from a disability.

Currently, prenatal testing followed by elective abortion is a widely recognized reproductive right. The constitutional status of the right not to reproduce protects abortion for a serious genetic anomaly, and this practice is deemed morally acceptable by a majority of citizens.[14] At the same time, abortion for nonanomalous genetic traits is considered to be morally reprehensible by many. For example, most doctors are hesitant to abort for sex selection (a nonanomalous trait that can be detected). However, legal scholar John Robertson argues that even this right is constitutionally protected.[15]

Support for prenatal diagnosis is sufficiently widespread that prospective parents may feel social pressure to abort fetuses with genetic anomalies. As a result, some advocates of prenatal testing call for restricting abortion to certain anomalous traits by limiting the availability of genetic information on fetuses. Ethicist Jeffrey Botkin suggests that we extend the current practice of patient privacy and confidentiality to fetuses in order to protect them from abortions for minor genetic problems or for "frivolous" reasons. Presently, patient confidentiality can be breached for the purpose of preventing serious harm to another party. Thus, "fetal confidentiality" would grant prospective parents the right to genetic information only in cases where the condition is considered serious enough to warrant harm to the family. The fetus would be protected from abortion for nonanomalous traits since being born with these traits would not meet this criterion.[16]

Robertson seeks to ensure that prospective parents retain a legal right both to reproduce and not to reproduce and therefore opposes state restrictions on abortion even for nonanomalous traits. He argues that state restrictions interfere with reproductive liberty. Moral restrictions such as notions of prenatal responsibility would be acceptable to Robertson to reduce the incidence of aborting for what some may consider "trivial" reasons. As an advocate of prenatal testing, Robertson also supports protection of the right to give birth to an anomalous fetus, but he discourages state provisions for prospective parents who lack the financial means to bear and raise a disabled child.[17]

In contrast to Robertson's support for the rights of prospective parents to reproduce children with genetic anomalies, other advocates of prenatal diagnosis claim that there is a moral duty not to "knowingly" reproduce an affected child. This perspective argues that the future person's right to not be born with genetic anomalies outweighs the prospective parents' right to give birth.

Currently, discussions on the legal rights of future persons are centered on wrongful-birth and wrongful-life torts. Wrongful-birth torts grant parents the right to sue medical practitioners for failure to disclose information on fetal anomalies.[18] The central claim in such cases, according to James Knight and Joan Callahan, is that "the wrongful error of the defendant resulted in a 'harmful birth,' which the woman, if properly informed, could have prevented by aborting."[19] The existence of wrongful-birth torts poses a serious dilemma for medical practitioners because it raises the question of how much genetic information they should be required to give to patients in order to protect themselves from wrongful-birth suits. As the capacity to identify a growing number of genetic traits—and now even susceptibility to various diseases—increases, this problem becomes more serious.

Where wrongful-birth torts are brought by parents against medical practitioners, wrongful-life torts would grant children who are born with genetic anomalies the right to sue medical practitioners for failure to conduct tests that are warranted or to disclose genetic information to parents. As Knight and Callahan point out,

> the action for damages is not brought because the defendant caused the injuries defeating hope for a reasonably high quality of life. Rather, the claim is that the defendant wrongly allowed the child to come into existence at all, given his or her afflictions.[20]

Conversely, if informed parents knowingly bring a disabled child into the world, then wrongful-life torts could open the door to suits against parents brought by children.[21] In a review of Joel Feinberg's theory of harm, Bonnie Steinbock and Ron McClamrock point out that wrongful-life torts are based on the idea that, from the child's perspective, existence itself can be an injury and that the child was harmed by being born.[22] According to Feinberg, harm can be defined as "the thwarting, setting back, or defeating of an interest" and assuming that a fetus will be born, certain future interests can be ascribed to it.[23] Wrongful-life torts have not been used to generate any explicit laws prohibiting the birth of an anomalous fetus; that is, wrongful-life torts do not require women to abort affected fetuses. And, as of this writing, courts remain unwilling to recognize these suits.[24] However, if wrongful-life torts are recognized at some point in the future, then the risk of such a suit will exert considerable pressure on prospective parents to seek abortion if they know their fetuses are anomalous.

In contrast to a legal approach to discourage reproduction of disabled children, the moral approach aspires to protect the rights of future persons through moral suasion. Moral principles that are grounded in an ethic of parental responsibility hold to the idea that future persons have a moral right to be born free from disabilities that seriously limit their lives. However, those who hold this view often hold the view that this right should not be captured in law.

In sum, most advocates of prenatal testing do not argue that people should be legally barred from reproducing a child with genetic anomalies, but some do contend that the decision to do so is not always morally justified—the harm to the child, the family, and society-at-large have an impact on the moral acceptability of these decisions.[25]

These advocates of prenatal testing and selective abortion who argue for moral as opposed to legal "rights of future persons" do so for two reasons. First, some, such as Steinbock and McClamrock, find the stringent conditions imposed by wrongful-life suits too arduous to meet. For instance, assessments of harm can only be met when

> a child's existence is so miserable that he would have been better off unborn, [he has] been both wronged and harmed. When, however, his condition is impaired, but not so seriously that nonexistence is preferable, he is neither wronged nor harmed.[26]

According to Steinbock and McClamrock, this assessment of harm narrowly restricts the capacity of the child to sue for wrongful life. As Steinbock and McClamrock suggest, no matter how miserable the life, there is no harm as long as the child prefers life to not being born at all.[27] Steinbock and McClamrock argue that an ethic of parental responsibility would incorporate the notion of fairness. For instance, they suggest that an ethic of parental responsibility ask parents to consider how a particular condition will have an impact upon the child's capacity to thrive. Choosing against abortion, without adequate consideration of the adverse conditions that the child will face, constitutes unfair treatment. Therefore, the authors claim that it is consistent to say that the child has been treated unfairly even though the child may prefer life to no life at all.[28] These authors recognize that the definition of a "good life" is subjective, and, as such, they recognize that their argument can be read as one that advocates giving birth only under ideal conditions. However, they support their argument by pointing out that

> the principle of parental responsibility says only that it is wrong to bring children into the world when there is good reason to think that their lives will be terrible. It does not suggest that people should not have children unless conditions are ideal.[29]

Aside from the limitations imposed by wrongful-life suits, the second reason some theorists argue for moral rather than legal restrictions is out of concern for reproductive freedom. For instance, some feminists are particularly troubled over legal mandates that could inadvertently open the door to other forms of state interference in reproductive freedom. Laura Purdy's work is an illustration of this position.[30] Purdy argues that there is a moral restriction on the right to reproduce on the grounds that a child's right to a healthy body outweighs potential parents' right to reproduce. The source of the right to a healthy body is left unclear. Purdy also cites financial and emotional costs as major reason to abort an anomalous fetus. She asserts that the lack of financial and emotional support can place great strain on families and that the stress of raising a seriously disabled child often leads to divorce and thus harms women (who are most often left responsible for the physical care of these children) as well as other children in the family. Finally, Purdy considers the cost to society as one of inefficient resource allocation (a matter to which we will return). Although advocates of abortion for fetal anomalies, such as Purdy, hold that there are strong moral limits on the right to reproduce, they are not advocating comparable legal mandates. Nor do they support the provision of state funding for prenatal testing and selective abortion.[31]

Wertz and Fletcher have taken a more empirical approach. Using data from a wide variety of sources to bolster their position, they maintain that prenatal testing and selective abortion are for the most part empowering for women. They point out that most women who use prenatal testing are more than 35 years of age. These women have delayed childbearing in order to empower themselves through educational and career opportunities. Thus, gains made from the early wave of the feminist movement have resulted in lifestyle changes for this group, and prenatal technologies allow women to adapt reproductive choices to these changes. While women did consider the cost of caring for a disabled child, considerations about the quality of the child's life, the potential effect of a disabled child on the marriage, and the effect of a disabled sibling on the existing children were all major factors in the decision-making process.[32]

While women's choice and reduction of human suffering are the ultimate goals of those who support genetic testing, such testing assumes that most women will selectively abort if anomolies are found. Nevertheless, advocates like to point out that prenatal diagnosis does not necessarily lead to selective abortion, even when serious anomalies are identified. It may simply be used as advance warning to prepare parents emotionally and practically. They argue that prenatal diagnosis is even responsible for preventing abortion in some unplanned high-risk pregnancies by reassuring prospective parents that certain anomalies are absent.

CRITICAL VIEWS ON PRENATAL TESTING AND SELECTIVE ABORTION

Some critics of prenatal testing categorically oppose the practice of aborting for fetal anomalies because they hold that all human fetuses are persons with attendant rights. This is the view of many religious groups. But opposition to prenatal testing is not limited to religious groups or those who hold an antiabortion position. Critics include disability-rights activists, feminists, and other scholars who are pro-choice. They support the right of women to control their own bodies but are concerned with issues of equality and are doubtful that an emphasis on individual rights is sufficient to override the eugenic implications of prenatal testing and selective abortion.

To the extent that advocacy of prenatal testing is grounded in a principle of individual autonomy, critics view this position as reflecting inadequate understanding of the contextual dimension of choice. They point out that persons positioned differently in the social order will have different experiences of medical institutions, share different historical memories, and will bring different values and resources to bear on childbearing, prenatal testing, and abortion.[33] They contend that the power of social structure and processes to determine individual behavior must be acknowledged and at least the most egregious injustices corrected if choice in human reproduction is to be meaningful. Some of the most obvious social characteristics that shape options and responses to prenatal diagnosis are religion, gender, race-ethnicity, class, and disability. It is from scholars and activists informed on these issues that many criticisms of prenatal testing arise.

Gender and Prenatal Testing

Mainstream discourse on the ethics of prenatal genetic technologies often discusses these practices in gender-neutral terms.[34] But critics point out that even though both men and women participate in procreation, biological differences in human reproduction and social constructions of motherhood and fatherhood create gendered experiences of reproduction.[35] For example, prenatal testing necessitates the conceptualization and treatment of the fetus as an entity that is separate from the woman. Increasingly, the fetus is seen as a medical patient in its own right—a patient whose *quality* of life can only be protected by recognizing its *individual* interests.[36]

Viewing the fetus as separate from the mother has important consequences for the relationship between them. Perhaps the most important consequence is that it sets up the conditions for an adversarial relationship. Since women's behavior may now be viewed as potentially harmful to their fetuses, greater control over women's bodies becomes justified. In this vein, epidemiologist and critic Abby Lippman suggests that genetic constructions of prenatal health define all women as "at risk." In other words, as women's bodies become increasingly defined as a threatening environment to the developing fetus, then pregnancy increasingly comes under the label of a health risk. As Lippman states, women are either at low risk or high risk, but the concept of no risk has dropped out of our reproductive vocabulary. Lippman adds that "by attaching a risk label to pregnancy, physicians reconstruct a normal experience, making it one that requires supervision."[37] Women who refuse prenatal testing and abortions are increasingly depicted as "irresponsible reproducers," a social construction that serves as a mechanism of social control.[38] Marteau and Drake studied attitudes of professionals and laypersons with regard to attributions of blame for disabilities in children in three countries (Germany, Portugal, and the UK). They found that in all groups a mother who declined prenatal testing was more likely to be blamed for her child's Down's syndrome than if she received no offer of testing.[39] Since the choice to abort is perceived as "in the hands of the woman," women who choose to give birth to a disabled child bear a greater share of this social stigma. Mary Mahowald et al. also express concern that women are the ones who will be challenged and criticized for continuing a pregnancy after prenatal testing confirms the presence of a fetal anomaly.[40]

As mentioned earlier, Wertz and Fletcher reject some feminist concern that prenatal testing is oppressive to women. Yet, their findings seem inadvertently to support the position that women's choices are increasingly constrained by third parties, such as immediate family, extended family, employers, and private insurance companies.[41] Empirical studies on this topic are scant. However, a study from Sweden by Sjogren and Uddenberg found that 15 percent of the women whom they interviewed reported that they did not feel that the choice to undergo testing was completely voluntary—they felt obliged to consent to the test. A majority of the women interviewed (75 percent) said that it was difficult to turn down a test once it was offered. These findings led the authors to hypothesize that the choice to be tested is often not completely voluntary.[42]

Even where testing is freely chosen, critics are concerned about unanticipated consequences. Those interested in women's experiences of technology are concerned that treating the fetus as a separate entity may impair the bonding process between mother and fetus. Where the psychological process of pregnancy was formerly a response to biological changes that was supported by social relationships, prenatal testing tends to make pregnancy a process whose stages unfold in response to the testing process. In a study of pregnant women, Beeson found that those who participated in amniocentesis experienced stress patterns that were imposed by the technology and that caused biological signals of development and attachment to be ignored or bracketed. The scheduling of testing and receipt of reports from the laboratory became more important determinants of the psychosocial experience of pregnancy.[43]

Sociologist Barbara Katz Rothman's empirical work on prenatal testing expands on this point. She observed that the separation of mother and fetus embodied in all new reproductive technologies reflects the male experience of attachment. For example, where men's experience of childbirth starts from separation and moves toward attachment, women's experience of pregnancy (in the absence of prenatal testing) begins with attachment, long before birth, and moves toward separation. The women undergoing prenatal testing in Rothman's study tended to delay bonding with the fetus, and they delayed identifying with the social process of pregnancy. For instance, women often hid the pregnancy from family and friends until the results of prenatal testing confirmed the absence of an anomaly, just as they did in Beeson's study. In a reassessment of her earlier work, Rothman states that "For many of the women I interviewed, a new state of pregnancy had been constructed: a pregnancy without a baby."[44]

A concern of critics that has particular relevance to women is that prenatal testing promotes a reductionist orientation to human reproduction in which women's bodies become instruments of production and children are viewed as "products." Rothman argues that new reproductive technologies are geared toward ensuring "quality" fetuses. The idea that future children can be regulated for quality promotes an instrumental approach to human reproduction driven by goals of calculated efficiency and cost reduction. As Rothman points out, technological ideology shifts our view of the body, self, and social organization away from one that centers on acts of doing and being—a self-reflexive orientation—to one of "making." Making captures the essence of the objectification of the body—the shift from relating to ourselves and others as interconnected subjects to treating ourselves and others as resources whose end goal is production.[45]

According to critics, prenatal testing promotes greater social control over all women's reproduction and, consequently, erodes "real" reproductive choice—a conclusion precisely opposite of the supporters' position that women's choice is enhanced by prenatal testing. However, all reservations about prenatal testing do not focus only on gender. Another source of concern is inequality resulting from the intersection of gender, race, and class.

Racial-Ethnic and Class Issues

Economic constraints and sociocultural differences are major factors influencing attitudes toward, and use of, prenatal testing. More empirical research on prenatal testing and selective abortion is needed across ethnicities and classes; however, the few studies that have been conducted report that there is less support for prenatal testing and abortion among African Americans, Hispanics, and poor white women than among white middle-class women.[46] A study conducted by E. Singer found race to be a significant predictor of attitudes toward genetic testing. Singer's study found that, after controlling for religion and education, African Americans were less likely to approve of genetic testing in general and were less likely to want prenatal testing for themselves or their partners when compared with whites.[47]

When actual utilization of prenatal diagnosis was assessed by racial-ethnic group in northern California, Kuppermann, Gates, and Washington found that Latinos and African-American women were much less likely to undergo these tests than were whites and Asians. They determined that socioeconomic factors explain some, but not all, of the differences.[48]

Regional differences in health care services may also have an impact upon the use of prenatal tests by poor women and women of color. For instance, in a study on the use of prenatal care services (prenatal testing was not examined as a specific form of prenatal care) in metropolitan and nonmetropolitan areas, Leslie Clarke et al. found that Hispanic residents living in nonmetropolitan areas had the highest rates of inadequate prenatal care, followed by African-American women living in nonmetropolitan areas.[49]

In a study on reproductive services for poor women and women of color, Nsiah-Jefferson indicates that many poor women do not use prenatal care because they lack health insurance. As she states, although state funding for prenatal testing provides some level of genetic testing services and prenatal care, most of these services impose eligibility requirements, such as minimum income requirements, that limit access to services. Nsiah-Jefferson is concerned that differential access to prenatal testing and abortion may result in a disproportionate representation of disabled persons among poor populations.[50]

Paradoxically, at the same time funds are becoming increasingly available for prenatal screening programs, the Supreme Court's finding in *Webster v. Reproductive Health Services* has worked to limit state funding for abortion.[51] Advocates of equal access to reproductive services point out that this places poor white women and poor women of color in a double bind. If they do obtain testing and decide to abort in cases of fetal anomalies, they may be financially prohibited from obtaining an abortion. Abortion restrictions imposed on a state-by-state basis, such as the level of funding that specific states allocate, may also produce regional variation in abortions among poor populations of women.

Some critics note that while disadvantaged women are underrepresented among those using prenatal testing and other forms of new reproductive technologies, such as in vitro fertilization, these groups are overrepresented among those who provide biological and social reproductive services, such as egg donors, contract mothers, child-care workers, and so on.[52] This reinforces critics' views that the capacity to exercise the right to reproduce or not reproduce is seriously complicated by social relations of privilege and power.

Unequal financial access to prenatal testing and selective abortion represents only one dimension of critical concern. Eugenic histories reflected in attempts to control reproduction among poor whites and persons of color are another aspect of race and class experiences of medical institutions, and these may shape responses to prenatal diagnosis.[53] Medical anthropologist Lisa Handwerker has drawn attention to the increasingly frequent reliance on medical testimony to prosecute poor women labeled "high risk" by definition of socioeconomic status for failure to comply with medical advice when their fetuses or babies die. She argues that they often do seek care but don't go through "normal" channels and that prosecution may result in greater numbers of poor women who fail to seek prenatal care through the standard channels.[54]

Some observers note that for the first time in history, the capacity to test for cystic fibrosis allows for a eugenic potential among privileged white populations.[55] However, the potential for eugenic control through testing for cystic fibrosis among whites cannot be equated with race and class eugenics, which have much stronger historical precedents throughout the world. In the United States, the birth-control movement of the early twentieth century was based on eugenic attempts to control reproduction among poor whites, "degenerate" populations such as criminals, and racially subordinated populations.[56]

African Americans and Hispanics have experienced particularly insidious attempts to control their reproduction—for example, forced sterilization of women. In contrast to Robertson's claim that eugenic practices are now widely discouraged, critics suggest that these attempts carry over into the present day, although they are now more typically expressed in covert forms of control.[57] For instance, Annette Dula points to examples of greater rates of sterilization and hysterectomies among women of color. Dula also points out that explicit forms of eugenic practices still occur. For instance, she reports that in 1973 a total of 13 young girls in Montgomery, Alabama, were sterilized, and 10 of them were African American.

The recent history of sickle-cell screening programs also may be of particular consequence to the formation of cultural attitudes toward prenatal testing and abortion. In some states, during the early phase of sickle-cell anemia screening programs, informed consent was violated and mandatory testing was proposed and, at times, enacted.[58] Violations of informed consent continued and were documented as recently as 1980. As Dula states,

> It may be tempting to assume that . . . medical abuses are part of the distant past. However, there is evidence that violations of informed consent persist. Of 52,000 Maryland women screened annually for sickle cell anemia between 1978 and 1980, 25 percent were screened without their consent.[59]

Racial eugenics, reflected in histories of medical abuse and attempts to limit reproduction among women of color, is woven into cultural views of prenatal testing.[60] A middle-class African-American woman who chose to forgo amniocentesis because of her husband's concern with medical abuse, illustrates the role of historical memory. Interviewed by anthropologist Rayna Rapp, this woman stated that the lab form contained a proviso to use discarded amniotic fluid anonymously for experimentation. As Rapp states, "Reading intensively, the husband was disturbed by this clause, citing the Tuskegee syphilis experiments and other examples of abusive research conducted on African Americans as his reason for rejecting the test."[61] An ongoing study by Duster and Beeson is a further illustration of this point. In interviews of families at risk for cystic fibrosis and sickle-cell anemia, they found that African Americans frequently were concerned about the social implications of testing. For example, one interviewee stated,

> You know, if I were confident that genetic testing would be used for the proper and righteous reasons, I probably would not have a problem with it. But I know that is not the case, and therefore, I do have a problem with it. I know people will be discriminated against. I know that! We can say anything we want, but the facts are, have been, and will be, that there will be discrimination. . . . I can see people being divided up into groups.[62]

Given the history of race and class discrimination and its consequences in the area of reproduction for poor and minority women, it is difficult to know to what extent racial-ethnic and class differences in current patterns of use of prenatal testing reflects lack of access and how much is an indication of mistrust of biomedicine.

The Meaning and Experience of Disability

The perspective of disability-rights activists provides additional insights to assumptions embedded in prenatal testing. Disability-rights leader Marsha Saxton has identified and challenged several of these assumptions. The first is that having a disabled child is a wholly undesirable thing. The second is that the quality of life for people with disabilities is less than it is for others. Finally, and most important, she challenges the assumption that we have the means ethically to decide whether some people are better off never being born. She maintains that these beliefs are prejudices that are a product of discriminatory attitudes and thoughtless behaviors. She admits that there are disabled people who "suffer" from their condition but points out that nondisabled people may also suffer from emotional pain and limitation of resources. The decisive factor, from her perspective, is not the disability but the lack of human caring, acceptance, and respect. Furthermore, she maintains that the deepest experiences of our humanness come not from denying or attempting to take flight from our human vulnerability but from confronting it.[63]

Two recent national conferences—one in Canada and one in the United States—have brought these and other concerns of disability-rights activists into the mainstream debate on prenatal diagnosis. The first, held in Vancouver in 1994 on New Reproductive Technologies, emphasized that a "dangerous void of information about disability is the context in which the public's attitudes about prenatal diagnosis and selective abortion are formed."[64] In the summer of 1996, Saxton convened the first national conference to foster dialogue between disability-rights activists and professionals in clinical genetics in the United States.[65] Both conferences addressed the fact that while the reproductive-rights movement has fought for the right of women to have abortions, the disability-rights movement has had to fight for the right of disabled women not to be coerced into having abortions.[66] This divergent experience highlights the importance of context in assessing the ethical and social implications of prenatal testing.

Adrienne Asch, another prominent disability-rights activist, acknowledges that there are biological impediments that diminish human capacities for the disabled. She also contends that, in large part, the difficulty of living with disability stems not from the disability itself but from the social response to disability. In asserting that disability is socially constructed, Asch is making two claims:

> First, . . . even those characteristics we label as "disabling" are at least partly socially determined; second, that disability's all-too-frequent consequences of isolation, deprivation, powerlessness, dependence, and low social status are far from inevitable and within society's power to change.[67]

Lippman's position is consistent with Saxton's and Asch's in emphasizing that disability is not a biological reality waiting to be discovered. Instead, social and cultural assumptions influence how we define disease and disability, and these definitions change over time.[68] This point is illustrated by the fact that in many parts of the world the primary "problem" prenatal diagnosis is used to detect and eliminate is femaleness, and that even in North America sex selection is practiced.[69]

The importance of social context is further illustrated by the fact that there are a number of genetic conditions whose desirability varies dramatically, including deafness and dwarfism. These conditions may be considered preferable to their absence in some families in which both prospective parents are affected. These parents may fear that they cannot be as effective as parents if their child does not share these characteristics with themselves and other members of their community.

The difficulty of providing prospective parents with "unbiased" information on which to base decisions related to abortion is further illustrated by the observations by Lippman and Wilfond. They have pointed out that even in medical settings "the *before*-birth information is largely negative" while "*after*-birth information tends to be more positive." The dominant message in the before-stories physicians and other health care providers tell (prospective) parents "appears oriented to avoiding the birth of a child with Down's syndrome or cystic fibrosis," while "*after*-birth stories" focus on compensating aspects of the condition, highlighting the availability of medical and social resources, and stressing hope for the future.[70] Not only do definitions of conditions change, but as Asch points out, some biological definitions of disability fail to recognize that the removal of physical and social barriers often enables those with disabilities to fill valuable roles in society.[71]

Disability-rights activists argue that prenatal testing and abortion for fetal anomalies express eugenic desires. By this they mean that the message behind the abortion of an otherwise-wanted fetus is that we seek to eliminate future persons with disabilities. In their view, not only does this message fail to recognize the social value of future persons with disability, it conveys a devaluation of the lives of those now living with disability.[72]

In response to arguments in support of genetic testing and selective abortion such as those raised earlier by Purdy, critics suggest that negative social constructions of disadvantaged groups work to effectively "blame the victim" and thereby support inequitable distributions of resources. Inequality is not an inevitable feature of our social system. Political struggles for equality have been formidable; and although gains have been limited, important changes have occurred, as evidenced in the 1990 civil-rights law prohibiting discrimination on the basis of disability, the *Americans with Disabilities Act.*

Critics of prenatal diagnosis point out that it is a mistake to think that identification and eradication of genetic disorders will reduce the cost of treating and caring for disabled people. As disability-rights activist Debra Kaplan points out, prenatal testing will only have a small impact on the number of persons with disabilities in the United States. Kaplan notes that there are an estimated 42 million persons in the United States with various disabilities and that few of these disabilities are genetic in origin; most result from trauma and age.[73] Insofar as disabilities do occur in infants, the major cause is poor prenatal care.[74] Kaplan and other critics contend that promoting prenatal diagnosis and selective abortion to solve problems related to disability occurs at the expense of a broader understanding of the relationship among genetics, the physical environment, and the social environment.

Only recently have encounters with disabled persons, who are also conversant with the civil-rights/minority view of disability, been systematically integrated into the training of genetic counselors. A small research and demonstration project conducted by Marsha Saxton cast them as consultants to genetic-counseling students. All participating students reported that these repeated encounters had a marked impact on their views of prenatal testing. The interactions stimulated intense ethical concerns in participants related to the questionable existence of unbiased counseling, the relationship between eugenics and reproductive choice, and the "technological imperative" to use tests because they exist.[75] Hopefully, this study marks the beginning of more forthright confrontation of perspectives and a deeper level of dialogue on the ethics of prenatal testing.

Diversity and Reductionism

While social relations of gender, race-ethnicity, and class exert strong influences on responses to prenatal testing, Rapp warns that we must be careful not to paint women's experiences within groups as monolithic.[76] For instance, while issues that are specific to particular groups do present unique challenges, not all white middle-class women experience prenatal testing in the same way. Nor do disabled women, poor women, or women of color have the same experience by virtue of disability, class, or race-ethnicity. Differences in religion, age, family experience, educational level, and region of the country may all influence decision-making processes as do direct experiences of health care provision and familiarity with persons with disabilities.

For instance, Nsiah-Jefferson points to variations of attitudes among women of color of different religions. As she indicates, "many Southeast Asians believe that amniocentesis interferes with the natural selection of the population, which is considered sacred." At the same time, Roman Catholicism, a religion represented among Latino populations, often views disability as God's will.[77]

Not only do various religions view disability differently, but individual experiences of religion mediate cultural experiences of religion. Rapp notes that differences in attitudes regarding the types of disabilities that individuals feel they can cope with also exist within cultural groups.[78] Rapp's study brings out another interesting point on diversity. She found that clinical experiences among women of color produce variation in decisions to have prenatal testing. Her field work led Rapp to conclude that clinical experience may override cultural differences in significance as a determinant of acceptance. For instance, women of color may be more likely to accept prenatal testing if their first experience with a clinic is positive.[79] Press and Browner's research on women who accept MSAFP screening supports Rapp's suggestion that the clinical experience can be pivotal in the decision to accept testing.[80] They suggest, however, that women collude with clinicians in constructing "collective fictions" of prenatal testing. These fictions situate testing within the domain of routine prenatal care and enable both parties to avoid discussions of abortion and its eugenic potential.[81] This work raises the question of how honestly and directly both women of various cultures and health care professionals are facing these difficult issues.

One way to simplify difficult human issues is to resort to reductionism. This is what biologist Ruth Hubbard describes as "breaking nature into smaller and smaller bits" and then ignoring, losing, and misreading their connections.[82] It is reflected, for instance, in the belief that human suffering can be identified in advance in our genetic codes. Reductionism, although a powerful force, has serious limitations in science as well.[83] It obscures the fact that "[d]isease . . . is a result of the organism's frustrated attempts to adapt phenotypically to a hostile environment or set of elements for which there is no adequate response basis."[84] Tremendous advances in life expectancy and improvements of the health and quality of life in recent years, even among those with single-gene disorders such as sickle-cell disease and cystic fibrosis, support this view.

A reductionist orientation to human reproduction, which critics believe is at the heart of positions in support of prenatal testing, advances a view of humans as machines and children as products that is most constraining for those at the bottom of the social and economic hierarchy. This mentality increasingly brings reproduction under the control of medical, corporate, and research institutions and under the control of persons and groups in positions of power and authority in those institutions. The choice to reproduce may become largely constrained by market forces and technical trends. For example, in some cases, insurance companies have attempted to refuse coverage of the birth, and future medical care, for defective children whose parents chose to give birth despite positive test results for fetal anomalies.[85] Examples of such cases continue to arise in spite of legal prohibitions against them. Critics are concerned that economic pressures may be brought to bear on policies that regulate reproduction.

Choices regarding prenatal testing may be influenced by the accumulation of stigmas. Decisions may reflect both oppression and resistance to oppression. The difference between these may not always be clear, but both may interact with culture and be reflected in responses to certain conditions. For instance, Rapp found that Puerto Ricans, Dominicans, and some other Spanish-speaking groups were fairly accepting of less visible problems such as mental retardation, but they were much less accepting of visible physical differences. In contrast, white women were more likely to consider mental retardation a justifiable reason for abortion.[86] Examples such as these indicate that variation in responses to prenatally detectable conditions arises from many factors in addition to biomedical ones.

Those in positions of wealth and power can avoid many of the problems related to prenatal diagnosis raised by critics, but for others who face multiple pressures or oppressions this is less likely. For example, the development of prenatal testing has serious consequences for prenatal care policies and for the distribution of social and financial resources. At the same time that genetic research is generously funded, there have been serious funding cuts for prenatal health care and nutrition programs that benefit less-privileged groups.

Culturally patterned variations in responses to prenatally detectable conditions, including those related to income and education, demonstrate that the extent to which people use prenatal testing and selective abortion is much more than an issue of personal preference. Critics urge us to pay more attention to the social context of prenatal diagnosis. Failure to do so, they fear, threatens to reduce human life to a production process and to compromise the meaning of choice.

CONCLUSION

In this chapter we have seen that there is broad support for the expanding applications of prenatal screening and testing. Much of this support is based on shared assumptions about the importance of biomedical intervention to prevent suffering and disability. The expansion of screening and testing is bolstered by a strong moral and legal tradition supportive of individual rights. Yet, the individual-rights argument can be reductionistic, failing to account for social diversity and unequal access to resources. A reductionist approach to human reproduction is reinforced by a consumer ideology that facilitates a view of children as products whose quality can be controlled through the employment of technical means.

As prenatal testing reaches an increasingly wide variety of women, however, a critical discourse is emerging that questions many of the assumptions on which these interventions are based. Questions are being raised about some of the consequences of prenatal testing for the experience of pregnancy, the relationship between mother and fetus, eugenics, and both the quality and commodification of human life. Treating potential children as products increasingly brings reproduction under the control of medical, corporate, and research institutions and professionals in positions of power and authority in those institutions. The choice to reproduce may become constrained by market forces and technological trends while ostensibly subject to individual choice. In an era of managed care, with decision making in the health arena increasingly determined by financial considerations, this is an issue worthy of more attention.

Marginalized groups such as ethnic minorities, poor women, and the disabled raise a particularly challenging array of concerns. They may be particularly inclined to experience these new prenatal tests as a smoke screen for yet another coercive experience. Another group, women from different language or cultural backgrounds, may experience language barriers or difficulty obtaining culturally sensitive genetic counseling services. Poor women, especially poor women of color, often lack the resources to provide their prospective children with adequate health care and supportive services—conditions that constrain their reproductive choices. They may find it particularly difficult to obtain accurate information on disability and access to services that support those with disabilities. On the one hand, they may feel compelled to have an abortion if genetic anomalies are diagnosed. On the other hand, they may find themselves without access to abortion when they decide to have one. Increased attention to the reproductive histories of these groups and their current standpoints is fostering deeper appreciation of the importance of social context in understanding the impact or value of reproductive technologies. We are only beginning to appreciate the complex relationship among individual choice, cultural values, and the distribution of resources in society. The dialogue between health care providers, policy makers, and ethicists on the one hand, and marginalized groups on the other, is still in the beginning stages. We hope this chapter has contributed to furthering that dialogue.

NOTES

1. J. C. Hobbins, "Amniocentesis," in *The Unborn Patient: Prenatal Diagnosis and Treatment,* ed. M. Harrison et al. (Philadelphia: W.B. Saunders, 1991), 60.
2. J. W. Larsen et al., "Second and Third Trimester Prenatal Diagnosis," in *Fetal Diagnosis and Therapy: Science, Ethics and the Law,* ed. M. I. Evans et al. (Philadelphia: J.B. Lippincott, 1989), 37.
3. M. I. Evans et al., "Report on the Council on Scientific

Affairs of the American Medical Association: Ultrasound Evaluation of the Fetus," *Fetal Diagnosis and Therapy* 6 (1991): 132–47.

4. R. S. Cowan, "Aspects of the History of Prenatal Diagnosis," *Fetal Diagnosis and Therapy* 8 (1993; suppl 1): 10–17.
5. G. G. Rhoads et al., "The Safety and Efficacy of Chorionic Villus Sampling for Early Prenatal Diagnosis of Cytogenetic Abnormalities," *New England Journal of Medicine* 320 (1989): 609–17; A. Lippman et al., "Canadian Multicentre Randomized Clinical Trial of Chorion Villus Sampling and Amniocentesis," *Prenatal Diagnosis* 12 (1992): 385–476.
6. L. Jackson and R. Wapner, "Chorionic Villus Sampling: 10 Years Experience" (paper presented at the Sixth International Conference on Early Prenatal Diagnosis of Genetic Disease, Milan, Italy, May 18–20, 1992).
7. F. J. Meany et al., "Providers and Consumers of Prenatal Genetic Testing Services: What Do the National Data Tell Us?" *Fetal Diagnosis and Therapy* 8 (1993; suppl 1): 18–27.
8. O. W. Phillips et al., "Maternal Serum Screening for Fetal Down Syndrome in Women Less Than 35 Years of Age Using Alpha-Fetoprotein, hCG, and Unconjugated Estriol: A Prospective 2-Year Study," *Obstetrics and Gynecology* 80 (1992): 353–58.
9. "Prenatal Testing Choices for Women 35 Years and Older," *California Department of Health Services, Genetic Disease Branch* (1995): 1.
10. J. Robertson, *Children of Choice: Freedom and the New Reproductive Technologies* (Princeton, N.J.: Princeton University Press, 1994), 155–56; Y. Verlinsky et al., "Preconception and Preimplantation Genetic Diagnosis of Genetic Diseases," *Journal of In Vitro Fertilization and Embryo Transfer* 1 (1990): 1–5.
11. For an assessment of in vitro fertilization costs and success rates see, E. Bartholet, "In Vitro Fertilization: The Construction of Infertility and of Parenting," in *Issues in Reproductive Technology,* ed. H. B. Holmes (New York: New York University Press, 1992).
12. J. Robertson, *Children of Choice: Freedom and the New Reproductive Technologies*, 157.
13. For a discussion of public attitudes toward genetic screening and selective abortion see, E. Singer, "Public Attitudes toward Genetic Testing," *Population Research and Policy Review* 10 (1991): 235–55.
14. Ibid.
15. J. Robertson, *Children of Choice: Freedom and the New Reproductive Technologies*, 159–60.
16. J. Botkin, "Fetal Privacy and Confidentiality," *Hastings Center Report* (September–October 1995): 32–39.
17. For a review of Robertson's position see, S. Sherwin, "The Ethics of Babymaking," *Hastings Center Report* (March–April 1995).
18. R. A. Charo and K. Rothenberg, " 'The Good Mother': The Limits of Reproductive Accountability and Genetic Choice," in *Women and Prenatal Testing: Facing the Challenges of Genetic Testing,* ed. K. Rothenberg and E. Thompson (Columbus, Ohio: Ohio State University Press, 1994); D. Knight and J. Callahan, *Preventing Birth: Contemporary Methods and Related Moral Controversies* (Salt Lake City, Utah: University of Utah Press, 1989), 261–62.
19. Knight and Callahan, *Preventing Birth,* 261.
20. Ibid., 262.
21. Charo and Rothenberg, "The Good Mother."
22. B. Steinbock and R. McClamrock, "When Is Birth Unfair to the Child?" *Hastings Center Report* (November–December 1994): 15.
23. J. Feinberg, *Harm to Others* (New York: Oxford University Press, 1984). Quoted in Steinbock and McClamrock, "When Is Birth Unfair to the Child?" 15.
24. Charo and Rothenberg, "The Good Mother," 112; Knight and Callahan, *Preventing Birth,* 262.
25. Steinbock and McClamrock, "When Is Birth Unfair to the Child?"; L. Purdy, "Loving Future People," in *Reproduction, Ethics, and the Law: Feminist Perspectives,* ed. J. Callahan (Bloomington, Ind.: Indiana University Press, 1995).
26. Steinbock and McClamrock, "When Is Birth Unfair to the Child?" 15.
27. Ibid, 19.
28. Ibid.
29. Ibid., 20.
30. Purdy, "Loving Future People."
31. M. Mahowald, "Reproductive Genetics and Gender Justice," in *Women and Prenatal Testing: Facing the Challenges of Genetic Technology,* ed. K. Rothenberg and E. Thomson (Columbus, Ohio: Ohio State University Press, 1994), 73.
32. D. Wertz and J. Fletcher, "A Critique of Some Feminist Challenges to Prenatal Diagnosis," *Journal of Women's Health,* 2, no. 2 (1993): 173–88.
33. For a discussion of gender as a social location see, D. Smith, *The Everyday World as Problematic* (Boston: Northeastern University Press, 1987). For a critique of feminist theory and a discussion of race, class, and gender as intersecting social locations see, P. Hill-Collins, *Black Feminist Thought* (New York: Routledge, 1990); B. Thornton Dill and M. Bacca Zinn, *Race and Gender: Re-Visioning Social Relations* (Memphis, Tenn.: Center for Research on Women, 1990); A. Dula, "Bioethics: The Need for a Dialogue with African Americans," in *The Ethics of Health Care for African Americans,* ed. A. Dula and S. Goering (Westport, Conn.: Praeger Press, 1994).
34. M. Mahowald et al., "The New Genetics and Women," *Milbank Quarterly* 74, no. 2 (1996).

35. D. Beeson, "Technological Rhythms in Pregnancy," in *Cultural Perspectives on Biological Knowledge,* ed. T. Duster and K. Garrett (Norwood: Ablex, 1984); Charo and Rothenberg, "The Good Mother"; E. Gates, "Prenatal Genetic Testing: Does it Benefit Pregnant Women," in *Women and Prenatal Testing: Facing the Challenges of Genetic Technology,* ed. K. Rothenberg and E. Thompson (Columbus, Ohio: Ohio State University Press, 1994); A. Lippman, "The Genetic Construction of Prenatal Testing: Choice, Consent, or Conformity for Women?" in *Women and Prenatal Testing: Facing the Challenges of Genetic Technology,* ed. K. Rothenberg and E. Thompson (Columbus, Ohio: Ohio State University Press, 1994); M. Mahowald, "Reproductive Genetics and Gender Justice"; C. Overall, *Human Reproduction: Principles, Practices, Policies* (New York: Oxford University Press, 1993); B. K. Rothman, *The Tentative Pregnancy: Prenatal Diagnosis and the Future of Motherhood* (New York: Norton Press, 1989); B. K. Rothman, *Recreating Motherhood: Ideology and Technology in a Patriarchal Society* (New York: Viking Press, 1986); B. K. Rothman, "The Tentative Pregnancy: Then and Now," in *Women and Prenatal Testing: Facing the Challenges of Genetic Technology,* ed. K. Rothenberg and E. Thompson (Columbus, Ohio: Ohio State University Press, 1994), 260–70.
36. Lippman, "The Genetic Construction of Prenatal Testing"; Overall, *Human Reproduction*; Rothman, "The Tentative Pregnancy."
37. Lippman, "The Genetic Construction of Prenatal Testing."
38. Charo and Rothenberg, "The Good Mother"; R. Hubbard, *The Politics of Women's Biology* (New Brunswick, N.J.: Rutgers University Press, 1990); Lippman, "The Genetic Construction of Prenatal Testing"; Mahowald, "Reproductive Genetics and Gender Justice"; Overall, *Human Reproduction*; Rothman, "The Tentative Pregnancy."
39. T. Marteau and H. Drake, "Attributions for Disability: The Influence of Genetic Screening," *Social Science and Medicine* 40, no. 8 (1995): 1127–32.
40. M. Mahowald et al., "The New Genetics and Women," *Milbank Quarterly* 74, no. 2 (1996): 241.
41. Wertz and Fletcher, "A Critique of Some Feminist Challenges to Prenatal Diagnosis."
42. B. Sjogren and N. Uddenberg, "Decision Making during the Prenatal Diagnostic Procedure: A Question of and Interview Study of 211 Women Participating in Prenatal Diagnosis," *Prenatal Diagnosis* 8 (1988): 263–73, in "The Council on Ethical and Judicial Affairs, American Medical Association, Ethical Issues Related to Prenatal Genetic Testing," *Archives of Family Medicine* 3 (1994): 637.
43. Beeson, "Technological Rhythms in Pregnancy."
44. Rothman, *The Tentative Pregnancy*; Rothman, "The Tentative Pregnancy."
45. Rothman, "The Tentative Pregnancy."
46. L. Clarke et al., "Prenatal Care Use in Nonmetropolitan and Metropolitan America: Racial/Ethnic Differences," *Journal of Health Care for the Poor and Undeserved* 6, no. 4 (1995): 410–31; F. John Meaney et al., "Providers and Consumers of Prenatal Genetic Testing Services: What Do the National Data Tell Us?" in *Fetal Diagnosis and Therapy Reproductive Genetic Testing: Impact upon Women* (Bethesda, Md.: NIH Workshop, Supplement 1, 1993), 18–27; L. Nsiah-Jefferson, "Reproductive Genetic Services for Low-Income Women and Women of Color: Access and Sociocultural Issues."
47. Singer, "Public Attitudes toward Genetic Testing."
48. M. Kuppermann, E. Gates, and A. E. Washington, "Racial-Ethnic Differences in Prenatal Diagnostic Test Use and Outcomes: Preferences, Socioeconomics, or Patient Knowledge?" *Obstetrics and Gynecology* 87, no. 5, Part I (May 1996).
49. L. Clarke et al., "Prenatal Care Use in Nonmetropolitan and Metropolitan America," 427.
50. L. Nsiah-Jefferson, "Reproductive Genetic Services for Low-Income Women and Women of Color," 237–38.
51. Charo and Rothenberg, "The Good Mother"; Dula, "Bioethics."
52. S. Boone, "Slavery and Contract Motherhood: A 'Racialized' Objection to the Autonomy Arguments," in *Issues in Reproductive Technology,* ed. H. B. Holmes (New York: New York University Press, 1992); Nsiah-Jefferson and Hall cited in, M. Mahowald, "Reproductive Genetics and Gender Justice," 76.
53. Dula, "Bioethics"; J. Bowman, "Genetic Screening: Toward a New Eugenics?: in *"It Just Ain't Fair": The Ethics of Health Care for African Americans,* ed. A. Dula and S. Goering (Westport: Praeger Press, 1994).
54. L. Handwerker, "Medical Risk: Implicating Poor Pregnant Women," *Social Science and Medicine* 38, no. 5 (1994): 665–75.
55. Lippman, "The Genetic Construction of Prenatal Testing."
56. Dula, "Bioethics," 16–17.
57. See, T. Duster, *Backdoor to Eugenics* (New York: Routledge, 1990).
58. Dula, "Bioethics"; Duster, *Backdoor to Eugenics*; D. Wilkinson, "For Whose Benefit? Politics and Sickle Cell," *The Black Scholar* 5, no. 8 (May 1974): 26–31.
59. Dula, "Bioethics," 18.
60. Bowman, "Genetic Screening"; Dula, "Bioethics"; Nsiah-Jefferson, "Reproductive Genetic Services for Low-Income Women and Women of Color."
61. R. Rapp, "Women's Responses to Prenatal Diagnosis: A Sociocultural Perspective on Diversity," in *Women and*

Prenatal Testing: Facing the Challenges of Genetic Technology, ed. K. Rothenberg and E. Thompson (Columbus, Ohio: Ohio State University Press, 1994), 224.

62. D. Beeson and D. Fullwiley, "Risk, Resistance and Relevance: Sickle Cell Testing and Issues of Control in the Lives of African Americans." Paper presented at 95th Annual Meeting of the American Anthropology Association, San Francisco, Calif., 21 Nov. 1996.
63. M. Saxton, "Prenatal Screening and Discriminatory Attitudes about Disability," in *Embryos, Ethics and Women's Rights: Exploring the New Reproductive Technologies,* ed. E. H. Baruch et al. (1988), 217–24.
64. M. Saxton, "Disability Rights and Selective Abortion," in *Abortion Wars: A Half Century of Struggle,* ed. R. Solinger (Berkeley, Calif.: University of California Press, 1998).
65. L. Hershey, "Choosing Disability," in *Ms.* July/August 1994, 26–32; A. Asch, "Reproductive Technology and Disability," in *Reproductive Laws for the 1990s,* ed. S. Cohen and N. Taub (1989): 69–117; M. Saxton, "Disability Rights and Selective Abortion."
66. M. Saxton, "Disability Rights and Selective Abortion."
67. Asch, "Reproductive Technology and Disability," 73.
68. Lippman, "The Genetic Construction of Prenatal Testing," 12–13.
69. T. Thobani, "From Reproduction to Mal[e] Production: Women and Sex Selection Technology," in *Misconceptions: The Social Construction of Choice and the New Reproductive and Genetic Technologies,* ed. Basen, Eichler, and Lippman (Hull, Quebec: Voyageur Publishing, 1993): 138–53.
70. A. Lippman and B. S. Wilfond, "Twice-told Tales: Stories about Genetic Disorders." *American Journal of Human Genetics* 51 (1992): 936–37.
71. Asch, "Reproductive Technology and Disability," 71–72.
72. Hershey, "Choosing Disability"; A. Asch, "Reproductive Technology and Disability."
73. D. Kaplan, "Prenatal Screening and Diagnosis: The Impact on Persons with Disabilities," in *Women and Prenatal Testing: Facing the Challenges of Genetic Technology,* ed. K. Rothenberg and E. Thompson (Columbus, Ohio: Ohio State University Press, 1994), 59.
74. Rothman, *Recreating Motherhood*; Hubbard, *The Politics of Women's Biology.*
75. M. Saxton, *Disability Feminism Meets DNA: A Study of an Educational Model for Genetic Counseling Students on the Social and Ethical Issues of Selective Abortion.* (Ph.D. diss. Cincinnati, Ohio: Union Institute, 1996).
76. R. Rapp, "Women's Responses to Prenatal Diagnosis."
77. Nsiah-Jefferson, "Reproductive Genetic Services for Low-Income Women and Women of Color," 251.
78. Rapp, "Women's Responses to Prenatal Diagnosis," 252.
79. Rapp, "Women's Responses to Prenatal Diagnosis," 222; L. Nsiah-Jefferson, "Reproductive Genetic Services for Low-Income Women and Women of Color."
80. N. Press and C. H. Browner, " 'Collective Fictions': Similarities in Reasons for Accepting Maternal Serum Alpha-Fetoprotein Screening among Women of Diverse Ethnic and Social Class Backgrounds," *Fetal Diagnosis and Therapy* 8 (suppl. 1, 1993): 97–106.
81. Ibid.
82. Hubbard, *The Politics of Women's Biology,* 4.
83. J. S. Alpers and J. Beckwith, "Genetic Fatalism and Social Policy: The Implications of Behavior Genetics Research," *Yale Journal of Biology and Medicine* 66 (1993): 511–524; R. Hubbard, *The Politics of Women's Biology,* 52–54; R. C. Strohman, "The Coming Kuhnin: A Revolution in Biology," *Nature Biotechnology* 15 (March 1997): 511–24.
84. R. C. Strohman, "Ancient Genomes, Wise Bodies, Unhealthy People: Limits of a Genetic Paradigm in Biology and Medicine," *Perspectives in Biology and Medicine,* 37, no. 1 (1993): 112–45.
85. Charo and Rothenberg, "The Good Mother," 112; E. Gates, "Prenatal Genetic Testing: Does it Benefit Pregnant Women," in *Women and Prenatal Testing: Facing the Challenges of Genetic Technology,* ed. K. Rothenberg and E. Thompson (Columbus, Ohio: Ohio State University Press, 1994), 190.
86. Rapp, "Women's Responses to Prenatal Diagnosis," 227.

Chapter 5

The Ethical Challenge of the New Reproductive Technology

Sidney Callahan

How should we ethically evaluate the new reproductive technologies developed to treat the increasing problem of human infertility? Our national debate over this troubling issue is just beginning. At this point, there are lacunae in law and regulatory procedures, while medical technological innovation and practice proceed without ethical consensus. This situation is due in part to the speed of recent developments, but we also find ourselves ethically perplexed because we, as a society, did not arrive at a consensus on the ethics of reproduction and responsible parenthood *before* the newest technologies appeared on the scene.

One obvious sign of the society's unresolved conflicts over the morality of reproduction can be found in the bitter debates over abortion and, to a lesser extent, contraception and contraceptive education in the schools. With no societal consensus on the ethical use of medical technology to plan, limit, or interrupt pregnancies, we are unprepared to evaluate the newest alternative reproductive technologies, which *promote* conception and pregnancies. At the same time as we have seen rapid advances in regulating fertility, we have experienced an evolution in attitudes toward women, children, sexuality, and the family. These intersecting social developments have produced the pressing need to develop a new ethic of parenthood and responsible reproduction.[1] My focus here, however, is on the most recent challenge. How should we ethically assess the innovative array of techniques developed to overcome infertility—egg and sperm donations, surrogate mothers, in vitro fertilization, and embryo transplants?

TWO INADEQUATE APPROACHES TO ALTERNATIVE REPRODUCTIVE TECHNOLOGY

Two inadequate approaches to the ethical assessment of the new alternative reproductive technologies are mirror images of each other in the narrowness of their focus and the limitations of their analysis. On the one hand, a conservative approach adopts as a moral standard the biological integrity of the marital sexual act. The married couple's marital sexual and reproductive acts must not be tampered with for any reason, and sexual intercourse and procreation must remain united in each marital act so that "lovemaking and baby making" are never separated. In this "act analysis," no technological intervention in the sexual act is countenanced or approved for any reason. Older arguments employed against artificial contraception are reiterated and applied to condemn any procedure separating functions that naturally occur together, and thus all reproduction by in vitro fertilization, artificial insemination, or third-party surrogacy is deemed immoral. The only ethical stance toward new reproductive technologies would be to absolutely cease and desist; such procedures should come to a full stop.

At the other end of the ideological spectrum, another form of act analysis narrows its own focus to a person's desire for a child and the individual acts the person might perform in carrying out private arrangements for reproduction. As long as due process and informed consent by competent adults is guarded by proper contracts, any adult should be able to engage in any alternative reproductive procedure that technology can provide or that persons will sell or procure. This permissive stance is held to be justified on the basis of individual liberty, autonomy, reproductive privacy, and reproductive right. The burden of proof supposedly lies with those who would limit alternative reproductive technology, and in the name of liberty and individual autonomy, potential regulators are enjoined to show that concrete harmful consequences will result from a particular practice (if it is to be rejected). Of course, when there are as yet no existing consequences, it is impossible to *prove* harm will result. Indeed, even when there have been relevant cases (e.g., the artificial insemination by donor (AID) children, no long-term in-depth studies have been done. Therefore, the ethical response to alternative reproductive technologies is to proceed full steam ahead (with consideration given to due process and informed consent).

The premature ethical foreclosure implied in either of the above approaches to reproductive technologies is not adequate. An ethic based solely on the natural biological integrity of marital acts will not serve, because the mastery of nature through technological problem solving is also completely natural to us—indeed, it is the glory of *homo sapiens.* Yet, because we are rational, we can also see that a fully permissive attitude toward reproductive technology presents serious problems as well. We are reminded that in the past, innovative uses of technology have resulted in ecological and ethical disasters. Abuses have been either fully intended, as with the Nazis, or inadvertent and accidental, as in countless innovative interventions, such as the use of diethylstilbestrol (DES) or thalidomide, which had bad side effects far outweighing the supposed advantages. There is a grain of truth in the warning that "control of nature" often ends up producing increased control (or oppression) of some people by other more powerful people. Technology itself has to be ethically assessed and rationally controlled. Faced with new reproductive technologies, we should not let the technological imperative (what can be done should be done), fueled in this case by people's desires, decide the question whether a course of action is right or good.

THE BASIS FOR DEVELOPING AN ETHICAL POSITION

In the case of reproductive technology, ethical positions should emerge from a consideration of what will further the good of the potential child and the family, as well as provide appropriate social conditions for childrearing and strengthening our commitment to moral principles concerning individual responsibility in reproduction. We should move beyond a narrow focus on either biology or people's desires for children. In this serious matter, which involves children's lives and the social structure of our society, it is more prudent to consider first the values and goods safeguarded and protected at present by the operating norms of reproduction and childrearing before countenancing radical alterations. In matters of such serious collective import, the burden of proof should rightly be upon those who wish to experiment with the lives of others. (An ethical problem also arises concerning the justice of allocating medical resources to increase individual fertility in an overpopulated, impoverished world. However, since the main issue here concerns the use of reproductive technology, I think the correct statement of the ethical question is whether, or how far, present norms should be altered.)

One troubling tactic used by those urging the permissive acceptance of all new reproductive technologies is to base their arguments upon analogies from adoption or other childrearing arrangements that arise from divorce, death, desertion, or parental inadequacy. Much is made of the cases in which persons cope with single parenthood or successfully adapt to other less-than-ideal situations. But the adequacy of "after the fact" crisis management does not justify planning beforehand to voluntarily replicate similar childrearing situations. Emergency solutions make poor operating norms. Even a child conceived through rape or incest might adapt and be glad to have been born, but surely it would be wrong to plan such conceptions beforehand on the grounds that the future child would rather exist than not or that the sexual abuser had no other means to reproduce. Similarly, and more to the point, heretofore we have not ethically or legally countenanced the practice of deliberately conceiving a child in order to give it to others for adoption, with or without payment. We have forbidden the selling of babies or, for that matter, the purchasing of brides, sexual intercourse, or bodily organs. Certain cultural goods, safeguards, and values have been preserved by these existing norms. How can ethical guidelines for employing alternative reproductive methods strengthen rather than threaten our basic cultural values?

A PROPOSED ETHICAL STANDARD

It is ethically appropriate to use an alternative reproductive technology if, and only if, it makes it possible for a normal, socially well-adjusted heterosexual married couple to have a child that they could not otherwise have owing to infertility. Infertility does not seem strictly classifiable as a disease, but for a married couple it is clearly an unfortunate dysfunction or handicap, one that medicine may sometimes remedy. It seems wonderful, almost miraculous, that medical technology can often overcome a couple's infertility to restore normal function with techniques such as artificial insemination by husband (AIH), in vitro fertilization (IVF), or tubal ovum transfer methods. But holding to a proposed ethical standard of medical remediation and restoration of a married couple's average expectable fertility implies that medical professionals should not aim to alter or contravene what would otherwise exist as the normal conditions for procreation and childrearing.

A remedial standard based upon operating cultural norms requires that the genetic parents, the gestational parents, and the rearing parents be identical and that the parents be presently alive and well, in an appropriate time in their lifecycle, and possess average or adequate psychological and social resources for childrearing. Helping the severely retarded, the mentally ill, the genetically diseased, the destitute, the aged, or a widow with a dead spouse's sperm to have children they otherwise could not would be ethically unacceptable by this standard. It would also be unacceptable to alter average expectable conditions by efforts to produce multiple births or to select routinely for sex (the latter practice producing a whole host of other ethical problems that cannot be dealt with here). The power to intervene in such a crucial matter as the procreation of a new life makes the medical professionals or medical institutions involved into ethically responsible trustees of a potential child's future. As trustees, medical professionals would seem to have an ethical duty not to take risks on behalf of unconsenting others.

Medical professionals should be guided by a form of communal judgment influenced by cultural values and norms. What would most responsible would-be parents deem ethically appropriate reproductive behavior in a particular case? Physicians or other health care personnel can hardly, in good conscience, agree to and make possible irresponsible or ethically inappropriate reproductive acts affecting innocent new lives. Socially informed ethical judgments on behalf of the society are unavoidable. The fact that medical professionals and medical resources must be employed for remedial infertility treatments, which will produce direct social consequences, justifies using standards of judgment that take into account the general social good. Ethical standards that protect and strengthen positive outcomes for children, childrearing conditions, and cultural norms of responsible parenthood should be used to judge the appropriateness of a particular request for treatment of infertility.

The claim that an individual's right to reproduce would be violated if fertility treatments are not made available to any individual who requests them seems wrongheaded. A negative right not to be interfered with (e.g., the right to marry, which itself is not absolute) does not entail a positive right (e.g., that society is obligated to provide spouses). Moreover, as a society, we have already decided that when adequate childrearing conditions and the well-being of children are in the balance, social and professional intervention is justified. Adoption procedures, custodial decisions, and the child abuse laws involve rights and duties of professionals to make judgments on the fitness of parents. And as child abuse and resulting deaths regularly attest, it is far better to err on the side of safety than take risks. Should not medical professionals be similarly responsible in carrying out the interventions that will in essence give to a couple a baby to rear? If a couple seems within the normal range of average expectable parents, then remedial techniques that maintain the identicalness of genetic, gestational, and rearing parentage, techniques such as AIH or IVF or tubal ovum transfer, would be ethically acceptable.

Employing third-party donors or surrogate mothers is not, in my opinion, ever an ethically acceptable use of reproductive technologies. Procedures using donors or surrogates separate and variously recombine the source of sperm, eggs, embryos, gestational womb, and rearing parents. Such a separation—whether through AID, embryo transplants, or surrogate mothers—poses too many ethical and social risks to the dignity and well-being of the future child, the donor, individual spouses, the family as a whole, and our cultural ethos. To argue the case against third-party donors, even for acceptable couples, we need to consider what values, goods, and safeguards have been inherent in the cultural norm: two heterosexual parents who are the genetic, gestational, and rearing parents of their child.

Many proponents of third-party donors in alternative reproduction—for single men and women, homosexual couples, or infertile couples—ignore what happens *after* a baby is conceived, produced, or procured. Focusing on an individual or on individual couples, the psychological and social dimensions of childrearing are separated from conception, gestation, and birth. Little account is taken of the fact that individuals live out their lifespans intergenerationally and in complex ecological and social systems.[2] No account is taken of the newest developments in family therapy and family systems analysis. The assumption seems to be that why and how one gets a baby makes no difference in what happens afterward. This may be true of hens or cows, but it is hardly true of complex, thinking, emoting, imaginative human beings functioning within social systems.

Another equally invalid line of argument cites the current trends toward the breakdown of the traditional family unit and jumps to the conclusion that since the nuclear family seems to be disintegrating anyway, and the society survives, why try to preserve the norms heretofore valued? Ominous cultural effects on children and women that correlate with the breakdown of the family are dismissed as having no application to individual cases.[3] But a growing body of psychological literature points to a less sanguine judgment. Having *two* rearing parents provides important advantages, and fathers play more of a role in the moral, social, and sexual-identity development of the child than has been recognized.[4]

Legitimizing and morally sanctioning third-party or collaborative reproduction or assisting single or homosexual conceptions can contribute directly to the specific negative childrearing conditions in the culture that *do* harm individuals and the larger community. The culture's operating norms concerning the family provide irreplaceable goods and safeguards—particularly for women and their children—that we come to truly value as we see them attenuated. Arguments for limiting reproductive interventions to remediation with no third-party interventions can best be made by considering what is at stake if we alter our norms. We put at risk the good of the family, the parents, the child, and the donor(s), as well as our sexual morality, with its focus on sexual responsibility.

THE FAMILY

The advantages and safeguards of having two heterosexual parents who are the genetic, gestational, and rearing parents are manifold and basic; this type of family was not accidentally selected for in biological and cultural evolution. Mammalian "in vivo" reproduction and primate parent-child bonding provide adaptive means for the protection, defense, and complex socialization of offspring. They far outperform reproduction by laying eggs that are then left floating in the sea or buried in the sand to take their chances with passing predators.[5] With the advent of long-living rational animals such as human beings, the basic primate models are broadened and deepened, which results in family units that include fathers and encompass additional kinship bonds.[6] Two heterosexual parents supported by kin and clan can engage in even more arduous parenting, including nurturing the young over an extended period. The nuclear family is founded on biology and may have originally evolved through natural selection, but it is as a cultural phenomenon, with its psychological and social effectiveness in generating responsibility, socialization, and deep altruistic bonds, that the family has achieved stability and universality.

Why has the nuclear family worked for so long and held first place in the cultural competition?[7] The Western cultural ideal, gradually becoming less patriarchal as it comes to recognize the equality of women and children, has ensured far more than law, order, and social continuity. As the heterosexual members of a couple freely choose each other, they make a loving commitment to share the vicissitudes of life. Bonded in love and legal contract, they mutually exchange exclusive rights, giving each other emotional and economic priority. Love and sexuality often result in procreation, and the children then have a claim to equal parental care from both their father and mother. In addition, the extended families of both parents are important as supplemental supports for the couple, especially in cases of death or disaster.

No act analysis of one procreative period of time in a marriage can do justice to the fact that the reproductive couple exists as a unit within a family extended in time and kinship. Grandparents, grandchildren, aunts, cousins, and other relatives are important in family life for both pragmatic and psychological reasons. Individual identity is rooted in biologically based kinship and in small cooperating social units. The family is one remaining institution where status is given by birth, not earned or achieved. The irreversible bonds of kinship over time and through space produce rootedness and a sense of identity. Psychologically and socially the family provides emotional connections, social purpose, and meaning to life. Those individuals who do not marry and found families or who achieve membership in larger communities are still strongly connected to others through their families.[8] Each human being exists within a social envelope and must do so to flourish; the family is one of the most important elements in a human life. But as a cultural invention, why must a family be based upon biological kinship? Cannot any persons who declare themselves a family be a family?

While the internalized psychological image of a family and the intention to belong to a family are part of the foundations of a family, there is no denying the bond created by genetic kinship. One definition of the family is that a family consists of people who share genes. Sociobiologists have not exaggerated the importance of gene sharing in human bonding.[9] In fact, the unwillingness of infertile couples to adopt and their struggles to have their own baby is testimony to the existence of what appears to be a strong innate urge to reproduce oneself. Culturally this is understood as the fusion of two genetic heritages, with the child situated within two lineages. Members of both lineages may be supportive, or one set of kin may by choice or chance be more important than the other, but having both sets provides important social resources. The child is heir to more than money or property when situated in a rooted kinship community.

The search by adopted children for their biological parents and possible siblings reveals the psychological need of humans to be situated and to know their origins.[10] When there are one or more third-party donors—of sperm, eggs, or embryo—the child is cut off from either half or all of its genetic heritage. If deception is practiced concerning the child's origins, then both the child and the extended family will be wronged. Since family secrets are rarely kept completely, the delayed revelations produce disillusionment and distrust among those deceived. When a child and relatives are not lied to, the identity of the donor (or donors) becomes an issue for all concerned.

Parents and Spouses

Psychology has come to see genetic factors as more and more important in parent-child interactions and childrearing outcomes.[11] When rearing parents and genetic parents differ and the donor is unknown, there is a provocative void. If the donor is known and is part of the rearing parents' family or social circle, there are other psychological problems and potential conflicts over who is the real parent and who has the primary rights and responsibilities. When the third-party donor is also the surrogate mother, combining genetic and gestational parenthood, the social and legal problems can be profound. The much discussed Whitehead-Stern court struggle indicates the divisive chaos, struggle, and suffering that is possible in surrogate arrangements.

In the average expectable situation, two parents with equal genetic investment in the child are unified by their mutual relationship to the child. They are irreversibly connected and made kin to each other through the biological child they have procreated. Their love, commitment, and sexual bond have been made manifest in a new life. Their genetic link with the child, shared with his or her own family, produces a sense of family likeness and personal identification, leading to empathy and affective attunement. The child's genetic link to each spouse and his or her kin strengthens the marital bond. But the fact that the child is also a new and unique creation and a random fusion of the couple's genetic heritage gives enough distance to allow the child also to be seen as a separate other, with what has been called its "alien dignity as a human being" intact.[12] (Cloning oneself would be wrong for its egotistic intent and for the dehumanizing effects of trying to deny the uniqueness of identity.) The marital developments that occur during pregnancy also unite the couple and prepare them for the parental enterprise.[13] Since we are embodied creatures, the psychological bonds of caring and empathy are built upon the firm foundation of biological ties and bodily self-identity.

When technological intervention without donors, such as AIH or IVF or tubal ovum transfer, is used to correct infertility, the time, money, stress, and cooperative effort required serve to test the unity of the couple and focus them upon their marital relationship and their mutual contribution to childbearing. The psychological bonding between them can transcend the stress caused by the less-than-ideal technological interventions in their sexual lives. The result of their joint effort will, as in natural pregnancy, be a baby they are equally invested in and equally related to. (In adoption, both parents also have an equal relationship to the child they are jointly rescuing.) Given the equal investment in their child, both parents are equally responsible for childrearing and support.

With third-party genetic or gestational donors, however, the marital and biological unity is broken asunder. One parent will be related biologically to the child and the other parent will not. True, the nonrelated parent may give consent, but the consent, even if truly informed and uncoerced, can hardly equalize the imbalance. While there is certainly no real question of adultery in such a situation, nevertheless, the intruding third-party donor, as in adultery, will inevitably have a psychological effect on the couple's life. Even if there is no jealousy or envy, the reproductive inadequacy of one partner has been made definite and reliance has been placed on an outsider's potency, genetic heritage, and superior reproductive capacity.[14]

Asymmetry in biological parental relationships within a family or household has always been problematic, from Cinderella to today's stepparents and reconstituted families. The most frequently cited cause of divorce in second marriages is the difficulty of dealing with another person's children.[15] Empathy, identification, a sense of kinship, and assurance of parental authority arise from family likeness and biological ties. In disturbed families under stress, one finds more incest, child abuse, and scapegoating when biological kinship is absent.[16] Biological ties become psychologically potent, because human beings fantasize in their intersubjective emotional interactions with one another and with their children. Parents' fantasies about a child's past and future do make a difference, as all students of child development or family dynamics will attest. Identical twins may even be treated very differently because parents project different fantasies upon them.[17] Third-party donors and surrogates cannot be counted on to disappear from family consciousness, even if legal contracts could control other ramifications or forbid actual interventions.

The Child

The most serious ethical problems in using third-party donors in alternative reproduction concern the well-being of the potential child. A child conceived by new forms of collaborative reproduction is being made party to a social experiment without its consent. While no child is conceived by its own consent, a child not artificially produced is at least born in the same way as its parents and other persons normally have been. A child who has a donor or donors among its parents will be cut off from at least part of its genetic heritage and its kin in new ways. Even if there is no danger of transmitting unknown genetic disease or causing physiological harm to the child, the psychological relationship of the child to its parents is endangered, whether or not there is deception or secrecy about its origins.

It should be clear that adoption (which rescues a child already in existence) is very different ethically from planning to involve third-party donors in procuring a child. An adopted child, while perhaps harboring resentment against its birth parents, must look at its rescuing adopters differently than a child would look at parents who have had it made to order. Treating the child like a commodity—something to be created for the pleasure of the parents—infringes upon the child's dignity. When one is begotten (not made), then one shares equally with one's parents in the ongoing transmission of the gift of life from generation to generation. The child procreated in the expectable way is a subsidiary gift arising from the prior marital relationship, not a product or project of the parental will.

Alternative reproductive techniques made available to single men and women or to homosexual couples will further endanger the child's status. Why should a child, at its creation, be treated as a property, a product, or a means to satisfy the wishes of adults? Even in natural reproduction, we now consider it ethically suspect to attempt to have a child not for its own sake, but because an adult wants to satisfy some personal need or desire.

Unfortunately, we are still saddled with residual ideologies that view children as a kind of personal property. Only gradually have we welcomed children as gifts—new lives given in trusteeship—and treated them as equal to adult persons in human dignity despite their dependency and their powerlessness.[18] Having a child for some extrinsic reason is now as generally unacceptable as marrying for money or some motive besides love and a desire for mutual happiness. Unfortunately, in the past some persons have wanted children to secure an inheritance, to prove sexual prowess, to procure a scapegoat, to gain revenge, to increase marital power, to secure social prestige, or to have someone of their own to love. The motives for conception influence the future relationship of the child to the parents. A couple absolutely and obsessively driven to have a child (as some couples become when faced with infertility) may not be prepared to rear the actual child once it is born. Being wanted and being well-reared are not identical. Parental overinvestment in "gourmet children" can be psychologically difficult for a child.[19] Every child must achieve independence and a separate identity. Adolescent problems of anorexia, depression, and suicide have been seen as related to the dynamics of parental control.[20] Growing up and leaving home becomes a problem for children who have been used to fulfill parents.[21] The child who was wanted for all the wrong reasons is pressured to live up to parental dreams of the optimal baby or perfect child. Outright rejection of imperfect or nonoptimal babies contracted for by alternative reproductive technology is possible and should be a matter of grave concern.

In the course of a child's development, psychologists note that thinking and fantasizing about one's origins seems to be inevitable. A child with a "clouded genetic heritage" has a more difficult time achieving a secure personal identity.[22] Yet a secure identity, self-esteem, and a sense of autonomy and self-control are crucial in children's growth.[23] Parental control is overwhelming to children. If they know or believe their parents contracted to fabricate them rather than merely received them, they feel more reduced in power.

In alternative reproduction, the question "Whose baby am I?" becomes inevitable.[24] "Why was my biological parent not more concerned with what would happen to the new life he or she helped to create?" The need to know about possible half-siblings and other kin may become urgent at some point in later development. From the child's point of view, the asymmetry of the relationship with the rearing parents is also a factor. Even if the Freudian psychoanalytic account of Oedipal family relationships is not correct in all its details, there still exist extremely complex fantasies and psychological currents that arise in the family triangle of mother, father, and child. Having two parents whom one can safely identify with, love, and leave behind is a great advantage. One's sexual origins and one's kin are important psychological realities to a child.

DONORS AND THE CULTURAL ETHOS

Procuring donors of sperm, eggs, embryos, or wombs is an essential component of collaborative reproduction. Yet encouraging persons to give, or worse, to sell, their genetic or gestational capacity attacks a basic foundation of morality—that is, the taking of responsibility for the consequences of one's actions. Adult persons are held morally responsible for their words and deeds. In serious matters, such as sex and reproduction, which have irreversible lifetime consequences, we rightly hold persons to high standards of moral and legal responsibility. To counter the tendency or temptation toward sexual irresponsibility or parental neglect, Western culture has insisted that men and women be held accountable for their contribution to the creation of new life.

A donor, whether male or female, who takes part in collaborative reproduction does not assume personal responsibility for his or her momentous personal action engendering new life. In fact, the donor contracts (possibly with payment) to abdicate present and future personal responsibility. The donor is specifically enjoined not to carry through on what he or she initiates, but instead to hand over to physicians or others, often unknown others, the result of his or her reproductive capacity. The generative power to create a new life is by design ejected from consideration. This genetic generative capacity is not like a kidney (or any other organ), but is part of the basic identity that is received from one's own parents. When a person treats this capacity as trivial or sells the use of it, he or she breaks an implicit compact. Parental responsibility is an essential form of the natural responsibility human beings have to help each other, and it gives rise to moral claims not governed by specific contracts or commitments.[25]

Persons who abdicate parental responsibility also deprive their own parents of grandparenthood and any other of their descendants of knowledge of their kin. Future children of the donor, or other children of a surrogate mother, will never know their half-brother or -sister. To so disregard the reality of the biological integrity of our identity and allow donors to engage in contractual reproduction is to have a mistaken view of how human beings actually function—or should function.

If we succeed in isolating sexual and reproductive acts from long-term personal responsibility, this moral abdication will increase existing problems within the culture. Do we want to encourage women to be able to emotionally distance themselves from the child in their womb enough to give it up? Do we wish to sanction male detachment from their biological offspring? Already epidemics of divorce, illegitimate conceptions, and parental irresponsibility and failures are straining the family bonds and the firm commitment that are necessary for successful childrearing and the full development of individuals. If we legitimize the isolation of genetic, gestational, and social parentage and regularly allow reproduction to be governed by contract and purchase, our culture will become even more fragmented, rootless, and alienated.

One of the foundations of a responsible ethic concerning sexuality is to see sexual acts as personal acts involving the whole person. Lust is wrong because it disregards the whole person and his or her human dignity. Another person is reduced to a means of selfish pleasure, and if money is involved, exploitation of the needy can occur. So, too, it seems wrong to isolate and use a person's reproductive capacity apart from his or her personal life. When it is a woman donating her egg and gestational capacity, there is a grave danger of exploitation, as feminists have warned.[26] The physiological risks attending the drastic intervention in a woman's reproductive system needed for surrogacy or embryo transplants are considerable. But perhaps more important is that pregnancy is not simply a neutral organic experience, but a time of bonding of the mother to her child.

If a great deal of money is offered for surrogacy, needy women will be tempted to sell their bodies and suffer the emotional consequences—and the experience of prostitution leads one to expect that many of these women will then hand over the money to males. Feminists rightly protest that allowing women to be surrogates will in fact turn women into baby machines bought and regulated by those rich enough to pay.[27] From another perspective, a surrogate mother could also be seen as deliberately producing and selling her baby. What will these practices do to other children of the surrogate or, for that matter, other children in the society? Can children comprehend, without anxiety, the fact that mothers make babies and give them away for money? The great primordial reality of interdependency and mutual bonding represented by mother and child is attacked. Contracts and regulations can hardly stem the psychological and social harm alternative reproductive technologies make possible.

CONCLUSION

Our society faces a challenge to its traditional ethics of reproduction and family norms. The cultural norm, based upon biological predispositions, is for the genetic, gestational, and rearing parents to be identical and for the nuclear family to exist within an extended family kinship system. The family should be seen as an intergenerational institution having an ecological relationship with the larger society.

As the range of ethics has broadened to include a concern for the dignity, worth, and rights of women and children, so has our understanding of morally responsible parenthood been refined and developed. The parental enterprise is rightly seen as basically an altruistic one—children should not be viewed as a form of personal property or as a means to satisfy adult desires or fulfill adult needs. When making reproductive decisions, the good of the potential child, along with the general cultural conditions that further childrearing and family support systems, should take precedence over other considerations, such as biologically integral acts or individual desires.

I have argued for an ethical position that limits alternative reproductive techniques to remedying infertility in expectable parental conditions that preserve the cultural norm, which includes the identity of genetic, gestational, and rearing parents. Collaborative reproduction will not serve the good of the potential child or the family, nor will it meet the need of the culture for morally responsible reproductive behavior.

It seems a sign of cultural progress that children are highly valued and infertility is acknowledged as a misfortune. It is also wonderful that medical reproductive technology can remedy the handicap of infertility. But as medical professionals and people in general confront these innovative interventions, the ethical, psychological, and cultural dimensions of technological procedures cannot be discounted. For the good of the child, the donors, the family, and our society, certain ethical limits must be set. Not everything that can be done to satisfy individual reproductive desires should be done. As Ghandi said, "Means are ends in the making."[28] Collaborative reproduction using third parties comes at too high a price.

NOTES

1. See S. Callahan, "An Ethical Analysis of Responsible Parenthood," in *Genetic Counseling: Facts, Values, and Norms,* Birth Defects: Original Article Series, vol. 15, no. 22 (New York: Alan R. Liss, 1979).
2. B. M. Newman and P. R. Newman, *Development through Life: A Psychosocial Approach* (Homewood, Ill.: The Dorsey Press, 1979); L. Hoffman, *Foundations of Family Therapy: A Conceptual Framework for Systems Change* (New York: Basic Books, 1981).
3. D. P. Moynihan, *Family and Nation* (New York: Harcourt Brace Jovanovich, 1986); L. J. Weitzman, *The Divorce Revolution* (New York: The Free Press, 1986).
4. The role of the father has been seen as critically important in both the female and male child's intellectual development, moral development, sex role identity, and future parenting; for a summary of relevant research, see R. D. Parke, *Fathers* (Cambridge, Mass.: Harvard University Press, 1981) and S. M. H. Hanson and F. W. Bonett, *Dimensions of Fatherhood* (Beverly Hills, Calif.: Sage Publications, 1985).
5. See J. Altman, "Sociobiological Perspectives on Parenthood," *Parenthood: A Psychodynamic Perspective* (New York: Guilford Press, 1984).
6. K. Gough, "The Origin of the Family," *Journal of Marriage and the Family* (November 1971): 760–68. P. J. Wilson, *Man the Promising Primate: The Conditions of Human Evolution* (New Haven, Conn.: Yale University Press, 1980).
7. G. P. Murdock, "The University of the Nuclear Family," in *A Modern Introduction to the Family,* ed. N. W. Bell and E. F. Vogel (New York: The Free Press, 1968); M. J. Bane, *Here to Stay: American Families in the Twentieth Century* (New York: Basic Books, 1976).
8. S. P. Bank and M. D. Kahn, *The Sibling Bond* (New York: Basic Books, 1982); G. O. Hagestad, "The Aging Society as a Context for Family Life," *Daedalus: The Aging Society* (Winter 1986): 119–39.
9. E. O. Wilson, *Sociobiology* (Cambridge, Mass.: Harvard University Press, 1975).
10. C. Nadelson, "The Absent Parent, Emotional Sequelae," in *Infertility: Medical, Emotional and Social Considerations,* ed. M. D. Mazor and H. F. Simons (New York: Human Sciences Press, 1984); A. D. Sorsky, A. Baron, and R. Pannor, "Identity Conflicts in Adoptees," in *New Directions in Childhood Psychopathology,* vol. I (New York: International Universities Press, 1982).
11. Twin studies and the recognition of inherited temperamental traits have followed studies showing a genetic component to alcoholism, manic-depression, schizophrenia, antisocial behavior, and I.Q. For a popular discussion of the findings in regard to schizophrenia and criminal behavior, see S. Mednick, "Crime in the Family Tree," *Psychology Today,* 19 (March 1985): 58–61. For a more general discussion by an anthropologist, see M. Konner, *The Tangled Wing: Biological Constraints on the Human Spirit* (New York: Holt, Rinehart & Winston, 1982).
12. H. Thielicke, *The Ethics of Sex* (New York: Harper & Row, 1964), 32ff.
13. A. Macfarlane, *The Psychology of Childbirth* (Cambridge, Mass.: Harvard University Press, 1977); M. Greenberg, *The Birth of a Father* (New York: Continuum, 1985).
14. The difficulties of undergoing AID are described in S. G. Collotta, "The Role of the Nurse in AID," in *Infertility*; see also R. Snowden, G.D. Mitchel, and E.M. Snowden, "Stigma and Stress in AID," in *Artificial Reproduction: A Social Investigation* (London: George Allen & Unwin, 1983).
15. B. Maddox, *The Half Parent: Living with Other People's Children* (New York: M. Evans and Company, 1975); R. Espinoza and Y. Newman, *Stepparenting: With Annotated Bibliography* (Rockville, Md.: National Institute of Mental Health, Center for Studies of Child and Family Mental Health, 1979).
16. See "Explaining the Differences between Biological Father and Stepfather Incest," and "Social Factors in the Occurrence of Incestuous Abuse," in *The Secret Trauma: Incest in the Lives of Girls and Women,* ed. D. E. H. Russell (New York: Basic Books, 1986).
17. D. N. Stern, *The Interpersonal World of the Infant: A View from Psychoanalysis and Developmental Psychology* (New York: Basic Books, 1985).
18. There is the beginning of a philosophical reassessment of the status of children in J. Blustein, *Parents & Children: The Ethics of the Family* (Oxford: Oxford Univer-

sity Press, 1982), and in O. O'Neill and W. Ruddick, eds., *Having Children: Philosophical and Legal Reflections on Parenthood* (New York: Oxford University Press, 1979).

19. See "The Child as Surrogate Self" and "The Child as Status Symbol," in David Elkind, *The Hurried Child* (Reading, Mass.: Addison-Wesley, 1981).
20. S. Minuchin, B. L. Rosman, and W. Baker, *Psychosomatic Families: Anorexia Nervosa in Context* (Cambridge, Mass.: Harvard University Press, 1978).
21. J. Haley, *Leaving Home: The Therapy of Disturbed Young People* (New York: McGraw-Hill, 1980).
22. B. J. Lifton, *Lost and Found: The Adoption Experience* (New York: Dial Press, 1979).
23. See "The Sense of Self," in E. E. Maccoby, *Social Development: Psychological Growth and the Parent-Child Relationship* (New York: Harcourt Brace Jovanovich, 1980).
24. L. Andrews, "Yours, Mine and Theirs," *Psychology Today* 18 (December 1984): 20–29.
25. H. Jonas, *The Imperative of Responsibility: In Search of an Ethics for the Technological Age* (Chicago: University of Chicago Press, 1984).
26. B. Rothman, *The Tentative Pregnancy* (New York: Viking Press, 1986); H. Holmes, B. Hoskins, and M. Gross, *The Custom Made Child* (Clifton, N.J.: Humana Press, 1981).
27. A. R. Holder, "Surrogate Motherhood: Babies for Fun and Profit," *Law, Medicine, and Health Care* 11 (June 1984): 115–17.
28. M. Gandhi, *The Essential Gandhi* (New York: Random House, 1962).

CHAPTER 6

Ethical Considerations of Preimplantation Genetic Diagnosis and Embryo Selection

Frank L. Barnes

Significant technological advances in molecular genetics and assisted reproduction have outpaced discussion and consensus on the ethical ramifications of such technology. Two techniques, advanced during the last 10 years, polymerase chain reaction (PCR) and embryo micromanipulation provide the framework for preimplantation diagnosis of genetic disease and alteration of the human genome. These technologies awaken our fear of eugenics; however, the equitable dissemination of this type of medical approach is of similar concern.[1] This discussion seeks to define these methodologies and provide a perspective on an evolving ethical debate.

TECHNOLOGY

Preimplantation embryo genetic diagnosis (PGD) consists of two basic steps: biopsy of the early cleavage-stage embryo and diagnostic assay. Embryo micromanipulation, or microsurgery, has been a popular tool in the study of embryogenesis since the middle of this century and is now the method of choice for obtaining cells from mammalian embryos. Prior to the elucidation of the DNA double helix, embryo microsurgery determined the totipotence of cells. Observation of embryos following microsurgery led to the concept of critical cell mass, or the number of cells required in the early embryo for successful growth and development. The eight-cell stage has proven to be optimal in the human embryo.[2] Earlier biopsy threatens embryo survival due to reduction in critical cell mass required for development. Later biopsy is technically more difficult due to cell compaction and threatens embryo viability due to trauma. The basic biopsy process consists of creating a hole called the zona pellucida in the outer layer of the ovum, either by acidic digestion at a specific site or by cutting with a glass needle. A small-bore pipette is introduced into the embryo and juxtaposed to a single cell. Gentle suction aspirates the cell up the pipette from which it is subsequently delivered for genetic analysis.

In cattle, where sex selection of embryos is routine, 5 to 10 cells are cut free with a glass needle from the trophoblast of a blastocyst-stage embryo. Embryo survival following this procedure is excellent with the small opening in the trophoblast annealing almost immediately following biopsy. An additional advantage of this approach is that more cells are available for analysis, thus reducing the risk of error. Current culture practices preclude this approach in human embryos; however, this will likely change in the near future.

In 1986, Mullis and coworkers described a process for amplifying DNA in vitro and termed the process *polymerase chain reaction* (PCR).[3] Utilizing Taq polymerase, a DNA enzyme isolated from bacteria found in the hot springs of Yellowstone National Park, known segments of DNA can be amplified as much as 10^{12} times after thermal cycling.[4] Brief exposure to high temperature denatures or unwinds a target sequence of double-stranded DNA into a single stranded DNA with a five-inch and a three-inch end. Temperature reduction allows DNA primers to attach to the five-inch end. The temperature is once again increased and Taq polymerase brings about the synthesis of DNA complementary to the target sequence. The amplified product may be visualized by electrophoresis on an agarose gel.[5]

PCR is an incredibly sensitive tool for amplifying small sequences of DNA, lending itself to the identification of single-gene defects regardless of their chromosomal location. This same sensitivity necessitates stringent laboratory conditions lest contamination from nonbiopsied cellular material result in misdiagnosis. PCR specificity dictates individual laboratory conditions and procedures for each genetic disease. Couples suspecting the presence of a genetic disease must first undergo DNA screening to determine their specific defect. Individualized PCR conditions are then applied to those identified as having single-gene defects, exemplified by cystic fibrosis, Lesch-Nyhan syndrome, Tay-Sachs disease, Huntington's disease, and familial breast-ovarian cancer syndrome.[6] Although new protocols are being developed rapidly, PCR is considered to be a qualitative, not a quantitative, procedure. Genetic diseases resulting from aneuploidies are better identified with alternative technology.

Fluorescent in situ hybridization (FISH) allows enumeration of chromosomes by fluorescently labeled chromosome-specific DNA probes. Currently the best procedure for detecting numerical chromosomal disorders, FISH protocols are more standardized than those for PCR. FISH allows the visualization of chromosomal domains within interphase nuclei mounted on glass slides and viewed with a fluorescent microscope. Direct visualization limits concerns of contamination: embryonic cells and their nuclei are much larger than other contaminating sources of DNA. FISH is indicated for embryos derived from women of advanced maternal age (> 35 years old) comprising the high-risk group for chromosomal aneuploidies, including Down's syndrome, Turner's syndrome, Klinefelter's syndrome, trisomy 13 and trisomy 18.[7] Utilization of X and Y chromosome-specific FISH probes can identify embryo sex, allowing the selection against a male embryo possibly affected by an X-linked disease. FISH technology cannot distinguish between affected and nonaffected male embryos; PCR should be applied to sex-linked disease when the gene sequence is known.

Both diagnostic technologies are best served when two cells are available for analysis, thus allowing two independent tests on a given embryo. Concerns regarding contamination during PCR are reduced when independent tests end in the same result. Moreover, the diagnostic value of FISH is enhanced by examining the possibility of genetic mosaicism. It would be better, in this particular scenario, to remove two cells not immediately opposed to each other to prevent biopsy of only one cell lineage.[8]

ETHICAL CONSIDERATIONS

Whether or not to abort a fetus with a severe genetic disorder is not a new dilemma posed to couples and bioethicists. The process of prenatal genetic diagnosis through amniocentesis and chorionic villus sampling has been available for many years. Providing an alternative to having an affected child, these procedures are not without risk to the maintenance of pregnancy with a nonaffected fetus. Many couples concerned with having an child with a genetic disorder are prepared to take that risk and proceed with termination when the fetus is genetically abnormal. The ability to select healthy embryos by preimplantation genetic diagnosis following in vitro fertilization (IVF) is seemingly a more desirable alternative although not without disappointments and risks. IVF is costly and many insurance carriers do not cover infertility services. The cost alone may be an insurmountable barrier to treatment.[9] Additionally, IVF is a process of percentages; a sufficient number of embryos need to develop before the opportunity of establishing a pregnancy is reached. Two to three healthy embryos may be transferred into the mother's womb with approximately a 15 to 25 percent chance of a full-term pregnancy. This frequency is similar to the natural fecundity rate of 25 percent per cycle.[10] Efficiencies of initiating a pregnancy being similar between IVF and natural intercourse, preimplantation genetic diagnosis eliminates concerns regarding pregnancy termination and risk of pregnancy maintenance associated with prenatal genetic diagnosis.

There are two groups of patients who may be interested in preimplantation genetic diagnosis: those who are fertile and those who are infertile. Fertile couples approach IVF and PGD with the suspicion or certain knowledge of being carriers for a serious genetic disorder. This is either from having an affected family member or as a result of already having an affected child. Infertile couples may approach IVF as a remedy to their childlessness and discover their infertility is secondary to their carrier status for a genetic disease. For example, male carriers of cystic fibrosis often have congenital absence of the vas deferens causing them to be azoospermic. Couples with a long history of infertility and/or advancing maternal age may seek IVF as a last option. PGD then becomes a consideration with regard to numerical chromosome disorders that occur *de novo* at this stage of reproductive life.

While PGD may appear to be a more palatable solution for the selection of genetically healthy offspring, it does not define who should have access to this technology. Clearly all couples do not have the same risk of carrying a genetic disorder, and all couples will not choose to undergo IVF to answer their childbearing needs. Does our ability to screen the population as a whole for serious genetic disorders necessitate that we do so, and as health care providers is it our responsibility to eliminate disease? This concern gives way to other ethical questions: If an individual is known to be a carrier of a genetic disorder, who will decide whether this individual may reproduce without the benefit of genetic screening of the embryo or fetus or should such screening be mandated? If the individual does produce an affected child that requires care beyond that which is normally anticipated, is society responsible for that child via insurance or government support?

The human genome project, an effort to provide a detailed gene map, is rapidly isolating late-onset genetic diseases, for example, the breast-ovarian cancer gene and familial polyposis gene. As the genetic links to many of our adult disorders become known, who will decide what is a serious genetic disorder? Will those diseases that are curable by advances in medicine such as kidney transplants be deemed to be less serious than something like Huntington's disease? As surely as disease genes are discovered, their presence in an embryo may be determined. What obligation do the parents, doctor, and society have to an unborn carrier of the breast-ovarian cancer gene should that embryo be selected for implantation? When, if ever, should individuals be told of their pending health status, and what will that knowledge do to their life choices? The resolution may not be as dark as it first appears; the ability to reduce risk by avoidance of compounding risk factors through tailoring of lifestyles and prophylactic surgery may provide the opportunity for a full and happy life.

As DNA methodology and microsurgery improve, physicians will likely choose to treat genetic disorders in the future. Genetic defects in eggs may be treated by microinjection of targeted replacement genes. Viral vectors carrying replacement genes may possibly be used to infect sperm during spermatogenesis in vivo. Pronuclear zygotes may be microinjected with gene repair sequences for specific defects. Diseases resulting from single-gene defects may potentially disappear if treated as theorized above. These strategies leave spontaneous and age-related aneuploidies as major genetic-disease issues. Different approaches may alleviate these problems; maturation of sperm and eggs may be carried out in vitro, bypassing environmentally induced nondisjunction events. Possibilities abound, and the future should focus on the treatment and eradication of disease. The approach to treatment should be compassionate and available to those in need and not suppressed due to concerns of inappropriate genetic manipulation.

NOTES

1. G. Sher and M. A. Feinman, "The Day-to-Day Realities: Commentary on the New Eugenics and Medicalized Reproduction," *Cambridge Quarterly of Healthcare Ethics* 4 (1995): 313–15.
2. S. Munne, K. Xu, J. Cohen, and J. A. Grifo, "Preimplantation Diagnosis," in *Reproductive Endocrinology Surgery, and Technology,* ed. E. Y. Adashi, J. A. Rock, Z. Rosenwaks (Philadelphia: Lippincott-Raven, 1995), 2385–99.
3. K. Mullis, F. Faloona, and S. Scarf et al., "Specific Enzymatic Amplification of DNA *in vitro:* The Polymerase Chain Reaction," *Cold Spring Harbor Symposia on Quantitative Biology* 5 (1986): 263–73.
4. D. Gelfand, "Taq DNA Polymerase," in *PCR Technology: Principles and Applications for DNA Amplification,* ed. A. Henry (New York: W. H. Freeman, 1992), 17–22.
5. R. Saike, "The design and organization of the PCR," in *PCR Technology: Principles and Applications for DNA Amplification,* ed. A. Henry (New York: W. H. Freeman, 1992), 7–16.
6. J. D. A. Delhanty and A. H. Handyside, "The Origin of Genetic Defects in the Human and Their Detection in the Preimplantation Embryo," *Human Reproduction* 1, no. 3 (1995): 201–15.
7. Ibid.
8. Ibid.
9. Sher and Feinman, "The Day-to-Day Realities."
10. Delhanty and Handyside, "The Origin of Genetic Defects in the Human and Their Detection in the Preimplantation Embryo."

Chapter 7

Abortion: The Unexplored Middle Ground

Richard A. McCormick

During the Republican National Convention in August 1988, I listened to an interview with fundamentalist minister Jerry Falwell and Faye Wattleton, president of Planned Parenthood, on the subject of abortion. Falwell kept insisting that unborn babies were the last disenfranchised minority—voiceless, voteless, and unprotected in the most basic of civil liberties. Wattleton's statements all returned to the concept of privacy and the woman's right to decide whether she would or would not bear a child. It was a tired old stalemate. Nether party budged an inch. The moderator identified their only common ground as the fact that this is a great country in which people are free to disagree.

Unfortunately, the Falwell-Wattleton exchange is an example of the way discussions on abortion are often conducted. One point is picked as central and then is all but absolutized. The discussion accomplishes nothing except perhaps to raise everyone's blood pressure. All remarks return to the single absolutized starting point and are interpreted in light of it. Thus Falwell sees nonviolent demonstrations at abortion clinics as signs of hope for a transformation of consciousness and a growing rejection of abortion. Wattleton sees them as unconstitutional and violent disturbances of a woman's exercise of her prerogative to make her own choice.

Are we doomed forever to this kind of dialogue of the deaf? Perhaps, especially if the central principles identified by both sides are indeed central. An important difference in these "central issues" should be noted here. Falwell and those who share his view are speaking primarily of the *morality* of abortion and only secondarily about public policy or the civil rights of the unborn. Wattleton says little about morality (though she implies much) but puts all her emphasis on what is now constitutional *public policy*. On his level, I believe Falwell is right. On her level, Wattleton is right (in the sense that *Roe v. Wade* does give women a constitutional right). Two planes passing in the night at different altitudes.

What rarely gets discussed in such heated standoffs is what public policy *ought to be*, especially in light of *which morality*. The linkage of these two in a consistent, rationally defensible, humanly sensitive way almost always falls victim to gavel-pounding. It never gets discussed. Unless this linkage is made more satisfactorily in the public consciousness than it has been, any public policy on abortion will lack supportive consensus and will continue to be seriously disruptive of social life. The terms *pro-choice* and *pro-life* will continue to mislead, label, and divide our citizenry.

Can we enlarge the public conversation so that a minimally acceptable consensus might have the chance to develop? I am probably naive to think so. But I have seen more unexpected and

---

Source: Reprinted with permission from R. A. McCormick, Abortion: The Unexplored Middle Ground, *Second Opinion,* Vol. 10, pp. 41–50, © 1989, The Park Ridge Center.

startling things happen—Vatican II, for example. Falwell and Wattleton could agree on a few things beyond the edifying puff that this is a great country because people are free to disagree. I call my proposed area of conversation "the unexplored middle ground." If we talked more about this middle ground, we could perhaps establish a public conversational atmosphere with a better chance at achieving a peaceable public policy. I say perhaps because I am not at all optimistic. Still, it is worth a shot.

Before listing possible elements for this unexplored middle ground, I want to make three introductory points. First, diverting attention to the middle ground is not an invitation to compromise. To attempt to discover what we might agree on is not to forfeit our disagreements. It is only to shift the conversational focus. It is to discuss one's convictions with a different purpose, with different people, in a different way.

Second, my own *moral* position is abundantly clear from previous writings.[1] So is my conviction that the policy set in *Roe v. Wade* does not adequately reflect the position of a majority of Americans. Although that conviction should in no way hinder the search for a middle ground, it does warn the reader that the "middle ground" I propose is influenced by these postures. The consensus I would like to see develop and be reflected in policy is not unrelated to my own beliefs. It will undoubtedly shape my identification and wording of the "unexplored middle ground." Indeed, some—from both sides—will undoubtedly see my middle ground as a poorly disguised presentation of only one point of view, hardly in the middle. I acknowledge the possibility in advance, but forge ahead nonetheless.

Third, when I speak of a common ground I do not mean that all or many now agree on these points. But I believe there is solid hope that they can be brought to agreement.

ELEMENTS OF A MIDDLE GROUND

1. *There is a presumption against the moral permissibility of taking human life.* This means that any individual or society sanctioning this or that act of intentional killing bears the burden of proof. Life, as the condition of all other experiences and achievements, is a basic good, indeed the most basic of all goods. If it may be taken without public accountability, we have returned to moral savagery. For this reason all civilized societies have rules about homicide, though we might disagree with their particulars.

I take the presumption stated above to be the substance of the Christian tradition. The strength of this presumption varies with times and cultures. Cardinal Joseph Bernardin has noted that the presumption has been strengthened in our time.[2] By that he means that in the past capital punishment was viewed as a legitimate act of public protection. Furthermore war, in which killing was foreseen, was justified on three grounds: national self-defense, the recovery of property, and the redressing of injury. Now, however, many people (including several recent popes) reject capital punishment and view only national self-defense as justifying violent resistance. While such applications remain controversial, they are not the point here. The key principle is the presumption against taking human life.

2. *Abortion is a killing act.* So many discussions of abortion gloss over the intervention as "the procedure" or "emptying the uterus" or "terminating the pregnancy." In saying that abortion is a killing act, I do not mean to imply that it cannot be justified at times; the statement does not raise that issue. I mean only that the one certain and unavoidable outcome of the intervention is the death of the fetus. That is true of any abortion, whether it is descriptively and intentionally direct or indirect. If the death of the fetus is not the ineluctable result, we should speak of premature delivery. To fudge on this issue is to shade our imagination from the shape of our conduct and amounts to an anesthetizing self-deception. All of us should be able to agree on this description, whether we consider this or that abortion justified or not.

(A final gloss. I here pass over—with no intention of ignoring it—a key issue: At what point does interruption of the reproductive process merit the name *abortion*? That is a legitimate question. Plausible reasons exist for saying that only interruption of an *implanted*, fertilized ovum deserves this name. Here, however, I wish not to distract from the main assertion—one that applies to the 1.3 to 1.5 million abortions done per year in this country.)

3. *Abortion to save the life of the mother is morally acceptable*. Readers may wonder why I bother to mention this point. I do so because those who are morally opposed to abortion frequently see their position caricatured into unrecognizability. Such a caricature only intensifies opposition and polarization.

Let me cite a recent instance. The *New York Times* is hardly celebrated for its serene objectivity in this realm (it has supported *Roe v. Wade* from the beginning). In an editorial on George Bush's supposed gender gap it reported the Republican platform as follows: " 'That the unborn child has a fundamental individual right to life which cannot be infringed.' In other words, given a choice between saving the fetus or the mother, the mother must die" (August 19, 1988).

The interpretation of a "fundamental individual right to life" is so distorted that it comes as close to editorial hucksterism as can be imagined. Those who formulate their convictions in terms of a "fundamental right to life" by no stretch of the imagination deny a similar right to the mother. Nor does such a general statement about fetal rights even address situations of conflict. The language is meant to restate for the abortion context the presumption mentioned in my first point.

Presumptions can at times be overcome. Here it would be useful to recall the statement of J. Stimpfle, bishop of Augsburg: "He who performs abortion, *except to save the life of the mother*, sins gravely and burdens his conscience with the killing of human life."[3] The Belgian bishops made a similar statement.[4]

Agreement on this point may seem a marginal gain at best. But in the abortion discussion, *any* agreement can be regarded as a gain, especially when it puts caricatures to rest.

4. *Judgment about the morality of abortion is not simply a matter of a woman's determination and choice*. Pro-choice advocates often present their position as though the woman's choice were the sole criterion in the judgment of abortion. But I believe that very few if any really mean this, at least in its full implications. It is simplistic and unsustainable. Taken literally, it means that *any* abortion, at *any* time, for *any* reason, even the most frivolous, is morally justified if only the woman freely chooses it. That is incompatible even with the admittedly minimal restrictions of *Roe v. Wade*. I know of no official church body and no reputable philosopher or theologian who would endorse the sprawling and totally unlimited acceptance of abortion implied in that criterion. It straightforwardly forfeits any and all moral presumptions protective of the unborn. In this formulation, the fetus becomes a mere blob of matter.

Conversation about the fourth point will not, I am sure, bring overall agreement on the abortion issue. But it might lead to a more nuanced formulation on the part of those identified with the pro-choice position. It might also lead to a greater sensitivity on the part of some pro-life advocates to the substantial feminist concerns struggling for expression and attention in the pro-choice perspective.

5. *Abortion for mere convenience is morally wrong*. This only makes explicit the above point. Once again, agreement on this point may seem to represent precious little gain. And even agreement might be fugitive because of the problem in defining the phrase "mere convenience." One person's inconvenience is another's tragedy, and so on. Yet for those not hopelessly imprisoned in their absolutisms, I think agreement is possible if discussion is restrained.

Furthermore, such discussion could be remarkably fruitful. Those who agree with the statement—and that would include some, perhaps many pro-choice advocates—eventually would have to say *why* such abortion is morally wrong. Such a discussion could go in one direction only: straight to the whys and wherefores of the claims of nascent life upon us.

6. *The conditions that lead to abortion should be abolished insofar as is possible*. I refer to

poverty, lack of education, and lack of recreational alternatives to sexual promiscuity among teenagers. Nearly everyone agrees with these prescriptions, but they should be emphasized much more. In other words, we have tended to approach abortion too exclusively as a problem of *individual choice*. Left at that, it tends to divide people. Were it also approached as a *social problem*, it could easily bring together those in opposition at the level of individual choice.

7. *Abortion is a tragic experience to be avoided if at all possible*. Regardless of one's moral assessment of abortion, I believe most people could agree that it is not a desirable experience in any way. It can be dangerous, psychologically traumatic, generative of guilt feelings, and divisive of families. And, of course, it is invariably lethal to fetuses. No amount of verbal redescription or soothing and consoling counseling can disguise the fact that people would prefer to achieve their purposes without going through the abortion procedure. It is and always will be tragic.

8. *There should be alternatives to abortion*. This is a corollary to the preceding point. Its urgency is in direct proportion to the depth of our perception of abortion as a tragic experience. It seems to me that the need for alternatives should appeal above all to those who base their approach on a woman's freedom of choice. If reproductive choice is truly to be free, then alternatives to abortion should be available. By alternatives I mean all the supports—social, psychological, medical, financial, and religious—that would allow a woman to carry her pregnancy to full term should she choose to do so. Expanding the options is expanding freedom.

9. *Abortion is not a purely private affair. Roe v. Wade* appealed to the so-called right of privacy to justify its invalidation of restrictive state abortion laws. In public debate, assertions about a woman's "control over her own body" often surface. Such appeals either create or reinforce the idea that abortion is a purely private affair. It is not—at least not in the sense that it has no impact on people other than the woman involved. It affects husbands, families, nurses, physicians, politicians, and society in general. We ought to be able to agree on these documentable facts.

I am proposing that the term *privacy* is a misleading term used to underline the primacy of the woman's interest in abortion decisions. Communal admission of this point—which is scarcely controversial—would clear the air a bit and purify the public conversation.

10. Roe v. Wade *offends many people. So did previous prohibitive laws*. On these matters those who acknowledge facts must agree. But to place these facts together invites people out of their defensive trenches. In other words, it compels them to examine perspectives foreign to their own.

11. *Unenforceable laws are bad laws*. Unenforceability may stem from any number of factors. For instance, a public willingness to enforce the law may be lacking. Or the prohibited activity may be such that proof of violation will always be insufficient. Or attempts to enforce might infringe other dearly treasured values. Whatever the source of the unenforceability, most people agree that unenforceable laws undermine the integrity of the legal system and the fabric of social life.

Our own American experience with prohibition should provide sufficient historical education on this point. Its unenforceability stemmed from all the factors mentioned above and more. It spawned social evils of all kinds. In this respect, Democratic Senator Patrick J. Leahy of Vermont once remarked that amendments should be used not to create a consensus but to enshrine one that exists. He added:

> The amendments that have embodied a consensus have endured and are a living part of the Constitution. But where we amended the Constitution without a national meeting of minds, we were forced to retract the amendment, and only after devastating effects on the society.[5]

This is an obvious reference to the Eighteenth Amendment.

12. *An absolutely prohibitive law on abortion is not enforceable*. By "absolutely prohibitive" I

mean two things. First, such a law would prohibit all abortions, even in cases of rape and incest and in cases where the life of the mother is at stake. Second, by "abortion" would be meant destruction of the human being *from the moment of conception*. The latter was the intent of the Human Life Statute (S.158) introduced by Jesse Helms on January 19, 1981. It sought by a simple majority of both houses to declare the fetus a human being from the moment of conception. Thus in effect it sought to redefine the terms *person* and *life* to bring them under the protective clauses of the Fourteenth Amendment.

I say that such an absolutely prohibitive law is unenforceable. First, it has no consensus of support, as poll after poll over the years has established. Even religious groups with strong convictions against abortion have noted its unenforceability. For example, the Conference of German Bishops (Catholic) and the Council of the Evangelical Church (Protestant) issued a remarkable joint statement on abortion some years ago.[6] After rejecting simple legalization of first-trimester abortions (*Fristenregelung*), they stated that the task of the lawmaker is to identify those conflict situations in which interruption of pregnancy will not be punished (*straflos lassen*). I mention the German example because of the apparently ineradicable American tendency to identify moral conviction with public policy ("There oughta be a law!"). This penchant is visible in the refusal of some pro-life advocates to admit any toleration into public policy.

The second reason an absolutely prohibitive law would not work concerns specification of legal protection *from the moment of conception*. If this were enshrined in the penal code and attempts made to enforce it, we would be embroiled in conspiracy law (the *intent* to abort). Why? Because in the preimplantation period there is no evidence of pregnancy. Lacking such evidence, one could not prosecute another for having performed an abortion, but only for having *intended* to do so. That is just not feasible.

13. *There should be some public policy restrictions on abortion*. This point may seem to lack bite: after all, those most polarized could agree on this "middle ground," and even *Roe v. Wade* admitted "some" control. This tiny island of agreement is not important in itself. By focusing on it, however, discussants will be forced to face these two questions: What kind of control? and Why?

I admit that discussing these questions could take us right back to square one. But it could also lead to a more nuanced and sophisticated notion of public policy in a pluralistic society.

14. *Witness is the most effective leaven and the most persuasive educator concerning abortion*. I do not mean to discredit the place of rational discourse. We abandon such discourse at our own risk, and very often the result is war. I mean only that genuine education is eye opening. The most effective way of opening eyes is often the practical way of witness. We come to understand and appreciate heroism much more by seeing heroic activity than by hearing or reading a lecture on it. Are we not more selfless when surrounded by people who are concerned for others? Are we not more fearlessly honest when friends we deeply admire exhibit such honesty?

Those with deep convictions about freedom of choice for women or about the sanctity of fetal life would be considerably more persuasive if they emphasized what they are for rather than what they are against and did so *in action*. Pro-life advocates (whether individuals, organizations, or institutions such as dioceses) should put resources into preventing problem pregnancies; when those pregnancies occur, they should support them in every way. Paradoxically, the same is true of those who assert the primacy of free choice. For if the choice is to be truly free, genuine alternatives must exist. In summary, putting one's money where one's mouth is can be done at least as effectively (and far more so, I believe) through means other than picketing.

15. *Abortion is frequently a subtly coerced decision*. Ethicist Daniel Callahan pointed out 15 years ago that "a change in abortion laws, from restrictive to permissive, appears—from *all data* and in *every country*—to bring forward a whole class of women who would otherwise

not have wanted an abortion or felt the need for one."[7] The most plausible interpretation of this phenomenon, according to Callahan, is that the "free" abortion choice is a myth. He states,

> A poor or disturbed pregnant woman whose only choice is an abortion under permissive laws is hardly making a "free" choice, which implies the possibility of choosing among equally viable alternatives, one of which is to have the child. She is being offered an out and a help. Nor can a woman be called free where the local mores dictate abortion as the conventional wisdom in cases of unmarried pregnancies, thwarted plans, and psychological fears.[8]

Interestingly, agreement that many abortion decisions are coerced might result in cooperation between pro-choice and pro-life advocates. The concern of pro-choicers for true freedom would lead them to attempt to reduce or abolish coercive forces by offering genuine alternatives. The pro-life faction should rejoice at this provision of alternate options because it would reduce the felt need for abortion and thus the number of abortions.

16. *The availability of contraception does not reduce the number of abortions.* I include this element because I have been exposed to discussions of abortion soured by the introduction of statements like the following: "The Catholic Church, being so staunchly opposed to abortion, should be in the forefront of those backing contraception to prevent it. By condemning contraception the church adds to the number of abortions." Someone making such a remark supposes that support for contraception will reduce the number of abortions performed.

One of a group of "minor" truths listed by Daniel Callahan in 1973 was the following: "There is no evidence yet from any country that, with enough time and [the] availability of effective contraceptives, the number of abortions declines."[9] Clearly the availability of effective means of contraception is one thing; official approval of their use is quite another. But as witnessed by the number of Catholics who depart from official church teaching on contraception, official disapproval does not seem to make much difference. Callahan's assertion should therefore serve as a rebuttal to the above statement about Catholic inconsistency. I do not attach much conciliatory significance to this rebuttal except that it clears the air of distracting and one-sided statements.

17. *Permissive laws forfeit the notion of "sanctity of life" for the unborn.* This is a hard saying, but that does not make it less true. Here Daniel Callahan is at his best—and most tortured. He grants a woman the right not to have a child she does not want. But he is unflinchingly honest about what this means. "Under permissive laws," he notes, "any talk whatever of the 'sanctity of life' of the unborn becomes a legal fiction. By giving women the full and total right to determine whether such a sanctity exists, the fetus is, in fact, given no legal or socially established standing whatever."[10] Callahan does not like being backed into this corner. But he is utterly honest. His legal position does not allow for any pious doublethink. The law "forces a nasty either-or choice, devoid of saving ethical ambiguity." I wish that all discussants, on both sides, were so honest.

18. *Hospitals that do abortions but have no policy on them should develop one.* I introduce this as a contribution to the unexplored middle ground because non-Catholic health care facilities have approached the problem almost exclusively in terms of patient autonomy. I know that some hospitals have grown nervous about this posture because it amounts to simple capitulation to patient preferences. They have begun to see that theirs is not a carefully reasoned moral stance on abortion but an abdication of the responsibility to develop one.

The counsel to develop a policy is relatively nonthreatening because it does not dictate what that policy ought to be. It is promising because it suggests that ethical complexity and ambiguity might become more explicit, which would represent an advance in the dialogue.

19. *The "consistent ethic of life" should be taken seriously.* I happily borrow the term *consistent ethic of life* from Cardinal Joseph Bernardin. Many have observed that the most vociferous about fetal rights are among our most hawkish fellow citizens. Something is amiss here. Abortions should be viewed within the larger context of other life-and-death issues, such as capital punishment and war making.

20. *Whenever a discussion becomes heated, it should cease.* This is the final piece of middle ground I propose. I am not suggesting that abortion is so trivial a concern that heat is inappropriate. Rather, I know from long experience that shouting sessions on abortion only alienate and divide the shouters. Nothing is illumined, not because the offerings are not illuminating but because nobody is either listening or being heard.

The idea of an unexplored middle ground and the invitation to explore it will please few. Yet the abortion problem is so serious that we must grasp at any straw. A nation that prides itself on its tradition of dignity and equality for all and the civil rights to protect that equality cannot tolerate a situation in which 1.3 to 1.5 million human fetuses are being denied this equality and these rights. We must at least continue to discuss the problem openly. Quite simply, the soul of the nation is at stake. Abortion's pervasiveness represents a horrendous racism of the adult world. When it is justified in terms of rights, all of our rights are endangered because their foundations have been eroded by arbitrary and capricious application.

For this reason (and for many others) I think it important that abortion continue to occupy a prime place in public consciousness and conversation, even though we are bone-weary of the subject. If we settle for the status quo, we may be presiding unwittingly at the obsequies of some of our own most basic, most treasured freedoms. That possibility means that any strategy—even the modest one of keeping a genuine conversation alive by suggesting a middle ground as its subject—has something to recommend it.

NOTES

1. See, for example, R. A. McCormick, "Public Policy on Abortion," in *How Brave a New World*? (Washington, D.C.: Georgetown University Press, 1981).
2. J. Bernardin, *Origins* 13 (1983–1984): 491–95; *Origins* 14 (1984–1985): 707–9.
3. F. Scholz, "Durch ethische Grenzsituationen aufgeworfene Normen probleme," *Theologish-praktische Quartalschrift* 123 (1975): 342.
4. Les évêques belges, "Déclaration des évêques belges sur l'avortement," *Documentation Catholique* 70 (1973): 432–38.
5. Cited in M. C. Segers, "Can Congress Settle the Abortion Issue?" *Hastings Center Report* 12 (June 1982): 20–28.
6. Conference of German Bishops and the Council of the Evangelical Church, "Fristenregelung" entschieden abgelehnt, *Ruhrwort*, 8 December 1973, 6.
7. D. Callahan, "Abortion: Thinking and Experiencing," *Christianity and Crisis*, 8 January 1973, 296.
8. Ibid.
9. Ibid., 297.
10. Ibid.

CHAPTER 8

Women, Fetuses, Physicians, and the State: Pregnancy and Medical Ethics in the 21st Century

Michelle Oberman

INTRODUCTION

Throughout the course of human history, healers have sought to secure the health and safety of pregnant women and their offspring. For much of that time, the threats to maternal and fetal well-being were so poorly understood that efforts at health promotion often were futile if not harmful. As medical science moves into a new millennium, it brings with it a comparatively thorough understanding of birth-related biological processes—one that is more than adequate to render pregnancy, labor, and delivery low-risk events. Nevertheless, pregnancy-related complications persist, and modern healers face new dilemmas in their struggle to ensure the health and safety of pregnant women. Increasingly it appears that many of the factors jeopardizing maternal and fetal health derive less from the physiological impact of pregnancy than from the pregnant woman's conduct and from the detrimental effects of the environment in which she lives. This greater awareness of the preventable harms suffered by pregnant women and their offspring serves to create a sense of urgency and frustration on the part of those who treat this population—a sense that has reconfigured the relationship between doctors and their pregnant patients and has generated a host of ethical dilemmas. These dilemmas may best be evaluated and resolved when viewed against the backdrop of the dynamic relationship between pregnant women and healers.

Over the course of the twentieth century, scientific understanding of pregnancy, and hence, the methodologies employed in the treatment of pregnant women, changed dramatically. In this brief 100-year period, the "typical" experiences of pregnancy, labor, and delivery were transformed several times over. In the early decades of the century, pregnancy was considered a private, natural, and uncontrollable phenomenon. Over the ensuing decades, pregnancy came to be seen as a medical condition, the treatment of which centered upon the physician-patient relationship. Later decades witnessed the arrival of the fetus as a second patient in this relationship, and still later decades have revealed the increasing presence of the state as a fourth party to the "treatment" and regulation of pregnancy.

At many points in the past 100 years, one could state without hesitation that the greatest sorts of medical achievements had been realized by the practice of obstetrics. At still other points in the century, however, it seemed that even the most wondrous of these achievements was marred by the disasters wrought by modern medical practices. As we stand on the brink of the new millennium and attempt to chart an ethically sound course for the dynamic and evolving relationship between doctors and pregnant women, we must remain conscious of past

I am indebted to Lisa Eckenweiler and Timothy F. Murphy for their insightful comments on an earlier draft of this chapter.

successes and failures and be ever cognizant of our limited ability to assess progress. With these goals in mind, this chapter will chart the rapid changes in the treatment of pregnancy over the course of the twentieth century. It builds a cautionary contemporary analysis and evaluation of the increasingly complex interrelationships between pregnant women, health care providers, fetuses, and the state.

PREGNANCY AND THE ADVENT OF THE MATERNAL-DOCTOR RELATIONSHIP

Until the twentieth century, pregnancy, labor, and delivery took place almost entirely outside of the health care setting.[1] Sometime near the end of her pregnancy, a pregnant woman would seek out the services of a midwife, who would be brought to her home as soon as labor began. The midwife stayed with the woman and her family throughout the labor and delivery. For the majority of women and infants, this treatment of pregnancy was an unqualified success. However, for those women who experienced any complications during pregnancy, labor and delivery, or recovery, reproduction became a life-threatening event. At the turn of the century, when fewer than 5 percent of women delivered their babies in hospitals, the maternal and infant mortality rates averaged 6.8 per 1,000 live births and 99.9 per 1,000 live births, respectively.[2]

During the early decades of the twentieth century, a number of factors converged to improve the health status and survival rates of pregnant women and infants. Perhaps most important among these were discoveries relating to the spread and the control of infection and infectious diseases. These discoveries yielded dramatic benefits for the health of the population as a whole and for pregnant women in particular. The discovery of antisepsis and, at midcentury, antibiotics dramatically reduced deaths due to puerperal fever, a generic term applied to the various postpartum infections that accounted for the majority of maternal deaths in the nineteenth and early twentieth centuries.[3] Additionally, over the course of the century, the age and parity of childbearing shifted, so that women had fewer children, with more space between pregnancies. Finally, women began obtaining prenatal care, using physicians rather than midwives, and in ever-expanding numbers, they opted to deliver their babies in hospitals rather than at home. By 1939, half of all women, and 75 percent of urban women were delivering in hospitals.[4]

It was this latter factor, the use of doctors rather than midwives as birth attendants, that most dramatically altered women's experience of pregnancy, labor, and delivery. Driven in large part by the fear of maternal and infant mortality and by the promise that proper medical supervision might eliminate these risks, doctors approached pregnancy from the perspective of pathology. Therefore, all pregnant women were viewed as potentially in danger, and pregnancy was transformed into a medical condition requiring a physician's supervision.

This statistically unreasonable approach (given that the overwhelming majority of pregnancies were healthy ones) might be viewed as logical and even necessary because medical science lacked any mechanism for predicting which pregnant women were at risk. In fact, until well into the twentieth century, doctors lacked the means to confirm pregnancy itself, let alone to identify women at risk of pregnancy-related complications. As a result of the limitations of scientific knowledge, the shift toward physician-provided prenatal care and hospital-based childbearing did not precipitate a dramatic decline in maternal and infant morbidity and mortality rates. Rather, these rates continued to decline gradually, as they had since the start of the century, due to general improvements in the population's overall health status.[5]

HIGH TECHNOLOGY AND THE EMERGENCE OF THE FETUS AS "PATIENT"

X-ray technology permitted the world its first glimpse of the fetus circa 1910. By 1920, X-rays were considered to be a valuable aid in detecting pregnancy as early as six weeks after a missed menstrual period. Ironically, this "advance" brought serious problems of its own, as the recommended length of exposure was one hour.[6] By the mid-1930s, doctors in Europe and the United States supported the routine use of X-rays in prenatal care. The primary use of this technology was to provide evidence regarding fetal size and growth. Despite the fact that, as early as 1920, there was evidence of long-term damage to humans exposed to X-rays, they continued to be utilized well into the 1950s, by which time approximately two-thirds of all pregnant women receiving prenatal care at maternity hospitals were given X-rays.[7]

In 1956, Oxford scientist Alice Stewart established the link between prenatal exposure to X-rays and childhood cancer.[8] Rather than resuming traditional methods of prenatal care, doctors sought alternatives to X-ray technology for visualizing the fetus. In the late 1950s, ultrasonography emerged as the safe alternative to X-rays. However, the early ultrasound apparatus was cumbersome and costly, so it was not until the mid-1970s that it became widely incorporated into routine prenatal care. In the interim, obstetricians had grown so accustomed to visualizing the fetus that a shocking number continued to use X-rays in their practices until the ultrasound became widely available. In fact, one study of British obstetricians reported that, in 1976, as many as 30 percent of all pregnant women received X-rays.[9]

Visualizing the Fetus

Visualizing the fetus had a profound effect on the practice of obstetrics: It provided absolute proof that a new life was growing inside the patient. Somehow, the impact of rendering the pregnant woman transparent made it possible to imagine the pregnant woman and the fetus as separate entities. Despite the physical impossibility of survival for the fetus apart from its mother, the notion that there were two lives transformed the relationship between doctor and patient, and obstetricians began to perceive their jobs as entailing the treatment of two patients, rather than one.

This revision of the doctor-patient relationship may be observed through the nomenclature surrounding obstetric practice. Originally, doctors interested in treating pregnancy specialized in obstetrics and gynecology—a field that involved the treatment of female patients for reproductive health care over the course of their lifetimes. They served on the staffs of hospitals within departments of obstetrics and gynecology. In the last decades of the twentieth century, these departments, and the doctors who work within them, have begun changing their names. Now it is common to refer pregnant women to departments of "maternal-fetal medicine," in which they might be treated by "maternal-fetal experts," or perhaps even by a "fetal medicine specialist."

The change in the obstetric doctor-patient relationship goes beyond mere nomenclature. As soon as doctors recognized the treatment of pregnancy as involving two patients, rather than one, they began to perceive "conflicts of interest" between the two. These conflicts of interest occur when pregnant women refuse to follow the medical advice of their doctors in regard to behavior, nutrition, and other factors considered favorable to the development of the fetus. Although they are, in essence, maternal-doctor conflicts, they commonly are termed *maternal-fetal conflicts.*

Maternal-Doctor Conflicts

As is evident from the rise and fall of X-ray technology's use during pregnancy, doctors' treatment of pregnancy has varied considerably over the course of the twentieth century. Likewise, medical advice to pregnant women has shifted, and on occasion, vacillated. For example, weight gain during pregnancy was considered good, then bad, then good again; breastfeeding was preferable to bottle feeding, then formula became the ideal food for babies, then breastfeeding reemerged as the best way to nourish a newborn. However, during the later decades of the twentieth century, not only the substance but also the tenor of medical advice changed. By the end of the twentieth century, a pregnant woman's failure to follow her obstetrician's advice might lead to an adversarial relationship between doctor and patient.

Medical advice to pregnant women necessarily took on a more urgent tone once the doctor began seeing the fetus as a second patient. The pregnant patient's lack of cooperation became more than merely a source of frustration to the physician—it became a threat to the fetus. Concern about fetal well-being grew along with the increasing evidence of the permeability of the placenta. During the middle decades of the century, a range of medical discoveries and disasters provided evidence that much of what pregnant women ingest can also affect fetal development. Drugs like thalidomide and diethylstilbestrol (DES), which were prescribed for therapeutic purposes during pregnancy, were shown to cause birth defects in the children exposed while in utero.[10] Even freely available and routinely consumed substances like nicotine, alcohol, and aspirin proved to be harmful to the developing fetus.

A combination of the growing awareness of teratogenicity and the sense that the fetus was a second patient led doctors, and society at large, to see pregnant women in a new light. Much of the historical awe and superstition surrounding pregnancy was displaced by moral perceptions that pregnant women were either "good" or "bad" mothers depending on the extent to which they cooperated with medical advice given on behalf of the fetus. Unlike popular notions of good and bad mothers, which are driven by community norms and cultural consensus and reflect a considerable range of permissible behaviors, the moral categorization of pregnant women seemingly depends entirely on the extent to which they comply with medical advice.

Evidence of this medicalized definition of good pregnant women may be observed in public responses to pregnant women who consume alcohol. For example, in 1991, the newspapers reported the story of a pregnant woman who was refused a daiquiri while dining in a restaurant. The waitress asked her if she was sure she wanted a drink. The patron stated that she was sure and said further that she had been "so good" throughout the entire nine months of her pregnancy (she was one week overdue). The waitress left the table and when she returned, rather than giving her the daiquiri, she slapped a warning label peeled from a beer bottle on the table and said, "In case you didn't know."[11]

This incident occurred during the era in which many alcohol manufacturers, in response to lawsuits, had begun placing warnings about drinking during pregnancy on the labels of alcoholic beverages.[12] Perhaps these notices are designed to assist pregnant women whose doctors neglected to warn them of the dangers of alcohol, or to remind those who were warned, but had forgotten, or to reach those women who lack access to care and have not yet seen a doctor.[13] But one must also wonder whether the notices serve the purpose, demonstrated so effectively by the Seattle waitress, of enlisting public support in an effort to protect fetuses from bad mothers.

In the medical setting, one finds evidence of the good-pregnant-woman and/or bad-pregnant-woman dichotomy in terms of patient compliance with medical interventions. One may observe this dichotomy in the attitudes of pregnant women toward the series of diagnostic tests that often accompany prenatal care. A fascinating example of this involves a study of women's responses to alpha-fetoprotein testing, a test designed to reveal evidence of neural tube defects. In the early 1990s, the state of California mandated that providers offer alpha-fetoprotein screening to all pregnant women as part of routine prenatal care.[14] As a diagnostic screen, by definition, the test has no bearing on fetal or maternal well-being. Instead, it provides information that the fetus may suffer from impairments—information that may lead some women to consider aborting the pregnancy.

Curious to see how women responded to prenatal diagnostic testing, two medical anthropologists observed women's responses to the California program. They elected to study a sample of Catholic women, hypothesizing that, because of their church's opposition to abortion, they might be more likely than other women to resist such testing. Instead, they found that these women behaved in precisely the same manner as did the overwhelming majority of those offered the alpha-fetoprotein test—when offered the test, they consented.[15]

What was perhaps the most fascinating finding of the study, however, was the explanation that the women gave for consent. In extensive interviews, the majority of participants expressed both their understanding that nothing could be done medically should their fetus be found to have a problem and also their conviction that they would not use the knowledge derived from the test as a basis for terminating the pregnancy. Nevertheless, they explained that they decided to undergo the test for reasons generally articulated along the lines of "want[ing] to do anything that could help me or my baby." The authors attribute these puzzling findings in large part to the manner in which the health care system approached the issue of testing. None of the 40 women interviewed reported having been informed of the choices they would face should they receive a positive test result. Instead, both their doctors and the state-mandated brochure designed to facilitate the consent process advised them that testing was "recommended" for all pregnant women. Wanting to be good mothers, they consented.[16]

The most striking evidence of the good-pregnant-woman and/or bad-pregnant-woman dichotomy is seen in physicians' responses to bad, or noncompliant, pregnant patients. Perhaps the quintessential example of this is the controversy generated when pregnant women reject a medically advised Caesarian-section delivery.

Many have noted that United States rates of Caesarian-section births far exceed rates of other First World nations. Moreover, these rates are not accompanied by higher rates of infant survival. In fact, the United States has a higher infant-mortality rate than virtually any First World country, and when factoring in racial variations, the infant-mortality rate for African Americans is comparable to that of many Third World nations.[17] Numerous authors have decried the interventionist mindset of American medicine that drives the Caesarian-section rates and the resultant high costs to the health care system. In addition to demonstrating an irrational allocation of scarce health care resources, the Caesarian-section phenomenon also reveals important information about the relationship between pregnant women and their doctors.

Virtually no pregnant woman wishes to have a Caesarian-section delivery. They are more risky to her own health, the recovery time is lengthier and more painful, the scarring is permanent, and many women report an intangible yet very real perception that a nonvaginal delivery is somehow "unnatural" and "a failure."[18] Additionally, Caesarian-section deliveries, whether because they involve blood transfusions or for other reasons, violate the religious beliefs of many women in the United States. Nevertheless, the overwhelming proportion of women for whom Caesarian-section deliveries are recommended comply with these requests. They do so because they believe the operation is medically necessary, and also because informal and formal sanctions brought to bear upon those pregnant women who refuse Caesarian sections are so overwhelming.

A woman who refuses to undergo a Caesarian-section delivery after being advised that it is necessary in order to protect herself or her baby is seen by her health care providers, and by society at large, as making a selfish choice. The urgency of her compliance with the Caesarian section will be impressed upon her by any or all of a number of individuals within the health care setting—doctors, nurses, social workers, ethicists, pastoral care workers, and even hospital attorneys. Ultimately, many institutions will resort to the law in an effort to compel the woman's compliance with the recommended course of treatment.[19] These cases highlight the stakes associated with the good-pregnant-woman and/or bad-pregnant-woman dichotomy and demonstrate the truly adversarial potential inherent in the relationship between doctors and their pregnant patients.

THE EMERGING RELATIONSHIP BETWEEN THE STATE AND THE FETUS: TURNING DOCTORS INTO PREGNANCY POLICE

As the example of court-ordered Caesarian sections demonstrates, the consequences of maternal-doctor conflict extend far beyond the classification of pregnant women into good and bad mothers. These conflicts bring a fourth party, the state, into the already crowded doctor-patient-fetus relationship.

There are at least two powerful reasons to be wary of an extensive state role in the treatment of pregnancy. The first is that scientific knowledge is inherently dynamic, and that one era's truths often emerge, in the next era, as falsehoods. From bloodletting to thalidomide, the history of pregnancy-related medical innovations is rife with treatments that ultimately have proven ineffective and even harmful to pregnant women and developing fetuses. David Grimes has chronicled the phenomenon whereby those practicing medicine repeatedly mistake "new" for "improved," and squander resources, and, in some cases, harm or kill patients, in the name of medical progress.[20] He notes that the problem of widespread utilization of unproved technologies is especially problematic in reproductive health, and cites electronic fetal monitoring, home uterine-activity monitoring, and routine episiotomy as contemporary examples of costly and unnecessary practices.[21] In view of this history, and in light of medicine's inherent inability to predict which, if any, contemporary procedures or practices may someday emerge as ineffective or disastrous, the willingness to seek state intervention in order to compel patients to undergo treatment is extremely troublesome.

The second reason to be wary of the state's growing role in the treatment of pregnant women is that it threatens the medical and ethical integrity of the doctor-patient relationship. Core ethical values of patient autonomy and privacy are necessarily threatened whenever the state seeks to influence a patient's choices. Once the fetus was rendered visible, it was perhaps inevitable that many would seek to lay claim to it—fathers, doctors, antiabortion activists, the state. Of these various contenders, only the state, which licenses doctors and grants them the privileges and powers associated with practicing medicine, has the power to radically redefine the obligations of physicians toward their pregnant patients. The following section will explore the manner in which the state's involvement in the treatment of pregnancy has begun to effectuate such a redefinition.

The State's Expanding Role in the Treatment of Pregnant Women

Despite the cautions outlined above, there are numerous contemporary examples of state-sanctioned interventions in pregnant women's health care decision making, ostensibly undertaken for the benefit of the fetus. Interestingly, these interventions not only limit the autonomy and privacy of pregnant women but also represent intrusions upon the relationships between the woman and her doctor, and the woman and the fetus's father. Two examples of such interventions are statutes limiting the applicability of advanced medical directives in the event that a patient is pregnant and laws governing the human immunodeficiency virus (HIV) testing of pregnant women and newborns.

Living wills and durable powers of attorney for health care represent the most powerful means by which an individual can ensure that her wishes regarding medical treatment will be followed in the event that she is no longer competent to express those wishes. Supported by state and federal laws, when properly executed, these documents permit decision making to take place at the end of life without forcing family members and doctors to resort to the courts. A surprisingly high number of these documents contain provisions rendering them unenforceable if the patient is pregnant.[22] Thus, doctors and family members are powerless to halt the treatment of a pregnant woman in the event of, e.g., irreversible brain injury, in spite of the fact that she has previously indicated her desire to be allowed to die should such circumstances occur, and in spite of knowledge by all parties to her treatment and by all those who knew her, that she never would have consented to such treatment.[23]

A more visible example of government intervention into health care decision making for pregnant women involves HIV-infected pregnant women. Following the 1994 discovery that zidovudine, taken by an HIV-positive woman during pregnancy, reduces the likelihood of maternal-fetal infection from approximately 25 percent to 8.3 percent, lawmakers at both the state and federal levels began calling for mandatory HIV testing of pregnant women.[24] At first blush, such a demand seems quite reasonable—it is difficult to imagine why a pregnant woman, upon learning that she was HIV-infected, would not take action to limit the possibility of harm to her fetus. Upon closer evaluation, however, there are at least two logical flaws in the assumption favoring mandatory testing.

First, there is the leap from the belief that it is desirable for a pregnant woman to know her HIV status to the conclusion that mandatory testing is the appropriate mechanism for achieving that goal. Mandatory testing has been vigorously opposed by public health officials and acquired immune deficiency syndrome (AIDS) advocates ever since the HIV tests were first developed.[25] The reasons for this opposition stem from the potentially devastating negative consequences that may follow from a positive test result. First, there are the obvious psychological consequences of receiving the news that one has a fatal disease. Evidence suggests that, when given the choice, many prefer not to know that they will die prematurely. Then there are all of the well-documented forms of discrimination exhibited by landlords, employers, insurers, family, and friends. Finally, the consensus against mandatory testing reflects our society's deep-seated belief in the legal and ethical rights to patient autonomy, liberty, and privacy. Competent individuals may refuse any and all medical treatment—even if it is necessary to save their own lives. In the past, these reasons were thought to outweigh any benefits gained by compulsory testing.

To justify making an exception to this strong consensus against mandatory testing in the case of pregnant women, there should be overwhelming evidence that the benefits of such testing so far outweigh the harms that no reasonable individual would decline to be tested. Yet, it remains the case that pregnant women who test positive for HIV are exposed to all of the above-noted risks, and more important, face an additional, and perhaps even more menacing threat: An HIV-positive test result may jeopardize a woman's access to her child. Given that a substantial majority of HIV-infected women acquire the virus through a combination of illicit drug use and/or sexual activity (which may itself be illicit) with a drug user, the state may question the ability of an HIV-positive woman to provide a safe environment for her children.[26] Thus, an HIV test may become far more than a prenatal diagnostic screen—indeed, it may be more of a proxy for a broad-scaled state intervention into a woman's life.

This does not mean that pregnant women never should be tested. Quite the contrary—all pregnant women should be counseled regarding the risks and benefits of knowing their HIV status. When such counseling takes place, evidence indicates that between 90 and 95 percent of pregnant women elect to undergo HIV testing. This result is unsurprising in light of evidence that women tend to perceive their assent to prenatal treatment, and even diagnostic tests, as a ratification of their identities as good mothers. Moreover, these rates of postcounseling testing are extraordinarily high. Indeed, no mandatory screening program in public health history has achieved rates approaching the 90 percent compliance rate reported in the settings utilizing mandatory counseling.[27]

The second logical flaw in the push toward mandatory testing is that it implicitly assumes that, once a woman tests positive for HIV, she will take zidovudine. The daily regimen of five doses, administered over the course of six months of pregnancy, requires patient compliance. What would happen if an HIV-infected woman, reasoning that her child stood a 75 percent chance of being born uninfected and that its health status could be jeopardized by the use of a destructive chemotherapeutic agent whose long-term effects are completely unknown, chose not to take zidovudine?[28] As of yet, there have not been any cases in which a state seeks a court order forcing an HIV-infected pregnant women to take zidovudine, but it takes only a passing familiarity with the issue of compelled Caesarian sections to imagine such an action being brought.

As one comes to understand the reasons why a pregnant woman might object to being tested for HIV, the devastating consequences for pregnant women and their fetuses should the state attempt to force compliance become apparent: Women who are sufficiently motivated to avoid HIV testing will opt to avoid prenatal care altogether. Thus, a mandatory screening program jeopardizes the well-being of the very population the state wishes to ensure. When one considers that at least 75 percent of children born to HIV-infected women would otherwise have been born uninfected and healthy, one cannot help but fear the folly and dangers inherent in such a policy.

In spite of this, physicians have been slow to recognize the threat to patients, fetuses, and health care providers posed by state interventions into the doctor-patient relationship. Indeed, at its 1996 meeting, the American Medical Association house of delegates voted to support mandatory HIV testing for pregnant women.[29] In so doing, physicians demonstrated a belief that government intervention will serve only to enhance the physician's authority in working toward maximizing the health of pregnant women and fetuses. The following section will describe the potentially negative ethical and practical implications of expanding the state's role in the doctor's relationship with a pregnant patient.

Ethical and Practical Implications of a State-Fetal Relationship for Doctors and Pregnant Women

To understand the reasons why doctors might welcome governmental intervention into the treatment of pregnant women, it is important to recognize the context that has given rise to a state role in the health care setting. In the present era, more than one in every five United States children lives below the poverty line.[30] Poverty is indisputably linked to diminished health status. For example, poor children often live in areas plagued by violence, which opens them to considerable risks to their health. As society's awareness of children's vulnerability increases, the number of reports of child abuse and neglect has grown exponentially. Yet, the state's capacity to help these children seems tenuous at best, and reports of ineffective state agencies, which routinely fail to protect these children, are commonplace.[31]

The consequences of poverty and/or neglect more often than not manifest in the health care setting. Health care providers are no better situated than any other members of society to solve these children's many problems, and yet, if they fail to take any action, they may feel as though they are perpetuating the harms suffered by such children. Because it is so difficult to identify the course of action appropriate for them as individuals, doctors increasingly look to the state to intervene. With expanding awareness of fetal vulnerability, this impulse toward intervention comes earlier, even while the patient is pregnant.

At the ethical core of the doctor-patient relationship lie several fundamental values, such as confidentiality, beneficence, and autonomy, which at minimum represent duties owed by the doctor to the patient. Virtually all of these values are jeopardized by governmental intrusion into the doctor-patient relationship. Although it is easy to understand why health care providers might tolerate or even welcome the state's intervention into the doctor-patient relationship, it is imperative to recognize the destructive potential represented by this intervention.

This potential may be illustrated by examining the duty of confidentiality. Among the oldest principles of medical ethics is the promise made by physicians to keep confidential any information obtained in the course of treating their patients. This duty serves a critical function in facilitating the doctor-patient relationship: It encourages the patient to disclose all information that may be relevant to his or her medical care. The duty of confidentiality is reinforced by laws creating a doctor-patient privilege, which prohibits doctors from disclosing information relevant to a patient's treatment absent the patient's consent.

When a doctor discloses information obtained from a patient, the relationship with the patient is forever altered. The trust upon which the patient relied may be replaced with a sense of betrayal, and the doctor who seeks to continue a relationship with that patient will find it challenging to regain the patient's confidence. The most familiar circumstance in which such disclosures occur is in the context of child abuse and neglect. Laws in virtually all jurisdictions mandate that physicians notify state officials whenever they have reason to believe that a child is being harmed. The justification for this breach of confidentiality reflects a policy trade-off: Because society places a primary value on child welfare, the confidential relationship between a doctor and a patient must be compromised when a child's safety is endangered. Until recently, this well-established duty to report child abuse represented a narrow exception to a universal rule of confidentiality. However, as policies regarding the HIV testing and drug testing of pregnant women and newborns demonstrate, a growing number of jurisdictions have begun to limit the confidentiality owed to pregnant women.

There are troubling implications that follow from stripping pregnant patients of their rights to confidentiality. As doctors work with the state to police the conduct of pregnant women, the trust that is thought to be the bedrock of the doctor-patient relationship necessarily is displaced. Instead, doctors offer women a conditional relationship—they will be accorded the rights taken for granted by other patients only insofar as they follow medical advice. This posture creates obvious disincentives for the patient in terms of full disclosure. Moreover, to the extent that screening or treatment is deemed mandatory, a patient may choose to delay or avoid any contact with the health care system. Precisely this result occurred in South Carolina, where rates of women delivering babies in abandoned buildings and bus stations soared following the implementation of a mandatory prenatal drug-screening policy, accompanied by criminal sanctions for those women who used drugs.[32]

Physicians are not alone in their frustration over the lack of easy answers to problems growing out of abusive and neglectful behavior by parents toward their children. Inadequate parenting causes harm that is felt not only by the children, but indirectly, by all of society. Nevertheless, to the extent that physicians permit the state to reestablish the terms of the doctor-patient relationship in order to control pregnant women, they will increasingly find themselves working against, rather than with, their patients. The adversarial posture not only is an unproductive one for promoting the health and well-being of patients, pregnant and otherwise, but also is likely to exacerbate many of the underlying problems that led to its adoption.

CONCLUSION

Over the course of the past 100 years, there have been great scientific strides forward in terms of understanding morbidity and mortality in pregnancy. Yet, increased scientific knowledge has not proven sufficient to guarantee healthy pregnancies and hearty offspring. To a large extent, this is because so many of the problems that lead to infant and maternal morbidity and mortality have their genesis outside of the health care setting in the broader context of a violent, impoverished environment. Thus it is that, at the dawn of the new millennium, the doctor's relationship to pregnant women, so new in terms of the scope of medical history, is poised for yet another transformation.

The prospect of doctors' working as agents of the state in an effort to protect fetuses from their mothers merits critical scrutiny. There is a profound irony inherent in the alignment of doctors and government against pregnant women. The vast majority of pregnant women would go to the limits of their abilities to secure the health and well-being of their future children. This is seen in women's willing compliance with medical advice, despite the history of medical disasters. The same impulse toward protectiveness also is demonstrated by many women whose actions are potentially threatening to their fetuses. For example, those who work with substance-abusing women report that, during pregnancy, they are particularly motivated to quit.[33] The prospect of having a child is perhaps the greatest possible motivation toward change. Thus, a state intervention predicated on punishment, rather than on health promotion, squanders a unique opportunity to maximize the well-being of fetuses and pregnant women alike.

Government efforts to intervene in the treatment of pregnant women also are ironic in that they are initiated by relative strangers to the fetus—persons who, once the child is born, will bear no responsibility for its care. Unless they are deemed unfit parents and are deprived of custody, the pregnant women who are the objects of critical scrutiny ultimately will be charged with the task of caring for their children. Therefore, even setting aside the human ties of love that generate their willingness to care for their children, without compensation, and at great cost to themselves, these women have at least as much incentive to attempt to enhance fetal well-being as do their doctors and the state.

The tendency to view "noncompliant" pregnant women as the single most important source of potential harm to the fetus flies in the face of scientific understanding regarding pregnancy. Access to care, good maternal health and nutritional status, stability, and safety are all at least as critical, if not more so, to fetal well-being. Doctors increasingly are left to pick up the pieces left behind by a violent, hostile society in which personal safety, housing, and jobs are scarce commodities; in which substance abuse provides a therapeutic reprieve from the pain of daily existence; and in which access to medical care, including substance-abuse treatment, is simply unavailable for many patients. From this vantage point, it is clearly imperative to the well-being of patients as well as the integrity of the medical profession, that twenty-first-century doctors assume a new role vis-à-vis their pregnant patients. But rather than an adversarial role, doctors must become advocates for their patients, helping to advance their struggles for day-to-day existence and demanding that the government assume its critical role in establishing a safe environment into which children can be born and thrive.

NOTES

1. For a description of the medicalization of the birthing process, see A. Oakley, *The Captured Womb* (New York: Basil Blackwell, 1984) and Pamela Eakins, ed. *The American Way of Birth* (Philadelphia: Temple University Press, 1986). Pregnancy was not atypical in this regard. For a description of the gradual process by which illnesses came to be treated by medical doctors in hospital settings, see P. Starr, *The Social Transformation of American Medicine* (New York: Basic Books, 1982).
2. U.S. Department of Commerce Bureau of the Census, *Historical Statistics of the United States: Colonial Times to 1970* (Washington, D.C.: U.S. Department of Commerce, 1975), Series B 136–47.
3. J. C. Bogdan, "Aggressive Intervention and Mortality," in *The American Way of Birth,* 88–94.
4. R. W. Wertz and D. C. Wertz, *Lying-In: A History of Childbirth in America* (New Haven: Yale University Press, 1989), 133.
5. In 1939, when 50 percent of women delivered in hospitals, the maternal mortality rate was 40/1,000 and the infant mortality rate was 48/1,000 live births. These rates had dropped approximately 10 points per decade from the start of the century, and although the maternal mortality rate dropped off more precipitously during the 1940s and 1950s, the infant mortality rate continued this slow pace of decline until it plateaued in the 1960s, in *Historical Statistics of the United States,* 136–147.
6. Oakley, *The Captured Womb,* 102.
7. Ibid., 98–105.
8. Ibid., 104–5.
9. Ibid., 279.
10. For a general discussion of medical interventions that proved harmful to pregnant women and developing fetuses, see J. Hanigsberg, "Power and Procreation: State Interference in Pregnancy," 23 *Ottawa L. Rev.* 35

(1991): 50–52. See also D. A. Grimes, "Technology Follies: The Uncritical Acceptance of Medical Innovation," 269 *JAMA* (1993): 3030.

11. See R. London, "2 Waiters Lose Jobs for Liquor Warning to Woman," *The New York Times,* 30 March 1991, Sec. 1, p. 7, Col. 3.

12. For a thoughtful discussion of the legal merits of such warnings, see M. S. Jacobs, "Toward a Process-Based Approach to Failure to Warn Law," 71 *N.C. Law Review* 121 (1992): 130–31.

13. Clearly, it is the latter group that represents the most plausible intended audience for this message. This somewhat singular focus on alcohol is ironic, given the grave health risks to the fetus and the pregnant women who lacks prenatal care. In many ways, alcohol is the least of the problems facing this population.

14. The following paragraphs draw heavily on the work of N. A. Press and C. H. Browner, "Collective Silences, Collective Fictions: How Prenatal Diagnostic Testing Became Part of Routine Prenatal Care," in *Women and Prenatal Testing,* ed. K. H. Rothenberg and E. J. Thompson (Columbus, Ohio: Ohio State University Press, 1994), 201–18.

15. Ibid., 216, n. 10, indicating approximately an 85 percent test rate.

16. Ibid., 212–13.

17. C. Beck-Sague, *U.S. Department of Health and Human Services Public Health Reports* 111, 2 (1996): 114.

18. For a comprehensive explanation of the emotional differences between women who have vaginal births and those who have a Caesarian delivery, see M. Samuels and N. Samuels, *New Well-Pregnancy Book* (New York: Simon & Schuster, 1996), 370–73.

19. For decades, court-ordered Caesarian sections were granted as a matter of course, and women were forced to undergo surgery to which they did not consent. V. Kolder et. al., "Court Ordered Obstetrical Interventions," *New England Journal of Medicine* 316 (1987): 1192–96; N. K. Rhoden, "Caesareans and Samaritans," *Law, Medicine & Health Care* 15 (1987): 118–25

    In the 1990s, several well-publicized judicial decisions have rejected this practice as legally unfounded and have upheld the woman's right to refuse treatment. (See, *In re A.C.,* 573 A.2d 1235 (D.C.App 1990) and *In re Baby Boy Doe,* 260 Ill. App. 3d 392, 632 N.E.2d 326 (1994). The practice of resorting to the law to force women to comply with medical advice emerges as particularly ironic in view of the widespread consensus that Caesarian sections are overutilized in this society, coupled with somewhat surprising informal evidence that an overwhelming number of the women allowed to refuse Caesarian sections ultimately deliver healthy babies.

    For example, in 1993, a married, competent, pregnant women was informed by her doctor that absent a Caesarian section, a placental abnormality could result in her child's being stillborn or severely retarded. The mother and the father refused the procedure due to personal and religious beliefs. The doctor and the hospital contacted the state attorney's office, which sought custody of the fetus in order to compel the Caesarean section. Included in their petition for custody was a medical expert's testimony that the fetus's chances of surviving a natural labor were close to zero. Nevertheless, the court denied the state's petition and reaffirmed the mother's autonomy rights. Two weeks later, the mother vaginally delivered a normal and healthy baby boy. For other cases with similar outcomes, see N. K. Rhoden, "Caesareans and Samaritans," *Law, Medicine & Health Care* 15 (1987): 118–25.

20. D. A. Grimes, "Technology Follies: The Uncritical Acceptance of Medical Innovation,'' 269 *JAMA* (1993): 3030.

21. Ibid., 3030–31.

22. For a comprehensive discussion of pregnancy clauses in living wills that terminate the woman's right to discontinue life support if she is pregnant and a thorough description of the variations of these restrictions by state, see T. J. Burch, "Incubator or Individual?: The Legal and Policy Deficiencies of Pregnancy Clauses in Living Wills and Advance Health Care Directive Statutes," *Md. L. Rev.* 54 (1995): 528.

23. This sort of state-mandated interventionist mindset is also reflected in recent reports of several brain-dead pregnant women whose bodies were maintained on life support until the fetus was capable of independent life. In one case, the brain-dead, pregnant woman's family told officials at the hospital that she once said that she did not want her life artificially prolonged if something were to happen to her. Regardless, her parents decided to continue life support until the fetus was sufficiently developed to be delivered. "Brain Dead Mother to Be Kept in Life Support," *U.P.I.* 7 January 1988. In another case, when the parents of a brain-dead, pregnant daughter requested that life-support machines be disconnected, the hospital refused and won a court-ordered guardianship of the pregnant woman over the objections of her parents. Further, when the woman began having contractions, while the legal dispute continued, the hospital performed a Caesarean section. The baby was seven weeks premature and suffered from hyaline membrane disease, appeared to have brain damage, and died three days later. J. Warren, "Girl Declared Brain Dead Has Premature Baby by Caesarean," *Los Angeles Times,* 12 May 1989, pt. I, p. 3, col. 4.

24. E. M. Connor et al., "Reduction of Maternal-Infant Transmission of HIV Type I with Zidovudine Treatment," *New Eng. J. Med.* 331 (1994): 1173. Proponents of this position include bioethicist Arthur Caplan, who asserts that, "[D]espite all the rhetoric . . . this isn't such

a complicated moral call. If you can prevent a young child from being infected, it would seem to me that you are under an obligation to take the steps necessary to prevent that harm." G. Kolata, "Debate on Infant AIDS vs. Mother's Rights," *New York Times,* 3 November 1994, A15.

25. The coalition of those opposing mandatory HIV screening included "an alliance of gay leaders, civil libertarians, physicians, and public health officials. . . ." R. Bayer, "Public Health Policy and the AIDS Epidemic: An End to HIV Exceptionalism," *New Eng. J. Med.* 324 (1991): 1501.
26. According to Mildred Williamson, the administrator of Chicago's first and largest hospital-based program for women and children with HIV, the majority of HIV-infected women have at least one child and have had at least one encounter with the state child-welfare agency. (Interview with Mildred Williamson, Program Administrator for Cook County Hospital Women and Children with AIDS Project, Chicago, November 15, 1995).
27. For a fascinating discussion on compliance rates with mandatory screening programs, see S. M. Rothman, "Seek and Hide: Public Health Departments and Persons with Tuberculosis, 1890–1940," *J. of L., Med. & Ethics* 21 (1993): 293.
28. A 1996 study found cancerous tumors in the offspring of mice exposed to zidovudine while pregnant. "AIDS Therapies (AZT) Experts Evaluate Line Between AIDS Drugs and Cancer," *AIDS Weekly Plus,* 27 Jan. 1997.
29. See J. Manier, "AMA Supports HIV Tests for All Pregnant Women; Critics Fear Some Will Avoid Prenatal Care," *Chicago Tribune,* 28 June 1996. Perhaps the delegates felt that mandatory testing was inevitable in light of recent governmental actions. On June 2, 1996, both the House and Senate mandated that by the year 2000, states that do not invoke mandatory HIV testing for pregnant women must demonstrate, (1) that they have reduced by 50 percent the number of newborns who develop AIDS as a result of parental infection or (2) that 95 percent of pregnant women who make at least two prenatal visits are seeking to be tested. If states do not satisfy at least one of these requirements, they will be required to test all newborns whose mothers' HIV status is unknown or risk losing their federal Ryan White AIDS funding. H. Dewar, "AIDS Testing Compromise Is Reached; Hill Negotiators Agree On Prenatal Program," *The Washington Post,* 2 May 1996. The President signed the Act on May 20, 1996. *United States Bill Tracking* (1995 United States Senate Bill No. 641 104th Congress).
30. More critically, American children have the highest poverty rate among the world's industrial countries. Children in other Western industrialized countries are at least a third better off than the average low-income American child. M. Rossi, "Rich Kids, Poor Kids: The Gap is Widening," *Syracuse Herald American,* 14 July 1996. This situation is even worse for African-American and Hispanic children, where 45.9 percent and 39.9 percent, respectively, live in poverty (compared to 17 percent of Caucasian children). P. McKeown, "Education Critical in Battling Poverty for Families," *Daily Oklahoman,* 15 July 1996.
31. See M. B. Muslin, "Unsafe Havens: The Case for Constitutional Protection of Foster Children From Abuse and Neglect," *Harvard Civil Rights–Civil Liberties Law Review* 23 (1988): 199 (chronicling the failure of state agencies and foster care systems to ensure the safety of their child-wards).
32. "Pregnant and Newly Delivered Women Jailed on Drug Charges," *Reproduction Rights Update* 6 (ACLU/Reprod. Freedom Project, New York, N.Y., Feb. 1, 1990).
33. See, e.g. W. Chavkin, N. Walker, and D. Paone, "Symposium: Drug Using Families and Child Protection: Results of a Study and Implications for Change," *U. Pitt. L. Rev.* 54 (1992): 295, describing successful treatment programs for substance-abusing women.

Part II

Adult Medicine

CHAPTER 9

The Family in Medical Decision Making

Jeffrey Blustein

Families have traditionally exercised, and continue to exercise, considerable control over medical treatment of minor children. In both law and morality, families (or more specifically, parents) are regarded not just as interested parties whose views should be solicited and taken into consideration, but rather as rightful surrogate decision makers to whose judgment the physician normally ought to defer. When the patient is an incompetent adult, physicians often consult with family members (that is, children or siblings, parents, or spouse) about specific medical interventions and even about continuation of treatment, and many physicians are guided by the family's decision if it is not obviously unreasonable and if it does not contradict any previously expressed wishes of the patient. Family involvement is also sought when the patient is a competent adult, not, of course, because the family is given the authority to decide for the patient, but because it is thought that patients may need the emotional support of family members during times of crisis.

The role of the family in treatment decisions for young children has been extensively discussed in the bioethics literature; I will not rehearse the familiar arguments for this general parental authority nor the reasons for preferring families as proxies for noncompetent adults. I want instead to turn to the case of competent adult patients and critically examine the current system of medical decision making and its legitimating ethos in light of the fact that patients are often cared for in the context of the family. I want to ask whether, in view of certain features of the relationship between patients and their families, the principle of patient self-determination at the core of contemporary medical ethics is in need of some serious rethinking. Might it be that family members, by virtue of their closeness to the patient, should not only have some special authority to speak on behalf of patients who are incompetent, but should also share decisional authority with patients who are competent?

A recent proposal that speaks to the family's role in medical decision making has been advanced by John Hardwig. In his provocative essay, "What about the Family?"[1] he contemplates far-reaching changes in medical practice based on a critique of our prevailing patient-centered ethos. My discussion of his proposal is chiefly designed to pave the way for what I call a communitarian account of the role of the family in acute care decision making. This account—which, I hasten to add, I do not endorse—has not to my knowledge been taken seriously as a

---

Reprinted with permission from J. Blustein, The Family in Medical Decisionmaking, *Hastings Center Report,* Vol. 23, No. 3, pp. 6–13, © 1993, The Hastings Center.

I want to thank John Arras, John Hardwig, Jonathan Moreno, Jim and Hilde Nelson, and several anonymous referees for the *Hastings Center Report* for comments on earlier drafts of this chapter.

theoretical possibility in the bioethics literature. Since the label "communitarian" is liable to be misunderstood, I should note at the outset that I am not interested in communitarianism as a political theory. Rather, I want to focus on the family as communitarian political writers sometimes think of it, namely, as a model for their concept of the larger society, and on the basis of this understanding of the family, to mount a challenge to the dominant patient-centered ethos that parallels the communitarian critique of liberal political philosophy. This communitarian position resembles Hardwig's proposal in that it does not regard the competent patient as the ultimate decision maker, but takes it as morally significant for the attribution of decisional authority that his or her life is intimately intertwined with the lives of close others. However, as we will see, the communitarian account is philosophically more radical than Hardwig's challenge to the dominant patient-centered medical ethos.

My own position is that the locus of decisional authority should remain the individual patient, but I also argue that family members, by virtue of their closeness to and intimate knowledge of the patient, are often uniquely well qualified to shore up the patient's vulnerable autonomy and assist him or her in the exercise of autonomous decision making. Families, in other words, can be an important resource for patients in helping them to make better decisions about their care. Recognition of this fact leads to a broader understanding of the duty to respect patient autonomy than currently prevails in acute care medicine.

FAMILY DECISION MAKING AND COMPETENT PATIENTS

According to Hardwig, even when the patient is a competent adult, it may be quite appropriate to empower the family to "make the treatment decision, with all competent family members whose lives will be affected participating" (p. 9). This is so because family members have legitimate interests of their own that are likely to be affected in dramatic and profound ways by whatever treatment plan is chosen by or for the patient. Their interests may be affected in these ways because "family," by definition, consists of "those who are close to the patient" and "there is no way to detach the lives of patients from the lives of those who are close to them" (p. 6). Since family members must often revise their own priorities and significantly alter their life plans to accommodate the needs of sick or dying relatives, and since the nature and extent of the adjustment depends on the treatment plan that is followed for the patient, it would be wrong categorically to deny family members a role in determining what the treatment will be, how it will be administered, where, and so forth. For one thing, there is a presumption that "the interests of patients and family members are morally to be weighed equally" (p. 7), and family decision making may be necessary to ensure that treatment decisions are fair to all concerned. Even when this is not necessary, the autonomy of other family members would be seriously undermined if the authority to make decisions that cut so deeply into their own lives belonged to the patient alone.

The interests of family members might be self-regarding or other-regarding. Particular choices about treatment can seriously affect the lives of family members in many ways, interfering not only with their own personal projects and individual lifestyles, but with their commitments to other family members as well. In any case, they are "separate" in the sense that they diverge from and possibly conflict with patient interests: they are not to be understood as interests in the interests of patients. Of course, those who love the patient also have a direct interest in the protection and promotion of the patient's interests, assuming that the patient has interests that can be protected and promoted. Indeed, this is part of the very meaning of love. But for Hardwig, there can be closeness without love, and even when there is love, there will usually be other interests of family members as well. When all of these interests are taken into account, it may turn out that what is best for the family as a whole is not what is best for the individual patient.

These other interests may be, and frequently are, quite legitimate, and treatment decisions should not be judged morally better or worse solely from the patient's perspective. Indeed, departures from optimal patient care may be justified "to harmonize best the interests of all concerned or to require significantly smaller sacrifices by other family members" (p. 7). Moreover, and very importantly, Hardwig expresses misgivings about the effectiveness of exhorting the patient to consider the impact of his or her decision on the lives of the rest of the family. Patients who seem to be ignoring their family's stake in the outcome of their decision-making process may sometimes respond appropriately to appeals from the physician or other family members, but many patients will be too self-involved to give the interests of others proper consideration or will use their illness as a kind of trump card to dominate the rest of the family. Because of this, Hardwig maintains, we must consider a more radical measure to ensure adequate protection of legitimate family interests, namely, rejection of the prevalent medical ethos according to which the competent patient is always the decisive moral agent. Under this ethos, it is certainly permissible for family members to offer information, counsel, and suasion to patients who must make treatment decisions. But the authority to make the decisions still resides with the competent patient alone, and this Hardwig finds untenable.[2]

The "ethic of patient autonomy" (p. 5) allows the competent patient, and the patient alone, to set the terms and conditions of care. Patients may be frightened and distracted by illness and hence in no position to give careful thought to the interests of others, but if their decision-making capacity is judged sufficient for the decision at hand, their wishes prevail. This troubles Hardwig because it amounts to giving patients permission to neglect or slight their moral responsibilities to other family members. Seriously ill patients tend to be self-absorbed and to make exclusively self-regarding choices about care, and in those cases where "the lives of family members would be dramatically affected by treatment decisions" Hardwig suggests that family conferences be "required" (pp. 9–10). These conferences would not merely have an advisory or supportive function: they would be decision-making forums. Patients and other family members would seek to reach a consensus that harmonizes the autonomy and interests of all concerned parties. Failing this, families would be forced "to invoke the harsh perspective of justice, divisive and antagonistic though that perspective might be" (p. 10).

Hardwig's proposal for greater family involvement in medical decision making, however, runs up against the problem of patient vulnerability: joint family decision making provides too many opportunities for the exploitation of patient vulnerability. Serious constraints on patient autonomy, such as anxiety, depression, fear, and denial, are inherent in the state of being ill.[3] Illness is also frequently disorienting in that patients find themselves thrust into unfamiliar surroundings, unable to pursue customary routines or to enjoy any significant degree of privacy. For these reasons, the ability of patients to assess their medical needs accurately and protect their own interests effectively is limited and precarious. But if those who are ill and those who are healthy already confront each other on an unequal psychological footing, then family conferences, as Hardwig conceives of them, seem especially ill-advised. Weakened and confused by their illness, patients are easy prey to manipulation or coercion by other family members and may capitulate to family wishes out of guilt or fear. (Given that Hardwig would allow even hateful or resentful family members to be included in family conferences, this is not an idle worry.) Family members will understandably not want to be seen by the physician as opposing the wishes of the patient, and so they might exert pressure on the patient to concur with their opinions about treatment. Of course, even as matters now stand, with decision making not generally thought to belong to the family as a whole, what seems like a patient's autonomous choice often only implements the choice of the others for him or her. But joint family decision making is likely only to exacerbate this problem and to make truly independent choice even more dubious.

Hardwig, it should be noted, does acknowledge that a seriously weakened patient may well need an "advocate" (p. 10), or surrogate participant from outside the family, to take part in the joint family decision. However, this hardly resolves all the difficulties his proposal presents. The presence of an outsider in what is supposed to be a deeply personal and private conference might only create (further) hostility and suspicion among family members. And if consensus in the conference cannot be achieved, the rest of the family could simply overrule the patient's proxy participant, just as it could overrule the patient himself.

From a theoretical point of view, we should, I think, agree with Hardwig about the inadequacy of any view that denies or overlooks the essential interplay between rights and responsibilities. But the practical moral problem as I see it is how to design procedures and structures of decision making that achieve an acceptable balance between rights and responsibilities, between the important values of a patient-centered ethos and the legitimate claims of other family members. If alternative approaches to medical decision making are judged in this light, as Hardwig wants them to be, and not solely in terms of overall happiness or preference satisfaction or the like, then family decision making for competent patients confronts serious moral obligations. For indications are that it will often result not in a mutual accommodation of the autonomy and interests of all affected parties, but rather in a serious erosion of patient autonomy and a subordination of patient interests to the competing interests of other family members.

THE COMMUNITARIAN DEFENSE OF FAMILY DECISION MAKING

I have focused on the problems that nonideal, less than fully harmonious families pose for Hardwig's proposal. Critics of the patient-as-primary-agent model might instead restrict their attention to those (admittedly infrequent) cases in which patients belong to close-knit and harmonious families, and with this as their concept of the family, offer a defense of family decision making that challenges the patient-centered model in a more radical way than Hardwig does. In ideal families, suspicions, resentments, disagreements, and the like, if they exist, are muted and do not set the tone of family life. But more important, it may be claimed, the concept of the person that underlies the theory of patient autonomy is patently inappropriate here. The patient is not, as this theory presupposes, an atomic entity, a free and rational chooser of ends unencumbered by communal and other allegiances. On the contrary, his or her identity is constituted by family relationships, and he or she is united with other family members through common ends and mutual understanding. In these circumstances, the patient is too enmeshed in a network of relations to others to be properly singled out as the one to make treatment decisions.

I call this the communitarian argument for family decision making to distinguish it from the argument from fairness and autonomy discussed in the previous section. When I refer below to what "communitarians" say about medical decision making, I am not thinking of any particular authors who have advanced this position.[4] Rather, I am suggesting that elements of the communitarian view can be taken out of their political context and that a challenge to the prevailing patient-centered ethos can be constructed on the basis of a communitarian concept of the ideal family. Let us look at this challenge more closely.

In acute care settings, the relationship between patients and physicians is, if not exactly adversarial, at least one in which patients should not normally suppose that they and their physicians are participants in a common enterprise with common values and goals. The values involved in medical decision making are by no means exclusively medical values, but also largely normative ones about which patients and physicians frequently disagree. In these circumstances, physicians may attempt to coerce compliance with their wishes, which they are in an advantageous position to do, or to control patient decisions by selective disclosure or nondisclosure of information. In recognition of normative diversity and in the face of various threats to patient autonomy in the caregiving relationship, we invoke the notion of patients' rights. Rights accord patients a protected space in which to make their own choices and pursue their ends free of inappropriate interference from others. Having rights, patients can confront caregivers with the demand that their (possibly conflicting) ends be respected.

Communitarian critics of the traditional ethos of patient autonomy need not deny that patients' rights and patient self-determination play an important role in the caregiving relationship. But, they note, the patient is not always to be thought of simply as the one who is sick or in need of medical attention. If the patient belongs to a close-knit and harmonious family, for example, it is the family as a whole whose values and goals may diverge from those of professional caregivers because such a family is a genuine community, not a mere collection of separate individuals with their own private and possibly conflicting interests. Members of a community have common ends, and these are conceived of and valued as common ends by the members. United by common ends and a common identity, the threats that work against the autonomy of some work against the autonomy of all. Moreover, in these cases the patient would not need to be protected from family pressures for inappropriate treatment. Rather, the family would act as advocate for the patient vis-à-vis the physician, and family decision making would put patients on a much more equal footing with caregivers.

For communitarians the ethics of acute care, focusing as it does on the individual who is the subject of treatment, rests on a concept of the self that is at odds with how persons define and understand themselves in a community. This is a concept for a world of strangers, where the content of each person's good is, to quote Michael Sandel, "largely opaque" to others, where persons have divergent and possibly conflicting plans and interests, and where their capacity for benevolence is extremely limited.[5] But in the community of a close and harmonious family these conditions do not obtain. Rather, the defining features of such a family are mutual sympathy, common ends, a shared identity, love, and spontaneous affection. Of course, it is sheer wishful thinking, and cavalier as well, to assume that all families are like this. Family life may instead be fraught with dissension and interests may diverge and conflict. In these situations questions of justice come to the fore and the importance of individual rights (and individual patient rights) is enhanced. But within the context of a more or less ideal family, the circumstances that make personal autonomy both an appropriate and a pressing concern prevail to a relatively small degree.

For communitarian philosophers, individual rights have no place in intimate harmonious communities. Charles Taylor, for example, suggests that "the whole effort to find a background for the arguments which start from rights is misguided,"[6] and according to Michael Sandel, in "a more or less ideal family situation . . . individual rights and fair decision procedures are seldom invoked, not because injustice is rampant but because their appeal is pre-empted by a spirit of generosity in which I am rarely inclined to claim my fair share."[7] Rights, as communitarians understand them, are conflict notions, and if they play any role in intimate communities, it is remedial only.[8]

Unlike Hardwig's argument for family decision making, the communitarian view I have constructed does not claim that families should make treatment decisions because this solves the problem of fairness or because this protects the autonomy of all those individual family members who have a stake in the outcome of treatment decisions. Rather, the argument proceeds from a picture of the family as a community of love where, it is alleged, questions of fairness and individual autonomy normally do not arise and are of minor importance. In the ideal family, there isn't enough of a distinction to begin with between self and others for these concerns to loom large. And this absence of a sharp line separating self and others is not a cause for alarm or a basis for moral criticism of family decision making but intrinsic to the nature of community, the experience of which, plainly, is an important good for humans.

The close-knit, harmonious family is a paradigm of community. Here the well-being of one family member does not just have an impact on the well-being of others, for this can happen in families that are no more than associations of individuals (like the ones Hardwig describes). Rather, in families that are genuine communities, individuals identify with one another, such that the well-being of one is *part of* the well-being of the other. This being so, the communitarian maintains, decisions that importantly affect the well-being of one family member are the province of the entire family. To be sure, in the medical cases there is only one family member, the patient, who literally bears the decision in his or her flesh and bones. But this fact alone, it is believed, does not confer upon the patient a unilateral decision-making right. The right to make the decision is still a right of the family in ideal circumstances—a group right rather than a right of individuals.

However, since the communitarian argument for family decision making applies only to families that are communities and not to those that are just collections of individuals whose lives affect each other in major ways, its implications for the practice of medicine will not be as significant as those of Hardwig's proposal. Many families, to acknowledge the obvious again, are not ideal. In addition, physicians frequently have only passing acquaintance with the patient's family and no reliable basis for judging the quality of the patient's relationship with other family members. Even if communitarians reveal genuine inadequacies in the prevalent ethos of patient autonomy and patient rights, physicians will often not be in a position to tell whether, in the particular case at hand, the family is harmonious enough to be entrusted with the authority to make decisions for one of its own. On the other hand, physicians will often have enough information to know that the lives of family members will be seriously affected by treatment decisions, and it is on this fact, not on the existence of a harmonious family, that Hardwig premises the case for joint family decision making.

Still, the communitarian critique of the dominant medical ethos of patient autonomy and individual patients' rights raises interesting and important philosophical issues. Practical implications aside, the theoretical challenge it poses deserves a response. In what follows, I will try to indicate why I think this challenge fails.

HOW THE COMMUNITARIAN CHALLENGE FAILS

Even in families that are true communities of love, the harmony that exists among their members may not be so thoroughgoing that invocation of individual decision-making rights loses its point. It is not necessary for community that there be complete identity of all ends and unanimity on all matters of value or the good. On the contrary, there is room for significant disagreement about how to rank different components of a common conception of the good, about the proper means and strategies for achieving it, and about whether certain risks are worth taking to achieve common goals. Even if the members of a family are in broad agreement about what is of most importance in life, for example, this does not ensure that they will assess the costs and benefits of particular medical treatments similarly. Indeed, given the diversity of human nature and experience, such disagreements are not just possible but to be expected. Absolute harmony in decision making and thoroughgoing convergence of values are only found in quite extraordinary communities. And this being the case, individual rights can be seen to have an importance the communitarian fails to acknowledge. They are not just claims we fall back on in the unhappy situation where community is lacking or faltering. Additionally, they serve to secure recognition of the diverse values and ends that persist even in intact and well-functioning communities. This lack of homogeneity is glossed over by talk of family rights.

Individual rights have an important place in community because the existence of community does not eradicate serious disagreement about ends, about the relationship between particular choices and shared ends, and so forth. Individual rights are needed because a significant degree of diversity may exist even in a group united by a common concept of the good. But what if, hard to imagine though it might be, there were a community without such diversity? Would individual rights have much importance in a perfectly homogeneous community like this? Would there be any point in ascribing rights to individual patients, rather than to families, if patients and their family members were in complete agreement about all matters pertaining to the good for themselves? Here if nowhere else, the communitarian would surely argue, individual rights are useless and irrelevant.

This is the conclusion we come to if we adopt a particular concept of rights. We find a clear and succinct statement of this concept in an earlier paper by Hardwig entitled, "Should Women Think in Terms of Rights?" The thrust of this essay, unlike that of "What about the Family?" is communitarian:

> Thinking in terms of rights rests on a picture, first sketched by Hobbes and then made more palatable by Locke, of the person as atomistic, primarily egoistic, and asocial—only accidentally and externally related to others. If we are lucky our independent interests may coincide or happily divide in a symbiotic relationship . . . but we should not expect this to be the normal state of affairs.[9]

The normal state of affairs in a genuine community is quite different, however. Here persons are not just "accidentally and externally related" to each other, but understand themselves as participants in a common enterprise and regard the well-being of others as part of their own. No wonder then that rights should seem alien or antithetical to community and, more specifically, ideal familial love.

But communitarians who think of rights only in these familiar legalistic terms underestimate the complexities and possibilities inherent in individual rights. To be sure, rights sometimes function to protect the individual in the pursuit of his or her independent self-interest. But this hardly exhausts their significance. Consider these remarks by Neera Badhwar:

> An ideal family or friendship may wipe out all differences of ends, both final and intermediate, but it cannot wipe out "the separateness of life and experience." *Au contraire,* it would seem that it is precisely ideal familial love and friendship that will appreciate the "distinction of persons," recognizing the interest of each individual in *pursuing* a shared good, and her right to do so within the constraints of justice.[10]

On this view, rights are important even in the most closely knit and harmonious community. Even if the lives of persons are inextricably intertwined and their concepts of the good agree in every respect, they remain numerically distinct persons with their own distinct perspectives on the world and an interest in expressing them. This interest in exercising one's agency in the pursuit of one's ends is not the same as an interest in seeing one's ends realized, for one's ends might be realizable quite independently of the operation of one's own agency. Nor is this interest contingent on one's ends being different from or in conflict with the ends of others.

By linking rights to this fundamental interest in one's own agency, we can explain what is wrong with the communitarian's antipathy to rights. Thinking in terms of rights, on the present account, does not rest either directly or by implication on a picture of the person as atomistic, egoistic, and asocial. It rests rather on a picture of the person as a separate being, with a distinctive personal point of view and an interest in being able securely to pursue his or her own concept of the good. This by itself entails neither that one's relationships to others are intrinsic to one's identity nor that one is only accidentally and externally related to others. In ascribing rights to individuals, we are responding to these basic and universal features of persons.

It may help here to distinguish between having a right and insisting upon or demanding it. The language of demands does seem ill-suited to harmonious families. If family members need to insist against one another that they have a right to make their own decisions, then we are probably dealing with a divided and quite antagonistic family. But these observations do not suffice to banish individual rights from harmonious families because the underlying supposition—that rights must always be linked to demands—is false. Rights can be expressed in different ways, and what is divisive and antagonistic to community is not the concept of rights, but only a certain way of expressing them. In harmonious families, rights are typically expressed "as reminders—gentle or forceful, matter-of-fact or emotional—of legitimate expectations and entitlements,"[11] and as such they play a vital role in the moral lives of families.

The implications of these remarks for a communitarian defense of family medical decision making are clear. Even in extremely close families, patients may have different priorities from their loved ones and assess life choices in disparate ways, and these differences may surface in disagreements about how and even whether patients should be treated. Patients need their own rights regarding choice of treatment not just because family members cannot always be trusted to have the patient's best interests at heart, but because, even in families where trust is not an issue and there is a remarkable measure of agreement on ends and deep mutual affection, other family members may not always concur with the wisdom of the patient's choices. Rights protect patient autonomy and patient interests in these circumstances.

Further, rights for patients would be appropriate and useful even in those quite unusual families where the minimal sort of disagreement just mentioned is absent. For decisions about treatment often have dramatic and far-reaching consequences for the shape, quality, and duration of a patient's life, and individuals have an interest in determining for themselves the course their lives take. The interest in directing how one's life will go in accordance with one's values and preferences exists whether these values and preferences are uniquely one's own or shared with other family members, and it calls for recognition even when there is no disagreement between patient and family over the correct treatment decision. This is why patients have rights as individuals even under the unlikely conditions of absolute intrafamilial harmony: These rights protect the interests that patients have in exercising their agency.

Important questions remain about how belonging to a harmonious intimate community creates a new identity for the parties involved and about the interplay, for those who belong to such communities, between their interests as single individuals and their interests as members of a community. But I believe enough has been said to establish the following, and this is all that is required for my purposes: community does not undermine the normative significance of the individual self nor does it render individual rights otiose.

FAMILY INVOLVEMENT IN THE PROCESS OF DECISION MAKING

These responses to the communitarian position do not show that patient choices about treatment always trump the choices of family members, and they do not cut against Hardwig's argument for joint medical decision making by all affected family members. What they show is only that the dominant patient-centered medical ethos cannot be refuted by the sort of all-out attack on the notion of individual rights the communitarian launches. To be sure, an adversarial and legalistic concept of individual rights is ill-suited to those cases where family relationships are nonadversarial and there are no deep conflicts of interests, preferences, or values among family members. But if this is the basis for the communitarian claim that community renders individual rights (including patient rights) useless or of minor importance, the communitarian betrays a distorted and incomplete understanding of rights.

Should the choices of competent patients trump the choices of family members, except in the rarest of circumstances? "It is an oversimplification to say of a patient who is part of a family," Hardwig notes, that "it's his life" or "after all, it's his medical treatment" (p. 6). Plainly, this by itself hardly shows that patient choices take priority over the choices of others, for when lives are so intertwined that one life cannot be shaped without also shaping the lives of others, it's their lives too. Another approach is to argue for a unilateral decision-making right for patients on the ground that patients have more to lose than their family members. That is, when we measure the sacrifices that family members must make for a patient's health care and the costs to the patient of not receiving the treatment that, other family members aside, he or she would select, the patient's sacrifices almost always outweigh the family's. Of course, the reverberations of patients' self-regarding choices can be so shattering to the lives of other family members that a calculation of relative costs favors the family instead. But familial hardship from this source is usually less of a burden than serious illness, and this difference would be sufficient to establish at least a presumption in favor of patient decision making.

But if the ethos of patient autonomy survives the challenges I have considered in this chapter, it is nevertheless the case that current medical practice and medical ethics can be faulted for not giving the family a more prominent place in medical decision making for competent patients, and that both family members and patients suffer as a result. For one thing, as we learned from our discussion of Hardwig, because treatment decisions often do have a dramatic impact on family members, procedures need to be devised, short of giving family members a share of decisional authority, that acknowledge the moral weight of their legitimate interests. For another, though patients might well benefit from family involvement in the process of formulating views about medical treatment, under the regime of patient autonomy patients tend to be treated for the most part as if they were solitary decision makers, isolated from intimate others.

The ethos of patient autonomy rightly understood takes seriously the impairments of autonomy that affect us when we are ill. Patients are not ideally autonomous agents but anxious, fearful, depressed, often confused, and subject to ill-considered and mistaken ideas. If we are genuinely concerned about ensuring patient self-determination, we will take these factors into account. Here it is necessary to distinguish, as Jay Katz does, between "choices" and "thinking about choices."[12] According to the dominant medical ethos, choices properly belong to the patient alone. At the same time, patients' capacities for reflective thought and effective action are limited and precarious, obliging them to converse and consult with supportive and caring others if they are to make their best choices. Patients' psychological capacities for autonomy can be enhanced by searching conversations with their physicians—the main point of Katz's book—and (I would add) by conversations with other family members.

To explain why this is so, we may turn to a characterization of the family found in Nancy Rhoden's influential law review article, "Litigating Life and Death."[13] Her argument, which focuses on decision making for incompetent patients, finds within family life features that warrant a legal presumption in favor of family choice. Family members are typically the best decision makers partly because of their special epistemic qualifications: they ordinarily have deep and detailed knowledge of one another's lives, characters, values, and desires. This knowledge might be based on specific statements made by one family member to another, for the intimacy of family life encourages and is partly constituted by the unguarded disclosure of one's most private thoughts and deepest feelings. But there may be nothing specific that was said or done to which family members can point as evidence of another member's preferences. Indeed, their knowledge, acquired through long association and the sharing of intense life experiences, is characteristically of the sort that "transcends purely logical evidence." In addition, family members are the best candidates to act as surrogates for an incompetent patient because of their special emotional bonds to the patient. This is important because possessing deep and detailed knowledge of another can put one in an especially good position to frustrate no less than fulfill this person's desires. Family members, however, can be presumed to have a deep emotional commitment to one another, and this makes it likely that they will put their knowledge to the right use—that is, that they will decide as the patient would have wanted.

Those features of families that, in Rhoden's view, justify a legal presumption in favor of family decision making for incompetent patients—intimate knowledge, caring, shared history—also provide good reasons for family involvement in the competent patients' thinking about choices. Family members would have no veto power over a patient's decision and would have to honor the choice ultimately made, no matter how foolish or idiosyncratic. But in family conferences, where the process of making a decision is shared, they could encourage the patient to evaluate different treatment options in terms of their impact on the interests of other family members, and could attempt to persuade the patient that the best choice is one that is fair to all affected parties. In some cases, understanding what a particular treatment decision would cost other family members might give the patient a compelling reason to alter an initial choice.

For the physician, the duty to respect patient autonomy has as its corollary a duty to engage in conversation with patients and to encourage and facilitate conversation between patients and other persons to whom they are close (including family members), unless the physician has reason to think that such conversation will not in fact assist the patient in making autonomous decisions. Current medical practice does not in general reflect a commitment to foster this sort of conversation as an integral part of the physician's professional responsibility. But if, as Katz suggests, genuine respect for patient autonomy is shown not merely in accepting patients' yes or no response to a proposed intervention, but rather in facilitating patients' opportunities for serious reflection on their choices, then promoting discussion and dialogue between patient and family is an important part of the physician's duty to satisfy the patient's right of self-determination.

A useful parallel can be drawn here with a central tenet of family medicine. Family physicians stress the importance of adopting a systems approach to health and disease in which the patient is seen as part of a family system. It is the individual patient, not the family unit, that is the primary focus of care, most family physicians will say, but since poor family dynamics can predispose to or cause disease and illness, effective treatment of the patient requires sensitivity to the multiple roles of faulty family relationships in the etiology of disease. In other words, to use language familiar to family physicians, if the physician is to treat "the patient in the family" appropriately, the physician must be cognizant of "the family in the patient."[14] My remarks about promoting and facilitating family involvement in the process of decision making make a similar point about the importance of physicians' generally extending their attention beyond the individual patient. Only now the rationale for doing so is not that family relationships may contribute to the illness the physician is trying to treat, but that family communication may assist patients in making autonomous decisions about how or whether to treat their illness. The family is the center of most people's lives, for better or for worse, and this means both that the health of individuals is most profoundly influenced by family relationships and that such relationships can play a vital role in restoring the autonomous functioning that illness undermines.

NOTES

1. J. Hardwig, "What about the Family?" *Hastings Center Report* 10, no. 2 (1990): 5–10.
2. Hardwig's proposal to "reconstruct medical ethics in light of family interests" (p. 10) is novel in that it rejects the model of patient-as-primary-agent for acute care. Others have argued, along lines similar to Hardwig's, that this is not the appropriate model for home care, where family members share heavily in the burdens of care on an ongoing basis. In the view of Bart Collopy, Nancy Dubler, and Connie Zuckerman, for example, "the ethical problem for home care becomes one of gauging the interplay of agents, the relative weight to be granted to the autonomy and interests of the family vis-à-vis those of the elderly recipient of care." While not disputing the value of the patient-centered model in acute care, these writers argue that decision making in home care should be "an interactive process, involving negotiation, compromise, and the recognition of reciprocal ties." See "The Ethics of Home Care: Autonomy and Accommodation," special supplement, *Hastings Center Report* 20, no. 2 (1990): 1–16, at 9, 10.
3. See T. F. Ackerman, "Why Doctors Should Intervene," *Hastings Center Report* 12, no. 4 (1982): 14–17.
4. One author who has advanced something like a communitarian position is James Lindemann Nelson. See his "Taking Families Seriously," *Hastings Center Report* 22, no. 4 (1992): 6–12.
5. M. Sandel, *Liberalism and the Limits of Justice* (Cambridge, England: Cambridge University Press, 1982), 170–71.
6. C. Taylor, "Atomism," in *Powers, Possession and Freedom,* ed. A. Kontos (Toronto, Canada: University of Toronto Press, 1979), 42.
7. Sandel, *Liberalism,* 33.
8. In a similar vein Alasdair MacIntyre, taking as his "moral starting point" the "fact that the self has to find its moral identity in and through its membership in communities," attacks the language of rights for its individualism and the ahistorical and asocial concept of the self it expresses. See *After Virtue* (Notre Dame, Ind.: University of Notre Dame Press, 1981), 1–5, 64–67, 204–5.
9. J. Hardwig, "Should Women Think in Terms of Rights?" *Ethics* 94, no. 3 (1984): 441–55, at 446.
10. N. Badhwar, "The Circumstances of Justice: Liberalism, Community, and Friendship," *The Journal of Political Philosophy* 1 (1993).
11. Badhwar, "Circumstances of Justice."
12. J. Katz, *The Silent World of Doctor and Patient* (New York: Free Press, 1984), 111.
13. N. Rhoden, "Litigating Life and Death," *Harvard Law Review* 102, no. 2 (1988): 375–446.
14. For a critical discussion of the distinctive orientation of family medicine, see R. J. Christie and C. B. Hoffmaster, *Ethical Issues in Family Medicine* (New York: Oxford University Press, 1986), 68–84.

Chapter 10

The Patient Self-Determination Act

David B. Clarke

The federal Patient Self-Determination Act (PSDA) became effective on December 1, 1991—more than 15 years after California became the first state to pass its Natural Death Act and more than 22 years after Louis Kutner coined the term "living will" in a law journal proposal.[1] Planning for and implementation of the PSDA began in 1990, shortly after the law was passed as part of the Omnibus Budget Reconciliation Act (OBRA) and continued throughout 1991. By now it is assumed that state agencies and health care providers affected by the legislation will have initiated programs and protocols designed to meet its basic requirements.

It is also presumed that programs initiated to meet PSDA requirements, either by states or institutions, will not be static. The PSDA is a dynamic process, intended to foster communication between health care providers and consumers and between persons and their chosen health care decision-making surrogates. While the core requirements of the PSDA can be implemented at a superficial level, the long-term benefits will only be realized through significant and fundamental changes in institutional policy, public and professional education, and social awareness.

The PSDA requires Medicare and Medicaid institutional providers to

1. provide written information to in-patients upon admission (or upon enrollment or initial entry into service) about:
   a. the person's rights under law to make health care decisions, including the right to accept or refuse treatment and the right to complete state-allowed advance directives, and
   b. the provider's written policies concerning implementation of those rights;
2. document in the person's medical record whether or not the person has completed an advance directive;
3. not discriminate or condition care based on whether or not the person has completed an advance directive;
4. ensure compliance with state laws concerning advance directives;
5. provide education for staff and the community on issues concerning advance directives.

In addition, each state (acting through a state agency, association, or other private nonprofit entity) must develop a written description of the law of the state—whether in statute or case law—concerning advance directives and distribute the document to local health care providers (see 1a above).

The PSDA, then, is a call to states and health care providers to educate professionals and the public about local laws concerning health care decision-making rights and advance directives. As such, it is a federal law necessitating broad agreement among legal and health care professionals on current rights and obligations in the health care arena and massive and persistent education efforts directed variously at medical professionals, administrators, social service providers, and the lay public.

The PSDA is *not* a law providing a universally accepted advance directive, though many would argue that that would certainly facilitate the process of public information and awareness. It is *not* a law to force health care professionals to talk more candidly with patients nor, in itself, to prompt consumers to initiate discussions with their providers. The PSDA will not resolve the issues arising from the provision of care to persons who have neither completed an advance directive nor expressed to others their wishes about treatment preferences or desired quality of life.[2] Nor does the PSDA deal directly with the developing issues of physician-assisted suicide and euthanasia. However, both supporters and critics of the PSDA believe that the new law will raise public awareness of these and related issues as health care decision making generally becomes more focused.

Since the PSDA relies on state law for the content of implementation efforts, the process of satisfying the PSDA will inevitably change in the months and years ahead. Legislation and court decisions at state and national levels will prompt states to revise and redistribute the "statement of state law" on health care decision-making rights and advance directives. As laws and institutional policies change, health care facilities will modify and reprint materials included in preadmission packets and provided to patients on admission. And professionals charged with patient and community education may develop effective teaching skills they never dreamed of using.

This chapter intends to address each of the major sections of the PSDA in light of the comments above. Attention will also be given to issues that have already arisen during this initial implementation period and to problems that are only tangentially related to the PSDA and its implementation.

BACKGROUND

Advance Directives

All states now have at least one kind of advance directive.[3] *Advance directive* is the general term for a variety of documents designed to enable competent adults to make health care decision-making plans in advance of future incapacity, including terminal illness. At present, advance directives are prescribed exclusively by individual state law. There is no federal legislation that allows for a uniform directive to be honored in all states, nor requires states to honor directives signed in other states. Efforts are under way, however, on both fronts.[4]

Advance directives are generally of two types: instructional and proxy. An instructional directive (most often called a living will or terminal care document) allows a competent adult to specify treatment wishes in advance of a terminal illness or condition during which the person is not capable of making sound health care decisions. Most living will laws specify a written form patterned loosely on the original document circulated widely by what is now the New York–based organization Choice in Dying. Whether called a natural death act, a rights of the terminally ill declaration, or a declaration of a desire for a natural death, most instructional directives share common features. They are written statements, to be signed by a competent adult, witnessed and perhaps notarized, that affirm that, in the event of terminal illness, the person wishes to forgo treatments that would serve only to prolong the dying process and would not effect a cure or recovery.

A proxy directive is very different. Patterned after a well-established legal document called a durable power of attorney, a health care proxy (or durable power of attorney for health care) allows a competent adult to choose another person to make health care decisions for him or her, according to his or her wishes, if—at any time and for any reason—the person becomes unable to make his or her own health care decisions. The chosen health care agent (or attorney-in-fact, in the case of a health care power of attorney) can make any health care decision that the person could him- or herself, except where the law or the person sets limits on the agent's authority to make certain kinds of decisions.

Some states have both directives, and in fact both might be needed in certain states to ensure that certain treatments are selected or avoided. No two states have the same laws, and no one form is accepted in each of the 50 states. The PSDA simply requires states and providers to give information about what is legally permitted in that state.

Researchers continue to express concern about the efficacy of advance directives, both instructional and proxy.[5] Typical was a letter to the *New England Journal of Medicine* in December 1991 signed by 16 physicians, nurses, lawyers, and ethicists.[6] The authors listed reservations about both forms of directive, including assertions that patients prefer to avoid discussions of future incapacity and death, patients cannot predict accurately their future preferences, patients may change their minds, an appointed agent might turn out to be a poor choice as a surrogate decision maker, and the documents or agents may specify treatments that the provider has sincere conscientious objections to using.

In many states, implementation of the PSDA has followed close on the heels of new or recently modified advance directive legislation. It is understandable that both providers and consumers will have to "feel their way" for the foreseeable future in assessing the value of both the PSDA and any state-specific advance directive legislation. And perhaps more than in the case of other kinds of legislation, the development of advance directives has been characterized by a high degree of modification and compromise. Concerted efforts of interest groups such as the professional medical community, institutional and agency providers, senior advocates, and religious associations have combined to produce legislation that may be virtually immune from legislative modification, at least in the near term. Those who favor extended trial implementation periods often get their wish, and more. Those who favor legislative "fine-tuning" of the law may have to be unusually patient. Answers to some questions will not come quickly, nor will they come as succinctly as advocates and critics might hope.

Almost everything known about the effect of advance directives—on professional practice, public opinion, patient preferences, courts, and consumer tendencies—is based on studies done *prior* to the PSDA. Advance directives have been in legal use since 1977. However, the PSDA has given the concept a "bump start" by requiring facilities to provide education to staff, patients, and the community. The professional literature has been disappointingly slow to indicate whether research studies were conducted before or after the wave of public and professional education on advance directives and the PSDA during 1991 and early 1992. It was encouraging in early 1993 to see articles emphasizing the need for empirical research in this complex field since passage of the PSDA.[7]

Patient Self-Determination Act

The PSDA was introduced in the United States Senate by John C. Danforth (R-Missouri) and Daniel Patrick Moynihan (D-New York) in October 1989, shortly before the case of Nancy Cruzan was first heard in a Missouri district probate court. Six months later, Representative Sander M. Levin (D-Michigan) sponsored a significantly revised version of the bill in the House. Many of the original provisions proposed by Danforth, Moynihan, and Levin were ultimately deleted from the "ambitious" legislation, including requirements that

- states have advance directive legislation (at the time, six did not)
- agencies "document the treatment wishes of such patient, and periodically review such wishes with the patient"[8]
- agencies "implement an institutional ethics committee which would initiate educational programs for staff, patients, residents and the community on ethical issues in health care, advise on particular cases, and serve as a forum on such issues."[9]

The PSDA was signed by President Bush in December 1990 as part of OBRA and it became effective December 1, 1991. In retrospect, political caution and expediency prevailed, though many of the excised provisions came to pass regardless. Passage of the PSDA itself prompted several states to enact advance directive legislation. Many providers willingly document patients' treatment wishes. And the education component was retained, though not as part of a specific obligation to establish an ethics committee.

As passed, the PSDA required the Secretary of Health and Human Services to "develop and implement a national campaign to inform the public of the option to execute advance directives and of a patient's right to participate and direct health care decisions," develop or approve nationwide informational materials, and assist state agencies to develop state-specific documents. To date, the federal government has provided little help to the states or health care facilities in this regard. There has been no coordinated "national campaign," and the offer of the Health Care Financing Administration (HCFA) to give assistance to states was sent out four months after the 1991 PSDA effective date. HCFA issued final interim regulations regarding the PSDA in early March 1992.[10]

The case of Nancy Cruzan brought national attention to the need for widespread education about the use of advance directives. Nancy Cruzan, a 23-year-old Missouri woman, was left in a persistent vegetative state as a result of a single car accident. After her parents accepted the fact that their daughter would never regain either consciousness or any level of meaningful existence, they petitioned a Missouri court for permission to have her removed from artificial nutrition and hydration. Nancy Cruzan had never completed an advance directive of any kind, had left no written evidence of her treatment preferences in case of future incapacity, nor had she legally appointed a surrogate decision maker for her health care. A local probate judge, accepting oral testimony from her parents and personal friends that Nancy would not have wanted her life to be sustained under such conditions, granted her parents permission to have her removed from life supports. The attorney general of Missouri appealed the matter to the Supreme Court of Missouri, and the case was eventually heard by the U.S. Supreme Court.

The only question put before the U.S. Supreme Court—the first time that court had considered the issue of the "right to die"—was: Can the state of Missouri require "clear and convincing evidence" of Nancy's own wishes in deciding whether to grant permission to Nancy's parents? "Clear and convincing" is one of the highest levels of evidentiary proof required by the law in order to prove as true a statement or event. In a criminal trial, for example, a person can be found guilty only if a judge or jury finds him culpable "beyond a reasonable doubt"—the highest standard required in a court of law. "Clear and convincing," a slightly lower standard, is often taken to mean written evidence, such as could be shown by an advance directive, letter, diary, or other document written by the person him- or herself.[11] The Supreme Court ruled that while such a high level of proof is not required in such cases, states are indeed permitted to set the standard at that level.

The case was returned to the trial court, where additional witnesses testified that Nancy herself had told them that she would not want to live in the condition she now was in. Finding that this new evidence met the clear and convincing standard, the judge ruled in favor of Nancy Cruzan's parents on December 14, 1990. No further appeal was filed. Nancy Cruzan died several days after her health care providers agreed to withdraw artificially supplied food and water.

In an important side note to the Cruzan case, Supreme Court Justice Sandra Day O'Connor wrote in her concurring opinion,

> Few individuals provide explicit oral or written instructions regarding their intent to refuse medical treatment should they become incompetent. States which decline to consider any evidence other than such instructions

> may frequently fail to honor a patient's intent. Such failures might be avoided if the State considered an equally probative source of evidence: the patient's appointment of a proxy to make health care decisions on her behalf. . . . These procedures for surrogate decisionmaking, which appear to be rapidly gaining in acceptance, may be a valuable additional safeguard of the patient's interest in directing his medical care.[12]

STATEMENT OF STATE LAW

The PSDA requires that states develop written statements of local law concerning advance directives that would be distributed by covered providers or organizations to patients, residents, members, or clients. Efforts to meet this requirement have varied considerably. In a recent evaluation of each state's response, researchers sought to identify the process used to comply, the difficulties encountered, and the effects of the PSDA on the effort itself.[13]

Most states read the language of the statute narrowly: The drafting effort was led by a state agency in 33 states and by a hospital or legal association in another 12. Massachusetts Health Decisions, a nonprofit health education and public opinion organization, was the sole consumer group taking a lead role by convening a statewide task force of 16 professional, provider, and education associations and state agencies. Most states worked collaboratively with a variety of concerned groups and organizations. Typical representation came from professional associations (hospital, medicine, nursing, hospice, long-term care, social work, chaplaincy, and law), interested state agencies (health and human services, attorney general, elder affairs), and, to a lesser extent, consumer organizations (illness support, aging, health promotion). It is interesting to note that only 1 state had a minority group involved, though 19 states had plans to translate the state law description.

While the statute requires only a description of advance directive law, most states included related information about informed consent, decision making in the absence of an advance directive, and competency (to complete a directive) and capacity (to make one's own health care decisions). Most also addressed the role of health providers in counseling patients' decisions to forgo or withdraw life-sustaining treatments, and the kind of information generally needed to make health care decisions.

In the survey, 40 states reported problems or concerns with their own state law. These fell into five categories: (1) concerns about living will laws, (2) concerns about durable power of attorney legislation, (3) decision making absent advance directives, (4) nutrition and hydration, and (5) witnessing procedures. Ten states introduced new legislation to remedy the problems or clarify ambiguities. Fifteen simply noted the uncertainty in their public description of the law (e.g., "If you have no family, or if there is disagreement about what treatment you would want, a court *may* be asked to appoint a guardian to make those decisions for you"). Other states did nothing or sought clarification from their attorney general.

Since all states now have a written statement, was the required process a total success? No, but all states will have the opportunity to modify their statement and must inevitably do so as federal and state laws change. For instance, only 10 states included information about updating the directive. Just over half advised discussion with family or friends. Only six described the process for determining incapacity (in order to invoke the advance directive). Less than half addressed the issue of having the directive honored in other states.

From a layperson's point of view, these omissions may be critical. Many, if not most, people will first learn about advance directives on admission, just as envisioned by the PSDA. Easy access and quick comprehensibility may determine whether the concept is worth a second thought—then or at a later time. Since health facilities are not required to distribute advance directives, the statement of state law may be the only introduction to advance directives offered by a facility to new patients. It is important, then, that the document convey not only the letter of the law but its spirit. The intent of the PSDA is to educate and foster communication. If the initial exposure to information does not promote those goals, then subsequent efforts may prove starkly ineffective.

Collaborative efforts to refine and improve the statement of state law may also point out inconsistencies and vague areas in the law. Rose Gasner, former legal director at Choice in Dying, points out that the law regarding treatment refusal has "developed very haphazardly in many states, as the legislatures and the courts have responded to the fast-paced development of the issue. . . . Coalition work can create opportunities for law reform and bring together those interested groups that need to be involved in the political process to ensure passage of amending or substitute legislation."[14]

"ON ADMISSION . . . "

Providers must give inpatients, on admission, written information about their health care decision-making rights, including the right to complete an advance directive. Presumably this statement will be taken verbatim or adapted from the statement of state law, also required by the PSDA and discussed above.

Providers must also give to inpatients, on admission, written information about the provider's policies respecting the implementation of patients' health care decision-making rights. In most cases, this has not required a burst of administrative development by institutions. Facilities have routinely added policies concerning informed consent protocols, advance directives, and decision making in the absence of family or advance planning documents. Where this has not yet been done at all, or has not been modified to reflect current law or practices, many professional associations and private organizations have excellent resources for developing policies.[15]

It is essential that policies reflect both the reality of professional interaction in the facility and the moral philosophy guiding the provision of care (conscientious objection to advance directives is covered in a later section). For example, most proxy laws require a determination of capacity to be made by an attending physician before the patient's named health care agent is legally authorized to act. If frequent or lengthy visits by an attending physician are not the general rule, as is often the case in long-term care facilities and hospice and home care, then policies should clearly indicate how the facility will honor advance directives completed by patients, residents, or clients.

Providers must document in the patient's medical record whether or not the patient has executed an advance directive. For most facilities, this also means filing a copy of the advance directive itself in the patient's medical record, according to state law. The PSDA is silent, as are most state laws, on the extent of the provider's responsibility to secure a copy of the directive once a patient says he or she has completed one. Providers should be encouraged to use reasonable efforts to emphasize the importance of having a copy of the directive in the medical record where the person is or is planning to be a patient or resident. Yet consumers have the final responsibility of making sure that their completed directive is filed and has been discussed with their provider, surrogate, and any other person who may have an interest in their health care.

For supporters and critics alike, the three required items above are the "heart and soul" of the PSDA. Without them, the act is all gums and no teeth. But it has become abundantly clear that providers will comply with the law in a variety of ways, from the marginally legal and painfully superficial to the exemplary. Anecdotal evidence has some providers handing out photocopies of articles about advance directives from the popular press. And that's all. Other providers have given directives and decision-making rights top billing in comprehensive preadmission packets, complete with state law, instructions, and blank forms plus a referral number for more information.

Facility staff should be encouraged to develop presentation skills that both meet the letter of the law and promote the kind of careful consideration needed to make advance directives work as intended. For example, nursing intake personnel at the University of Minnesota Hospital asked patients on admission the following questions:

1. Have you discussed your current medical condition with a family member or close friend?
2. Has a family member or close friend been told what medical treatment you want or do not want if you are unable to speak for yourself?
3. Have you told your doctor what medical treatment you want or do not want?
4. Have you written a living will? If yes, have you discussed it with your doctor?[16]

Who will present the required information is an important concern in many facilities and organizations. Typically, information is included in preadmission packets for people voluntarily admitted into service. This is especially true of health maintenance organizations (HMOs), nursing homes, and hospice and home care agencies. It is important to note that every Medicare and Medicaid provider has the obligation to query patients and provide information, even though many patients will have been exposed to the information from a previous provider.

In large institutions, however, the task has proven more difficult. Admissions clerks are often the first employees to give out information, with information or counseling backup provided variously by social service staff, chaplains, patient care representatives, or nurses. Unless patients are already familiar with the facility and its staff, they may find it very difficult to make the necessary connection between printed information received as a small part of a typical admissions packet and an identified staff resource. Both printed information and initial information providers should point to further sources of information and conversation.

Whoever provides required information and asks patients if they have completed an advance directive should stress that completing an advance directive is a voluntary act by patients. It is too easy for advance directives to be included in a stack of forms to sign, and most experts agree that admission is an inappropriate place to complete advance directives. Admission personnel must also be familiar with

- the process for completing advance directives under state law
- institutional policy on having employees witness advance directives as well as other legal documents
- the general elements of a valid advance directive under state law
- institutional policy on honoring or dishonoring advance directives
- the answers to the most commonly asked questions or the name and phone number of the person identified as a primary resource on advance directives (see also "Staff Education" below)

ENSURING COMPLIANCE

The PSDA requires that covered providers will ensure compliance with state laws on advance directives. Compliance will be a logical extension of efforts to educate thoroughly the medical and professional staff involved with implementing advance directives in any facility. Rose Gasner believes that "this section of the PSDA may serve as a basis for a new federal legal argument placing responsibility on the facility for knowledge of the law, as well as holding facilities responsible for the actions of staff."[17] She cites the example of a physician who refuses to comply with the decision of an authorized agent. In this case, many state statutes require the physician to transfer the patient to another physician who *is* willing to honor the request. Gasner argues that the PSDA compliance section may put the burden on the facility as well as the physician to ensure the prompt transfer of the patient.

OBJECTION ON THE BASIS OF CONSCIENCE

The PSDA, as it was passed as part of OBRA 1990, does not "prohibit the application of a State law which allows for an objection on the basis of conscience for any health care provider . . . which, as a matter of conscience, cannot implement an advance directive." Most state directives do, in fact, include provisions for conscientious objection on religious, moral, or professional ethical grounds.

The interim final regulation issued by HCFA in March 1992 tries to clarify the provider's obligation to alert patients on admission of any conscientious objection—as a matter of written policy—by the facility. It states that the provider must inform the person in writing of state laws regarding advance directives and of the policies of the provider regarding the implementation of advance directives, including a *clear and precise* explanation of the provider's conscientious objection to implementing an advance directive.

Charles Sabatino, assistant director of the American Bar Association's Commission on Legal Problems of the Elderly, points out that providers and consumer advocates have very different views of the "clear and precise" requirement. Providers contend that it is better to adopt general, flexible policies so that objections can be handled on a case-by-case basis and that the standard itself is unrealistic. A facility's policies rarely take into account the personal values of each member of the professional staff. Consumers, on the other hand, feel that the requirement doesn't go far enough: The too-general language can be used to thwart any treatment option raised by a patient or agent that the facility objects to—whether or not as a matter of conscience.

The Commission suggests that provider policies

1. clarify any differences between institution-wide conscience objections and those that may be raised by individual physicians
2. explain the basis for any facility objection (e.g., religious, moral, professional)
3. identify the state legal authority permitting the objection
4. describe the range of medical conditions or procedures affected by conscience objections
5. describe what steps will be taken to transfer or otherwise accommodate people whose wishes are impeded by the institution's policy[18]

NONDISCRIMINATION

Under the PSDA, providers may not condition care or otherwise discriminate against a person based on whether or not he has completed an advance directive. Indeed, many state statutes and statements of state law have already made note of this requirement. The Massachusetts statement, for example, reads, "You are not required to complete a Health Care Proxy on admission or at any other time in order to receive medical care from any health care providers. You have the right to receive the same type and quality of health care whether or not you complete a Health Care Proxy."[19]

Providers are cautioned that this provision may inadvertently be violated if admissions staff give the impression that an advance directive, included as just one of a number of required forms to be completed at or before admission, is part of the regular admissions routine. Staff must alert patients that advance directives are voluntary documents that require significant prior thought and conversation to be truly effective.

Some providers have the mistaken impression that the requirements of the PSDA apply only to Medicare or Medicaid patients rather than to all admitted inpatients in facilities that accept Medicare or Medicaid payments.

Some people will never sign an advance directive, and that right must be respected. Patients may have family constellations upon whom they depend utterly and may have confidence in the family's efforts to make appropriate decisions. Some may come from cultures where naming as an agent someone other than a family leader would be an unforgivable affront. And still others may be resigned to live and die fatalistically, either unwilling or unable to choose a surrogate. These are strictly personal choices for the patient, however frustrating or burdensome they may be for ultimate decision makers.

It is altogether appropriate, however, to let patients know that if they don't make choices about their future health care and health care decision makers, the choices may still have to be made. But they may be made by total strangers.

EMERGENCY ADMISSIONS

Nonvoluntary admissions may require special consideration in the development of facility policy, professional practice, staff education, and statewide protocols. Emergency admissions are addressed in the HCFA final regulations, but only with regard to the timing of informing patients of decision-making rights:

> If a patient is incapacitated at the time of admission . . . , then the facility should give advance directive information to the patient's family or surrogate to the extent that it issues other materials about policies and procedures. . . . This does not, however, relieve the facility of its obligation to provide this information to the patient once he or she is no longer incapacitated or unable to receive such information.[20]

Anecdotal evidence indicates that institutional emergency departments will not honor an advance directive unless it is absolutely clear that the incapacitated patient's preference would have been to refuse emergency care. Some emergency departments have begun keeping card files or other records of advance directives, though this is practical only in smaller facilities. Most difficult are emergency admissions where an appointed health care agent has accompanied the now-incapacitated patient to the facility and demands that his authority be honored in directing treatment on behalf of the patient. Many emergency medical staff believe that the emergency room is not the time or place to make a critical judgment call: Either spend time making a written determination of patient incapacity, validate the integrity of the written advance directive, verify the identity of the authorized agent, and engage in the required informed consent procedures with the agent *or* treat the patient. Supporters of this view argue that they would opt to treat the patient under typical implied consent protocols, at least to the point of stabilization, and then follow advance directive procedures—even if that meant withdrawing life-sustaining treatment.

Some consumer groups, as well as providers, have already begun efforts to educate consumers about the appropriate use of emergency services. Most laypersons are unaware of the legal requirements to "activate" a health care agent's decision-making authority, assuming that simply being a holder of a validly signed document is sufficient to direct treatment decisions. In addition, most laypersons are unaware of state laws that require emergency medical service staff to provide life support at the scene. Hospice home care presents a typical situation. A person cares for a dying spouse at home, supported by hospice services. Though counseled about the actual events of dying and death, the caregiver and appointed health care agent (who is, however, not yet authorized by a physician's determination of incapacity) panics at the onset of a terminal seizure and calls emergency services. Emergency personnel arrive and begin treatment despite the caregiver's protests that the dying patient wanted no heroic measures.

In response to frequent episodes like the one above, several states have taken the lead in establishing preadmission "do not resuscitate" (DNR) procedures, either through legislation, regulation, or statewide adoption of protocols.[21] While the situations covered by DNR orders are far fewer than usually addressed in advance directives, emergency service personnel nevertheless believe the new guidelines help to recognize patient autonomy in treatment preferences. Several states now employ a dated DNR bracelet as a way of notifying emergency service staff. It is hoped that these tentative steps will encourage wider observance of more comprehensive advance directives among emergency services and institutional emergency departments.

PSYCHIATRIC ADMISSIONS

At admission, some patients are not capable of receiving or comprehending information, nor of completing advance directives. Many, as described above, are emergency admissions and can receive the required information at a later time. Other people, however, are neither emergency admissions nor adjudicated legally incompetent. Such cases are common in long-term care facilities, where up to one-half of all admissions may be persons who are mentally and functionally incompetent but who have not been declared so by a court and do not have a legal guardian. Since the law assumes that all persons are competent to conduct their own affairs until a court determines otherwise, and since many advance directive laws presume the validity of signed directives, facilities with significant admissions of "questionably competent" persons will need to get good counsel in developing effective but legally sound policies.

It is useful to remember that, as a general rule, competency is something determined by a judge in an impartial court hearing. The law presumes competence until proven otherwise. Capacity to make health care decisions is frequently determined (as allowed and required by law) by an attending physician in following an advance directive state statute. Indeed, the two concepts may be quite separate and distinct: A person involuntarily committed to a psychiatric facility may still be legally capable of making his or her own health care decisions—so long as he or she can participate meaningfully in the traditional informed consent or refusal process.[22] To the extent that any person can engage in significant discussion about his or her own health care, treatment preferences, quality of life, or personal values, he or she can not only help shape future options but also help providers become aware of his or her wishes.

Most proxy and durable power of attorney statutes do not specify a time period during which an attending physician must determine that a person has either lost or regained decision-making capacity. The danger exists that the act of determining capacity can be misused as a management tool. For example, if a physician is uncomfortable with treatment preferences being expressed by a still competent patient, or if dealing with the designated agent seems to be easier or more consistent with his or her own values, then the physician has the option—albeit unprofessional, illegal, and unethical—to determine the patient incapacitated for the purpose of seeking consents or refusals from the agent. Conversely, if the physician believes that the designated agent will make treatment choices inconsistent either with his or her professional values or the known wishes of the patient, already incapacitated, the physician may postpone making a determination of incapacity and rely temporarily on other vehicles for securing treatment consents or refusals.

To be sure, these are gross abuses of professional authority and would open the physician to substantial liability. Yet in the often hazy area of capacity determination, where hesitation, caution, and prudence are more the rule than the exception, the law provides little direction for physicians, who may be guided at a practical level by their good professional instincts and their desire to take "the long view." In becoming familiar with advance directives, many physicians are still uncomfortable dealing with designated agents, who are often strangers to them but who hold the authority of consent and refusal no less certainly than their competent patients. The obligation of a physician to get to know an agent should be shared by both the physician and the patient. The agent deserves to be brought into conversations between doctor and patient well before the agent may be required to consult with the doctor in making choices on behalf of the patient. Should misuses of capacity determination as a management tool become anything more than isolated incidents, legislatures might consider modifying statutes to require that patient assessments and reassessments be made within specified time periods.

STAFF EDUCATION

Throughout 1991 and early 1992, health care facilities, education and training organizations, lawyers, bioethicists, and others held thousands of seminars, conferences, video-linked teleconferences, and in-service sessions concentrated on advance directives and the PSDA. By late 1992, however, the bloom was clearly off the rose. Staff development personnel typically reported, "We did that last year. All our staff know about the living will; we had an in-service and put a sample will in everyone's mailbox."

Regular and periodic education should be provided to all health care staff with direct patient contact, including physicians, nurses, social service professionals, patient care representatives, chaplains, admissions clerks, and others who may be in a position to talk with inpatients about directives. Even if their obligation is only to refer the patient to a more knowledgeable resource, staff should be aware of the basics. Because of staff turnover, especially among physicians, nurses, and nursing aides, facilities should include information on advance directives and policy in the basic orientation process.

Passage of the PSDA has prompted a deluge of clinical articles and educational information on advance directives as well as on the law itself. Much of this material is generic and not specific to any one state's law. Health care professionals are obliged to have not just a general knowledge of advance directives but a solid understanding of their own state's law and their facility's policies to implement it. Educational materials for staff and the public should contain information specific to the state and facility.

Many physicians have been reluctant to honor advance directives for fear of liability. Some simply ignore directives entirely.[23] Even the advantage of having an identified decision maker was not enough to persuade them to accept a surrogate, legally appointed or not. Because most education efforts have been aimed at consumers, not providers, some physicians are still unaware that state statutes offer full immunity from criminal or civil prosecution if the physician follows the wishes of a validly appointed health care agent in good faith. While this does not totally insulate providers, it does give some assurance that a physician's reasonable efforts to secure informed consent through conversations with an agent will not lead to the devastating consequences of a successful suit for malpractice or, worse, wrongful death.

Admissions and records staff should be aware of basic form requirements as specified or allowed by state law. Many providers believe that the only advance directives submitted to them will be the ones they themselves distribute to patients and the public. This certainly is not so and will become less true as time passes. People will be introduced to directives from a variety of sources: lawyers, doctors, financial planners, insurance agents, senior organizations, illness support groups, religious organizations, and libraries, to name a few. In states with a prescribed form, nonconforming documents may be less of a problem than in states with either no form or only suggested language. Gatekeepers of the medical record ought to be able to spot a faulty document before it is filed and flag it without referring the document to the legal department or administration.

Patients will naturally assume that if they complete a document in good faith and submit it to the facility for filing, they can depend on the terms of the document being honored. While the PSDA does not address the issue of filing the form itself, many state statutes do. I believe that facilities that do not object to honoring advance directives (by conscience and as an explicitly stated policy) have a moral obligation to tell patients whether the form submitted will be honored in the event of future incapacity. There can be no guarantees, understandably. But of what use to a patient is a directive dismissed as nonconforming or defective when pulled from a medical record just at the time it might be of use—that is, after the patient has become incapacitated and is unable to redo the directive?

Should facility staff help patients complete advance directives? This may depend, in part, on whether the facility has formal policies that support conscientious objection to advance directives. In general, however, facilities should be encouraged to provide the means for a patient to complete an advance directive while in the facility. The facility should have an adequate supply not only of the required materials to provide at admission but additional information to be considered at a later time, appropriate and state-specific forms, a personal resource person, and at least several people who can serve as witnesses to signing (if allowed by local law).

PUBLIC EDUCATION

Long-term health education campaigns, like those on smoking cessation, substance abuse, human immunodeficiency virus (HIV) prevention, nutrition, and women's health, have taught us a valuable lesson. We know that education works . . . but it takes a long time. The legal requirements of the PSDA will certainly result in many people being given information on their rights to accept or refuse recommended treatment and on advance directives. But the real change occurs when completing a living will or health care proxy comes to be perceived, quite simply, as the right thing to do, like giving up smoking or cutting back on prime rib and pizza in favor of grilled chicken and pasta salad. Systemic changes cannot be forced. They can be facilitated by persuasion, perhaps eased by suggestion. But transformations happen when all participants in the system begin to operate as if the change had already taken place. In the case of PSDA, the 15–20 percent advance directive completion rate will jump to 50–60 percent when both providers and consumers of health care agree that having a directive makes life easier and more certain for everyone.

The PSDA requires health care facilities to provide information to patients, residents, clients, or members on admission. Real change will occur when physicians in private practice routinely ask their 18-year-old patients, "Say, now that you can vote and you have your own place, did you ever give any thought about who would make health care decisions for you if you got in a skiing accident and were unconscious for a few weeks?" Real change will occur when lawyers give out free copies of advance directives to clients, perhaps as part of an overall estate planning discussion. Real change will occur when colleges and universities include advance directives in admission packets sent to incoming frosh. "Dear Frosh Parent: We look forward to welcoming Carmen to our beautiful campus in early Fall. During these summer months, we hope you and your daughter will give some thought to what it means for a young person to make the transition into adulthood. Moving away from home into a new environment is certainly part of that change. But making one's own choices, especially about matters as personal as health care, is also a matter for adults. We have enclosed a pamphlet on the Massachusetts Health Care Proxy . . . "

Physicians can be the best primary source of information. Written materials for the professional office are now available in every state from a variety of sources. Virtually every professional health care association in the country has some kind of PSDA or advance directive publication for general use. There are videos on advance directives, health care power of attorney forms available in Braille, large type, and dozens of non-English languages, and books sold in shopping mall bookstores on all facets of health care decision making for the lay as well as professional reader.[24] Trained medical office staff can be good sources of information and responsive to patient questions. But nothing will substitute for the sincere suggestion from a trusted doctor to consider the issue. Physicians must reclaim their roles as teacher and counselor in this regard.

Any public education program must emphasize the importance of talking with one's chosen health care agent and family members. Most advance directive forms are easy to complete and take little time. The discussions needed to give substance to those forms are not. But there are good resources here as well. The values history—an in-depth assessment of personal values, activities, goals, and preferences—has become a useful teaching tool as well as personal supplement to any kind of advance directive.[25] Initiating a discussion with family members is perfect for role play exercises, and especially useful in settings where family members are actually present. The American Hospital Association, American Medical Association, American Association of Retired Persons, and most of the community Health Decisions programs have suggested guidelines for holding conversations with one's family, chosen agent, or physician.[26]

Any print materials distributed by your facility should be in a language, format, and style appropriate to your community.[27] If you have the chance to develop your own materials, make sure the drafting committee represents a cross section of interested people. Members might include a physician, a nurse, a lawyer, an ethicist, a clergyperson, a records administrator, the lay community, and maybe even a visiting English or humanities professor. Before you go to press, test a draft with your own staff, patients, and community members.

In the past two years, many providers have discovered that inviting the public into a health care facility to hear a talk about advance directives rarely attracts an overflow crowd. Following are suggestions for fulfilling the PSDA community education requirement.

1. If you invite the public, do whatever you need to ensure your facility is known to be the sponsor—but unless you have a well-established reputation for holding lively, community-based meetings and events at your facility, hold the event somewhere else.
2. Work with other health care or social service providers in your area to present programs. If you work for a long-term care facility, join with staff from other nursing homes, a local hospital and hospice, or the local town nurse. A shared program will attract more people, reduce the staff burden on each facility, and provide economies of scale for print materials. It also reassures laypeople that this is not a competition for new clients: If several institutions and agencies are working together, with common materials, it *must* be okay.
3. Develop a linguistic or cultural minority outreach program in collaboration with other neighborhood organizations.
4. Work with local secondary schools, junior and community colleges, and universities to present programs to the 18- to 24-year-old crowd. Remember, many of the major cases of health care decision making and incapacity involved young people, not elders (Karen Ann Quinlan, Nancy Cruzan, Paul Brophy, and Elizabeth Bouvia). Teachers in civics, health, health care administration, social work, and even government would appreciate your willingness to help with an occasional class.
5. Offer your help to classes of entering students in local medical schools, nursing schools, and schools of the allied health professions.
6. Adopt the "train the trainers" model of education. Develop a program to train office staff of physicians in your area. And make sure the physicians are invited too.
7. Develop a program to train local parish clergy on the use of advance directives.
8. Develop a program to train a group of your best facility volunteers—the people who make you feel guilty because you never seem to have enough challenging tasks for them. Many facilities are using their volunteers rather than paid staff to provide community education.
9. Offer an intergenerational program, or one for your patients and their families, or for family members only. Offer a program for patients and their chosen agents.
10. Offer a program for employee assistance professionals in your area. How about benefits managers or staff in human resources?
11. Develop a program that provides "brown bag" seminars for employees in local corporations. (California and Massachusetts Health Decisions both have active programs for corporate employees. Almost

without exception, employees are grateful to have the opportunity to consider the topic when they are healthy and making other kinds of future plans.)

12. If your facility does not have its own video production studio, do a program for your local community access cable station. Six months later, you can sponsor a repeat showing.
13. Invite your board president, mayor, governor, or one of your legislators to sign an advance directive at a public event.
14. At every public event, make sure two items are given out without fail: free copies of an advance directive and a simple three- or four-question evaluation to be returned anonymously. If you do not know what went wrong, you will never get it just right.

The Patient Self-Determination Act is one of those rare pieces of legislation that gives us a good sense of things as we know they ought to be in the best of all worlds but few specifics on how to construct that world. No health care facility runs quite like another, and no two health care professionals share identical values. In a health care system strained by legislation and public opinion from all sides, the requirements of the PSDA remind us that the enduring value of good health care comes not from legislated procedures but from the quality of human relationships born and nurtured in the system. The PSDA encourages health care providers and consumers to talk candidly with each other about matters of consequence: Will I get well? How will you treat me? What do you do here? Who will speak for me? Can I trust you? In a perfect world, all such questions merit straight and honest answers. Let us hope that the PSDA succeeds in encouraging both providers and consumers to ask the right questions and answer honestly.

FIVE-YEAR IMPLEMENTATION UPDATE

Five years have passed since the PSDA became effective in December 1991, a half decade during which the health care industry has undergone extraordinary change. During this period, there has been an unprecedented and largely unsuccessful effort to reform the very nature of the delivery system, a refocusing of attention on the issue of physician-assisted suicide and euthanasia at state and national levels, and a massive shift toward managed care in both the private and public sector. Many smaller community hospitals have had to close their doors, unable or unwilling to form alliances with other organizations. Extended care facilities have been assimilated by large national chains. Home care agencies have merged, and merged again, often as part of multisetting provider networks. And health care professionals—once among the most independent of workers—have either had their jobs "re-engineered" into extinction, or become employees of newly formed corporations. In short, the PSDA quickly became overshadowed by apparently more pressing issues.

Has the PSDA fulfilled its promise? Is it working? It depends where you look and whom you ask. It is important, however, to ask even more basic questions, some generated by the federal law itself, others stemming from the administrative changes required by the regulation (and by associated state laws), and still others emerging from case law and health professional practice. Certainly not all of these will be dealt with in this update, but the following questions warrant significant empirical research in their own right:

- How effective were state agencies in circulating the statement of state law required by the PSDA? Did every facility receive a copy, along with information about its use? If there have been subsequent changes in the statutory or case law, have state agencies been successful in notifying all covered organizations of the change(s)?
- What percentage of organizations covered by the PSDA have fully institutionalized the requirements of the PSDA? That is, are facilities giving patients, residents, and clients copies of their health care decision-making rights, including the right to complete an advance directive? Have all

facilities developed written policies? Are facilities training *all* staff with relevant patient contact, including physicians? Are facilities providing education to the wider community-at-large?
- Are advance directives being recognized and honored?
- Is there an effective evaluation program in place? If there are flaws in the advance directive administrative system, who would know? How effective is the ongoing process of remediation? How are organizational policies being enforced, and by whom?

In the absence of any large-scale studies, some assessment must be limited to anecdotal evidence, though that itself is considerable. In general, the basic legal mandates of the PSDA have become institutionalized in health care agencies and institutions nationwide. To a greater or lesser degree, people admitted to facilities are asked, "Do you have an advance directive?" And there is some effort to provide information about health care decision making to admitted patients, residents, clients, and members.

It is far less certain, however, that the other PSDA requirements are being satisfied by organizations in any care setting. In my experience, few facilities have developed protocols for patient education beyond handing out a sheet of state law decision-making rights, though systematic follow-up has become a requirement of the Joint Commission on Accreditation of Healthcare Organizations (Joint Commission). This will be discussed later in the update. Given the large rate of staff turnover in health care generally, it has been surprising that staff education—at least among patient care representatives, nurses, social workers, and clergy—appears to have been consistent. Among professionals, physicians, however, seem to be the least knowledgeable about advance directives. This may be due to the "point of contact" established by the PSDA itself. According to the regulation, persons are to be informed and queried on admission, which most often puts the responsibility for program administration on admissions clerks or social workers. Unless a person becomes terminally ill or incapacitated, it is highly likely that a physician would not even be alerted to the existence of an advance directive, much less its instructions or appointed agent. One of the lessons of the SUPPORT project is that communication between physicians and other professional care providers, especially with regard to prognostic information and family interaction, needs substantial improvement.[28]

Other than anecdotes and observations, what has happened to the PSDA in the past five years? This update will focus on three areas of movement: (1) the Interim Final Rule (1992) and the Final Rule (1995) of the PSDA itself as published by HCFA, (2) new standards regarding advance directives established by the Joint Commission for all care settings, and (3) known case law challenges involving advance directives.

PSDA Interim Final Rule (Effective April 1992)

In March 1992, HCFA issued the Interim Final Rule of the PSDA. It officially implemented sections 4206 and 4751 of OBRA '90, also known as Public Law 101–508. It described in general terms the provisions of the PSDA that had already become effective on December 1, 1991—several months previously. It also announced a 60-day public comment period, the results of which formed the basis for the Final Rule issued in 1995. And finally, the Interim Final Rule gave brief suggestions on how providers might meet the requirements of the PSDA, offered sample text for a public information document on advance directives, listed print and video resources, and assured providers that HCFA would provide technical assistance for providers in the PSDA implementation process.

PSDA Final Rule (Effective July 1995)

The Final Rule restates the original OBRA regulation with several minor changes based on HCFA's review and consideration of 85 comments submitted during the 60-day public comment period. The Rule reports on a public-education campaign conducted by HCFA in 1992, primarily by means of print materials, public-service announcements on television and radio, and a toll-free Medicare hotline. The Rule specifically notes that

> the Office of the Inspector General (OIG) conducted an early implementation study in December, 1992, to determine compliance with the advance directive provision and facility and patient responses (OEI-06-91-01130 and OEI-06-91-01131). This study found that at that time two-thirds of the patients in the facilities studied had some understanding of advance directives. We believe that this finding indicates that HCFA, in concert with other members of the health care industry, has made significant strides towards educating the public on advance directives.

The large majority of the Final Rule, however, consists of the comments submitted by citizens and HCFA's responses. While these are too numerous and lengthy to summarize, it is instructive to read the document if only to appreciate the caution and concern clearly shown by all parties to the document. Issues range from conscientious objection to patient or agent treatment requests, facility exemption from PSDA requirements, public-education definitions, and costs of program administration. In general, HCFA tactfully disagrees with most commenters—many of whom wrote to seek exemption, modification, or simplification of the general rule. To critics of the regulation, the PSDA was yet another administrative requirement loaded onto an overburdened and overregulated industry. To supporters, it was reassuring to see the government say, as it does in several places: "While we recognize that preparing this material may be a challenge, the law requires that it be done. . . ."

Following are synopses of key issues discussed in the Final Rule, often at length. Where the Final Rule either affirms or modifies the regulation as it was first circulated in 1991, I note it at the end of each synopsis.

Information To Be Provided Patients

The PSDA requires providers to give each adult individual admitted information concerning his or her rights under state law to make decisions concerning medical care, including the right to accept or refuse medical or surgical treatment and the right to formulate, at the individual's option, advance directives.[29] By December 1991, the effective date of the PSDA, almost all states had developed and circulated to providers statewide the required "statement of state law" regarding health care decision-making rights. In most cases, this statement is a brief summary of statutory and case law *specific to that state* describing the elements of informed consent, advance directives, and perhaps involuntary treatment, emergency care, and protective services. Many facilities, however, seem to have neglected this statement and, instead, opted to inform patients that they have a simple but unexplained right to accept or refuse treatment and complete an advance directive. This is insufficient to meet the requirements of the PSDA, and providers should secure copies of the statement of state law for their state to incorporate or modify as appropriate.

In addition, many providers, especially those serving large populations of elders, seem to have confused the PSDA-required statement of state law with the statement of patient's rights required separately under Medicare provisions. The two are not the same, and both are required. (Affirm)

Informing on Admission

Each organization or facility bears responsibility for informing patients of their health care decision-making rights, including the right to complete an advance directive. If a patient is being transferred from one care setting to another, it is suggested that the transferring facility include copies of completed directives in order to ensure a smooth coordination of care. The receiving facility, however, still has the responsibility of informing the newly admitted patient or resident and asking whether a directive has been completed.[30] (Affirm)

In the case of hospitals, information must be given to patients on admission, unless they are incapacitated. Information is not required for patients in an outpatient setting, except for home health, hospice, and personal care services.[31] (Affirm) For these providers, it is permitted to give information at the time of the first home visit so long as the information is given before actual care is provided.[32] (Affirm)

Incapacitated Admissions

If a patient or resident is incapacitated at the time of admission, the facility should give information to the family or surrogate. However, the facility is still obliged to inform the patient once he or she regains capacity.[33] (Modify) Providers will need to develop appropriate follow-up procedures (see also Joint Commission update, below). There is no "good faith" exception for persons involuntarily admitted for psychiatric treatment. Such a determination must always be made on a case-by-case basis.[34] (Affirm)

Community Education

Providers must now be able to document their community-education efforts. This could be done by maintaining copies of any materials used as part of its community-education programs.[35] (Modify)

Educational materials used to inform the community about advance directives must be written and must include a description of a person's rights under state law to make health care decisions, including the rights to accept or refuse treatment and to complete an advance directive. The materials must also include the provider's or organization's implementation policies concerning an individual's advance directive.[36] (Affirm)

Providing written materials to individuals who come to a facility to investigate admission or to visit family members is *not* sufficient to meet the community-education requirement.[37] (Affirm)

In response to one commenter who asserted that enforcement of the community-education requirements would violate a provider's First Amendment rights to freedom of religion, and hence would warrant an exemption from the requirement, HCFA responded:

> We believe it would be appropriate for a provider to register that objection as it conducts its community education requirement. That is, the provider must meet its obligation to conduct community education on advance directives, but may inform the community that the State law offers a choice that, because of a conscientious objection, it would not honor. We believe that this information is valuable for community members to have since it may affect their choice of a provider.[38]

Facility or organization public-relations offices may be used to inform the community about advance directives, and the associated costs generally would be related to patient care rather than to advertising to the general public. As such the costs of advance directives activities could be considered an allowable cost related to patient care under existing Medicare policy. And to the extent that states make additional payments to providers for their costs of advance directives, federal financial participation is available at the federal Medicaid Assistance Percentage.[39] (Affirm)

What is "the community"? It relates to the catchment area of the individual providers, which means that an HMO and a hospital, for example, would likely have community areas very different in scope. For managed care plans, community is defined as the organization's service area.[40] (Affirm) For all other organizations—hospitals, home care agencies, extended care facilities, and personal service organizations—the definition of community is left to the discretion of the organization but is generally meant to be the catchment area and community-at-large. (Affirm)

Providers should distribute materials that are clear and understandable to each patient. If the patient's knowledge of English or the common language of the facility is inadequate for clear understanding, then a means to communicate the information concerning patient rights and providers' responsibility and practices *must* be available and implemented. For foreign languages commonly encountered, the provider should have written translations of its description of state law and its statement of protocols, and should, when necessary, make the services of an interpreter available.[41] (Affirm)

In the same vein, providers should be sensitive to cultural differences that may make a discussion of even the remote possibility of death awkward or difficult. The law does *not* make any exception, however, for these cases: patients must still be offered information about their rights to enhance control over medical treatment decisions. (Affirm)

Conscientious Objection

Where a provider, as a matter of conscience, cannot implement an advance directive, the provider must now provide in its written policies (and, hence, to patients) a "clear and precise statement of limitation." Regardless of any religious affiliation, that statement should (1) clarify any differences between institutionwide conscience objections and those that may be raised by individual physicians, (2) identify the state's legal authority permitting such objection, and (3) describe the range of medical conditions or procedures affected by the conscience objection.[42] (Modify)

It is important to note that many states adopted language found in the first statutory advance directive, the California Natural Death Act of 1976, which said that if providers could not, as a matter of conscience, honor an advance directive, the physician bore responsibility for facilitating the patient's transfer—not just to another health care provider, but to one who *would honor* the request. Providers are encouraged to check state law before assuming either that the patient's desire for transfer is the patient's sole responsibility, or that it is sufficient for the physician or facility to arrange transfer to any other willing provider.

Enforcement Procedures

Providers must now inform individuals that complaints concerning noncompliance with the advance directives requirements may be filed with the state survey and certification agency. To comply, providers could post a notice of an individual's rights and the name, address, and telephone number of the appropriate state survey and certification agency. This information must also be included in the written description of a resident's rights. The Medicare Hotline (1-800-638-6833) and the home health hotline may also be used to lodge complaints.[43] (Modify)

Joint Commission Standards

Effective June 10, 1996, the Joint Commission clarified the Advance Directive standard RI.1.2.4. Previous Joint Commission standards on advance directives—based on the PSDA and most state statutes—required facilities and agencies only to ask patients on admission or enrollment into service whether they had completed an advance directive. If so, and if presented, the facility was required to place a copy in the patient's medical record. The new standard applies when a patient reports *not* having an advance directive. The Joint Commission now gives facilities three options:

1. the facility may make arrangements to immediately obtain a copy of the existing—but not currently present or available—advance directive; or
2. the facility may offer assistance to complete a new written advance directive; or
3. a facility/agency designee may inform the patient that she or he may verbally specify treatment preferences, explaining the substance of any original advance directive, including preferred surrogate decision maker and specific wishes. If the patient

chooses this option and verbalizes the information, the conversation must be documented in the patient's record, and the physician must be informed.

Facilities are strongly cautioned about the third option since most state advance directive statutes require written documents with formal witnessing and possible notarization for either living will or proxy-type directives. But certainly the facility ought to be as proactive as possible in either seeking out an existing directive or offering to help complete (but not requiring) a new directive.

It is also clear that Joint Commission inspectors have been unusually forthright about encouraging facilities to develop follow-up strategies. Reasonable policies might describe ways to remind or encourage patients to bring copies of directives for scheduled inpatient stays, number and timing of follow-up phone calls to family members, and clear protocols for facilitating on-site completion including providing persons who can serve as witnesses and, if required, a notary public. Many facilities, especially in extended care, have policies prohibiting any employee from serving as a witness to a resident's will or other legal matter. Advance directives ought to be given special consideration. It is to mutual benefit that a facility can provide the conditions under which a person can thoughtfully and calmly complete an advance directive.

Case Law Challenges to Advance Directives

In the more than 20 years since California enacted the first statutory advance directive, there have been very few cases involving advance directives in the courts. And if they made it to court at all, the matter may have been resolved through mediation or settlement before proceeding to trial. Trial court cases are rarely published except as reported in the popular press because they do not set precedent: Cases that do not go on to appeal or to the state's highest court do not make law. Nor is it easy to go back and review the case.

Disputes frequently occur around a very narrow range of issues:

- Is the document valid and binding? Was the person who signed it mentally competent at the time of signing to do so? Was the signing forced in some way? Has the document been revoked, either through an automatic statutory revocation such as divorce or by some statement or action of the person?
- What does the document say? What is the appointed agent authorized to do, either by law or by the terms of the document? What treatment choices has the person made, as spelled out in the document or as told to the named surrogate?
- If legal and valid, is the document being honored? Has a facility or agency produced the document entrusted to it in the medical record? Is a health care provider abiding by the terms of the document or following the directions of the named agent? Is there a valid conscientious objection by a provider to follow the directions of the patient or surrogate? Is there any other reason for a provider to ignore the directions of the patient or surrogate?

Generally speaking, most of the questions above are resolved in discussions between the patient and provider, or between surrogate and provider. An administrator or risk manager may become involved, perhaps even a lawyer for the agency or family. But cases specifically involving advance directives that proceed to open court usually follow one of very few courses:

1. the patient's request for treatment has been ignored or overridden, and as a result of a failure to treat, the patient is now dead; or
2. the patient's request to forgo treatment has been ignored or overridden, and despite having requested to die, the patient is still alive and charged for treatment given over his or her objection; or
3. the patient's request to forgo treatment has been ignored or overridden, and as a result

of unwanted treatment, the patient is still alive, but is either in a worse condition or simply doesn't want to be alive.

The first case, exemplified by *Gilgunn v. Massachusetts General Hospital,* indicates that medical professionals may refuse to provide requested care when that care is clearly not medically appropriate or is actually harmful to the patient.[44] Persons do not have a right to demand what a provider honestly believes will not be a benefit. But providers must be open and proactive in developing so-called futility policies so that honest respect for the limits of the medical profession is not construed as a shield of professional arrogance or economic advantage. In developing such policies, it may prove very useful to involve other organizational providers and residents of the community, as has been done in several metropolitan areas nationwide.[45] Among the three examples, this appears to be most easily resolved through traditional actions for professional malpractice, or through more recent discussions of "medically inappropriate care."

The second and third examples are more difficult, primarily because courts have traditionally ruled that being alive is always better than being dead, no matter how burdensome or unwanted the living. The trend may be changing, however.

In *Elbaum v. Grace Plaza of Great Neck, Inc.*, the second example, a nursing home resident sued when the home billed the family for care provided after the patient specifically refused that treatment.[46] An early decision favoring the family was later reversed on appeal.

The third example is taken from a distressing Michigan case reported on the front page of the *New York Times* in 1996.[47] In that case, a young woman developed a seizure syndrome. Advised by her physician that the condition would only become progressively worse, she named her mother as her health care surrogate in a valid Michigan Health Care Proxy. When she later became fully incapacitated from an unusually strong seizure, the mother instructed the attending physician and hospital to do what her daughter wished: forgo the extraordinary treatment, the ventilator, and allow her to die. The directive and mother were allegedly ignored, and the daughter remains profoundly disabled following a two-month coma during which time she was tube fed and on a ventilator. In a suit against the hospital and physician on behalf of the young woman, a jury awarded her $16.5 million.

A recent Ohio case, however, indicates that the consequences of failing to honor valid advance directives are far from settled and certainly not uniform across the country. In 1988, an 82-year-old man entered a hospital for treatment of a coronary problem. Despite a valid DNR order, the man was resuscitated when tachycardia caused him to stop breathing. He later suffered a stroke that left him partially paralyzed and in a nursing home. He sued for damages for his pain, suffering, emotional distress, and medical and other expenses of his "wrongful life." He died two years after entering the hospital.

The trial court initially held for the defendant hospital, stating that Ohio did not recognize a cause of action for wrongful life. After several appeals, the case was heard by the Ohio Supreme Court, which finally dismissed the action. It ruled that even though the hospital might be accused of committing a battery (legally defined as any unconsented touching, such as unrequested medical treatment), unless the plaintiff could show that the battery actually caused a further impairment such as the man's stroke and paralysis, there was no harm from treating a person against his wishes.[48]

Other cases are presently in the courts, and many have gone before, each seeking to confirm what many scholars and attorneys often take for granted: that competent persons have the constitutionally protected right to accept treatment or to refuse any unwanted treatment.[49] Causes of action (the legal basis on which a lawsuit can be brought to court) vary somewhat: battery, right of privacy, common law right to refuse treatment, negligence, wrongful death, wrongful life, as well as simple medical malpractice. But the issues under consideration are even more complex: persons who are competent, incompetent but conscious, never competent, semicomatose, or permanently comatose; substituted judgment; and the clear and convincing standard for evidence brought before the court. Even with 97 advance directive laws—at least 1 in each of the 50 states—and the PSDA, it seems to remain questionable whether those rights can be exercised in advance of incapacity and with confidence.

If the intent of the PSDA was to *introduce* a concept to the general public by means of an education program having little oversight of content, delivery, evaluation, and enforcement, then the regulation is working. As the Inspector General found, many people have "some understanding" of advance directives. And health care professionals and organizations have largely institutionalized protocols designed to meet minimum thresholds set by the law. But if the intent of the law was to increase substantially the number of advance directives completed, discussed, submitted, and honored, then it can be described as a law that has had a good beginning with the better part of the race yet to be run. Both empirical research and anecdotal evidence indicate that the percentage of persons with signed advance directives remains somewhat constant at 15 to 20 percent.[50]

As with preventive medicine, education leading to behavioral change is a long-term enterprise. Just ask the folks in the smoking cessation movement who have worked and waited for almost 50 years for positive feedback from one of the longest education efforts in history. Not smoking is, at last, becoming the norm. Will it take 50 years for the PSDA to have more than a superficial effect on how health care providers and their patients relate to each other? One hopes not.

Further regulation and promotion of the education process, either by the Joint Commission or by changes in state law, will inevitably result in greater adherence to the prescribed PSDA regimen. So, too, may lawsuits like the ones described above. But legal remedies for violations of distinctive state laws will have only a gradual effect on behavior in other jurisdictions. So far as we know, there have been no suits filed alleging violation of the federal PSDA requirements, only violation of state advance directive laws or federal constitutional law regarding the right to refuse treatment. With the PSDA modified by the Final Rule to require notification to patients of a state-based complaint process, it will be interesting to see whether this path to enforcement will be used by persons who believe their advance directive rights have been violated.

Will providers be the primary source of information about health care decision making and advance directive rights? They may be in a good position to do so, but many people argue that admission to a health care facility is a profoundly poor time to think carefully about one's treatment preferences, possible incapacity, and naming a surrogate decision maker. Better to consider those weighty issues when healthy and curious. The more effective efforts will likely come through innovative education programs developed by professional associations, nonprofit organizations, and voluntary associations who want to promote wider use of advance directives and interact more frequently with healthy constituents.

Will the PSDA ever result in having *all* persons complete advance directives, just as we all apply for driver's licenses and credit cards? Doubtful. Many citizens find the concept of personal autonomy strange, even highly objectionable. Self-disclosure, one of the necessary components of completing any of the proxy documents, is not a valued skill to many people. And is it, in fact, desirable that as many people as possible exercise as much control as possible over their health care? What is to lose? What is at risk if we do not? Skeptics will answer that we do not need to have control over treatment options that we may not be offered anyway. And they will argue that health care is so technologically advanced that the choice we are authorized to make is illusory: Our doctor cannot explain the choice in words we know, and we cannot comprehend the true range of options we really have. So why choose at all?

Choice is, after all, one of the enduring American values. Pity the grocer who stocks only one brand of anything. That grocer will soon be out of business. Put choice on the shelves, and the register will ring all day. And so it is with the PSDA. At the insistent request of the American public, the federal government has enacted legislation that urges, encourages, pushes, and nudges us to be choosey. Inspect, assess, evaluate, weigh, discuss, deliberate. Then choose. I will not settle for health care that someone *else* selects for me. I want to choose it myself, in my own time. It has to suit me. I will have *that* one, please.

NOTES

1. L. Kutner, "Due Process of Euthanasia: The Living Will, A Proposal," *Indiana Law Journal* 44 (1969): 537–554; Omnibus Budget Reconciliation Act of 1990, Sections 4206 and 4751, Public Law 101–508, signed by President Bush on November 5, 1990, and effective December 1, 1991.
2. However, as of June 1992, 30 states had passed "family consent" statutes that give a priority by which certain family members (e.g., one's spouse, adult children, etc.) are authorized to act for the incapacitated person. Only four states—Arizona, Florida, Illinois, and New York—include "close friend" in the list of permissible surrogates. Traditional guardianships and protective service proceedings are available, though courts are reluctant to become involved in large numbers of health care decisions. For a complete listing, see C. P. Sabatino, "Surrogate Decision Making in Health Care," in *Health Care Decision-Making in the 1990s: The Surrogate and Advance Directives at the Bedside* (Chicago: American Bar Association Section of Real Property, Probate and Trust Law, 1992). For full discussion of the issues, see New York State Task Force on Life and the Law, *When Others Must Choose: Deciding for Patients Without Capacity,* 1992: 304. Order from Health Education Services, PO Box 7126, Albany, NY 12224.
3. Choice in Dying, *Refusal of Treatment Legislation: A State by State Compilation of Enacted and Model Statutes* (New York: Choice in Dying, 1991; with annual updates).
4. See, for example, the draft "Health-Care Decisions Act" proposed by the National Conference of Commissioners on Uniform State Laws, 676 North St. Clair Street, Suite 1700, Chicago, IL 60611. See also T. A. Eaton and E. J. Larson, "Experimenting with the 'Right to Die' in the Laboratory of the States," *Georgia Law Review* 25 (1991): 1253–1326.
5. In "the battle of the forms," a number of articles have appeared in which authors not only urge the use of a particular kind of advance directive over another, but also question the effectiveness of the PSDA in achieving its goals by means of promoting advance directives. For a sampling, see G. J. Annas, "The Health Care Proxy and the Living Will," *New England Journal of Medicine* 324 (1991): 1210–13; A. S. Brett, "Limitations of Listing Specific Medical Interventions in Advance Directives," *JAMA* 226 (1991): 825–28; L. Emanuel and E. Emanuel, "The Medical Directive: A New Comprehensive Advance Care Document," *JAMA* 261 (1989): 3288–93; R. S. Olick, "Approximating Informed Consent and Fostering Communication," *Journal of Clinical Ethics* 2, no. 3 (1991): 181–95.
6. S. M. Wolf et al., "Sources of Concern about the Patient Self-Determination Act," *New England Journal of Medicine* 325 (1991): 1666–71.
7. J. Lynn and J. Teno, "After the Patient Self-Determination Act: The Need for Empirical Research on Formal Advance Directives," *Hastings Center Report* 23, no. 1 (1991): 20–24.
8. M. M. Handelsman, "Federal Policy Regarding End of Life Decisions," in *Euthanasia: The Good of the Patient, the Good of Society,* ed. R. Misbin (Frederick, Md: University Publishing Group, 1992).
9. Ibid.
10. Department of Health and Human Services, Health Care Financing Administration, Medicare and Medicaid Programs, Advance Directives, 42CFR Parts 417, 431, 434, 484, 489, 498.
11. The "clear and convincing" standard, adopted by Missouri and New York, has prompted concern that relatives or caregivers of persons in persistent vegetative states might never be able to have treatment withdrawn, no matter how futile the present or proposed treatment.
12. *Cruzan v. Director,* Missouri Department of Health, 110 S.Ct. 2841 (1990), concurring opinion.
13. J. M. Teno et al. (Center for Evaluative Clinical Science, Dartmouth Medical School; and American Bar Association, Commission on the Legal Problems of the Elderly), Evaluation of the Impact of the Patient Self-Determination Act: State Response to Write Description of State Law, presented at Choices and Conversations (National PSDA conference sponsored by the Pacific Center for Health Policy and Ethics, University of Southern California Law Center, Pasadena, Calif., January 8–9, 1993).
14. M. R. Gasner, "The PSDA: A Next Logical Step," *Journal of Clinical Ethics* 2, no. 3 (1991): 173–77.
15. See, for example, American Association of Homes for the Aging, Patient Self-Determination Act of 1990: Implementation Issues (Washington, D.C.: American

Association of Homes for the Aging, 1991); California Consortium on Patient Self-Determination, *The PSDA Handbook,* hospital edition (Los Angeles: Pacific Center for Health Policy and Ethics, University of Southern California Law Center, 1991); J. F. Monagle and D. C. Thomasma, *Medical Ethics: Policies, Protocols, Guidelines and Programs* (Gaithersburg, Md.: Aspen Publishers, 1992).

16. R. Jackson and A. Carlos, "Getting Ready for the PSDA: What Are Hospitals and Nursing Homes Doing?" *Journal of Clinical Ethics* 2, no. 3 (1991): 177–81.
17. Gasner, "The PSDA."
18. C. P. Sabatino, "Surely the Wizard Will Help Us, Toto? Implementing the Patient Self-Determination Act," *Hastings Center Report* 23, no. 1 (1993): 12–16.
19. Massachusetts Health Care Proxy Task Force, Consensus Report (Sharon, Mass.: Massachusetts Health Decisions, 1992).
20. Department of Health and Human Services, Health Care Financing Administration, Medicare and Medicaid Programs, Advance Directives, 42CFR Parts 417, 431, 434, 484, 489, 498.
21. Examples of programs designed to recognize preadmission DNR orders include Connecticut (Emergency Medical Services), Virginia (EMS-initiated legislation), North Carolina (county-by-county adoption of EMS guidelines), California (EMS; guidelines adopted county by county; legislation introduced), New York (State Department of Health; 1992 legislation), and Montana (legislation). Also, MedicAlert® (2323 Colorado Avenue, Turlock, CA 05380) has initiated a national preadmission DNR project.
22. For a model policy for implementing living wills and medical durable powers of attorney for the Virginia Department of Mental Health, Mental Retardation and Substance Abuse Services, see K. H. Swisher, "Implementing the PSDA for Psychiatric Patients: A Commonsense Approach," *Journal of Clinical Ethics* 2, no. 3 (1991): 199–205. See also New York Task Force on Life and the Law, *When Others Must Choose: Deciding for Patients without Capacity* (New York: New York Task Force on Life and the Law, 1992; order from Health Education Services, P.O. Box 7126, Albany, NY 12224). On the nature of competency in general, see especially B. Chell, "Competency: What It Is, What It Isn't, and Why It Matters," in *Medical Ethics: A Guide for Health Professionals*, ed. J. Monagle and D. Thomasma (Gaithersburg, Md.: Aspen Publishers, 1988).
23. M. Z. Solomon et al., "Decisions Near the End of Life: Professional Views on Life-sustaining Treatment," *American Journal of Public Health* 83, no. 1 (1993): 14–23.
24. In my experience, three of the best are G. J. Annas, *The Rights of Patients: The Basic ACLU Guide to Patient Rights, 2d ed.* (Carbondale, Ill.: Southern Illinois University Press, 1989); N. Dubler and D. Nimmons, *Ethics on Call* (New York: Harmony Books/Crown Publishers, 1992); and T. Scully and C. Scully, *Making Medical Decisions* (New York: Fireside Books/Simon & Schuster, 1989).
25. P. Lambert et al., "The Values History: An Innovation in Surrogate Medical Decision-Making," *Law, Medicine and Health Care* 18 (1990): 202–12. The values history is published without copyright and may be reproduced and adapted as necessary.
26. See, for example, B. Mishkin, *A Matter of Choice: Planning Ahead for Health Care Decisions* (Washington D.C.: American Association of Retired Persons, 1986); American Hospital Association, *Put It in Writing: A Guide to Promoting Advance Directives* (Chicago: American Hospital Association, 1991).
27. T. C. Davis et al., "The Gap between Patient Reading Comprehension and the Readability of Patient Education Materials," *Journal of Family Practice* 31 (1990): 533–38; J. Klessig, "The Effect of Values and Culture on Life-Support Decisions," *Western Journal of Medicine* 157 (1992): 316–22.
28. SUPPORT Principal Investigators. "A Controlled Trial to Improve Care for Seriously Ill Hospitalized Patients: The Study to Understand Prognoses and Preferences for Outcomes and Risks of Treatments (SUPPORT)." *JAMA* 274, no. 20 (Nov. 22/29, 1995):1591–98.
29. United States Department of Health and Human Services, Health Care Financing Administration, 42 CFR Parts 417, 430, 431, 434, 483, 484, 489. Medicare and Medicaid Programs—Advance Directives (Patient Self-Determination Act, Final Rule). Federal Register 60 (June 27, 1995): 33262–92, 33264.
30. Ibid., 33265.
31. Ibid., 33277.
32. Ibid., 33278.
33. Ibid., 33265.
34. Ibid., 33279.
35. Ibid., 33274.
36. Ibid., 33266.
37. Ibid., 33274.
38. Ibid.
39. Ibid., 33275.
40. Ibid., 33290.
41. Ibid., 33277.
42. Ibid., 33280.
43. Ibid., 33285.

44. *Gilgunn v. Massachusetts General Hospital,* et al., Suffolk (Mass.) Superior Court, 92–4820, April 1995.
45. See, for example, *ECHO (Extreme Care, Humane Options): Community Recommendations for Appropriate, Humane Medical Care for Dying or Irreversibly Ill Patients* (Sacramento, Calif.: Sacramento Healthcare Decisions, 1997). Similar projects have been carried out in Denver and other urban areas.
46. *Elbaum v. Grace Plaza of Great Neck, Inc.,* 148 AD2nd 244, 544 NYS2nd 840 (2d Dept 1989).
47. "Ignoring 'Right to Die' Directives, Medical Community Is Being Sued," *New York Times,* 2 June 1996.
48. *Anderson v. St. Francis—St. George Hospital, Inc.*, No. 95–869 (Ohio, Oct. 10, 1996), as reported by Choice in Dying, New York.
49. *Cruzan v. Director, Missouri Department of Health,* 497 US 261 (1990).
50. E. J. Emanuel, et al., "How Well is the Patient Self Determination Act Working?: An Early Assessment," *American Journal of Medicine* 95, no. 6 (Dec. 1993): 619–28.

ADDITIONAL RESOURCES

American Bar Association, Commission on Legal Problems of the Elderly. *Patient Self-Determination Act State Law Guide*, Washington, D.C.: Commission on Legal Problems of the Elderly, 1991.

Barnette, C. "Advance Directives: Implementing a Program that Works." *Nursing Management*, Oct. 1994, p. 58–65.

Brett, A.S. "Limitations of Listing Specific Medical Interventions in Advance Directives." *JAMA* 266 (1991): 825–28.

Brunetti, L.L. et al. "Physicians' Attitudes toward Living Wills and Cardiopulmonary Resuscitation." *Journal of General Internal Medicine* 6 (1991): 323–29.

Buchanan, A.E., and D.W. Brock, *Deciding for Others: The Ethics of Surrogate Decision-Making*. New York: Cambridge University Press, 1990.

Burke, M. "Implementing the Patient Self-Determination Act." *Nursing Management* (Ambulatory Surgery Edition, Nov. 1993): 80B–80H.

Danis, M.M. et al. "A Prospective Study of Advance Directives for Life-sustaining Care." *New England Journal of Medicine* 324 (1991): 882–88.

Emanuel, E.J. et al. "Advance Directives for Medical Care—A Case for Greater Use." *New England Journal of Medicine* 324 (1991): 889–95.

———. "How Well is the Patient Self Determination Act Working?: An Early Assessment." *American Journal of Medicine* 95, no. 6 (Dec. 1993): 619–28.

Emanuel, L.L. "Advance Directives: Do They Work?" *Journal of American College of Cardiology* 25 (Jan. 1995): 35–38.

Emanuel, L.L. et al. "Advance Care Planning as a Process: Structuring the Discussions in Practice." *Journal of the American Geriatrics Society* 43 (1995): 440–46.

———. "Advance Directives: Stability of Patients' Treatment Choices." *Archives of Internal Medicine* 154 (Jan. 24, 1994): 209–17.

Gieszl, H.C., and P.A. Velasco, "The *Cruzan* Legacy: Legislative and Judicial Responses and Insights for the Future." *Arizona State Law Journal* 24 (1992): 719–99.

Hastings Center. "Advance Care Planning: Priorities for Ethical and Empirical Research" (Special Supplement). *Hastings Center Report* (Nov.–Dec. 1994): 1–36.

———. "Dying Well in the Hospital: Lessons of SUPPORT (Special Supplement)." *Hastings Center Report* (Nov.–Dec. 1995): S1–34.

Hoffman, D. et al. "The Dangers of Directives or the False Security of Forms." *Journal of Law, Medicine & Ethics* 24, no. 1 (Spring, 1996): 5–17.

Loewy, E., and R. Carlson, "Talking, Advance Directives, and Medical Practice." *Archives of Internal Medicine* (Oct. 24, 1994): 2265–67.

Malloy, T.R. et al. "The Influence of Treatment Descriptions on Advance Medical Directives." *Journal of the American Geriatrics Society* 40 (1992): 1255–60.

Markson, L. et al. "Implementing Advance Directives in the Primary Care Setting." *Archives of Internal Medicine* (Oct. 24, 1994): 2321–28.

McIntyre, K.M. "On Advancing Advance Directives: Why Should We Believe the Promise (Editorial)." *Archives of Internal Medicine* 155 (Nov. 27, 1995): 2271–73.

Meisel, A. "Legal Myths about Terminating Life Support." *Archives of Internal Medicine* 151 (1991): 1497–1502.

Menikoff, J.A. et al. "Beyond Advance Directives: Health Care Surrogate Laws." *New England Journal of Medicine* 327 (1992): 1165–69.

Morrison, R.S. et al. "The Inaccessibility of Advance Directives on Transfer from Ambulatory to Acute Care Settings." *JAMA* 274, no. 6 (Aug. 9, 1995): 478–82.

———. "Physician Reluctance to Discuss Advance Directives: An Empiric Investigation of Potential Barriers." *Archives of Internal Medicine* (Oct. 24, 1994): 2311–18.

Neumark, D. "Providing Information about Advance Directives to Patients in Ambulatory Care and Their Families." *ONF* (April 1994): 771–75.

Oleson, K. et al. "A Quality Improvement Focus for Patient Rights: Advance Directives." *Journal of Nursing Care Quality* (April 1994): 52–67.

National Health Lawyers Association. *The Patient Self-Determination Directory and Resource Guide*. Washington, D.C.: National Health Lawyers Association, 1991.

New York State Task Force on Life and the Law. *Life-Sustaining Treatment: Making Decisions and Appointing a Health Care Agent*. New York: New York State Task Force on Life and the Law, 1987.

———. *When Others Must Choose: Deciding for Patients Without Capacity*. New York: New York State Task Force on Life and the Law, 1992.

Orentlicher, D. "The Illusion of Patient Choice in End-of-Life Decisions." *JAMA* 267 (1992): 2101–4.

———. *Making Health Care Decisions: The Ethical and Legal Implications of Informed Consent in the Patient-Practitioner Relationship*. Washington, D.C.: U.S. Government Printing Office, 1982.

President's Commission for the Study of Ethical Problems in Medicine and Biomedical and Behavioral Research. *Deciding to Forgo Life-Sustaining Treatment: Ethical, Medical and Legal Issues in Treatment Decisions*. Washington, D.C.: U.S. Government Printing Office, 1983.

Reilly, B. et al. "Promoting Inpatient Directives about Life-Sustaining Treatments in a Community Hospital." *Archives of Internal Medicine* 155 (Nov. 27, 1995): 2317–23.

Reilly, B. et al. "Can We Talk? Inpatient Discussions about Advance Directives in a Community Hospital: Attending Physicians' Attitudes, Their Inpatients' Wishes, and Reported Experience." *Archives of Internal Medicine* 154 (Oct. 24, 1994): 2299–2308.

Seckler, A.B. et al. "Substituted Judgment: How Accurate are Proxy Predictions?" *Annals of Internal Medicine* 115 (1991): 92–98.

Smucker, W. et al. "Elderly Outpatients Respond Favorably to a Physician-Initiated Advance Directive Discussion." *Journal of American Board of Family Practitioners* (Sept.–Oct. 1993): 473–82.

Sugarman, J. et al. "Catalysts for Conversations about Advance Directives: The Influence of Physician and Patient Characteristics." *The Journal of Law, Medicine, & Ethics* (Spring 1994): 29–35.

Sulmasy et al. "More Talk, Less Paper: Predicting the Accuracy of Substituted Judgment." *American Journal of Medicine* 96 (1994): 432–38.

Uhlmann, R.F. et al. "Physicians' and Spouses' Prediction of Elderly Patients' Resuscitation Preferences." *Journal of Gerontology* 43 (1988): M115–121.

United States Department of Health and Human Services. Omnibus Budget Reconciliation Act of 1990, Sections 4206 and 4751, Public Law 101–508 (Patient Self Determination Act).

———. Health Care Financing Administration, 42 CFR 417, 431, 434, 483, 484, 489, and 498, Medicare and Medicaid Programs—Advance Directives (Patient Self Determination Act, Interim Final Rule). Federal Register 57 (March 6, 1992): 8194–204 .

———. Health Care Financing Administration, 42 CFR Parts 417, 430, 431, 434, 483, 484, 489. Medicare and Medicaid Programs—Advance Directives (Patient Self Determination Act, Final Rule). Federal Register 60 (June 27, 1995): 33262–92.

Virmani, J. "Relationship of Advance Directives to Physician-Patient Communication." *Archives of Internal Medicine* 154 (April 25, 1994): 909–13.

Wanzer, S.H. et al. "The Physician's Responsibility toward Hopelessly Ill Patients." *New England Journal of Medicine* 310 (1984): 955–59.

———. "The Physician's Responsibility toward Hopelessly Ill Patients: A Second Look." *New England Journal of Medicine* 320 (1989): 844–9.

Zweibel N.R., and C.K. Cassel. "Treatment Choices at the End of Life: A Comparison of Decisions by Older Patients and Their Physician-Selected Proxies." *Gerontologist* 29 (1989): 615–21.

Chapter 11

Competency: What It Is, What It Isn't, and Why It Matters

Byron Chell

A competent adult has the absolute right to refuse medical treatment—even lifesaving medical treatment! Can there be any doubt that this is a correct statement of principle, medical ethics, and law?[1]

In spite of this clear and seemingly straightforward declaration, however, when a patient refuses to accept needed medical care, we yet find much concern and confusion. This is especially true when the treatment is lifesaving.

The rule that a competent adult has the right to refuse any and all medical treatment emphasizes the importance of the concept of *competency*. In fact, if we are uneasy about a decision to refuse treatment, we immediately retreat to the thicket of competency.[2] Such a retreat is appropriate, however, because when confronted with a refusal of needed medical care, the first and key question we should ask is whether the patient is competent to make the required decision.

Yet difficulties regarding competency remain, because the concept is confusing. What is a competent adult? What is the definition of *competency*? Are those who refuse lifesaving treatment on religious grounds really competent? How do we find the proper answers to these questions when evaluating patients? Anyone involved in bioethics and medical decision making regularly confronts such questions.

This chapter discusses what competency is and is not. It also discusses what we should and should not be doing in making determinations of competency for the purpose of deciding whether to allow a patient to refuse medical treatment. If we have a clear understanding of what competency is, why we seek it, and why it matters, we will know how to approach and complete the task of determining competency without unnecessary anxiety and confusion.

WHAT COMPETENCY IS AND IS NOT

Competency is not a thing or a fact. It is not something we can look for and find if only we know how. Determinations of competency are not medical judgments. Clinical training is not required. Being competent does not necessarily mean being rational. We find many persons competent to make medical care decisions even though their refusal of treatment is based upon irrational beliefs. When we make determinations of competency we are not seeking truth or facts. We are not assessing the patient in light of a clear and neutral standard upon which we can make a definitive finding. It is not that easy.

Competent is simply a label we apply to persons after we examine various aspects of their physical and mental condition. Decisions relating to competency are legal and social decisions. They are legal decisions in that they are determinations of an individual's legal capacity to exercise the right to self-determination. No legal education is required, however. They are social decisions in that the statutory definitions we apply in the search are societal decisions. Additionally, when we make determinations of competency, we are doing so with imprecise criteria, vague notions, and personal beliefs and prejudices, all of which affect the outcome.

Considering the importance of the concept of competency in making determinations relating to, respecting, or overriding the patient's refusal, it would at first appear necessary that we fix upon *the* definition of the term *competency.* But despite our attempt as a society to define it, we have failed to find an adequate definition.

THE SEARCH FOR THE DEFINITION OF *COMPETENCY*

Fortunately, we do not need to find the definition of *competency* to fulfill our task. This is fortunate because there is no pre-existing single definition of the term. We can only create a definition—or various definitions.

No standard definition of *competency* is to be found. No statutory consistency or line of cases can be uncovered that would allow the simple discovery of the meaning of the terms *competent* or *incompetent.* Definitions of competency can be found in a number of different and specific situations where society and the law have always had to deal with the concept. We generally recognize that people can be competent to do one thing and not another or can be competent to some extent and not another. For example, we have laws regulating a person's competency to make a will, to enter into contracts, or to stand trial.

Definitions of incompetency have generally fallen into two categories: definitions that emphasize end results and definitions that emphasize thought processes. Both types of definition, however, are intimately and necessarily related in light of what we actually do in making determinations of competency.

Definitions in terms of end results essentially ask us to look at how persons live. What is their condition? What are the consequences or the end results of their thinking? For example, a former definition of the term "incompetent" for mental health commitment purposes is as follows:

> As used in this chapter the word incompetent shall . . . be construed to mean or refer to any adult person who . . . is unable properly to provide for his own personal needs for physical health, food, clothing or shelter, (or who) is substantially unable to manage, his own financial resources.[3]

A definition emphasizing end results tells us to look at what is happening to persons as a result of their thinking. Examine the physical consequences that follow from their mental status. An incompetent person is one whose mental processes lead to bad or serious consequences. A competent person simply would not live like that or be in that situation.

While such definitions work adequately in the context of mental health civil commitment proceedings, they are not very helpful in many cases of refusals of medical care. We question the competency of many persons who refuse medical treatment even though they are quite capable of providing for their own food, clothing, and shelter and can manage their daily affairs very well.

Because definitions in terms of living conditions or end results are not always adequate to the task, we also use definitions of "competency" that emphasize thought processes. A definition of "incompetency" in terms of thought processes involves determining if someone is competent by looking at how he or she relates to and decides things. One essentially tests the person's comprehension of reality, understanding, and ability to make rational judgments. One example of this type of incompetency definition is as follows:

> Several tests of competency might be applied, e.g., patients may be considered competent if 1) they evidence a choice concerning treatment, 2) this choice is "reasonable," 3) this choice is based on "rational" reasons, 4) the patient has a generalized ability to understand, or 5) the patient actually understands the information that has been disclosed. . . . [T]he courts have not settled on any single test of competency; in practice, doctors seem to

> apply an amalgam of some or all of these tests.[4]

A definition emphasizing thought processes involves listening to the patient and judging whether what is said "makes sense." Is the patient rational? The point is not to examine the physical consequences that follow from the patient's mental state but rather to examine the mental state itself.

There are currently many competing definitions of competency, and this is simply a reflection of the fact that competency can be properly defined in many different ways.

> The search for a single test of competency is a search for the Holy Grail. Unless it is recognized that there is not a magical definition of competency to make decisions about treatment, the search for an acceptable test will never end. 'Getting the words just right' is only part of the problem. In practice, judgments of competency go beyond semantics or straightforward applications of legal rules; such judgments reflect social considerations and societal biases as much as they reflect matters of law and medicine.[5]

Competency is, of course, whatever we define it to be. The trick is to define it so that it best helps us to do the job that needs to be done. The job in this context is to make decisions involving decision making. We must decide whether or not we will allow the patient to decide. Thus, what are the proper considerations we must keep in mind in making our decisions? What is the essence of competency? What criteria should be reflected in a proper definition?

THE ESSENCE OF COMPETENCY

Competency is essentially the ability to make a decision. Regardless of the particular definition used, determining competency in a given situation basically involves answering one question: Should we allow this person to make this decision under these circumstances?

Generally, but not always, the answer to this question is yes and a person is labeled competent if (1) he or she has an understanding of the situation and the consequences of the decision, and (2) the decision is based upon rational reasons.

Determining whether the person does or does not understand his or her condition is usually not the troublesome part. Sometimes it is difficult to determine the seriousness of the patient's condition and sometimes physicians will disagree. But if the medical conclusion is that intervention is required to prevent death or serious harm, it is normally not too difficult to determine whether the patient understands what the doctors are saying and whether the patient appreciates the consequences of his or her choice. This aspect of determining competency does not create philosophical and conceptual confusion. It can do so, however, in some cases of religious refusals, which are discussed below.

Determining whether or not the patient's decision to refuse treatment is based upon rational reasons can cause us much concern. While "rational" may appear redundant, its meaning in this context is "sensible," "sound," "reasonable," or "lucid." The term *reasons* is used in the sense of "reasons why," "motive," or "explanation." Thus, the reason why or the explanation of the decision to refuse treatment is to be considered rational if it is sensible or sound, lucid and not deranged, and it conforms to reason. In other words—it makes sense! In lieu of rational reasons, we might require sound explanations, sensible motives, or even reasonable reasons why.

There is no way to specifically define terms such as *rational reasons, sound explanations,* or *sensible motives* or to definitively measure what is rational or reasonable. These determinations will necessarily vary from person to person. We can set out cases where most persons would conclude that the reasons for the refusal are rational or sensible under the circumstances, and such examples can be instructive.

Suppose, for example, that an older patient is informed that her leg is gangrenous and that an amputation is necessary to save her life. Understanding the situation, she replies, "I refuse the amputation. I am not afraid of death. It is the natural end to life. I am 86 and I have lived a good and full life. I do not want a further operation, nor do I want to live legless. I understand that the consequence of refusing the amputation is death and I accept that consequence."

This woman understands both her situation and the consequences of her choice. Additionally, her decision is understandable. It is based on facts and logic. Although we might wish her to choose otherwise (or we might choose otherwise), her reasons and reasoning are sane, sound, and sensible. She is competent.[6]

If she were to say, however, "I understand the consequences but I refuse the operation because the moon is full," it is not likely she would be considered competent. Although she understands her situation and chooses death to medical treatment, her decision is not understandable. Her decision does not rationally or reasonably follow from her premise. Her explanation doesn't make sense. She would be labeled incompetent.[7]

A thousand reasons for refusing treatment could be set out. Regarding each, we could ask the question, "Is this a rational or sensible reason?" On some we might all agree. On others, there would be great disagreement. It is simply important to recognize that it can be no other way. Understanding this fact relieves the anxiety that accompanies the attempt to find out what competency is or to apply the proper definition of *competency* or *rationality*.

The fact that there can be neither a "true" finding of reasonableness nor a single test that will lead to uniform results should not, however, lead us to abandon our responsibility to make these judgments. Yet, when we weigh the reasons for the patient's choice, we many times discard the requirement of reasonableness and label persons competent even though their refusal is founded upon irrational beliefs. Patients who refuse necessary medical care based upon religious beliefs are often labeled competent even though their beliefs may be quite "irrational."

COMPETENCY IS COMPATIBLE WITH "IRRATIONALITY"—RELIGIOUS REFUSALS

We face many difficult questions when we confront a person who is refusing lifesaving medical care on the basis of religious belief.[8] If the patient is going to die because he or she is refusing a readily available medical procedure, we are puzzled, and we necessarily question the patient's competency. We find it difficult to accept that a rational and competent person would die when a simple act would save his or her life.

In considering competency and making judgments regarding those who refuse necessary medical treatment on the basis of religious belief, we can apply the above general definition of competency with a slight modification.

In cases of religious refusals, a person is competent if (1) he or she has a proper understanding of the situation and the consequences of the decision, and (2) the decision is based upon religious beliefs ("irrational" beliefs) that are within our common religious experience or common notions of religion and do not appear to us "crazy" or "nonreligious." If this definition seems vague, it is because it *is* vague.

To demonstrate how to apply this definition of competency, consider the following four examples of religious refusals. In each of these cases, suppose that the patient is refusing a lifesaving blood transfusion. Suppose also that each patient expresses sincerely held beliefs.[9]

Patient A states, "I refuse the blood transfusion because I am a Jehovah's Witness and I believe it is a violation of God's law to accept such blood. I understand that the consequence of my refusal is my death and I accept that result." Patient B states, "I refuse the blood transfusion because I am one of Yoda's Children and, based upon Luke Skywalker's teachings, I believe the acceptance of blood is a violation of Yoda's law and the work of the dark side of the Force. I understand that the consequence of my refusal is my death and I accept that result." Since we must make a determination relating to competency in these cases to decide if we are going to respect or override the patient's refusal, what will be the likely result?

The first patient will be judged competent and he will be allowed to refuse treatment and die. The second patient, while a more troubling case, will be labeled incompetent, and some other person will be allowed to give substituted consent to the treatment necessary to prevent his death.

Now, why is this the case? If we ask what is the difference between the statement of patient A as opposed to the statement of patient B, the answer must be none. Both are identical as statements of "irrational" religious belief or faith.

Belief and faith *are* irrational in at least one sense. In the context of this discussion, the term *irrational* means not derived logically from facts, data, or circumstances—outside the scope of reason. Faith is essentially belief based upon that which is incapable of proof. It does not involve logic, facts, or proof; it is trust and belief in a matter empirically unknowable. If it were knowable through facts or proof, we would speak in terms of knowledge and truth and not faith and belief. Theologians should know this.

A discussion that would attempt to label patient A's belief in Jehovah a religious belief and patient B's belief in Yoda a religious delusion would go nowhere. A conclusion in this situation that A's faith is based upon a belief as opposed to a delusion would depend entirely on the beliefs, experiences, and prejudices of the person drawing that conclusion. In these cases the label applied to the belief and the determination of competency depend on the novelty of the belief and on whether we want to give priority to the individual's continued life or to respecting the individual's choice. If the former, we would conclude that the decision is "crazy" and label the individual incompetent. If the latter, we would conclude that his belief is "religious" and label him competent.

In these two cases, the only difference is that patient A has voiced a religious belief held by organized and recognized groups within our society while patient B has voiced a belief totally outside our common religious experience. The Jehovah's Witness's belief relating to the refusal of blood is now well within our society's general "religious belief experience." Because of our concurrent societal belief in the free exercise of religion, we "respect" the Jehovah's Witness's belief even though it is irrational.[10] We recognize the belief as religious and we label patient A competent. As far as patient B is concerned, sincere or not, religious or not, we conclude that his belief is too "crazy" to determine a life and death decision, and we label him incompetent.

But what about the protections afforded by the First Amendment? If we do not accept patient B's belief, are we not unlawfully discriminating against this Yoda's Child and denying him his right to the free exercise of religion? While it is true that our constitution guarantees certain rights relating to the free exercise of religion, it is emphasized that only "religious beliefs" are protected.[11] And while it is often asserted that the courts will not assess or inquire into the truth or validity of individual religious beliefs,[12] the courts most certainly do decide what constitutes a "religion"[13] and what amounts to a "religious belief."[14] And in making such decisions, the courts also apply imprecise criteria and vague notions.

In determining whether a belief is a religious belief entitled to protection, the courts have at various times required that the belief be "truly held"[15] or that it be "sincere and meaningful,"[16] and judges have often emphasized the helpful test of orthodoxy.[17] The courts have also noted that some beliefs may simply be "too crazy" to qualify for protection.[18] In sum, the courts do judge the validity of religious beliefs, and they do it in a manner similar to the method of determining competency described above. That is, if a belief is "too crazy," there is sufficient room within our law to conclude that the belief is "nonreligious," not "sincere and meaningful," not "truly held," or not sufficiently similar to orthodox religious beliefs. This is the conclusion that ought to be reached about patient B's belief in Yoda.[19] Because his belief is too crazy, we would label him incompetent, and the courts would label his belief as one not entitled to First Amendment protection. In doing so, both we and the courts would be acting properly.[20]

There may be objections to making such judgments, but, despite objections and difficulties, we ought and will continue to do so.[21] The only alternative to making such distinctions is to accept *any* statement of belief as consistent with competence and sufficient to support a life and death decision regardless of its apparent "craziness." Few would feel comfortable with such a rule.

Next, consider the following patients, who express slightly different reasons for refusing the lifesaving medical care. Patient C states, "I refuse the blood transfusion because the full moon, properly understood, is the source of the human spirit and the key to human happiness and cures all disease. When the moon rises in full next week you shall see that it will cure me without the need of your medical procedure."

This is the easiest case. As with patient B, patient C has based her choice upon a belief quite outside our common religious experience. Additionally, she clearly does not appreciate either the nature of the situation or the consequence of her decision. She does not understand that her death is imminent. She fails both tests and is clearly incompetent. Is there any doubt that this patient's refusal would be overridden and action taken to provide the lifesaving care?

Patient D states, "I refuse the blood transfusion because I am a Jehovah's Witness and I believe it is a violation of God's law to accept such blood. God will heal me without the need of your medical procedures." This is a more difficult case. Would you allow this patient to refuse the lifesaving care?

This Jehovah's Witness has based her refusal upon a belief within our common religious experience. However, it is also evident that she does not appreciate either the nature of her situation or the consequences of her decision. She does not understand that without the blood transfusion, her death is imminent. While we may accept this patient's belief relating to the prohibition of blood, her religious beliefs go too far. Her belief in a cure without medical intervention in this situation does amount to a religious delusion.

Patient D is similar to the patient in a recent Ohio case where treatment was allowed in spite of the patient's "religious refusal." The patient refused to consent to treatment because she believed that she was the wife of an evangelist who would arrive to heal her. The court noted the rule that a patient's honestly held religious belief must be respected, but it decided that when those beliefs amount to a religious delusion, they may be disregarded.[22]

This may at first appear to be a subtle distinction, but it is a very important one. Carefully consider the difference between patient A and patient D. Patient A states, "I believe accepting blood is against God's will and I will not accept blood even though I will die because of my belief." Patient D states, "I believe accepting blood is against God's will and I will not accept blood. I also believe God will cure me and I will not die."

In failing to understand and recognize the consequences of her decision, patient D is *not* making the life and death decision required here. She is not deciding between the two, because she does not recognize one as being a consequence of her decision. The decision here is not simply to either accept blood or refuse blood. The decision that needs to be made involves the choice of either accepting blood *and living* or refusing blood *and dying*. In patient D's mind, she is simply choosing between life with treatment as opposed to life without treatment. One cannot freely decide between two choices if one does not understand what the choices actually are. If one cannot freely decide, one is not competent to decide.[23]

Since patient D is in fact not making the required decision between the two alternatives of life and death, in failing to respect her "nonchoice" we are neither denying the principle of personal autonomy nor freedom of religious expression. We are obligated only to respect a decision. In refusing treatment, patient D is not making the required decision based upon a religious belief. Rather, her religious belief prevents her from understanding that her death is imminent and what the decision is that we require her to make. Her belief in this situation is a delusion—religious or not—in that it has adversely affected her ability to understand.

In summary, in religious refusal cases and following the general definition of competency set out above, we ought only label a patient competent and respect a refusal of medical treatment when (1) the patient is not deluded and he or she understands the situation and appreciates the consequences of the decision, and (2) the patient's refusal is founded upon a religious belief that is within our common religious experience or our common notions of religion and is not perceived as extremely unreasonable, crazy, or nonreligious.

Some concepts involved in the issue of competency, the manner in which we should evaluate competency, and the conclusions that should be reached concerning patients A–D can be set out as in Table 11–1.

CONCLUSIONS RELATING TO COMPETENCY

The above view of how to determine competency in cases involving understanding, appreciation, rationality, and religious belief can be summarized in another fashion. As with the cards used by police officers to assist in giving *Miranda* warnings, a medical decision-making card might state the following:

Process for Determining Competency of Patients Who Refuse Medical Treatment

Answer the following questions concerning the patient:

1. Does the patient understand his or her medical condition?
2. Does the patient understand the options and the consequences of his or her decision?
3. Is the patient's refusal based upon rational reasons?
4. If the refusal is based upon religious beliefs, are the religious beliefs acceptable and entitled to First Amendment protection, i.e., beliefs held by a sufficient

Table 11–1 Competency among Patients A–D

	Proper Understanding	*Acceptable Belief*	*Competent*
Patient A (Jehovah's Witness)	Yes	Yes	Yes
Patient B (Yoda's Child)	Yes	No	No
Patient C (Moon Child)	No	No	No
Patient D (Jehovah's Witness)	No	Yes	No

Proper Understanding: The patient understands his or her condition and the consequences of the decision. In these cases, the patient understands he or she is going to die without medical intervention. His or her understanding is not "deluded" by religious belief.

Acceptable Belief: The person's decision is based upon a belief that is within our common religious experience. It is a belief that has been held by a sufficient number of persons for a sufficient period of time or is sufficiently similar to other orthodox beliefs so that we label it a religious belief and not nonreligious, unsound, or insane.

Competent: The label we apply in the various situations.

> number of persons for a sufficient period of time or sufficiently similar to other orthodox beliefs such that we do not label the beliefs crazy or nonreligious?

If the answers to (1), (2), (3), and (4) are all yes, then the patient's refusal will be respected. He or she should be labeled competent. If the answer to either (1), (2), (3), or (4) is no, then the patient's refusal should not be respected and action should be taken to obtain substitute consent. He or she is incompetent.

Using this procedure, one will reach a proper result in all cases, no matter who makes the determination, be it physician or judge, or what the particular statutory definition might be. If the answer to all four questions is yes, any proper statutory definition of competency will be fulfilled. If the answer to any of the four is no, any proper definition of incompetency will be met.[24] This is not to say that in any given case there is a proper conclusion or that different persons asking these same questions will not reach different conclusions. This is also not to say that such questions can be easily answered in all cases. Sometimes it is easy to answer these questions and we feel quite confident in our conclusions. Sometimes it is terribly difficult. Nevertheless, following this type of procedure will give a proper result simply because these questions are based on the essence of the concept of competency. They contain the necessary considerations, vague and slippery as they may be, to make the required decision. Such a procedure simply allows us to reach a conclusion in a straightforward manner and this is all we can hope to do.

WHY IT MATTERS

It is always important to emphasize the significant ethical and moral issues involved in labeling a person incompetent. Such emphasis underscores our need to work hard at making proper determinations.

Consider just what it is we are saying when we exercise the power of the state to override a patient's specific refusal of medical care because the patient is incompetent. We are, most assuredly, judging the validity of the patient's reasoning and the truth of the patient's beliefs. We do so without precise criteria or objective standards. We decide which reasons expressed by the patient are acceptable and which are proper religious beliefs entitled to protection.

As a society, we simply think that some persons, for one reason or another, should not be allowed to make certain decisions. We reach this conclusion for the same reason that we think certain defendants should not be held responsible for otherwise criminal actions. Based on our experience, some persons just do not appear to be rational, responsible, or competent human beings.

In medical decision making, we must distinguish between rational and irrational reasons and between acceptable religious beliefs and craziness (or whatever one wishes to call it). If we do not make such distinctions, then we must allow the refusal of any patient no matter what the basis, even though the patient's beliefs are such that they delude the patient's understanding of the situation and prevent him or her from making the required decision. What if the patient's beliefs seem clearly senseless and unacceptable, as nonsensical as the beliefs of an acutely psychotic person who chooses death based on "commands" from the television set?

As a further matter, consider this aspect of judging a person to be incompetent. In spite of the person's stated choice, we make a different choice and force our choice upon the person. We do so claiming that we have the right (and the duty) to force our decision on the person—we do so for his or her "own good." We do so because, in spite of the person's choice (an incompetent choice), the person has a right to the benefits of our decision (a competent choice). We reason the person has a right to the benefits of the choice that he or she would have made if competent. If the person were competent to decide and had reached a different conclusion, he or she would be, in effect, a different person. When you change a person's understanding, beliefs, thoughts, conclusions, and choices, you have changed the person. In forcing our choice upon the patient, we are claiming that the patient has a right to the benefits of being a different person. Indeed, we are insisting that he or she be a different person. It is not difficult to understand and appreciate the ethical and moral problems involved in negating personal autonomy under such circumstances and in using power and force, if necessary, to insist that a person be another person.

Of course, most persons are aware that good intentions and the exercise of power for another person's own good can bring about horrendous results. Controversial decisions and disagreements have always and will always result from determinations of competency. Such is our condition, however, and the nature and consequences of these decisions simply underscore the weight of our obligations.

SUMMARY AND CONCLUSION

While more needs to be said, this discussion has attempted to explain what competency is and to set out a fairly straightforward process for making determinations of competency.

The patient's competency is the first and foremost question that must be resolved in deciding whether or not we will respect or override the patient's refusal. There is no single definition of *competency,* and there are many different ways of stating the concepts involved in that term.

The term *competent* is nothing more than a label we place on a person when we conclude that we should allow him or her to make the decision at issue. Generally, we apply the label to the person who understands his or her condition and the consequences of the choices and whose reasons make sense to us. Sometimes, however, especially in cases of religious refusals and First Amendment considerations, we apply the term *competent* to persons who base their refusal upon irrational beliefs as long as those beliefs are within our common religious experience and do not seem too strange.

In making determinations of competency and in forcing treatment on others, we are engaged in serious matters. These are decisions that should not be avoided, however. We must use our experience of the human condition and our best judgment in the attempt to make proper decisions. As long as they are made with proper motives and a proper understanding of the task, they are properly made. And although these decisions may yet be difficult in individual cases, they should be made without unnecessary concern or doubt because in doing so we are doing all that can properly be done. We are, after all, simply human beings attempting to make very difficult decisions relating to other human beings.

NOTES

1. Judge Cardoza stated it this way: "Every human being of adult years and sound mind has a right to determine what shall be done with his own body. . . ." *Schloendorff v. Society of New York Hospital* (1914) 105 N.E. 92,93. See also Matter of Spring (1980) 405 N.E.2d 115; *Superintendent of Belchertown v. Saikewicz* (1977) 370 N.E.2d 417; *Bartling v. Superior Court* (1984) 163 Cal.App.3d 186; *Barber v. Superior Court* (1983) 147 Cal.App.3d 1006.
2. "On balance, the right to self-determination ordinarily outweighs any countervailing state interests and competent persons generally are permitted to refuse medical treatment, even at the risk of death. Most of the cases that have held otherwise . . . have concerned the patient's competency to make a rational and considered choice of treatment." *Matter of Conroy* (1985) 486 A.2d 1209,1225.
3. Cal. Welf. & Inst. Code Sec. 1435.2 (repealed Jan. 1, 1981).
4. R. Meisel and L. Meisel, "Toward a Model of the Legal Doctrine of Informed Consent," *American Journal of Psychiatry* 134 (March 1977): 285, 287.
5. R. Meisel and L. Meisel, "Tests of Competency to Consent to Treatment," *American Journal of Psychiatry* 134 (March 1977): 279, 283.
6. See *Lane v. Candura* (1978) 376 N.E.2d 1232 for a decision respecting a patient's refusal of an amputation under similar circumstances.
7. *Matter of Schiller* (1977) 372A.2d 360 is another case where the court struggled with the refusal of an amputation. In the *Matter of Schiller,* the patient was found incompetent and a guardian was appointed primarily

because Mr. Schiller failed to properly evidence an understanding of his medical condition and the reality of death, the more likely situation in such cases.

8. Our additional concern is occasioned, of course, by the First Amendment to the Constitution of the United States. "Congress shall make no law respecting an establishment of religion, or prohibiting the free exercise thereof. . . ."
9. Of course, in making determinations of competency one would always want to know more and would question the patient carefully and thoroughly.
10. It should be emphasized that the beliefs of Jehovah's Witnesses are not used to single out those beliefs as being less rational than or deserving of less respect than any other religious beliefs. The Jehovah's Witness examples are used solely because the beliefs of Jehovah's Witnesses form the most widely known religious basis for the refusal of medical care in this country.
11. "Only beliefs rooted in religion are protected by the Free Exercise Clause, which, by its terms, gives special protection to the exercise of religion." *Thomas v. Review Board* (1981) 450 U.S. 707,715.
12. "Men may believe what they cannot prove. They may not be put to the proof of their religious doctrines or beliefs. Religious experiences which are as real as life to some may be incomprehensible to others." *United States v. Ballard* (1944) 322 U.S. 78,86. "[R]eligious beliefs need not be acceptable, logical, consistent, or comprehensible to others in order to merit First Amendment protection." *Thomas v. Review Board* (1981) 450 U.S. 707,714.
13. See *Engel v. Vitale* (1962) 370 U.S. 421 (school prayer); *Loney v. Scurr* (1979) 474 F.Supp. 1186,1194. "[T]he Church of the New Song qualifies as a 'religion.'" *Theriault v. Silber* (1978) 453 F.Supp. 254, 260. "The Church of the New Song appears not to be a religion." *Malnik v. Yogi* (1977) 440 F. Supp. 1284 (transcendental meditation).
14. See *Wisconsin v. Yoder* (1972) 406 U.S. 205, which contrasted the "religious beliefs" of the Amish with the "philosophical and personal" beliefs of Thoreau; also, *United States v. Seeger* (1965) 380 U.S. 163, which determined whether or not the beliefs of a conscientious objector qualified as "religious beliefs" to allow an exemption.
15. "[W]hile the 'truth' of a belief is not open to question, there remains the significant question whether it is 'truly held.'" *United States v. Seeger* (1965) 380 U.S. 163,185.
16. "We believe that . . . the test of belief 'in a relation to a supreme being' is whether a given belief that is sincere and meaningful occupies a place in the life of its possessor parallel to that filled by the orthodox belief in God of one who clearly qualifies for the exemption." *United States v. Seeger* (1965) 380 U.S. 163,166.
17. "[D]oes the claimed belief occupy the same place in the life of the objector as an orthodox belief in God holds in the life of one clearly qualified for exemption?" *Seeger* supra at 184. "[I]t is at least clear that if a group (or an individual) professes beliefs which are similar to and function like the beliefs of those groups which by societal consensus are recognized as a religion, the First Amendment guarantee of freedom of religion applies." *Loney v. Scurr* (1979) 474 F.Supp. 1186,1193 citing *Welsh v. United States* (1970) 398 U.S. 333,340. "While recently acquired religious views are worthy of protection, the history of a religious belief and the length of time it has been held are factors to be utilized in assessing the sincerity with which it is held." In re *Marriage of Gove* (1977) 572 P.2d 458,461, citing *Wisconsin v. Yoder*.
18. "One can, of course, imagine an asserted claim so bizarre, so clearly nonreligious in motivation, as not to be entitled to protection under the Free Exercise Clause . . ." *Thomas v. Review Board* (1981) 450 U.S. 707,715.
19. If a professed belief in *Star Wars* characters and making a life and death decision based upon faith in Yoda and Luke Skywalker is not sufficiently "crazy" for you, create your own patient. Consider, for example, a refusal by the patient who tells you he is "Serumzat, believer in the teachings of the Prince of Liquids and Tabletops; I believe that accepting blood is wrong and will prevent my passage to the afterlife, which I am destined to rule."
20. As a further example of how courts make these decisions, see *Powell v. Columbian Presbyterian Medical Center* (1966) 267 N.Y.S.2d 450. The facts presented the classic case of the Jehovah's Witness who did not want to die but who refused a lifesaving blood transfusion. In a most candid decision that demonstrated the reality of the difficulty, vagueness, and room for legal discretion involved in these matters, the court stated in part: "This matter generated a barrage of legal niceties, misinformation and emotional feelings on the part of all concerned—including the Court personnel. . . . Never before had my judicial robe weighed so heavily on my shoulders. . . . I, almost by reflex action subjected the papers to the test of justiciability, jurisdiction and legality. . . . Yet, ultimately, my decision to act to save this woman's life was rooted in more fundamental precepts. . . . I was reminded of 'The Fall' by Camus, and I knew that no release—no legalistic absolution—would absolve me or the Court from responsibility if I, speaking for the Court, answered 'No' to the question 'Am I my brother's keeper?' This woman wanted to live. I could not let her die!" 267 N.Y.S.2d at 451,452.
21. It should be noted that in all cases of refusals of medical care, religious or not, as our certainty in the prognosis decreases, our willingness to allow the refusal increases. See, for example, *Petition of Nemser* (1966) 273 N.Y.S.2d 624, which contains an interesting discussion

of these issues, although in some areas the court's analysis is incomplete or incorrect.

22. In re *Milton,* 505 N.E. 2d 255 (Ohio 1987). What would we do if this patient was Mrs. Oral Roberts?
23. Consider how terribly subtle these distinctions can be, however. Does it make a difference if the patient says "I leave my fate to Jehovah," as opposed to "I believe Jehovah will cure me"? Or if the patient states "God will save me" as opposed to "God may save me"? Again, we would explore this patient's understanding and beliefs carefully.
24. It should also be remembered that if the answer to any of these questions is no, the patient is also unable to *consent* to treatment.

Chapter 12

Domestic Violence: Changing Theory, Changing Practice

Carole Warshaw

Despite widespread recognition of domestic violence as a public health problem, many clinicians still have difficulty integrating routine intervention into their day-to-day practice. This is in part because domestic violence raises a distinct set of challenges for both providers and the institutions that shape clinical practice. Domestic violence is a complex social problem rather than a biomedical one; addressing it means asking clinicians to step beyond a traditional medical paradigm to confront the personal feelings and social beliefs that shape their responses to patients and to work in partnership with community groups committed to ending domestic violence. In addition, addressing domestic violence raises important challenges to the health care system itself—to its theoretical models, to the nature of medical training, and to the rapidly changing structure of clinical practice. If we truly want to play a role in preventing domestic violence, rather than just treating its consequences, we must work together to transform both the individual and social conditions that create and support this kind of violence in the first place.

It has become increasingly clear over the past 20 years that domestic violence carries not only serious health consequences for women, but many hidden social costs as well. As clinicians we see the profound effects of this violence on a daily basis[1] and are often deeply affected when we allow ourselves to listen, understand, and grapple with issues that require far more than our medical expertise.

Through the combined efforts of the domestic violence advocacy community, individual practitioners, and a growing number of professional societies, standards of care have been developed and major initiatives have been launched to increase provider awareness, to establish and distribute clinical guidelines, and to offer strategies for improving institutional responses to domestic violence.[2] Innovative hospital-based advocacy programs are increasing in number, and medical schools and residencies are beginning to develop models for incorporating training on family violence into standard curricula.[3]

Yet despite widespread recognition of domestic violence as a public health problem, many clinicians still have difficulty integrating routine inquiry about domestic violence into their day-to-day practice.[4] Understanding the difficulties faced by health care providers as they attempt to address this issue can help not only to improve clinical practice but also to develop more realistic strategies for prevention and social change.[5]

Domestic violence raises a distinct set of challenges for both providers and the institutions that shape medical practice. Because domestic violence is, in fact, a complex social problem rather

---

Source: Reprinted with permission from C. Warshaw, Domestic Violence: Changing Theory, Changing Practice, *Journal of the American Medical Women's Association,* Vol. 51, No. 3, pp. 87–91, © 1996, The American Medical Women's Association.

than a biomedical one, addressing it requires more than simply adding new diagnostic categories to differential diagnoses or new technical skills to clinical repertoires. It means asking clinicians to step beyond a traditional medical paradigm to confront the personal feelings and social beliefs that shape their responses to patients, and to work in partnership with community groups committed to ending domestic violence. In addition, the health care system itself, through its theoretical framework, the nature of its training process, and the rapidly changing structure of clinical practice, presents another set of barriers that profoundly affect the ability of individual providers to respond to women who have been abused.[6]

PERSONAL AND SOCIAL BARRIERS

As Holtz et al. have reported, most health care providers do not learn about domestic violence during their training.[7] Consequently, "clinical" responses are often shaped by an interplay of the physician's own personal experiences and his or her social, cultural, and religious beliefs.[8] Many factors combine to shape the ways we interpret and respond to life events, including both our individual experiences and the social contexts in which they take place. Koss et al.,[9] Johnson,[10] Brown,[11] Rieker and Carmen,[12] and Miller[13] have described the psychological impact of gender socialization, the traumatic effects of social disenfranchisement, and the ways in which the denial of intolerable feelings can distort our perceptions and lead to protectively rationalized ways of viewing ourselves, other people, and the world. For instance, the psychological need to deny or avoid certain feelings or emotional experiences in order to ensure psychic survival often combines with social explanations to solidify into beliefs that may then appear to us as "givens."[14] Clinicians absorb a range of societal views regarding gender and power, around which their own identities are constructed. Assumptions about gender, race, and class so permeate our culture that they often provide an unconscious backdrop through which we come to understand our own experiences and interpret those of others.

In addition, listening to women describe the violence in their lives can have a significant psychological impact on providers.[15] When physicians are not specifically trained to deal with psychological trauma, they are forced to rely on their own capacities to address painful and potentially overwhelming issues. And, given the prevalence of violence against women in this society, a significant number of physicians will have experienced or witnessed abuse in their own lives.[16] These issues touch too close to home for many health care providers, who may be understandably reluctant to have their own painful experiences evoked while trying to function in a professional capacity.[17]

SYSTEMIC BARRIERS

Impact of Medical Training

Once they enter the health care arena, clinicians are faced with a new set of forces that shape their perceptions and responses.[18] A number of authors have described the gaps in medical education that influence psychosocial aspects of care.[19] Not only is medical training often lax in equipping physicians to deal with difficult social and personal issues, but more insidiously, the process of professional socialization can actually extinguish the capacities they already have. Pain, anger, frustration, and sadness are common responses to hearing about abuse. Without specific training and support, many clinicians find themselves dealing with these situations through a variety of techniques designed to protect and distance themselves from potentially distressing encounters. In a field where competence and mastery are highly valued, it is difficult to risk venturing into areas that make clinicians feel less competent. They may find it easier to focus on problems where interventions lead to more predictable outcomes or where it is possible to retain a greater sense of control. These difficulties are only magnified by increasingly time-pressured working conditions.[20]

Professional Socialization and the Integenerational Transmission of Abuse

Extrapolating from the work of Richman et al.,[21] Baldwin et al,[22] and others,[23] we can see how abusive training environments may also affect clinicians' abilities to deal with abuse among the women they see as patients. Medical training can be physically punishing, emotionally draining, and socially isolating. Trainees often report feeling humiliated and controlled as well as anxious, exhausted, depressed, overwhelmed, and traumatized.[24] Over time, students and house staff begin to reorient their identities in terms of medicine's values, to internalize its constructs and judge themselves by its terms. Thus, medical training itself can create some of the same dynamics as abuse. In addition, the structure of medicine is hierarchical and as such, reflects the gendered power arrangements of the larger society. In their review of the sexual harassment literature, Schiffman and Frank found that sexual harassment and gender discrimination were common experiences among women physicians, adding yet another layer of abuse for women working within that system.[25] Clinicians' inabilities to recognize abuse in their own lives, whether personal, social, or professional, or to tolerate acknowledging their own vulnerability, make it more difficult for them to empathize with a woman who is struggling in an abusive relationship. The need to maintain a sense of power and control in order to be recognized as competent within that system and the pressure to avoid feelings that may arise when one cannot, reinforce this dynamic on both individual and systemic levels. While there has been much discussion about how abuse is transmitted intergenerationally in families, the process of professional socialization within the current structure of medicine can also serve as a vehicle for the intergenerational transmission of abuse.[26]

IMPACT OF THEORY ON CLINICAL PRACTICE

Medicalization of Social Problems

One aspect of medicalization involves the reduction of complex social problems into distinct clinical diagnoses.[27] One of the clearest illustrations of the need to shift from a standard problem-oriented framework to a more comprehensive model involves our evolving understanding of the role domestic violence plays in the lives of women with human immunodeficiency virus (HIV). Several studies have reported that many HIV-positive women either are or have been abused by partners.[28] Many "discrete" medical problems are, in fact, intimately connected to domestic violence, but because we think of them as separate issues, their interrelationships are more likely to be missed. For instance, one might easily generate a problem list that includes HIV infection, substance abuse, pregnancy, depression, and domestic violence without necessarily seeing the connections among them. Initial recognition of domestic violence among HIV-positive women led to appropriate concerns about reducing risk for further violence, particularly around partner notification.[29] It took longer for domestic violence education and intervention to be incorporated into risk reduction counseling for HIV, pregnancy, and substance abuse. There are significant implications for funding, education, and prevention if coerced sex within the context of an abusive relationship also proves to be a major risk factor for HIV transmission and the other consequences of unprotected sex. And substance abuse among women, the other major risk factor for HIV, also increases in the context of domestic violence.[30] In fact, recognition of these connections has led a number of comprehensive HIV programs to integrate screening and counseling for domestic violence into the preventive as well as treatment services they provide.[31]

Limitations of Mental Health Models

The process of stripping away context and transforming lived experience into disorders also occurs within the major mental health models and affects the nature of both diagnosis and intervention. For example, clinicians who work within a purely biological or disorder-specific framework run risks similar to medical and surgical colleagues of failing to recognize and respond to the ongoing violence in a patient's life. Or they may see the abuse as being caused by a particular woman's increased vulnerability or as only a secondary problem—a social stressor affecting the course of her primary biological or developmental disorder.

Traditional psychoanalytic theory presents a different set of limitations. The context of ongoing violence and danger that creates and perpetuates a woman's symptoms may not be addressed, or may be regarded as symptomatic rather than etiologic. In addition, a clinician bound by the constraints of remaining true to the neutrality of a psychodynamic framework may find it difficult to play a more active role in advocating for safety and in helping women gain access to community resources. There are, however, newer models—both feminist and psychodynamic—that do recognize the importance of social and intersubjective contexts.[32]

A family systems approach can present even greater dangers to battered women. Assuming equal power within and responsibility for relationship dynamics, it inadvertently holds a battered woman responsible for her partner's criminal behavior and keeps her engaged in the countertherapeutic task of trying to change herself in order to get him to change. In addition, sessions often precipitate further threats or violence. Andersen et al.[33] and Walker[34] have described the dynamics of battering as a term of ongoing domestic terrorism, akin to hostage situations. In that kind of setting, particularly when her partner continues to engage in violence, controlling behavior, or threats, it is not safe for a woman to be honest or to assert herself. Nor is she likely to be free to make her own choices.[35]

These models are limited precisely because they are clinical models. They do not provide a framework for recognizing that it is the combination of the abuser's use of violence, threats, and intimidation *with* the social conditions that support gender inequality and limit options for safety that keeps women trapped in abusive situations and restricts their possibilities for change.[36]

Inadvertent Retraumatization

Inadvertent retraumatization of patients through disempowering interactions with the health and mental health system is another crucial issue. The pressure under current practice arrangements, particularly in managed care environments, to make rapid assessments, diagnoses, and treatment recommendations can push clinicians into taking a more controlling stance in their clinical encounters. For someone whose life is already controlled by another person, the subtly disempowering quality of many clinical interactions can serve to reinforce the idea that adapting to another's controlling behavior is both expected and necessary for survival.

Changing Theory and Incorporating Context

Clearly, a purely clinical framework limits our ability to respond to abuse. In fact, maintaining such a stance would require that we "diagnose" and find ways to "treat" a pervasive, longstanding form of normative social pathology characterized by a gender socialization process that (in its most polarized form) has taught women to focus their identities on meeting men's needs and on maintaining relationships at all costs, while teaching men that it is both necessary and legitimate to sustain their sense of self at the expense of those with less power, often women and children.[37] This belief is produced within the context of a socioeconomic system that frequently leaves women, particularly those with small children, increasingly fewer options for living independent lives[38] and a criminal justice system that often fails to protect. While the health care system is finally beginning to face the consequences of a problem rooted in centuries of social and legal tradition, it is also important for us to address the more difficult task of transforming gender socialization patterns and to recognize that gender equality is an essential component of primary prevention.

We also stretch the boundaries of the health care system when we work with the domestic violence advocacy and criminal justice systems. For example, many women are in danger at the time they seek health care, yet the danger itself is not something amenable to "medical" intervention. By becoming informed of options available in their communities for increasing women's safety, clinicians can help women get the services they need and begin to understand the complexity of their situations. Will a woman risk losing her children in a custody battle? Will she risk losing her means of providing for them? Will she risk losing someone she loves and who may act loving to her much of the time? Will she risk being killed if she leaves? A more comprehensive model provides a framework for understanding responses not only to trauma, but more significantly, to ongoing danger, and for mobilizing the social and legal resources that can increase safety, expand options, and ultimately prevent further violence.[39]

STRUCTURAL CONSTRAINTS

Health care providers also face a number of structural constraints that affect their ability to provide appropriate care to women dealing with ongoing abuse. In the current health care climate, cost containment is often achieved at the expense of care, and clinicians' needs are placed in conflict with patients' for access to diminishing resources.[40] This is a problem for primary care providers, who are often penalized for spending too much time with patients and for making too many referrals. This is even more problematic for patients, however, at a time when reimbursement for social and mental health services is rapidly diminishing.

Micromanagement strategies devised by insurance companies to reduce "unnecessary" mental health care utilization (e.g., continuous intrusive demands to justify treatment) can be disruptive and traumatic in themselves. They create an environment in which short-term medication management or potentially retraumatizing directive treatments focused on symptom reduction rather than healing are rapidly becoming the standard of care, making the consistency and safety required for long-term trauma recovery nonreimbursable. It is unfortunate that, just when an expanding body of research is clearly delineating the impact of trauma on the human psyche and the need for more intensive treatment for many survivors,[41] market forces are decreasing the likelihood that these kinds of services will be available. This becomes increasingly true as managed care further erodes the possibility of choosing one's provider and type of treatment, removing even the consumer-based economic power from individuals seeking care. For low-income women whose only access to services has been through the public mental health system, this lack of choice has been the norm.[42]

While providing short-term reductions in cost, these policies do not address the long-term personal, financial, and, ultimately, social costs of failing to provide appropriate intervention.[43] In this rapidly proliferating type of system, cost containment is seen only in terms of direct individual costs to a given health care corporation whereas the exponential but indirect personal and social costs that could be prevented by early intervention are not considered part of the relevant financial equation.

A diagnosis-driven reimbursement system poses yet another set of problems for battered women. In order for a woman to use mental health services, she has to be given a diagnosis. But for battered women, the very diagnosis itself may create new dangers.[44] Batterers often use their victims' psychiatric diagnoses to "prove" that they are right, that the problems are her fault, that she is crazy, or that she is an unfit mother. In seeking treatment, a battered woman potentially risks losing her children in custody battles and losing her credibility in court. For some women, "psychiatric" symptoms disappear once they are out of danger, but many women continue to be threatened and stalked long after they have left the relationship.[45] For others, symptoms of posttraumatic stress disorder may not begin until they are relatively safe.[46]

Women have been refused health insurance for having the pre-existing condition of being battered and disability or life insurance because they are considered at higher risk for injury and death.[47] In addition, if a woman is insured on her husband's policy and the bills are sent to him, she is likely to be placed in further jeopardy when he discovers she is seeking outside help.

In some states, laws that require mandatory reporting of domestic violence may again place the clinician's legal obligations in conflict with the wishes and the safety of his or her patients. Not only do these policies potentially destroy the ability of clinicians to provide a safe place for women to discuss their most pressing concerns, they violate women's rights to choose what they feel will be safest and most helpful to themselves and their children. Under these conditions, both clinicians and patients may avoid raising concerns about abuse, thus losing important opportunities to intervene.[48]

Listening to patients, learning about the repercussions of our interventions, and working to prevent systemic revictimization become important components of our roles as physicians practicing preventive medicine. Without a clear institutional commitment to address these issues, however, the pressures to continue practice as usual may be greater than the ability to change.

IMPLICATIONS FOR TRAINING AND PRACTICE

Experience has led many clinician-educators to realize that new training strategies must be developed in order to change attitudes and behavior on the scale that is required to address domestic violence.[49] Standard didactic formats, for example, do not provide sufficient opportunity to address the attitudes and feelings that may interfere with a clinician's ability to provide appropriate care, nor do they offer room to acquire the interviewing skills necessary for an optimal response. Training environments that offer the emotional safety to explore personal and cultural responses to abuse and the opportunities to discuss individual, professional, and institutional obstacles may also provide a vehicle for generating change within the health care community. While one-time trainings may raise awareness, ongoing feedback and support are necessary to sustain provider response.[50]

Providing quality health care involves integrating routine inquiry about domestic violence into ongoing clinical practice. This means asking all women patients, including women in lesbian relationships, about abuse and violence in their lives. Whether or not a woman chooses to use services or leave her partner, our intervention is very important. Women often return to violent partners many times before they feel safe enough to leave, feel that they can survive on their own, or can accept that the person they love will not change. When we fail to ask about abuse, we inadvertently isolate women who are living in danger.[51] Just by inquiring and expressing concern, we begin to build bridges, decrease isolation, and create hope. For a person who lives in an atmosphere of ongoing threats, intimidation, and violence, being treated with respect and taken seriously and feeling free to make her own choices lets her know supportive experiences are possible. By asking women to describe the pattern of their abuse and level of danger and to discuss their options for safety, we provide a place for women to reflect on their situations and consider their choices. By providing access to resources and by facilitating a woman's own decision-making process rather than attempting to direct her to change, we help her shift the balance of power in her life. When we work collaboratively with other members of our communities, we not only help individual women rebuild their lives, but also help change the conditions that allow domestic violence to exist.

In order for clinicians to develop and sustain appropriate responses to domestic violence, however, they must also have the support of the institutions in which they practice. Thus, addressing this issue requires some fundamental changes in the nature of most medical training and in the culture of medical institutions. Creating practice environments and policies that model nonabusive ways of interacting, that support clinicians' efforts to address complex issues with skill and compassion, and that reimburse the more labor-intensive tasks of listening and advocating for change, are important components of institutionalizing effective responses to domestic violence.[52] Refocusing our priorities is particularly important in the rapidly changing health care climate where administrators, insurers, and those who influence health care policy must begin to recognize that the long-term consequences of nonintervention far exceed the costs of investing in appropriate intervention and prevention.[53]

In addition, providers acting alone, no matter how motivated, cannot meet all the needs of battered women and their children. An optimal response requires the efforts of all members of the community. Developing interdisciplinary teams within the health care setting and creating collaborative partnerships between the domestic violence advocacy community, the health care system, the child protective system, and the legal system serves a number of functions. It not only provides referral networks for patients, but also creates support networks for providers. More important, it is only by working together that we can begin to develop the kinds of intervention strategies that will be appropriate for and respectful to all victims of domestic violence, while laying the groundwork to develop effective prevention strategies as well.

CONCLUSION

When we ask what battered women need from individual providers, we must also ask what providers need from their training institutions and practice environments in order to respond to those needs. When we do not address the denial of intolerable feelings at a personal level, we are in danger of recreating them not only in individual relationships, but also on social and political levels. Further, when socially sanctioned abuses of power are not acknowledged, they are often internalized and reproduced through individual interactions. If we truly want to play a role in preventing domestic violence, rather than just treating its consequences, we must work together to address the social conditions that create and support this kind of violence in the first place. A social structure sustained through abuse of power cannot end domestic violence. We know that. We need to use that knowledge.

NOTES

1. E. Stark and A. Flitcraft, "Violence among Intimates: An Epidemiologic Review," in *Handbook of Family Violence,* ed. V. N. Van Hasselt et al. (New York: Plenum, 1988), 293–317; D. Dossman et al., "Sexual and Physical Abuse in Women with Functional or Organic Gastrointestinal Disorders," *Ann. Intern. Med.* 113 (1990): 828–33; J. Domino and J. Haber, "Prior Physical and Sexual Abuse in Women with Chronic Headache: Clinical Correlates," *Headache* 27 (1987): 310–14; M. Koss and I. Heise, "Somatic Consequences of Violence against Women," *Ach. Fam. Med.* 1 (1992): 53–59; M. Koss et al., "Deleterious Effects of Criminal Victimization on Women's Health and Medical Utilization," *Ach. Intern. Med.* 151 (1991): 342–47; J. Fildes et al., "Trauma: The Leading Cause of Maternal Death," *J. Trauma* 32 (1992): 43–45; L. McKibben et al., "Victimization of Mothers of Abused Children: A Controlled Study," *Pediatrics* 84 (1989): 531–35; E. Stark and A. Flitcraft, "Women and Children at Risk: A Feminist Perspective on Child Abuse," *Int. J. Health Serv.* 18 (1988): 97–118; E. Stark and A. Flitcraft, "Killing the Beast Within: Woman Battering and Female Suicidality," *Int. J. Health Serv.* 25 (1995): 43–64; A. Jacobsen and B. Richardson, "Assault Experiences of 100 Psychiatric Inpatients: Evidence of the Need for Routine Inquiry," *Am. J. Psychiatry* 144 (1987): 908–13; L. S. Brown, "The Contribution of Victimization as a Risk Factor for the Development of Depressive Symptomatology in Women" (paper presented

at the 97th Annual Convention of the American Psychological Association, New Orleans, La., August 1989); J. A. Hamilton and M. Jensvold, "Personality, Psychopathology and Depression in Women," in *Personality and Psychopathology: Feminist Reappraisals,* ed. I. S. Brown and M. Ballou (New York: Guilford Press, 1992); J. Herman, *The Aftermath of Violence: from Domestic Abuse to Political Theory* (New York: Basic Books, 1992); B. M. Houskamp and D. Foy, "The Assessment of Posttraumatic Stress Disorder in Battered Women," *Journal of Interpersonal Violence* 6 (1991): 367–75; A. Kemp et al., "Post-traumatic Stress Disorder (PTSD) in Battered Women: A Shelter Sample," *Journal of Traumatic Stress* 4 (1991): 137–48; L. E. Walker, "Post-traumatic Stress Disorder in Women: Diagnosis and Treatment of Battered Woman Syndrome," *Psychotherapy* 28 (1991): 21–29; J. C. Campbell, "Battered Woman Syndrome: A Critical Review," *Violence Update* (December 1990): 1, 4, 10–11; J. C. Campbell, "Post-traumatic Stress in Battered Women: Does the Diagnosis Fit?" *Issues Ment. Health Nus.* 14 (1993): 173–86; C. R. Figley, "Posttraumatic Stress Disorder Part 2: Relationships with Various Traumatic Events," *Violence Update* (May 1992); C. Warshaw and S. Poirier, "Case and Commentary: Hidden Stories of Women," *Second Opinion* 17 (1991): 48–61.

2. Flitcraft et al., *Diagnostic and Treatment Guidelines on Domestic Violence* (Chicago: American Medical Association, 1992); C. Warshaw et al., *Improving the Health Care Response to Domestic Violence: A Resource Manual for Health Care Providers* (San Francisco: Family Violence Prevention Fund and Pennsylvania Coalition Against Domestic Violence, 1995); C. J. Scott and N. Matricciani, "Joint Commission on Accreditation of Health Care Organizations Standards to Improve Care for Victims of Abuse," *Md. Med. J.* 43 (1994): 891–98; W. K. Taylor and J. C. Campbell, "Treatment Protocols for Battered Women," *Response* (1992): 1–21; A. Flitcraft, "Commentary: Physicians and Domestic Abuse: Challenges for Prevention," *Health Aff.* 12 (1993): 156–61.
3. *Curricular Principles for Addressing Family Violence: Conference Report* (Oklahoma City, Okla.: Robert Wood Johnson Foundation, 1995); S. Hadley, "Working with Battered Women in the Emergency Department: A Model Program," *J. Emerg Nus.* 18 (1992): 18–23; C. Warshaw et al., "An Advocacy-Based Medical School Elective on Domestic Violence" (class offered at the National Conference on Cultural Competence and Women's Health, Curricular in Medical Education, Washington, D.C., October 1995).
4. Chambliss et al., "Domestic Violence: An Educational Imperative?" *Am. J. Obstet. Gynecol.* 172 (1995): 1035–38; I. S. Friedman et al., "Inquiry about Victimization Experiences: A Survey of Patient Preferences and Physician Practices," *Ach. Intern. Med.* 152 (1992): 1186–90; E. Gondolf, *Psychiatric Responses to Family Violence: Identifying and Confronting Neglected Danger* (Lexington, Mass.: Lexington Books, 1990).
5. N. K. Sugg and T. Inui, "Primary Care Physician's Response to Domestic Violence: Opening Pandora's Box," *JAMA* 267 (1991): 3157–60; D. H. Gremillion and G. Evins, "Why Don't Doctors Identify and Refer Victims of Domestic Violence?" *N. C. Med. J.* 55 (1994): 428–32; C. Warshaw, "Limitations of the Medical Model in the Care of Battered Women," *Gender and Society* 3 (1989): 506–17; id., "Domestic Violence Challenges to Medical Practice," *J. Women's Health* 2 (1993): 73–80.
6. Warshaw, "Domestic Violence."
7. H. A. Holtz et al., "Education about Domestic Violence in US and Canadian Medical Schools: 1987–88," *MMWR* 38 (1989): 17–19.
8. S. K. Burge, "Violence against Women as a Health Care Issue," *Fam. Med.* 21 (1989): 368–73; A. Kramer, "Attitudes of Emergency Nurses and Physicians about Women and Wife Beating: Implications for Emergency Care," *J. Emerg Nurs.* 19 (1993): 549, D. R. Langford, "Consortia: A Strategy for Improving the Provision of Health Care to Domestic Violence Survivors," *Response to the Victimization of Women and Children* 13 (1990): 7–18; N. S. Jecker, "Privacy Beliefs and the Violent Family: Extending the Ethical Argument for Physician Intervention," *JAMA* 269 (1993): 776–80; D. Kurz and E. Stark, "Not-so-Benign Neglect," in *Feminist Perspectives on Wife Abuse,* ed. K. Yllo and M. Bograd (Newbury Park, Calif.: Sage, 1988), 249–66.
9. M. Koss et al., *No Safe Haven: Male Violence against Women at Home, at Work and in the Community* (Washington, D.C.: American Psychological Association, 1994).
10. K. Johnson, *Treating Ourselves: The Complete Guide to Emotional Well-Being for Women* (New York: Atlantic Monthly Press, 1990).
11. L. S. Brown, "A Feminist Critique of Personality Disorders," in *Personality and Psychopathology: Feminist Reappraisals,* ed. L. S. Brown and M. Ballou (New York: Guilford Press, 1992).
12. P. Rieker and E. Carmen, "The Victim-to-Patient Process: The Disconfirmation and Transformation of Abuse," *Am. J. Orthopsychiatry* 56 (1986): 360–70.
13. A. Miller, *Prisoners of Childhood: The Drama of the Gifted Child and the Search for the True Self* (New York: Basic Books, 1981); id., *Thou Shalt Not Be Aware: Society's Betrayal of the Child* (New York: Farrar, Straus & Giroux, 1984).
14. Rieker and Carmen, "The Victim-to-Patient Process"; Miller, *Prisoners of Childhood*; Miller, *Thou Shalt Not Be Aware.*
15. Herman, *Trauma and Recovery*; M. A. Dutton, *Empowering and Healing the Battered Woman: A Model for Assessment and Intervention* (New York: Springer,

1992); M. Koss, "The Women's Mental Health Research Agenda: Violence against Women," *Am Psychol.* 45 (1990); 374–80; L. Goldman et al., *American Medical Association Diagnostic and Treatment Guidelines on Mental Health Effects of Family Violence* (Chicago: American Medical Association, 1995).

16. Sugg and Inui, "Primary Care Physician's Response to Domestic Violence."
17. Warshaw, "Domestic Violence"; Koss et al., *No Safe Haven*; Johnson, *Treating Ourselves*; Brown, "A Feminist Critique of Personality Disorders."
18. Warshaw, "Domestic Violence."
19. P. Williamson et al., "Beliefs That Foster Physician Avoidance of Psychosocial Aspects of Health Care," *J. Fam. Pract.* 13 (1981): 999–1003; R. Fox, "Training in Caring Competence: The Perennial Problem in North American Medical Education," in *Education: Competent and Humane Physicians,* ed. H. C. Hendrie and C. Lloyd (Bloomington, Ind.: Indiana University Press, 1990), 199–216.
20. Warshaw, "Domestic Violence"; Williamson et al., "Beliefs That Foster Physician Avoidance of Psychosocial Aspects of Health Care."
21. J. A. Richman et al., "Mental Health Consequences and Correlates of Reported Medical Student Abuse," *JAMA* 167 (1992): 692–94.
22. D. Baldwin et al., "Student Perceptions of Mistreatment and Harassment during Medical School: A Survey of Ten United States Schools," *Western J. Med.* 155 (1991): 140–45.
23. T. M. Wolf et al., "Perceived Mistreatment and Attitude Change by Graduating Medical Students: A Retrospective Study," *Med. Educ.* 25 (1991): 182–89.
24. Warshaw, "Domestic Violence"; Richman et al., "Mental Health Consequences and Correlates of Reported Medical Student Abuse."
25. Richman et al., "Mental Health Consequences and Correlates of Reported Medical Student Abuse"; Baldwin et al., "Student Perceptions of Mistreatment and Harassment during Medical School: A Survey of Ten United States Schools"; Wolf et al., "Perceived Mistreatment and Attitude Change by Graduating Medical Students: A Retrospective Study"; M. Schiffman and E. Frank, "Harassment of Women Physicians," *JAMWA* 50 (1995): 207–11; D. A. Charney and R. C. Russell, "An Overview of Sexual Harassment," *Am. J. Psychiatry* 151 (1994): 10–17; M. Komaromy et al., "Sexual Harassment in Medical Training," *N. Engl. J. Med.* 328 (1993): 322–36.
26. Warshaw, "Domestic Violence"; Kurz and Stark, "Not-so-Benign Neglect": Koss et al., *No Safe Haven*; Johnson, *Treating Ourselves*; Brown, "A Feminist Critique of Personality Disorders"; Fox, "Training in Caring Competence": C. S. Widom, "Does Violence Beget Violence: A Critical Examination of the Literature," *Psych. Bull.* 106 (1989): 437–47.
27. K. Johnson and E. Hoffman, "Women's Health and Curriculum Transformation: The Role of Medical Specialization," in *Reframing Women's Health: Multidisciplinary Research and Practice,* ed A. Dan (Thousand Oaks, Calif.: Sage, 1994), 27–39.
28. M. Cohen et al., "Prevalence of Domestic Violence in Women with HIV" (paper presented at the Midwest Society of General Internal Medicine, Chicago, October 1995); K. Rothenberg et al., "Domestic Violence and Partner Notification: Implications for Treatment and Counseling of Women with HIV," *JAMWA* 50 (1905): 87–93.
29. Rothenberg et al., "Domestic Violence and Partner Notification: Implications for Treatment and Counseling of Women with HIV."
30. Stark and Flitcraft, "Violence among Intimates."
31. Cohen et al., "Prevalence of Domestic Violence in Women with HIV"; Rothenberg et al., "Domestic Violence and Partner Notification: Implications for Treatment and Counseling of Women with HIV"; V. Breitbert et al., "Model Programs Addressing Perinatal Drug Exposure and HIV Infection: Integrating Women's and Children's Needs," *Bull. N. Y. Acad. Med.* 71 (1994): 236–51.
32. Miller, *Thou Shalt Not Be Aware*; G. Atwood and R. Stolorow, *Structures of Subjectivity: Explorations in Psychoanalytic Phenomenology* (Hillsdale, N.J.: The Analytic Press, 1984); L. Brown, *Subversive Dialogues: Theory in Feminist Therapy* (New York: Basic Books, 1994).
33. S. Andersen et al., "Psychological Maltreatment of Spouses," in *Case Studies in Family Violence,* ed. R. Ammerman and M. Hersen (New York: Plenum, 1991): 293–328.
34. L. Walker, "The Battered Woman Syndrome," in *Family Abuse and Its Consequences,* ed. G. T. Hotaling et al. (Beverly Hills, Calif.: Sage, 1988), 139–48.
35. Brown, "A Feminist Critique of Personality Disorders"; M. Bograd, "Family Systems Approaches to Wife Battering: A Feminist Critique," *Am. J. Orthopsychiatry* 54 (1984): 558–68.
36. A. Jones and S. Schechter, *When Love Goes Wrong: What To Do When You Can't Do Anything Right* (New York: Harper, 1993); A. Ganley, "Understanding Domestic Violence," in *Improving the Health Care Response to Domestic Violence: A Resource Manual for Health Care Providers,* ed. C. Warshaw et al. (San Francisco: Family Violence Prevention Fund and Pennsylvania Coalition against Domestic Violence, 1995), 15–45.
37. Miller, *Prisoners of Childhood.*
38. A. Brown, "Violence, Poverty, and Minority Races in the Lives of Women and Children: Implications for

Violence Prevention," Bridging Science and Program Centers for Disease Control Violence Prevention Conference, Des Moines, Iowa, October 1995.

39. Jones and Schechter, *When Loves Goes Wrong*; Ganley, "Understanding Domestic Violence."

40. S. Woodhandler and D. Himmelstein, "Extreme Risk—The New Corporate Proposition for Physicians," *New England Journal of Medicine* 33 (1995): 1706–8; S. Glied and S. Kofman, *Women and Mental Health Reform* (New York: Commission on Women's Health, Commonwealth Fund, 1995).

41. L. Mellman and R. Bell, "Consequences of Violence against Women," in *Violence Against Women in the United States: A Comprehensive Background Paper* (New York: The Commonwealth Fund Commission on Women's Health, 1995), 33–40; L. Innes and L. Mellman, "Treatment for Victims of Violence," in *Violence Against Women in the United States: A Comprehensive Background Paper* (New York: The Commonwealth Fund Commission on Women's Health, 1995), 41–54.

42. E. Carmen, "Inner City Community Mental Health: The Interplay of Abuse and Race in Chronically Mentally Ill Women," in *Mental Health, Racism, and Sexism,* eds. C. Willie, B. Kramer, and B. Brown (Pittsburgh: University of Pittsburgh, 1995).

43. T. Miller, M. Cohen, et al. *Crime in the United States: Victim Cases and Consequences* (Washington, D.C.: National Institute of Justice, 1995).

44. Warshaw, "Domestic Violence."

45. Walker, "The Battered Woman Syndrome"; Jones and Schechter, *When Love Goes Wrong*; Ganley, "Understanding Domestic Violence."

46. Warshaw, "Domestic Violence"; Burge, "Violence against Women as a Health Care Issue."

47. Women's Law Project and Pennsylvania Coalition against Domestic Violence, *Insurance Discrimination against Victims of Domestic Violence* (Harrisburg: Pennsylvania Coalition against Domestic Violence, 1995); L. Kaiser, *Survey of Accident and Health and Life Insurance Relating to Insurance Coverage for Victims of Domestic Violence* (Harrisburg: Commonwealth of Pennsylvania, Pennsylvania Insurance Department, 1995).

48. A. Hymes, D. Schillinger, and B. Lo, "Laws Mandating Reporting of Domestic Violence: Do They Promote Patient Well-Being?" *JAMA* 272 (1995): 1781–87.

49. Warshaw et al., *Improving the Health Care Response to Domestic Violence: Curricular Principles for Addressing Family Violence*; Hadley, "Working with Battered Women in the Emergency Department"; S. McLean, "Education Is Not Enough: A Systems Failure in Protecting Battered Women," *Annals of Emergency Medicine* 18 (1989): 651–53.

50. Warshaw et al., *Improving the Health Care Response to Domestic Violence*; McLean, "Education Is Not Enough: A Systems Failure in Protecting Battered Women."

51. Jones and Schechter, *When Loves Goes Wrong.*

52. Warshaw et al., *Improving the Health Care Response to Domestic Violence: Curricular Principles for Addressing Family Violence.*

53. Warshaw et al., *Improving the Health Care Response to Domestic Violence: Curricular Principles for Addressing Family Violence.*

CHAPTER 13

Bioethical Dilemmas in Emergency Medicine and Prehospital Care

Kenneth V. Iserson

Emergency medicine is at once the oldest and the newest of medical specialties. Stemming from the aid given to injured comrades from time immemorial, the modern domain of emergency medicine describes care that is given in hospital emergency departments (EDs), urgent-care centers, and areas outside of medical facilities via ambulance and medically trained flight crews (prehospital care). Emergency medical practitioners, physicians, nurses, and prehospital personnel not only face the traditional ethical dilemmas but also newer ethical dilemmas stemming both from these practitioners' added responsibilities in the health treatment system and from the unique nature of emergency medical care.

The relatively new ethical dilemmas that emergency medical practitioners face stem both from the changing nature of the health treatment system and alterations in the technical practice of medicine. The United States health treatment systems increasingly fail to meet the needs of the medically indigent, and EDs have attempted to take up this slack; however, they often lack resources to perform both this task and their primary task of treating the acutely ill and injured. Eight key ethical dilemmas face emergency medical practitioners. These are, how to

- continue to care for the critically ill and injured while also acting as a medical safety net for the medically indigent;
- best advocate for their patients who are in managed care systems;
- aggressively treat critical patients and yet not be paternalistic toward those who can participate in their own health care decisions;
- respond to failed physician-assisted suicides;
- preserve patient autonomy while implementing prehospital advance directives;
- keep emergency medical providers safe while not ignoring their patients;
- respect both the living and the dead and yet keep current in necessary lifesaving skills;
- ethically perform research to advance the entire field of emergency care while safeguarding patients.

Each of these topics will be discussed in more detail below.

SAFETY NET

The United States health treatment system is in shambles and EDs have been described as the system's *safety net.*[1] Medically indigent patients who often cannot access the United States health treatment system in any other way, do so through the ED.[2] EDs have taken up this slack, but they often lack the resources to perform both this task and their primary task of treating the acutely ill and injured. This poses a significant dilemma: whether to skimp on emergency medicine's primary duty to treat the acutely ill and injured, or to provide a major source of care to medically indigent patients.

In the main, EDs still try to do both tasks. At the profession's edge, however, and gaining ground quickly, are emergency physicians who advocate turning away patients who seem to have minor complaints.[3] While triage, the sorting and prioritizing of patient treatment by the seriousness of their illness, is a common practice in all EDs, they have traditionally never refused treatment to people who come seeking their help. As is clear to anyone who has gone to an ED on a Friday or Saturday night, however, the wait for care for a nonemergent condition may be lengthy. In some instances, to speed the process and save resources, patients with minor complaints are seen in adjacent clinics, rather than in the ED. Yet all patients receive evaluation and, where appropriate, treatment.[4]

Recently, however, a new trend is taking hold—refusing treatment. Some EDs now refuse treatment to patients who present with what are considered minor problems. Rather than being sent to adjacent clinics, they are simply given phone numbers for clinics where they can try to make appointments to be seen. Researchers have shown that most of these patients will never see a health care provider for their problems. While some of these problems pose serious health risks, others are self-resolving or so minimal that any delay in care is not deleterious. What then is the dilemma?

Emergency medicine, in all of its manifestations, has been held out to the American public over the past two decades as an unfailing source of medical treatment at any time and for any problem. Practitioners are reneging on this promise.[5] The EDs refusing care are not those in the posh suburbs, but those in the crowded inner cities where the greatest percentage of medically indigent people reside. Yet, changes in health care treatment systems have produced a value conflict between refusing medical treatment to those seeking care (often in EDs as their last resort) or supplying EDs with enough resources to both act as a safety net and continue to treat the acutely ill or injured.[6]

Paradoxically, as EDs see increasing numbers of patients for a wider spectrum of problems (many nonemergent), they are being seen as a convenient site to access socially underserved populations. Emergency medical personnel are being castigated for not providing general medical screenings, preventive care, and public medical education programs. Social problems are being "medicalized" to put the onus of the remedy for multifactorial problems on medicine—and increasingly on emergency medicine. In part, this is due to the crumbling of our social supports; in part it is due to confusion about how to solve some serious social ills. With its scientific basis, our culture expects medicine to scientifically solve all problems (except, perhaps, increasing costs). The ethical dilemma facing emergency medicine is whether to assume these roles and dilute (or change) their primary mission, or to take a hard line and ignore these ills—as have most others in our society.

EMERGENCY MEDICINE AND MANAGED CARE

Managed care organizations (MCOs) continue to devour ever more of the health care market. And, while claims abound that physician self-interest drove medical testing and treatment under the fee-for-service system, most physicians had at least the patina of patient welfare guiding their actions (and for most, this was their primary motivator). Although MCO supporters claim idealistic motivations (which may have been true for some long-established MCOs), most must now concede that their primary loyalty is to their stockholders/owners, to whom they owe a fiduciary responsibility. In theory and in practice, patients come (a distant) second. Nowhere is this felt more acutely than in the ED, where patients are routinely deprived (payment for) treatment by the MCOs' "gatekeepers." For many individuals, this effectively denies them treatment, since they can ill-afford to pay any ED bill they may incur. MCOs also cause patient and family hardships by requiring transfers to other hospitals for admission. To say that patients "bought into" the MCO system denies the fact that it is usually their employers, rather than they, who choose the plan and provided services.

Emergency physicians have an ethical responsibility to advocate for their patients in every possible manner. This includes providing mechanisms for patients to personally and immediately challenge gatekeepers' decisions (by calling the MCO's medical director at home, for example); by taking a hard line, when it is in the patient's best interest, on the "patient stability" criteria mandated by federal law for interhospital transfers; and by demanding that gatekeepers take personal and professional responsibility for their telephonic decisions (such as requiring that they actually exam ED patients if they disagree with the on-site emergency physician about whether to discharge a patient).[7] These situations will not go away, and will, in fact, increase as MCOs face stiffer competition, regulation, and financial pressures. As the only independent advocate for many of these patients, emergency physicians must steer a firm moral course by strongly and consistently working in their patients' best interests.

PATERNALISM

The major resource in emergency medical care is time. The time an ED's limited personnel allocate to any patient is a lost resource; the split-second decisions they make are often immutable. Time pressures to make critical decisions are nowhere as intense or as constant as in emergency medicine. This constant pressure to maximally use time and resources combined often with critically ill or injured patients who lack decision-making capacity frequently imbues emergency medical practice with paternalism. This paternalistic attitude may put practitioners' values and their patients' desire to exercise autonomy in direct conflict.

Emergency medicine in its most basic form, seen during wars and disasters, is one provider's making an immediate decision about who gets treatment and who is allowed to die. In the common hospital and prehospital scenario, this translates into immediate unilateral decisions about intervening to save lives or limbs with tubes, fluids, medications, electrical shocks, and surgery. These practitioners' actions are generally desired and beneficial, rather than paternalistic. Patients want and expect aggressive and immediate action by emergency medical teams. Too easily, however, especially given medicine's (and nursing's) traditional attitudes, this transforms into paternalism toward the non–critically ill patient. ED and prehospital patients commonly complain that "things are done to them" without prior discussion or acquiescence once they enter the emergency medical system. Significantly, these "things" often commit patients to large expenses for tests or procedures. In cases where patients lack decision-making capacity and patient benefit can be expected from the medical team's actions, aggressive intervention is not only reasonable, it is essential. Transferring this attitude to other patients who maintain decision-making capacity is what causes problems.

Paternalism can also arise in the guise of "futility." In emergency medicine and prehospital care, two questions are closely linked: What constitutes futility for the emergency patient? And when should life-sustaining measures be withheld or withdrawn? As advanced cardiopulmonary life support and newer techniques in trauma resuscitation increase practitioners' capacity to extend biological life, the patient benefits remain uncertain. Yet few guidelines exist to aid either prehospital or ED practitioners in deciding to abandon therapeutic interventions other than their lack of success in a "reasonable" amount of time. Prehospital advance directive orders are, unfortunately, still rarely seen. The clinicians are, therefore, usually forced to make unilateral decisions about further care—often paternalistically giving unwanted treatments.

ASSISTED SUICIDES AND EMERGENCY DEPARTMENT RESUSCITATIONS

As assisted suicide laws spread throughout the United States, experience shows that the number of partial or failed suicides will increase—perhaps dramatically. Will this change the role of the entire emergency medical services (EMS), and of emergency physicians in particular? At present, all emergency medical personnel operate under the general rule to, when in doubt, preserve life. This rule stems from their frequent lack of information about the patient, circumstances surrounding the incident bringing the patient to the ED, and any wishes or values the patient may have. (This precipitated the introduction of prehospital advance directives (PHADs), discussed elsewhere in this chapter.)

This rule includes committing to psychiatric hospitals those patients who pose a danger to themselves. While this is, in fact, at odds with patient autonomy, both legal and ethical thought agree that protecting suicidal patients is a necessary, if sometimes perverse, medical function. In other settings, where physicians (and sometimes EMS through a PHAD or prehospital do not resuscitate [PHDNR] order) know that a patient does not want resuscitation, they generally follow these wishes.[8] Yet, how will they behave when the need for resuscitation was caused by the patient? What if there is an underlying condition that also precipitated signing a PHAD? (Patients without a serious medical illness generally will not fall under current assisted-suicide statutes, although whether or not they have such a condition may be difficult for EMS or ED personnel to initially determine.) Sporadic cases have already appeared in the bioethics literature.[9] They indicate that another complicating factor may be interference (perhaps self-motivated) from the physician who prescribed the almost-lethal drugs. Emergency medical personnel may well be caught between several very unacceptable options—maximal resuscitative efforts, no resuscitative efforts, or providing temporizing measures while gathering information.

The only indication of how emergency physicians will respond was an Oregon study, suggesting that many emergency physicians will abstain from aggressively resuscitating such patients only if they have clear proof that the patients desired and tried to die.[10] In itself, this should markedly increase the use of PHADs by terminally ill patients.

Until this issue can be analyzed and discussed and an ethically rational policy can be set, most emergency physicians will undoubtedly continue to attempt to preserve life, when possible—leaving the details to be sorted out when time permits.

PREHOSPITAL ADVANCE DIRECTIVES vs. PREHOSPITAL DNR ORDERS

Virtually all EMS systems have a rule that ambulance personnel, if called to the scene of a patient in cardiac arrest, must attempt resuscitation unless it is physiologically futile (generally meaning rigor mortis, decomposition, burned beyond recognition, or other situations incompatible with life). Over the past decade, an increasing number of systems have adopted rules or state laws whereby patients (or their surrogates) can plan to *not* have resuscitation if an ambulance is erroneously requested. Ethicists and emergency medical personnel have jointly helped to eliminate the tragedy of unwanted resuscitations through the development of PHADs. A danger, however, has arisen.

While some states have successfully maintained patient autonomy by using patient- or surrogate-initiated PHADs, others have rigidly attempted to preserve physician prerogatives by changing the nature of these laws and rules to mimic in-hospital DNR orders.[11] While PHDNR orders must be requested by (or at least discussed with) patients or their surrogate decision makers, physicians must approve and sign the orders.[12] This eliminates patients' autonomous decisions for what is perhaps the most important decision of their life—deciding how they will die.

Although initially the laws and EMS rules governing PHDNR orders stemmed from concerns about the misuse of and possible criminal activity using patient-initiated forms, experience with patient-initiated PHADs has shown that these concerns are unwarranted. Although physicians espouse patient autonomy, the widespread and continued use of primarily physician-initiated PHDNR rules belies this attitude.

Emergency medicine has three significant issues regarding prehospital directives: increasing the locales where these programs are available, increasing patient awareness of these programs, and ensuring that patient autonomy is preserved.

PROVIDER SAFETY AND SECURITY

Increasingly, EMS and ED health care providers must concern themselves with safety issues. Gang-related and other violent individuals no longer think of the EMS and ED as sanctuaries or "neutral zones" but rather, as sources of additional victims. Ethical dilemmas arise when the provider's desire to be beneficent conflicts with the innate need to be safe. This starts with access to the system. Should EMS personnel enter unsecured (no police) scenes to provide aid to victims of violence, or wait and possibly jeopardize their patients' well-being?[13] Similar, but not as obvious, are the restrictions on ED entry (or entering the patient-care areas) that are now much more common than in the past. Self-preservation can be justified both because it is a natural instinct that professionalism does not abolish and because the EM health provider is a valuable societal resource that should not be frivolously endangered.

The underlying theme here is that EM personnel must guard their own safety first. This includes not "playing cop" in the ED with violent patients. (Such behavior also distorts their roles, so that patients see them as security guards and may no longer willingly trust them as physicians.)

Next, emergency medical practitioners must protect their teams. As leaders, they must, whenever possible, safeguard their coworkers' well-being by actually preventing them from putting themselves in harm's way. Only once that is accomplished may emergency medical providers protect their patients.[14] Ideally, this situation rarely arises, but in a crisis, the ethics of resource conservation, if nothing else, dictates this order of priorities.

PRACTICING AND TEACHING ON THE NEWLY DEAD

The public demands and expects all emergency practitioners to be skilled in critical lifesaving skills and to teach these skills to new practitioners. The most efficient and practical way for them to remain proficient in these sometimes little-used, technically difficult skills is for them to practice and teach on the newly dead.

For many years, physicians learned technical skills such as intubation and central-line placement on patients who had recently died. Recently, however, it has been suggested that postmortem procedures are only permissible if prior consent is obtained from relatives. This position, though, ignores the nature of and purpose for informed consent, contravenes patient altruism, and disregards society's interest in having an optimal number of medical care providers experienced in lifesaving techniques.[15]

The process of obtaining informed consent stems from the concepts of patient autonomy and ultimately, a respect for others. In theory, the process increases communication between the physician and patient prior to dangerous, disfiguring, or seriously invasive procedures. Requiring prior consent by emergency medical personnel to practice or teach lifesaving procedures on the newly dead misapplies informed consent and misrepresents the concept of patient autonomy.

The dead, of course, have no autonomy claim. Autonomy, based on the principles of freedom and liberty, is a function of personhood. But the dead are no longer persons, although by societal consent they can still implement their wishes for the disposition of their bodies through advance directives or a legal will—neither of which are normally available in the ED. Nevertheless, the former patients' wishes should be respected, which generally means respecting an altruism not found as readily in their relatives.[16] The relatives' "quasiproperty rights" to a corpse are strictly limited and do not give relatives either moral or legal authority to counteract stronger competing claims.

Society also has a substantial interest. That interest is to maintain an optimal number of ED and EMS personnel proficient in lifesaving procedures. The medical professions recognize that both primary instruction and continued practice is necessary for proficiency in lifesaving skills. This instruction and practice is best done on fresh cadavers, since the available alternatives are not adequate. But while they recognize that unreasonable barriers to this training should not exist, there should be some limits. These limits should include the respectful treatment of the body, limiting the training to those who must use these procedures, and eliminating from use any corpses where the person had an available document declining use as a organ or tissue donor or obviously from a culture that does not permit this.

Alternatives to using fresh cadavers are inadequate—or dangerous. Although models, animals, and donated embalmed cadavers are useful ways to learn or practice some aspects of critical-care techniques, they poorly simulate the critical patient. The use of animals, aside from being logistically ever more difficult, is itself ethically problematic. Donated, preserved cadavers are less realistic, are expensive, and have limited availability. Models have been shown to have even less utility.[17] (In two decades, we will use virtual reality models for this training at larger training centers, and this discussion will be moot.) The commonly used alternatives are to use patients who are undergoing anesthesia for this teaching or to prolong resuscitations beyond the point where the clinicians know it to be futile so that procedures can be done.[18]

If a legal or ethical requirement exists for consent prior to postmortem ED instruction, it decreases the number of clinical personnel trained in lifesaving procedures. A need to request this permission from distraught relatives raises significant emotional barriers for clinicians to overcome in order to practice and teach the procedures. In a survey of medical personnel involved in organ harvesting, a dislike of "adding to relatives' distress by asking permission for donation" was the single biggest barrier to organ procurement.[19] This barrier is unlikely to be breached, especially for the seemingly more trivial request to teach or practice procedures. Any impediment is further compounded by the stringent time limitations imposed by the onset of rigor mortis, by the rapid transport of bodies to the morgue, and by the press of duties for the ED staff once a resuscitation attempt has ended.

In summary, patient autonomy plays an appropriate and vital role in keeping modern medicine from overstepping individual interests. However, its inappropriate extension to requiring consent for ED postmortem practice and teaching cannot be justified. The concept of autonomy would not be advanced, and future patients, the medical profession, and society would be harmed.[20]

RESEARCH UNDER UNUSUAL CIRCUMSTANCES

Lastly, emergency medicine cannot remain static. If it is to progress, research on the treatment of critical patients in the prehospital arena and the EDs is necessary. The outcome of this research will be beneficial to society. Yet, societal strictures on informed consent prohibit much of this work.[21]

Research in acute care is a troubling area for institutional review board (IRB) approval and informed consent. Confusion about ethical and legal requirements has hampered research efforts and subsequent patient benefits. These critical, acute care patients seen commonly in EDs and prehospital care are the relatively few patients who have suffered unexpected events that carry a high probability of mortality or severe morbidity unless immediate medical intervention is provided. Due to the lack of substantive research on their medical and surgical problems and the difficulty in implementing research protocols, thousands of individuals receive at best untested, and at worst inappropriate care each day in the United States. They deserve better. Acute-care research can be implemented more widely and still satisfy both bureaucratic mandates and the ethical requirements to protect patients and research subjects.

It has been previously argued that acute-care research is justified if the usual ethical requirements for research are modified to reflect the uniqueness of the situation. The recommendations are to (1) use an explicit definition of acute care as distinct from other modes of critical care, (2) eliminate the requirement for informed consent (as usually understood), and (3) require stringent IRB oversight regarding the unique ethical problems raised by this research. It has been further suggested that IRB oversight include review of the protocol by a panel of individuals who represent possible enrollees in the proposed study.[22]

Toward the end of 1996 the National Institutes of Health (NIH), Food and Drug Administration (FDA), and similar governmental agencies loosened a few of their restrictions on critical care research. Consequently, this caused a significant lag time until vital research could be designed, approved, funded, evaluated, published, and disseminated to benefit critical patients. But at least the first steps have been taken.

OTHER TROUBLESOME AREAS

Although the dilemmas described above epitomize some of emergency medicine's unique ethical conundrums, many other ethical dilemmas exist. Daily, emergency medicine practitioners face the question of whether to override patient autonomy when they question a patient's decision-making capacity. Not only must they base their decisions on little information, in the prehospital arena this must be done by physician extenders (EMS personnel) with variable amounts of education and experience and under the worst possible conditions.

In the ED, the basic beneficent value of alleviating pain runs up against two other values—to patients' detriment. The physicians' stricture against doing harm keeps adequate analgesia from many patients who are suspected of "drug-seeking" behavior. This includes many patients with migraines and back pain, and some with kidney stones (all classic complaints of drug seekers). Of course, the majority of patients with these complaints are only seeking relief for an acute problem. Similarly treated, but for different reasons, are patients who need pain relief before they are taken to operating or procedure rooms. Many physicians want the patient to be coherent rather than comfortable when they sign an operative or procedure permit. Therefore, many of these same patients wait hours without adequate analgesia, especially those with fractures and abdominal catastrophes requiring surgery, due to an ethical (or more likely legal) necessity for the patient's signature on an operative permit.

One other dilemma commonly faces emergency physicians, for which there does not seem to be an adequate answer. In most clinical situations, a patient's decision-making capacity is easily determined. If there is a question, clinicians test the patient's understanding.[23] There is a significant question about decision-making capacity under the severe stress of an acute and unexpected illness, compounded by the strange surroundings of the ED. Patient autonomy governs much of modern United States biomedical ethics. It is unclear, however, what it takes to be autonomous in crisis. The patient gasping for breath who refuses intubation, the acquired immune deficiency syndrome (AIDS) patient who at the last moment verbally changes a well-thought-out advance directive, or the patient agreeing to take a risky medication or undergo a major operative procedure under these circumstances may be exhibiting panic behavior rather than autonomy in any accepted sense. Even in these scenarios, many patients continue to want to make their own health care decisions.[24] Is this appropriate? We just do not know.

NOTES

1. American College of Emergency Physicians, "American College of Emergency Physicians: Emergency Care Guidelines," *Ann. Emerg. Med.* 20 (1991): 1389–95.

2. K. V. Iserson and T. Kastre, "Are Emergency Departments a 'Safety Net' for the Medically Indigent?" *Am J. Emerg. Med.* 14, no. 1 (1996): 1–5.

3. R. W. Derlet et al., "Triage of Patients Out of the ED: Three Year Experience," *Am. J. Emerg. Med.* 10 (1992): 195–99.
4. T. A. Schmidt et al., "Ethics of ED Triage: ASEM Position Statement," *Acad. Emerg. Med.* 2 (1995): 990–95.
5. K. V. Iserson, "Assessing Values: Rationing ED Care," *Am. J. Emerg. Med.* 10 (1992): 263–64; *id.,* "Limits of Health Care Resources," *Am. J. Emerg. Med.* 10 (1992): 588–92.
6. R. K. Knopp et al., "An Ethical Foundation for Health Care: An Emergency Medicine Perspective," *Ann. Emerg. Med.* 21 (1992): 1381–87.
7. Schmidt et al., "Ethics of ED Triage."
8. R. Byock, "A Slight Postmortem Disagreement," in *Ethics in Emergency Medicine,* 2d ed., ed. K. V. Iserson et al. (Tucson, Ariz.: Galen Press, 1995), 80–87.
9. K. V. Iserson et al., "Willful Death and Painful Decisions: A Failed Assisted Suicide," *Cambridge Quart.* 1, no. 2 (1992): 147–58.
10. T. A Schmidt, "Oregon Emergency Physicians' Experiences, Attitudes, and Concerns about Physician-Assisted Suicide," abstract in *Acad. Emerg. Med.* 3, no. 5 (1996): 490.
11. K. V. Iserson, "A Simplified Prehospital Advance Directive Law: Arizona's Approach," *Ann. Emerg. Med.* 22, no. 11 (1993): 1703–10.
12. K. V. Iserson, "If We Don't Learn from History . . . : Ethical Failings in a New Prehospital Directive," *Am. J. Emerg. Med.* 13, no. 2 (1995): 241–42.
13. R. A. Lazar, "Prehospital Personnel's Safety vs. A Duty to Treat," in *Ethics in Emergency Medicine,* 2d ed., ed. K. V. Iserson et al. (Tucson, Ariz.: Galen Press, 1995), 412–16.
14. K. V. Iserson, "Ethics of Wilderness Medicine" in *Wilderness Medicine: Management of Wilderness and Environmental Emergencies,* 3d ed., ed. P. Auerbach (St. Louis: Mosby, 1995), 1436–46.
15. K. V. Iserson, "Postmortem Procedures in the ED: Using the Recently Dead to Practice and Teach," *J. Med. Ethics* 19 (1993): 92–98; id., "Life versus Death: Exposing a Misapplication of Ethical Reasoning," *J. Clin. Ethics* 5, no. 3 (1994): 261–64; id., "Law versus Life: The Ethical Imperative to Practice and Teach Using the Newly Dead ED Patient," *Ann. Emerg. Med.* 25, no. 1 (1995): 91–94.
16. R. M. Oswalt, "A Review of Blood Donor Motivation and Recruitment," *Transfusion* 17 (1977): 123–35; A. Spital and M. Spital, "Living Donation: Attitudes outside the Transplant Center," *Arch. Int. Med.* 148 (1988): 1077–80.
17. R. D. Stewart et al., "Effect of Varied Training Techniques on Field Endotracheal Intubation Success Rates," *Ann. Emerg. Med.* 13 (1984): 1032–36.
18. K. V. Iserson, *Death to Dust: What Happens to Dead Bodies?* (Tucson, Ariz.: Galen Press, 1994), 98.
19. R. E. Wakeford and R. Stepney, "Obstacles to Organ Donation," *Br. J. Surg.* 76 (1989): 435–39.
20. K. V. Iserson, "Requiring Consent to Practice and Teach Using the Recently Dead," *J. Emerg. Med.* 9, no. 6 (1991): 509–10.
21. K. V. Iserson and D. L. Lindsey, "Research on Critically Ill and Injured Patients: Rules, Reality, and Ethics," *J. Emerg. Med.* 13, no. 4 (1995): 563–67.
22. K. V. Iserson and M. Mahowald, "Acute Care Research: Is It Ethical?" *Crit. Care Med.* 20 (1992): 1032–37.
23. A. E. Buchanan, "The Question of Competence," in *Ethics in Emergency Medicine,* 2d ed., ed. K. V. Iserson et al. (Tucson, Ariz.: Galen Press, 1995), 61–65.
24. A. Davis et al., "Impact of Patient Acuity on Patient Preference for Medical Decision-Making Autonomy and Information," abstract in *Acad. Emerg. Med.* 3, no. 5 (1996): 491.

CHAPTER 14

High-Technology Home Care: Critical Issues and Ethical Choices

Allen I. Goldberg, Eveline A. M. Faure, and John J. O'Callaghan

This chapter highlights and explores critical issues and ethical choices facing those concerned about high-technology home care (HTHC). The discussion focuses on medically fragile, technology-dependent (MF/TD) children.

The intended audiences of this chapter include:

1. health care consumers: patients and families, employers, and other purchasers of health care services;
2. health care, educational, social service professionals and all service providers participating within integrated community delivery systems of care;
3. public policy experts and agencies; managed care organizations and other sources of health care funding associated with a new phase of health and social service delivery: managed care.

This chapter is structured to accomplish the following intended outcomes:

1. Assess the past: Understand *the past* background of issues resulting from the creation of the initial and subsequent populations of medically fragile/technology-dependent children who required HTHC
2. Analyze the present: Describe the complexity of *the present* concerns of parents, professionals, and organizations involved in providing services to meet the health care, psychosocial, educational, and developmental requirements of these children with special needs
3. Apply for the future: Consider ethical issues and choices to plan for *the future* strategies to develop and manage comprehensive/integrated approaches for these children/families who require HTHC that will consider ethical choices and operate within the framework of managed care.

INTRODUCTION AND BACKGROUND

All peoples of the world face rapidly growing health care expenditures that compete for restricted resources that are needed for other political, social, and economic priorities. This demand for increasing health finance confronts industrial nations responding to global market pressures and changing societal forces as well as developing countries and former Communist nations undergoing economic transformation. Rapid discovery and application of life-sustaining diagnostic and therapeutic technologies provide one major explanation for this cost escalation.[1]

All nations must also meet the challenge to adapt traditional health care delivery to demands from unanticipated needs. Specifically, growing numbers of elderly, persons with disabilities, and those with previously unforeseen health issues (addicted babies, people with acquired immune deficiency syndrome [AIDS], technology-dependent persons) require care for chronic conditions, while the health systems in place are based on an industrial era model focusing on acute care. These systemic challenges represent outcomes of progress: successes of modern medical science and advanced medical technology. Evidence suggests that current systems and their focus may not be appropriate to meet these evolving demands.

A global search has begun for innovative, nontraditional approaches to health systems as a result of these concerns. In November 1990, the MaxPlanckInstitut held a health care summit to analyze alternative delivery models suitable for the elderly and persons with chronic conditions. Participants reviewed the evolution of different community-based models—including home care—in national health systems, national health insurance systems, and evolving market-oriented systems.[2] In addition to analyzing health care finance systems, invited health service research experts analyzed national delivery systems to determine differences between countries using the same health finance approach.

Among the concerns raised were: (1) What are suitable models for persons with long-term requirements for health care and medical technology? (2) What can other nations' experiences tell us about optimal economic/finance systems to avoid limited access to care?

The conclusions researchers reached were fundamental to understanding global health system reform. No matter what organizational model they described (traditional hospital, home care, community centers, nursing homes, other long-term care alternatives), the experience of each nation is based on two factors: (1) *Funding.* The finance system does not matter. What matters is that money is available as an incentive to develop an organizational model; and (2) *Culture:* Differences between nations with the same health care finance system can best be understood in the context of cultural differences between nations, even more so at the regional/local level. At the local level, innovative health care solutions are accomplished and encouraged by, or despite, national health care policy.

The Home Care Matrix: The Scope of Home Care Practice

Home care stands as one appealing organizational model competing with others for limited financial resources in global health care reform. Home care growth is driven by the increasing percentage of older persons in the total population, although children with chronic disease/disability are the fastest growing segment.[3]

Home care can be defined as the provision by one or more organizations of physician-prescribed nursing care, social work, therapies (physical, occupational, nutritional, speech), vocational and social services, homemaker, home health aide, and/or personal assistance services to disabled, sick, or convalescent persons in their home. Home care has three dimensions[4]: (1) duration of time, (2) support by others, and (3) application of technology.

The duration of time is as follows: Acute (zero to seven days); Subacute (one to six weeks); Long term (more than six weeks).

The level of professional/personal support ranges from: none (self, family member); to intermittent skilled professional visits; to continuous (private duty nursing/personal attendant).

The involvement of technology ranges from: none; to low technology (aids for daily living, communication, mobility); and to high-technology (life-sustaining devices).

People who require prolonged use of HTHC must anticipate dramatic changes in public policy and new dynamics of marketplace forces early in the twenty-first century. The population at greatest risk for service denial are MF/TD children.

The Home Care Culture: How It Differs from the "Medical Model"

Home care should not be considered an extension of the medical model into the home. In the medical model, the physician commands the situation, with the patient/family dependent on professional authority for decisions and actions. Thus, when receiving care in a hospital or ambulatory care setting, the patient and family are at a power disadvantage and are not in control. Technical and scientific information predominates in the making of decisions, and these decisions may not take into account the patient's and family's wishes. In these settings, physicians and other health professionals control decisions and plan implementation subject to patient compliance. The goal is the reversal of illness and, when possible, a cure.

All service providers involved with home care must accept a different mind-set from this institutional way of thinking and relating to patients. Home care represents a culture with attitudes, beliefs, values, and norms of behavior that differ from the more traditional medical model. Home care demonstrates a person-centered social concept typified by the independent living of persons with disabilities. In this model, physicians serve as collaborators of care and are invited partners with a patient/family active in decision making, plan implementation, and outcome evaluation. In family-centered care, the patient/family is central and in charge; properly prepared patients/families consider multiple options since they have been empowered and have the resources necessary to make good decisions. Much of their information comes from self-help and mutual aid groups. The patient/family focus more on wellness and desire to improve their health status and life situation rather than expecting a total cure. They are active participants taking responsibility for their own health. Patients/families have important management insights and can make decisions enhancing safety, reducing risk, improving quality, and reducing costs. This makes them essential participants in catastrophic care management (see Table 14–1).

UNDERSTANDING THE PAST

The Polio Era: Creation of the First Population of MF/TD Children

Technological Advances

Technological breakthroughs in health care result from catastrophic events. Many advances in modern medicine, surgery, and anesthesia were in response to the carnage of World War II. However, it was another global crisis that provided the stimulus to the life-supportive technology that is the concern of this chapter.

During the pandemic of poliomyelitis in the 1950s, countless numbers of infants, children, and young adults were stricken with paralytic respiratory polio. Universal panic ensued, and the medical community faced a plaguelike crisis of catastrophic proportions.[5] The polio crisis

Table 14–1 Health Care Models

	Medical Model	*Home Care Model*
Process:	Command/Control	Collaboration
Focus:	Professional focus	Person-centered
	Patient-focus	Family-centered
Emphasis:	Illness (episodic)	Health-wellness (continuous)
		Health promotion/prevention
Goal:	Curing	Caring
Fosters:	Dependency	Independency
Decisions:	Receptive	Participatory
Communication:	One-way	Two-Way
Response:	Reactive	Proactive
Respect:	Professional wisdom	Person/family insights
Environment:	Clinical, invasive	Dignified, private
Ethical foundation:	Beneficence	Autonomy

stimulated medical advances in upper airway management (tracheostomy) and mechanical ventilation.[6] Technology reduced mortality of bulbar polio from 90 percent to 20 percent.[7]

Organizational Advances

Significant organizational response to the polio pandemic of the 1950s included the creation of designated respiratory polio centers.[8] In the United States, the National Foundation for Infantile Paralysis, a voluntary organization, established these centers. Americans gave millions of dollars of support through the March of Dimes. Polio centers were unique because they featured interdisciplinary teams of health care professionals including physicians, nurses, social workers, and therapists—all working together. Among the new professions were rehabilitation (physical) medicine and respiratory (inhalation) therapy born during World War II. These centers focused not only on acute survival but on long-term rehabilitation and education. Hence, the team included physical, occupational, speech, vocational as well as social support, and educational professionals.

Community-Based Solutions

The leadership begun by Franklin D. Roosevelt and the research efforts of Dr. Jonas Salk at the National Foundation resulted in communitywide immunization and eradication of the threat of polio in 1956. Leaders also established HTHC made possible with the invention of portable home respirators. Engineers designed these life-sustaining devices in response to thousands of polio victims with respiratory insufficiency who preferred life in the community with families as an alternative to long-term institutions. Consumers working with their doctors and manufacturers helped design technology and the home care programs from which they benefited.[9] Gini Laurie, noted historian of the poliomyelitis era, stated, "the centers and home care resulted in tremendous financial savings and a greater degree of independence and self-sufficiency than was ever dreamed possible for people so severely disabled. The average hospital time was cut from more than a year to seven months; the home care costs were one-tenth to one-fourth hospital costs."[10]

Home care was not a new concept in America. From colonial times, the home was the traditional site of health care.[11] Furthermore, the United States had long experience with home visiting to support the health, social, educational, and other needs of children.[12] However, with HTHC, life could be sustained/supported on a prolonged basis at home by augmenting or replacing a person's ability to breathe with a machine. *Partnerships involving patients/families, physicians and other health care professionals, and organizational leaders all working together on a local basis developed these home care programs.* Creative people designing cost-saving solutions made HTHC less expensive and more desirable than institutional care (e.g., the use of personal care attendants/alternative care providers).[13]

The Critical Care Era: Creation of the Next Generation of MF/TD Children

Advances in Neonatology, Critical Care, and Rehabilitation Medicine

The technological and organizational advances of the polio era laid the foundation for the development of neonatology, critical care, and rehabilitation medicine. After the polio era, many physician leaders began to apply their new knowledge and skills to other challenges. Founders of intensive care units for neonates and children actually were often those with polio experience. Other leaders developed neonatology or critical care due to advances in their specialties and the need for units to concentrate technology and interdisciplinary teams. In the 1960s at the Children's Hospital of Philadelphia, C. Everett Koop, M.D., established the first neonatal intensive care unit (NICU) in the United States and Jack Downes, M.D., created one of the nation's earliest pediatric intensive care units (PICUs).[14] Advances in pediatric medicine, surgery, and anesthesia led to remarkable results such that critically ill neonates, infants, and children could recover from life-threatening acute illness with dramatically improved survival rates and recovery.

Meanwhile, in the late 1950s, the National Foundation ended support for the respiratory polio centers and redefined its focus to birth defects.[15] Some centers remained with support of public monies: Goldwater Memorial Hospital (NY), Texas Institute for Research and Rehabilitation (Houston), Rancho Los Amigos (Downey, CA).[16] Although acute care physicians no longer had experience with long-term mechanical ventilation, physicians at these former polio centers applied long-term mechanical ventilation for chronic ventilatory insufficiency to patients with spinal cord injuries and other neuro-muscular-skeletal disorders in the hospital and even at home.

Initial Hospital-Based Solutions

The "price to pay" for the miracles in the intensive care unit (ICU) turned out to be simultaneous survival of a small number of infants and children who could not be removed from medical technology. Almost all concerned considered such ventilator-dependent patients "failures of treatment," and the setting of their care received much criticism. The children also failed to thrive. When taken off technology, they became medically unstable, decompensated, or died in the hospital or at home.

Attempts to wean these children from mechanical ventilation failed. Occasionally, some pediatric residents just "let a month go by without weaning." This resulted in medical stability, enhanced energy and vigor, and improved eating and participation in therapy and play due to augmented functional reserve. Furthermore, autopsies of some of these children sent home without mechanical ventilation revealed potentially reversible narrowing of small pulmonary blood vessels usually observed "at high altitude," suggesting that such children needed ventilation. Evidence from young laboratory animals (anatomical studies) and humans (functional studies) suggested that the pediatric lung had potential for growth and development during the first decade of life. Children with chronic respiratory insufficiency, if provided optimal ventilation, might not only do better (become more active, alert, aware) but also might even grow and develop to the point that they would no longer require life support at all.

The initial hospital-based efforts to address these children with special needs focused on creation of "step-down" units. Solutions required an integrated team approach involving patients and families in self-care. *Optimal support* (optimal ventilation, pharmacology, nutrition, and developmental stimulation) changed the outcome and proved that special needs children could thrive. The first specialty-designated units featured patient-centered team approaches led by primary-care nurses. They emphasized child development and organization with team interaction. Families took an active position learning skills, adapting procedures, providing care, making management decisions, and, eventually, *if they chose,* planning transitional care. It was in these units that the parents and other family members could be *thoroughly* prepared for roles and responsibilities as caregivers, which one day would help them feel ready for care at home.

Over time, evidence suggested that additional solutions were necessary for other transitional care settings. Several pediatric centers with expertise in chronic illness/disability considered medically fragile technology-dependent children a challenge worthy of the extension of their mission and devoted part of their resources to their needs, including: Seashore House, Philadelphia; AI DuPont, Wilmington, DE; LaRabida, Chicago; Mt. Washington, Baltimore, MD; Hospital for Sick Children, Washington. In these centers, physicians focused on chronic care and the family as a social unit; professionals addressed long-term developmental, social, and educational needs.

Initial Home Care Experiences

Parents encouraged the first home-care initiatives for MF/TD children as a better option for families with children who required prolonged mechanical ventilation; physicians saw this as a way to reopen limited ICU capacity for more acute-care needs. By the mid-1980s, the pediatric literature reported several home-care discharge experiences.[17] The first reports came from the earliest developed units responsible for major advances in neonatology and critical-care pediatrics. Each report described organizational and funding concerns. Hospital care for MF/TD children was reimbursed (retrospective cost-plus); home care was not. However, early demonstrations determined that resources could be found and "creative financing" arranged by establishing working relationships among health care providers, administrators, and funders as colleagues.

The Recent Past

Bringing Public Attention to the Population of MF/TD Children

U.S. Surgeon General C. Everett Koop, MD (1981–1989), believed in care for life-supported children at home. Moreover, he shared the vision that responding to needs of technology-dependent children and their families stimulated more global solutions for all special-needs children with disabilities and/or chronic illness. As a result, the U.S. Public Health Service, Division of Maternal Child Health, sponsored the "Surgeon General's Workshop on Children with Handicaps and Their Families: Case-Example—The Ventilator-Dependent Child."[18] Conference planners invited a broad spectrum of actors who had been impacted by the issues at hand. The planners thought that if all stakeholders of a system could be present, they would become participants in planning and implementing that system and ensuring its success. A small task group format encouraged interaction among national leaders of relevant programs/policies, health care professionals and organizational leaders, and, most important, informed consumers (parents and ventilator users).

Public Policy Responses To Meet the Needs of Medically Fragile, Technology-Dependent Children

By the early 1980s, ventilator-dependent children were not rare. One example was Katie Beckett, a young child from Cedar Rapids, Iowa, being evaluated in Illinois for medical technology special needs. Julie Beckett, mother of Katie Beckett, had learned that home care for children like hers was possible in Illinois. Katie's mother and own pediatrician sought funding support for home care, but they came across bureaucratic red tape with Iowa Medicaid. With resourcefulness, determination, and conviction, Katie's mother contacted the appropriate politicians who brought the plight of these children and the barriers created by government policy and practice to the attention of then–Vice President Bush. President Reagan highlighted the case of Katie Beckett at a 1981 press conference; Katie was sent home as "an exception to policy."[19]

When the President makes an exception to policy, it may stimulate urgency to deal with anticipated future cases. Thus, U.S. Health and Human Services Secretary Schweiker established an ad hoc task force and Congressman Henry Waxman charged his health care committee staff members to design a public policy response: community-based "waivers" to existing policy determined by strict criteria with financial risk limited to a defined number of children. Ever since 1982, public funding for MF/TD children has been obtained as a waiver from Medicaid policy. States can apply to the Health Care Finance Administration for approval of a community-based waiver for a limited number of beneficiaries. The waiver provides a mechanism to utilize Medicaid funds without requiring a copayment by families that essentially reduces their financial assets to poverty level. However, not all states applied for waivers, and those that did were as relevant as the insights and understanding of the authors who submitted them. Furthermore, waivers limited the number of beneficiaries and took an excessive amount of time for approval. Once waivers were approved, restrictive policies and procedures replaced what had been more innovative creative financing negotiated for individual cases.

Private Reimbursement Practices

Not all technology-dependent children required Medicaid funding. Some had limited private indemnity benefits, often with major medical insurance. Although these policies did not cover this new category of patient, insurance company administrators (medical directors) and employers who determined benefit selection were open to direct dialogue for creative solutions to utilize remaining funds that they were obligated to spend. They were less restricted by rules and regulations and permitted more flexibility to meet the individual needs of their employee's family. However, physicians still thought it wise to involve all public payers (especially Title V agencies) who were knowledgeable about both community-based resources and access to public funds to supplement private benefits.

Service Delivery

When the first attempts were made to discharge MF/TD children to their homes, home care equipment providers and home health agencies were hesitant to provide high-technology devices and supportive personnel in the home due to potential medical liability risk and lack of funding. But as insurance companies and waiver cases began to provide a potentially limitless funding stream, home care agencies and vendors began to develop pediatric programs. Families could obtain equipment, supplies, and support, but they faced fragmented service programs in the community. Payers soon realized that HTHC, previously delivered at significant cost savings compared to hospitalization, started to approach or exceed costs of care in institutional alternatives. This resulted, in part, from inadequate coordination or integration of service delivery and from funding approaches that did not incorporate any mechanisms to manage costs. The availability of funding without adequate control encouraged development of an HTHC industry, causing an explosion in costs/utilization.[20] The excessive growth has become a major public policy concern.[21] Families are at risk for denial of home care since public policy requires that home care *must* by law be less expensive than institutional care.

ANALYZING THE PRESENT

Parents and professionals concerned about MF/TD children today face a disorganized array of fragmented sources of funding/services meeting health care, social, educational, and developmental needs. The cost of this lack of integrated management of services required by these children is high. With a nonsystem, needs of these children may not be met or, if met, the actual expenditures may be excessive. Children and families are victims of cost/operational inefficiencies that may put at risk home care as a viable option since cost might exceed institutional alternatives. The situation will become more critical with managed care/capitation.

Current Reimbursement Policies and Practices for HTHC

Public Sector

Not all MF/TD children at home require Medicaid (Title XIX). However, with time, those with finite private indemnity insurance will require a public funding alternative. Over a lifetime, insurance policy limits are commonly exceeded and home care benefits will be restricted by Medicaid policy with or without waiver exceptions. Community-based waivers are highly variable from state to state.

Each state also has a designated program for "children with special needs" (Title V). These funds have defined categorical criteria with or without additional Social Security benefits. Compared to funds available from Medicaid, Title V funding is far more restricted. Title V programs provide involvement by concerned professionals who want to meet the comprehensive needs of these special children. In Illinois, for example, Title V has been a valuable resource for information about community-based services and as a case manager of Medicaid waiver funds.

Other public funds have been identified and applied toward MF/TD children. For example, underutilized budgeted state funds identified by resourceful parents have funded a statewide case-management program for ventilator-dependent children in Pennsylvania. This was accomplished by a family who had chosen home care on a ventilator for their developmentally delayed MF/TD child as a preferable situation to prolonged institutionalization.

Private Sector

Private sector funding from traditional indemnity insurance commonly pays for health care costs retrospectively "at cost." "Cost shifting" by health care providers has placed an added burden upon private insurers to compensate for underfunded public payment. For private insurers, a MF/TD child represents a "catastrophic cost" case. As early as 1983, private insurers (Aetna and later Blue Cross/Blue Shield) responded with case-management strategies that required a health care professional (nurse/physician) to review and approve costs for these exceptional cases. Despite policy restrictions, these case managers have been approachable as colleagues to develop flexible, individualized programs. Employers who have developed self-insurance Employee Retirement Income Security Act (ERISA) programs both with and without third-party administrators also utilize case management for exceptional cases.

Health maintenance organizations (HMOs) assume full financial risk for enrolled members by accepting premiums for total comprehensive care. They attempt to locate and contract with hospitals and health care providers who will agree to financial arrangements that assume part or all of the financial risk for providing services. The line between funder and provider may become fuzzy, depending on the contract. Arrangements vary among contracts, which incorporate exceptions to deal with catastrophic cost situations. Funding systems are not designed for many of the health needs or the social support and educational/developmental needs for MF/TD children. Costs, not care, drive these financial considerations.

HMOs also have designed programs incorporating case management as a strategy to limit financial exposure that might exceed anticipated expenditures. In some cases, "benefit management" is interpreted very narrowly, limiting or rejecting payment for needed services for MF/TD children. However, some HMOs have demonstrated remarkable innovations in case management/program design that has led to significant cost saving *and* enhanced quality for MF/TD children.[22]

Alternative Funding Sources

Managed Care Practices. Managed care organizations (MCOs) apply funding practices that will become more prominent for MF/TD children and their families. Many states today are considering MCO management of Medicaid. Presently, all MCOs attempt to manage care by managing costs. Up to now, MCOs have tried to contain costs by using volume discount contracts with providers and by favoring provider networks that can provide comprehensive services. In some cases, MCOs can transfer all financial risk to providers by capitation: paying providers a payment "per patient per month" for *all* health care needs. Although the intent is to provide incentives for health promotion/prevention, it also provides incentives to limit expenditures since cost overruns are liabilities to the provider. Providers then may consider health promotional costs for MF/TD children not medically necessary.

MCOs attempt to control costs by determining "medical necessity" and requiring approval of all benefits by a gatekeeper, who is often a primary care physician (family physician/generalist). Since MF/TD children potentially represent catastrophic costs, MCOs also utilize case managers. Both gatekeepers and case managers may or may not be sensitive to the medical necessity of many services that would improve the well-being and promote the health of their beneficiaries. However, they are educable and will work with families and professional advocates as colleagues.

Family Contributions. Families are exposed to both direct and indirect costs for their MF/TD children. Many reimbursement programs require annual deductibles and copayments for covered benefits that may also have finite limits requiring major medical coverage, which also may be limited. (MF/TD children and families may find even million-dollar coverage insufficient.) Furthermore, the family must face many uncovered health-related expenses that are not often considered: need to expand/modify the house, increased energy costs/taxes, loss of earnings due to providing direct care, need to buy new means of transportation and mobility, and payments for technical aids for education/developmental purposes. Although these may not seem medically necessary, they promote health and indirectly affect health care expenditures. They permit continuity of home health care that, properly designed and managed, can limit health care costs and/or extend benefits.

Voluntary/Community Agencies. There exist nonprofit and voluntary/community agencies that could potentially provide funding for "categorical" needs. For example, organizations that address a particular medical condition raise funds for research/services directly or via the United Way (e.g., Muscular Dystrophy Association, United Cerebral Palsy, Easter Seals). Such agencies will not fund catastrophic health costs; rather, they may choose to provide supplementary funding for designated purposes (purchase of devices). Community agencies have been more helpful in responding to developmental and educational (health-affecting) needs. Some charitable organizations (Rotary International) have raised funds designated for individual children and special populations.

Creative financing (combining funding from private, public, community sources) designed by concerned professionals, organizations, and parents working together has funded extraordinary costs of MD/TD children on an individual case basis.

Current Service Provision

Services for complex chronic conditions are provided without a coordinated, integrated management approach. The fragmentation frustrates all participants and actors involved.

Health Care

MF/TD children at home require a variety of services for their medical, psychosocial, developmental, and educational needs that all promote health. However, until recently, few resources have been available that were targeted only to pediatrics or intended to provide "one-stop shopping," including case management. Thus, families and professionals must work with a fragmented and uncoordinated service system with gaps, duplications, and inefficiencies.

Psychosocial/Developmental

Psychosocial/developmental needs of MF/TD children affect health. Services that meet these needs may be at times available from home health agencies, but they may also may be found in other community agencies designated for other purposes. Many community agencies have "home visiting" as part of their programs.[23] However, they are not integrated with services provided by home health agencies.

Families have often found that they can get more support for health and related needs by turning to other families and concerned persons who join together as self-help and mutual aid groups.[24] Self-help groups such as SKIP (Sick Kids [Need] Involved Persons) are a major source of support for families; these groups supplement professional care and provide necessary assistance not available in the professional sphere. Other self-help groups (Family Voices) provide advocacy and serve as catalysts for social change.

Educational

As MF/TD children have become more prevalent in the community, educational systems have found these children to be a major challenge beyond current special-educational programming. In some school districts, developmental therapies (physical, occupational, and speech therapy) prepare children for school; these services do *not* depend on health insurance. Recently, MF/TD children have benefited from federally mandated early intervention programs for birth to three and three- to five-year-old children. In Illinois, families, health, and funding agencies have joined together in local area councils to facilitate case finding, system design, and coordination of services to prepare children for entry into the school system.

APPROACHING THE FUTURE

The future of MF/TD children is closely tied into the future of HTHC. Due to unconstrained growth of the home care industry and costs of HTHC, the future of HTHC has now been questioned appropriately on ethical grounds.[25]

The Ethical Framework

Ethical conflicts result when multiple ethical principles reflecting different perspectives must be considered. In terms of HTHC, there may be conflict regarding what the professional wants to do, what the patient/person/family wants to have done, and what society can afford to do. Since one option demands tradeoff with another, HTHC can give rise to an ethical debate.

Before engaging in that debate, it will be worthwhile to lay out groundwork for considering the ethical issues involved here, to avoid the trap of giving ready answers to objections whose implications brook no such answers. Judgments about right and wrong must always be arrived at by (1) considering the various human values involved in a complex life-situation, (2) assessing their proper weight with the help of agreed-upon criteria, and (3) resolving value-conflicts in light of that assessment. Each of those steps needs clarification.

Considering Human Values in a Complex Life Situation

Precisely because life situations are complex, we need to analyze them carefully for what is really at issue. Sorting out the underlying problems within the global presenting problem calls for rigorous analysis of the various physical, spiritual, psychological, and social realities present. It is important to know precisely what are the medical facts in a case and what conclusions may be validly drawn from them. Hunches or guesses, much less wishes, cannot validly ground ethical decisions. The spiritual and psychological state of a person must be questioned carefully, which can make a profound difference in the weight assigned to various values. Relationships, family attitudes, finances, and the larger social situation are all factors needing investigation before any decision can be prudently made.

Assessment of Values with Agreed-Upon Criteria

Values are of varying importance in common human estimation. Survival is more crucial than comfort; good health is more valued than material possessions. But "common human estimation" can also be controverted, hence the need for agreed-upon criteria to assess the relative importance of human values.

In Western tradition, the so-called natural law was for many people the norm for behaving in line with correct human values. It was thought to be inscribed in the heart of every human being, and it based conscience as the individual's practical judgment of right and wrong. For some, it is still the surest criterion of true value.

Resolving Value Conflicts

Values may be, or seem to be, sometimes in conflict. Safeguarding one value may entail risk for another value or values. When this is the case, we need criteria for deciding which value should be given priority.

In recent discussions of values in the medical field, there has been widespread use of some value-based principles that, many would agree, provide guidance for deciding the correct resolution of ethical dilemmas. They have to do with the overall welfare of the patient (*the principle of beneficence*), the appropriate freedom of the patient for self-determination (*the principle of autonomy*), and the rights of everyone connected with the patient's care (*the principle of justice*).

HTHC poses some ethical questions that differ in detail, but not in substance, from questions posed by health care in general. So we may find it helpful to use these principles in making ethical value judgments about various aspects of HTHC.

PRINCIPLE #1: Principle of Beneficence. *This principle asserts that the health care giver should always act in the best interest of the patient. Not only should the caregiver do the patient no harm (something often formulated in a separate principle of "non-maleficence" but in fact included in this principle implicitly) but always strive to achieve the overall good of the patient.*

Home health care is intended to further the patient's overall good. It is, when properly administered, care for the whole person: psychological, spiritual, and social as well as physical well-being. The very notion of the word *home* implies this. Home is commonly thought of as the place where we feel most comfortable: in the midst of family, surrounded by familiar things that call up memories of past happiness, with easy access to friends and the normal business of everyday life, and with none of the institutional trappings and timetables that are necessary in hospitals.

Applying Ethical Principles Using Adult Case Examples

Technological breakthroughs have made it possible to care at home for patients who, until recently, would have had to be hospitalized in order for their medical needs to be attended to. In itself this is obviously a good thing for patients. Of course, in concrete instances, such high-tech care at home may entail aspects that call into question its being the ethically correct thing to do.

A case in point is Fred Marks, a 49-year-old victim of non-Hodgkins lymphoma, diagnosed as terminal, who has been released from the hospital so that he can live out his remaining days at home, in accord with his and his family's wishes. Now bedridden, for the moment he needs, besides personal care, periodic injections, dressing changes, and enteral feeding.

His wife, Mary, has learned to manage all this, with the help of a married daughter who comes in from some distance away every other day for a few hours. But Mary is very worried about what may be in the offing as Fred's condition worsens: catheter tubes that will need unclogging, the suctioning of secretions, perhaps even monitoring a portable ventilator if her husband needs help in breathing, and so forth. Doctors assure her that the technology is available to enable Fred to stay at home as they both wanted, and as he desperately hopes to—but Mary secretly dreads the responsibilities this will impose on her: She's not sure she can cope. Just the other day the feeding tube was almost jarred loose, and she panicked until she managed to get it stabilized.

Meanwhile her two younger sons, 12 and 16, are spending more and more time out with their friends. They tell Mary they can't bear to be around their father for more than a short time, don't want to bring their buddies over, feel ashamed of themselves for this, but. . . . What used to be a lively, happy home for them is a real downer now.

So far, HTHC has been a helpful means to ensure the best interests of the patient (Principle #1). If Mary manages to master the intricacies of further technology as it becomes necessary, then this will continue to be the case. If not, then Fred's best medical interests may be in jeopardy. But there is a further complication with ethical ramifications: the possibility that Mary and Fred may end up disagreeing about what is in fact possible with regard to his care. This brings in the second basic principle.

PRINCIPLE #2: Principle of Autonomy. *According to this principle, the patient's responsible freedom should be respected in all decisions about the care of his or her health. Not only should doctors not impose treatment or measures that are not absolutely indicated medically, or otherwise preempt the patient's own choices (behavior often spoken of in terms of paternalism), but all caregivers should acknowledge the patient's right to decide the direction and extent of her/his care within the parameters of medical correctness and real possibility.*

Up to this point, everyone concerned has been able to respect Fred's wishes without any difficulty: They were precisely what doctors judged reasonable, and just exactly what Mary wanted for the husband she dreaded losing and wanted to stay close to as long as she could. Now the situation may be changing.

Fred insists that he is not bothered by the possibility that Mary will not be able to manage further technology with perfect assurance: He would rather be less well-cared for but at home, he says, than perfectly cared for in a hospital. Mary can't make him understand the absolute panic she feels at the thought of being responsible for something that harms her husband. She doesn't even want to mention the strain she knows the situation is putting on their younger children.

It is clear that Fred's freedom is beginning to be a problem in the larger picture of things because Fred is not the only person involved in his illness, though, of course, he is the central figure. There are other persons to consider, starting with his family, who have certain rights as well. These rights, among others, are what the third principle looks to.

PRINCIPLE 3: Principle of Justice. *Human situations always involve relationships, and relationships entail mutual rights and responsibilities. The balancing of rights and responsibilities is, at its most basic level, the sphere of justice: giving to each person that person's due. There are microrelationships like those in a family, and macrorelationships involving a person and society at large.*

In this case, Mary is owed some consideration that Fred may not be giving her. She has a right to her own health, physical and psychological, and the latter may be endangered by Fred's demands. And then there are the younger children: On the one hand, learning to care for their father can be a maturing factor for them and stand them in good stead when they assume adult responsibilities. On the other hand, it can be unjust to ask of them more than adolescents can bear. Clearly the situation needs discussion.

The case of Mary and Fred is one possible scenario for HTHC. It shows the tensions that can be involved and highlights the sensitivity needed to be aware of danger spots. But there are other scenarios that emphasize other dimensions.

Take the situation of Priscilla Smith, for example. At the age of 13, Priscilla, who was a good swimmer, dove headfirst into what she thought was fairly deep water. It turned out to have large rocks in it, and she hit one solidly, breaking her neck. Saved from drowning by the quick thinking of her companions, she came to in a hospital bed to find herself a quadriplegic for the rest of her life. She is able to move only her head, nothing else. From the hospital she was transferred to a nursing facility, where she lived for the next 15 years. She needed total care; she could do nothing for herself. Even her breathing was difficult, but she refused any thought of a ventilator: She wanted no part of a machine that would, she felt, create the ultimate dependency.

Fighting a continual battle with despair, at age 28, Priscilla had the good fortune to meet a doctor who was convinced that she could live outside an institution, given new technological possibilities for home care. With the help of friends, she found a suitable apartment and soon discovered that she was able to do much more than the limitations of the nursing facility had ever let her imagine. A motorized wheelchair that she learned to control by puffing and sipping on a plastic straw gave her new mobility; the clinic she visited for occupational therapy put her in touch with people looking to develop new technologies for home care, and she was able to help them understand what the needs of a consumer like her really were as well as what forms of technology were actually practical for her situation. Out of that came a job as a consultant that, in turn, expanded into speaking engagements: She was actually a wage earner!

Moreover, though still in need of 24-hour care, she found no lack of volunteers willing to take a turn helping her. Even if her apartment was equipped with sophisticated devices that enabled her to turn the TV on and off, unlock the door, even activate and use a computer—it looked like a cozy apartment, not a clinic! When one visits her today, there is no machinery evident apart from the motorized wheelchair in which she spends most of her day. A portable ventilator (recognized, in the end, as a means of independence, rather than its opposite) is neatly tucked under its seat, and her tracheostomy tube is artfully concealed by a lovely silk scarf. Priscilla is living a life amazingly close to normal, thanks to the miracles of HTHC.

This case gives us another view of HTHC: mirrored by a life enabled to be productive and happy despite fearful physical limitations because technology has found a way to compensate for such limitations. If we apply the same ethical principles to Priscilla's situation, we come to the following conclusions: There is no question that the ethical principle of beneficence is at work here, exercised by the volunteers Priscilla has attracted; by the doctors and therapists who have helped her achieve so much; by the public sector, various programs of which contribute to the costs of maintaining her; and by the private sector, which has found ways of using and paying for her services; thus enabling her to provide in good part for herself.

In terms of autonomy, Priscilla has been able to make choices about how to live her life that no one could have imagined at the beginning of her quadriplegia. Despite her dependence on caregivers—or perhaps because of her willingness to accept such dependence consciously and without resentment—she lives a dignified, useful, and fulfilling life. Without the technology to support her decisions, this would remain forever a pipe dream.

How is the justice principle addressed? In terms of family, there is no issue: She is not asking for care from them. The volunteers who help her do so because they want to, not out of any sense of obligation. What about society at large? Are the costs involved in giving Priscilla the care she needs an imposition on other taxpayers? Given her ability to work and make a contribution to society, it is not difficult to answer "no" to this question in Priscilla's case. But the question is a valid one, and in other situations the answer may be more difficult to formulate.

Pinpointing Ongoing Ethical Issues

These two cases begin to illustrate the variety of ethical choices to be found in situations of HTHC. Each individual variation needs its own special analysis; generalizations are, as always, dangerous. In a recent book, edited by John D. Arras, we can see the broad spectrum of HTHC in the results of a project that involved a working group of clinicians, scholars, and policy analysts reviewing specially commissioned papers and listening to the narratives of patients, health care professionals, family caregivers, and involved friends, as they related their own experiences of HTHC.[26] Five of the major papers have been published in abridged versions in a special Supplement to the Hastings Center Report (September–October 1994) furnishing a convenient collection of reflections on various aspects of HTHC, both *positive and negative.*[27] Most are thoughtful and many would seem correct, but some raise questions from the viewpoint of this chapter.

For instance, it is said that the really novel element of HTHC is "the hyper-medicalization of the home, the extension of medical dominion to the heretofore private sphere of family and friends."[28] This is based on an assumption about the nature of HTHC that we would question. If the mind-set of service providers is institutional and the model for home care is medical, then perhaps the statement stands. But we contend that proper home care represents a social concept that is person-centered and that is best understood from the independent living model of persons with disabilities (see Table 14–1 for the ramifications of these two models); home hypermedicalization then is not appropriate.

In the independent living model, it is rather the radically changed roles, relationships, and responsibilities of physicians, patient/family members, and care partners that is the truly novel element. The home is not hypermedicalized; there is no question of medical dominion's invading the private sphere of the home. Or if in a given case there is, then precisely for that reason ethical questions must be raised about the true good of the patient and his/her autonomy as well as about justice to everyone concerned.

Arras describes HTHC as "a complex social phenomenon that improves life for many while threatening to erode for others the conditions that tend to foster important social goods and opportunities. . . ."[29] Some of the antinomies involved include home versus miniature ICU; the gift of easy breathing versus being tethered to a machine; the real importance to caregivers of being given the opportunity to care versus the sometimes crushing burden for laypeople of having to perform functions that were once the exclusive province of trained medical personnel; important cost-containment factors for hospitals versus escalating (and sometimes highly inflated) costs at home; efficient high-tech versus human high-touch for patients. Arras raises the immensely complex issue of public costs and national priorities, noting that while the distinction between high-tech and low-tech is not necessarily important for public policy, there is an anomaly apparent in pouring huge sums of money into HTHC when "the basic needs of many patients for nonmedical community support often go unmet."[30]

There may well be an anomaly in the cost of HTHC, and the question needs continual investigation and monitoring. But as mentioned earlier in this chapter, the reasons for the escalation of costs from initial experiences with pediatric HTHC to the current situation raise a whole other category of ethical questions regarding public policies of control, regulation, and integration of production and delivery. The principle of justice can be useful in assessing when profits ought to be subject to governmental control to ensure that the consumers of HTHC not become victims of a kind of "blackmail" made possible by the dire need in which they find themselves, together with the monopolistic character of the industry that is serving that need. Are excessive costs due to lack of system design, operational inefficiencies, fragmentation of service delivery, and lack of coordination of the continuum of care just?

All these points need consideration in our assessing the ethical aspects of decisions about a given case involving HTHC. They may helpfully be looked at under the categories of beneficence, autonomy, and justice—but such categories can only structure our analysis of what is at stake; they cannot promise easy, preset solutions to complicated human situations. Beyond that, the considerations raised by examining HTHC point to the increasing necessity of public-policy decisions about health care in general, including such thorny questions as whether we need to create a whole category of intermediate-care institutions, whether we need to institute more effective monitoring and control of the health-technology industry as well as technology assessment, and whether we need to impose global limits on health care spending, even rationing quotas about who gets what kind of care.

These are not new issues, but they grow in importance and assume ever-new complexity as HTHC becomes a more prominent aspect of our health care landscape. People, both lay and professional, with a stake in HTHC—and we are increasing exponentially—must continue to wrestle with the issues, attempting to hold in proper tension their many, varied aspects that clamor for recognition and respect if we are to be able in the future to shape a society in which HTHC's obvious benefits can be reaped in a way that enables us to be truly human and responsible in caring for one another.

What Will the Future of Reimbursement Look Like?

Health care cost expansion exceeding the general rate of inflation cannot continue unabated. For over a decade, various strategies have been attempted in the United States to control costs (cost-plus retrospective reimbursement, case-mix average prospective payment for diagnosis-related groups [DRGs], volume discount contracting with preferred providers, catastrophic complex care case management, regulation of physician fees determined by resource-based relative value scales [RBRVS]) that limit expenditures, and potentially, quantity and quality of care. All of these tactics are part of the universal rubric of managed care that up to now has focused more on managing costs than maintaining or improving quality.

The recent attempt at federal health care reform will not end. Instead of being comprehensive, political health care reform will likely be incremental, focusing more on financial reform than system delivery. Instead of federal reform, states are likely to be the sites of experimental programs. Managed care is on the drawing board for many states' Medicaid programs. MCOs are now preparing strategies in response to states' Medicaid requests for proposals.

Market-driven health care reform has really been taking place for some time and will intensify. Many of the players are publically traded (investor-financed) private sector organizations that are developing the means to deliver basic health care services and financing. To realize potential return on investments, rigorous cost management will be put in place. Ultimately, all payers—and the public—will realize that capitation is inevitable. All health care will be delivered within a total finite amount of expenditures (global budget). Those receiving HTHC represent complex expensive care that are "outliers" to any managed care approach, and payment for their health care costs will be at risk without special "carve out" considerations.

Needs of MF/TD children include family social support as well as developmental and educational services. The constraints on public health care expenditures extend to social and educational budgets as well. All politicians are conscious of the need to reduce government expenditures. Although not specific, budgets for all federal programs are at risk. State and local budgets will also be strained as never before. State/local governments have responded to public referenda to limit debt and tax financing and have already put in cost controls (balanced budget requirements) that demand fiscal responsibility. Public sector funding for all services will be constricted and growth will be limited.

What Organizational Strategies Make Sense in This Future Funding Environment?

Market/political health care reform, proposed or real, has already resulted in market-driven responses that can help predict future realities. Health care in the future will be delivered by comprehensive community-based integrated delivery systems (IDSs). These systems will provide acute, subacute, and long-term care in institutional settings and non–facility-based alternatives including the home. All system components will have to operate within financial constraints that will encourage cost saving (e.g., replacement of professionals with paraprofessionals, nonprofessionals, and volunteers; substitution of human resources with advanced medical information and communication technologies).

There will be variations of IDSs with different strategic partners. Currently, physician hospital organizations (PHOs) are developing despite the uncertainty of future antitrust and other federal agency concerns. PHOs are being driven by hospitals (with deep pockets) or large physician group practices (independent practice associations [IPAs]) that are willing to compete within the constraints of partial/total assumption of risk (i.e., capitation). IDSs employ components of managed care: primary-care focus with generalist gatekeepers to restrict access to specialists, for example. Cost-management approaches provide disincentives to approval of services that are not considered medically necessary.

Health care is not the only need of MF/TD children. Other community-based services (social support, developmental, and educational), also under funding/budgetary constraints, must also consider integration and cost-limiting strategies. Voluntary and self-help organizations should realize the value of resource sharing and the synergy that is possible by organizational interdependency. Case management and home visiting, today used by many agencies, will be an essential component of future organizational growth. Many community-based service organizations that already utilize cost-management approaches (e.g., case management) will coordinate services, meeting multiple needs simultaneously. In the future, they will find that integration of services from multiple sources enhances client benefit and maximizes resource utilization. Public funders providing oversight will contract with social agency preferred providers that implement these strategies (public sector integration of social agency funding).

What Organizational Planning Approaches Will Make Them Happen?

Organizations wanting to serve MF/TD children and their families in the future will require systems thinking. The complexity of changes in the political, market, and public-policy environments will require our responding as learning organizations that are utilizing systems approaches. Meeting the multiple needs of MF/TD children with fragmented, isolated, and competing services will no longer be a possibility. Today HTHC is a nonsystem. Tomorrow, a systems approach will be mandatory. Organizations will entertain considerations of strategic alliances in a variety of forms, including joint ventures on a program/organizational basis, staged mergers, or provider-payer-consumer system development. In this way, complementary services can be better coordinated and managed (e.g., home visiting can serve multiple purposes, including medical/social service delivery, technical support, and case management).

Future action planning should consider a process whereby all stakeholders *in* systems development, *including* consumers, will be identified and invited into the process of system planning, implementation, and evaluation; outcome analysis will be used as feedback for further system development. These systems will be in the form of stakeholder partnerships, each representing unique perspectives essential for the successful operation of the system. The ultimate paternership will link health care consumers (patients), providers, and payers who design, use, and develop the systems together.

CONCLUSION

What will the future for MF/TD Children and HTHC be like? Will they survive in a managed care world? What can be established; how will it be established?

1. *An integrated family-centered service delivery system will operate within finite predetermined financial constraints.* The financial risk to manage available resources and respond to the multiple needs of all beneficiaries will be the burden of the system. Community-based alternatives (e.g., HTHC) cannot survive if they cost more than institutional-based alternatives.
2. *The system must be operated by an integrated management approach that involves and links all stakeholders in system development.* Stakeholders include health care, social service, developmental and educational professionals, patients/families, payers, community-based providers/agencies, and lenders. Ethical/management conflicts can be resolved by a process of planning, implementing, evaluating, and modifying the system that respects and incorporates multiple perspectives. In this way, the evolution of the system will be flexible, meeting needs of each individual participant and group while maximizing the utilization of resources. The system will not survive if it is fragmented or unable to innovate.
3. *The system must be designed "smartly," utilizing available technologies of*

management-information systems and advanced communications that can extend the impact of each player. The central role must be given to the people/families at home who have valuable insight and skills in self-management and management of their own program needs.

4. *The system must integrate a variety of services targeted to meet multiple needs.* The system must present a total service package that will offer options, depending on the needs of each individual situation. Such an integrated system must be designed and operated locally because its success will be based on dedicated collaborative efforts of professionals and parents, providers and payers who will all benefit if given the opportunity to work together within the constraints of managed care/capitation.
5. *The system must responsibly accomplish multiple goals: universal access, medical necessity as determined by system criteria, quality improvement, and cost containment.* It must prove itself by presetting desirable outcomes and acceptable indicators of variance. Only by achieving desired results as determined by rigorous outcomes research will the system justify the resources required for survival.

NOTES

1. Institute of Medicine, *Assessing Medical Technology* (Washington, D.C.: National Academy Press, 1985); U.S. Congress, Office of Technology Assessment, *Life Sustaining Technologies and the Elderly* (OTA-BA-306) (Washington, D.C.: U.S. Government Printing Office, 1987); B. A. Weisbrod, "The Health Care Quadrilemma: An Essay on Technology Change, Insurance, Quality of Care, and Cost Containment," *Journal of Economic Literature* 29 (1991): 523–52.
2. J. R. Hollingsworth and E. J. Hollingsworth, *Care of the Chronically and Severely Ill: Comparative Social Policies* (New York: Aldine de Gruyter, 1994).
3. B. C. Vladeck, "Home-Based Care for a New Century" (keynote address given at the Arden House Milbank Memorial Fund and Visiting Nurse Service of New York, Harriman, N.Y., 1993).
4. A. L. Goldberg, "Can High-Technology Home Care Survive in a World in Search of Health Care Reform?" in *Home Mechanical Ventilation,* ed. D. Robert et al. (Paris: Arnette-Blackwell, 1995).
5. G. Laurie, "Introductory Remarks," in *Whatever Happened to the Polio Patient? Proceedings of an International Symposium,* ed. A. L. Goldgery and E. A. M. Faure (Chicago: Yearbook, 1981).
6. C. G. Engstrom, "Treatment of Severe Cases of Respiratory Paralysis by the Engström Universal Respiratory," *British Journal of Medicine* 2 (1954): 666.
7. H. S. Kristensen and F. Neukirch, "Very Long-Term Artificial Ventilation (Twenty-eight Years)," in *Clinical Use of Mechanical Ventilation,* ed. C. C. Rattenborg and E. Via-Reque (Chicago: Yearbook, 1981).
8. Laurie, "Introductory Remarks."
9. "Roundtable Conference on Poliomyelitis Equipment" (paper presented at the National Foundation for Infantile Paralysis, New York, May 28–29, 1953).
10. Laurie, "Introductory Remarks."
11. E. Ginsberg et al., *Home Care: Its Role in a Changing Health Services Market* (Totawa, N.J.: Roman and Allanhead, 1984), 6.
12. D. S. Gomby and C. S. Larson, eds., *The Future of Children: Home Visiting,* vol. 3, no. 3 (Los Altos, Calif.: The David and Lucile Packard Foundation, Center for the Future of Children, 1993).
13. Laurie, "Introductory Remarks."
14. A. L. Goldberg, "Pediatric High-Technology Home Care," in *Intensive Homecare,* ed. M. N. Rothkopf and J. Askanazi (Baltimore: Williams & Wilkens, 1992), 199–214.
15. Laurie, "Introductory Remarks."
16. A. L. Goldberg, "Home Care for a Better Life for Ventilator-Dependent People," *Chest* 84 (1983): 365–66.
17. B. H. Burr et al., "Home Care for Children on Respirators," *New England Journal of Medicine* 309 (1983): 1319–23; A. L. Goldberg et al., "Home Care for Life-Supported Persons: An Approach to Program Development," *Journal of Pediatrics* 104 (1984): 785–95; R. G. Kettrick and M. Donar, "The Ventilator Dependent Child: Medical and Social Care," in *Critical Care, State of the Art,* vol. 4 (Fullerton, Calif.: Society of Critical Care Medicine, 1985), 1–38; R. C. Frates et al., "Outcomes of Home Mechanical Ventilation for Children," *Journal of Pediatrics* 106 (1985): 850–56.
18. Report on the Surgeon General's Workshop, *Children with Handicaps and Their Families: Case Example—*

The Ventilator-Dependent Child (PHS-83-50194) (Washington, D.C.: U.S. Department of Health and Human Services, 1993).

19. "Girl Cited by Reagan Received Medicaid under a Special Rule," *The New York Times,* 11 November 1981.
20. J. D. Arras, *Bringing the Hospital Home: Ethical and Social Implications of High-Technology Home Care* (Baltimore: The Johns Hopkins University Press, 1995).
21. "Caring for an Aging World—Allocating Scarce Resources. The Technology Tether: An Introduction to Ethical and Social Issues in High Technology Home Care," *Hastings Center Report,* September–October 1994, S1–S28.
22. A. L. Goldberg and M. J. Trubitt, "An Integrated Approach to Home Health Care," *Physician Executive* 20, 1 (1944): 45–46.
23. Gomby and Larson, eds., *The Future of Children.*
24. A. H. Katz, H. L. Hedrick, D. H. Isenberg, L. M. Thompson, T. Goodrich, and A. H. Kutscher, *Self-Help: Concepts and Applications* (Philadelphia: The Charles Press, 1992).
25. Goldberg and Trubitt, "An Integrated Approach to Home Health Care"; Katz et al., *Self-Help: Concepts and Applications.*
26. Arras, *Bringing the Hospital Home: Ethical and Social Implications of High-Technology Home Care.*
27. "Caring for an Aging World—Allocating Scarce Resources. The Technology Tether: An Introduction to Ethical and Social Issues in High-Technology Home Care."
28. J. D. Arras and N. N. Dubler, "Bringing the Hospital Home: Ethical and Social Implications of High-Technology Home Care," in *Hastings Center Report,* Special Supplement, September–October 1994, S20.
29. Arras, *Bringing the Hospital Home: Ethical and Social Implications of High-Technology Home Care,* S20.
30. Ibid., S27.

CHAPTER 15

The Plight of the Deinstitutionalized Chronic Schizophrenic: Ethical Considerations

George B. Palermo

Deinstitutionalization and noninstitutionalization of the mentally ill are complex issues from both a practical and an ethical point of view. Deinstitutionalization was suggested and implemented with the unanimous support of the antipsychiatry movement of the 1960s and of those citizens who were primarily interested in civil liberties. The opinions of the recipients of this new revolutionary reform in the field of psychiatry, the patients and their families, were not researched prior to its application. During the past three decades the implementation of the programs has taken place so rapidly that the goals originally proposed have been only partially achieved. Their ethics have come under frequent scrutiny as their failures are increasingly becoming more apparent. Because of this, confusion and ambivalent feelings have been experienced by professionals involved in the care of the mentally ill, the patients themselves, and the families of the patients.

At the basis of this drastic reform of the mental health care system in the United States and abroad was a long-standing controversy regarding the nature of mental illness—whether its main cause is organic (hereditary) or environmental. The so-called nature-versus-nurture issue has existed for centuries in the medical psychiatric field. Over the years, great psychiatrists and humanistic scholars who held diverse and at times opposite theoretical views tilted the balance toward one explanation of mental illness or another. Nonetheless, both approaches have, alternately, greatly benefited the mentally ill by promoting better understanding of the psychodynamics and pharmacotherapy of mental disorders.

The popularity of each side of the controversy has waxed and waned depending on changes in the social, historical, and political context. In order to better understand the strong impetus that deinstitutionalization had during the 1950s and 1960s and the early 1970s and its trickle-down effect, which still continues, one needs to analyze many of the factors involved. It should not be difficult to recognize that after the defeat of some of the European totalitarian regimes at the end of the World War II a new wave of commitment to freedom spread throughout Europe and the United States. Assuming that the sociopolitical context of any nation usually has a substantial influence on important social issues and decisions, it is easy to understand why human and civil rights were viewed the world over as essential and inalienable and why the concept of human dignity was acclaimed as the most important value to be taken into account in decision making. A new sensitivity and a humanitarian approach to social problems came to prominence. Self-criticism paved the way to new solutions to social problems.

The decision to deinstitutionalize the mentally ill was influenced by the fact that the hospitals housing them were generally antiquated and the conditions were often extremely poor. The leaders of society became attentive to this humane problem, and they decided, helped by chain discoveries of major antipsychotic and antidepressant drugs and in the United States by a concomitant shift of the financial burden from the states to the federal government, to tear down the old asylums and rapidly discharge the chronic patients to their families or to halfway houses and homes for the elderly.[1] Gradually, even the acutely ill were directed to outpatient care in mental health centers or in fragmented outposts called catchment areas. The above decision to deinstitutionalize, theoretically interesting even though utopian, lacked a holistic, objective appreciation of the diseases affecting the mentally ill—diseases whose treatment has baffled people for centuries. However, overenthusiasm, which usually diminishes sound reflection, took over.

The mentally ill have long been the object of societal attention. They are people affected by a disease of the mind, usually schizophrenia and manic-depressive illness, that is thought to impair their wholesome social functioning, making them helpless and unable to make decisions for themselves; prey to perceptual distortion in how they view the surrounding world; fearful of being in the midst of crowds; deeply tortured by unusual unconscionable thoughts, at times paranoid; and occasionally dangerous to themselves and others. Hospitalization is frequently an essential step in the care of patients who have a severe mental illness—the psychotic ones or those who are depressed and dangerous to themselves or others—and care and treatment cannot be delivered with conscience and expertise in any alternative setting.

Utilitarian and deontological theories have supported different practical approaches to the plight of the mentally ill and the ethics involved in the search for the solution to their problems. However, no solution has yet been found. The patient, in the meantime, continues to be a suffering being, a victim of frequent rejection, poor experimentation, and lack of humane concern. The Alliance for the Mentally Ill, which addresses the patients' humane needs, their civil rights, and the needs and rights of their families, is vociferous in its support of their welfare. It is interesting to note that a loud cry for a more humanitarian approach to the welfare of mentally ill comes from their families. They obviously speak from both their hearts and their minds.

The patients, for their part, often seem to apathetically disregard the rejection of the present-day system of care and its frequent and dehumanizing delivery. They become noncompliant with treatments and reject attempts to help them. They have apparently lost trust in the professionals caring for them. They may feel that they were pushed out of their old places of refuge, or they may feel abandoned and resent the new therapeutic dispositions. They feel unwanted and occupy the streets, open spaces in buildings, and the waiting rooms of bus or train stations, testimony to their unintended victimization. One wonders, at times, whether they, the sick and the weak, are showing an attitude of passive aggression.

In trying to apply the Hobbesian view of contractarian social morality to the plight of the mentally ill, one realizes that it may allow some form of exploitation of the weak. It would be better to see people as self-originating sources of valid claims and implicitly consider them as moral persons. John Stuart Mill stated that civil libertarians "conceive liberty to be so important a value to society that it transcends other values."[2] "Everyday morality, however, tells us that mutual beneficial activities must first respect the rights of others including the rights of those too weak to defend their interests."[3] Only then does morality equate with impartiality. Ethically, there is no doubt that the autonomy of any individual and his or her right to make a free choice should always be upheld, but one may question whether the majority of the mentally ill, especially those who roam the streets, still retain their capacity to decide on their own behalf. Many psychotic people have a great deal of difficulty in making serious decisions and in preserving their human dignity.

The principle of beneficence applies not only to interpersonal encounters such as between a doctor and patient but also within any normal intrapsychic-intrapersonal system. A healthy person possessing a moral and autonomous self should be able to function in such a way that any decision made by him or her, especially relating to his or her physical and mental health, will ultimately be beneficial and will not lead to a worsening of his or her condition. If the mentally ill are unable to decide about their welfare, should it not be up to an ethically interested social group, beyond partisanship, to decide what is good for them? Optimally, such a group should be formed by the representatives of the families of the mentally ill, the recovered mentally ill, mental-health professionals, and political legislators. Freedom from hospitalization and treatment is not always the expression of one's right to freedom of choice. At times, it even prevents freedom of choice.

HISTORICAL SKETCH

It is reasonable to assume that mental illness and/or insanity have been present in the world since shortly after the appearance of homo sapiens. Since our ancient progenitor had not yet reached the stage of mind-body development of present-day humans, and since the development of society was at its beginning, it can safely be argued that the manifestations of mental illness or insanity then were different from those confronting us today. Without doubt, early humans must have reacted in a primitive way to the particular psychosocial factors of their rudimentary community. It is also reasonable to think that humans gradually began to define, through progressive refinement of their knowledge and understanding of their biological and psychological natures, the significance, the boundaries, and the manifested behavior of what later came to be called mental illness and/or insanity. Throughout the centuries, humans slowly jettisoned (1) naive, magical, and superstitious thinking due to ignorance or misunderstanding of natural phenomena and (2) unconscious projections (primitive attempts to understand inner feelings and emotions) onto a mythological cosmos, where the forces of nature were soon supplanted by anthropomorphic gods. As human insight into the human psyche grew through the centuries, humans began to appraise the feelings and behavior of the people around them and slowly defined and redefined their significance and described behaviors as well as the difference between the unusual and the common. Humans eventually grouped together the unusual, the strange, and the abnormal on one side and the common and normal on the other. That applied to feelings and behavior as well, as the dichotomies between good and bad, evil and holy, mad and sane saw their beginning.

Indeed, as people became more inquisitive and more rational as well as more observant of human behavior, a clear dichotomy in the description of human conduct appeared on the social horizon, and soon the concepts of mad and sane became commonplace. The concept of madness carried and unfortunately still often carries the connotation of unusual, evil, irrational, aggressive, violent, and disruptive. The terms *mens sana* or *mens insana* were coined, and *insanity* usually meant psychosis and/or schizophrenia or mania.

Through the centuries, society approached the unusual and disruptive mad and their madness in different ways. The emotions of fury, revenge, and grief were well-described in Homer's *Iliad* and *Odyssey.* The heroes appeared to be at the mercy of the good- or bad-natured gods of Olympus or of the Furies or of fate itself. It was only with the Greek philosophers and playwrights that both men and mythological heroes began to possess a psyche of their own. The madness and despair of Oedipus, described by Sophocles, is, perhaps, the best-known example. It ushered in a period when reason was trying to understand nature, society, and human behavior.[4] Plato and his followers thought of madness as irrational and as the antipode of human dignity, and irrational madness was seen as a menace that reason should combat.[5] Even though the Hippocratic tradition denied that madness was due to supernatural visitations but held that it was essentially due to physical and natural causes, including heart, brain, blood, and humor dysfunctions, madness continued to remain, through the centuries, an inexplicable and feared manifestation. Later, Augustinian philosophy reflected upon the spiritual disharmony at the basis of humans' emotional ills, especially in their relationship to God, a thought that psychotherapists should be reminded of today.

The Roman Empire categorized the manifestations of the major mental illnesses as *furiosus, insania, amentia,* and *dementia.* During the reign of Justinian (483–565 A.D.), understanding and a humane attitude were shown toward the mentally ill. They were admitted to institutions for the poor and the infirm, perhaps as a result of the influence of Christianity. The mad were viewed as children—and were treated with compassion.[6]

In the early medieval period, a small number of homes for the insane were built, and some monasteries sheltered a few lunatics each.[7] The majority of the mentally ill, however, lived with their families, were kept under continuous scrutiny by the villagers, or were left to themselves as forgotten people. (This type of treatment still exists in present-day society, although it is rare.) Leprosy, a deadly and disfiguring illness, became pandemic in Europe during the medieval period, and from the high Middle Ages to the end of the twelfth century, leprosariums and lazarets multiplied at a rapid pace. As leprosy gradually declined, the physical structures that had been used for the care of the lepers were used to house vagabonds, criminals, and people who were different and thought to be mad. The psychotics were even denied basic human and spiritual support. "Access to churches was denied to madmen, although ecclesiastical law did not deny them the use of the sacraments."[8] The mad were mistreated, mocked, expelled from towns, or forced to live at the periphery of cities. The rejection of the mad became so extensive that they were eventually confined on ships that would deliver them to different lands where they would be partially and for an undetermined period protected by their anonymity. Water and navigation certainly played a role in this rejection. "Confined on the ship, from which there is no escape, the madman is delivered to the river with its thousand arms, the sea with its thousand roads, to that great uncertainty . . . prisoner in the midst of what is the freest."[9] Brant's *Narrenschiff,* Bosch's *Ship of Fools,* and other works served to immortalize that curious historical period during which human folly was seen as sinful and as something to be rejected. A few people, however, thought that the voice of folly might be a medium for the voice of God or have some recondite benefit (e.g., Erasmus's *Praise of Folly*).

Eventually, an attempt to care for the insane was made. The Hôpital Général in France and the first houses of correction in Germany and England became the forerunners of future asylums.[10] However, the plight of the schizophrenic and the manic continued. "One-tenth of all the arrests made in Paris for the Hôpital Général concern the insane, demented men, individuals of wandering mind and persons who have become completely mad."[11]

Later, during the eighteenth and nineteenth centuries, Europe was inundated with the establishment of a great number of schools, prisons, houses of correction, workhouses, and madhouses that dealt with the insane who were felt to be a social threat. An attempt was made to confine and shut away the different, the weird, the peculiar, and the mad. This continued for many years, during which time the mad were housed in antiquated hospital structures. Tuke had already reported on the sad condition of the insane at Bethlehem Hospital. The Salpêtrière was no different. There, the mad (schizophrenic or manic) were chained to their cell doors and to the walls, like beasts, living in filth. At times they even had an iron ring around their necks. Eventually, the mad were freed from real chains by the humane approach of people like Chiarugi, Pinel, Tuke, and Dix, and the birth of the asylum took place. The mad were no longer subjected to restraints, segregation, unusual diets, and even opium (to calm their agitation and soften their physical constitution). Eventually, Kraeplin, Pinel, Esquirol, Bleuler, and others better appraised the schizophrenias and freed the mad from the aura of evilness. The revolutionary ideas of Freud further assisted the sane in their attempt to properly address the problem of the mad by stressing that madness is the outcome of inner psychological conflicts and that any possible resolution comes from the intensive application of the old Socratic dictum—know thyself.

The above historical sketch indicates the vicissitudes of the mad through the centuries, their plight, and the defensive mass hysteria of the sane during various periods of social change. More recently there has been a focus on the potential powers of humans and their abilities to be both artists and masters of their destinies. Thus, the mad began to be viewed as humans in search of themselves or of a new self, and the sane were finally willing to help and to understand their plight in a compassionate way.

LIFE, LIBERTY, AND THE PURSUIT OF HAPPINESS

One of our constitutional axioms is that each individual has an inalienable right to life, liberty, and the pursuit of happiness. Even though the interpretation of the concepts of life and liberty may vary from one individual to another, it is unquestionable that the range of interpretation has definite boundaries. In other words, there are certain basic features that are common to any reasonable interpretation of the concepts. Life, in a social context, is not a mere vegetative state or a bizarre, disorganized type of existence. Optimally, life is the expression of the rational and reasonable behavior of an individual who has sufficient mental capacity to care for him- or herself and to be alone or with others in a way neither injurious to the self or to others, and who is usually productive and beneficial to him- or herself and others. It is a state where free choice, autonomy, self-interest, and willpower exist in a condition of social communion, not in a vacuum, and where the same basic principles of reasonable ethical thinking and behavior are accepted by the majority of people involved.

Autonomy and liberty are similar concepts, and both encompass one of the most natural human rights: the right to freely decide in matters that only involve oneself. It is a right that should be exercised by all citizens in a responsible way; the right, not to license but to liberty, usually goes hand in hand with responsibility. Responsibility is a state of "moral, legal, or mental accountability" and being responsible is being "able to choose for oneself between right and wrong, . . . able to answer for one's conduct and obligations."[12] All too often the acute and chronic mentally ill exercise the right to choice in way that is harmful to them, physically or mentally, and therefore in an irresponsible way. They have often lost their discriminatory capacity, and they may not be aware of the moral consequences of their decisions.

The essence of what is called mental illness is not changed by social, economic, or political theorizing. Indeed, mental illness, regardless of the philosophical approach to it, will continue to be a condition of the mind that manifests itself as confusion of thinking, inability to appreciate the surrounding reality, fluctuation of mood, lack of interest, poor judgment, and occasionally delusional or hallucinatory thinking and behavior. Based on the above, it is hard to accept that the acute and chronic states of mental illness do not interfere with ethical choice making and the mental capacity to freely choose, as well, moral accountability and responsibility toward self and others. The mentally ill cannot be expected to exercise their inalienable right to liberty when their state of mind does not allow them to do so. Consequently, it is unethical to permit the aimless vagabondage of homeless schizophrenics, and to force a nonhospitalization law on sick persons incapacitated by a disorganizing mental condition and in need of treatment in a supervised asylum. The frequent and insistent demands of the families of the mentally ill that their sick relatives be hospitalized for appropriate treatment and possibly custodial care instead of being left in the streets in their psychotic and disruptive state are objective, humane, and moral. Can a self-appointed group of guardians, upholding libertarian or utilitarian views, make decisions for the mentally ill and exclude from a decisional forum their voices and those of their families? Can they refrain from taking action when viewing how the homeless, chronic mentally ill live?

Last, in considering the last prong of the constitutional axiom—the pursuit of happiness—one must recognize that it, too, does not seem to be reflected by the way of life of the homeless mentally ill. The deranged homeless schizophrenics, whose rational thinking is highly disrupted, are obviously pursuing, if anything at all, a state of socioethical abasement, an outcome of their mental confusion. The exercise of civil rights or liberties should not call for personal, self-injurious consequences. Can the behavior of the mentally ill be seen as the dramatization of their need for adequate care—their cry for help? If the behavior of the homeless mentally ill is accepted as their right to self-expression and free choice, it must be noted that it certainly contrasts with the rights of the majority who consider it offensive to human dignity, contrary to the welfare of the mentally ill.

In conclusion, the old constitutional axiom does not seem consistent with the life of the homeless mentally ill. This realization makes it even more evident that the well-intended reform of our mental health system has not achieved its goals. Libertarian philosophy, stressing freedom from hospitalization and freedom from treatment for the mentally ill at any cost, has created social confusion and raised ethical and legal issues that need to be confronted. "The most conspicuous misdirection of psychiatric practice—the precipitate dismissal of patients with severe, chronic mental disorders such as schizophrenia from psychiatric hospitals—certainly required a vastly oversimplified view of mental illness . . . as though it were not their illnesses but society that deprived them of freedom in the first place."[13]

SOCIOETHICAL CONSIDERATIONS

The primary objective of the President's Commission on Mental Health consisted of "maintaining the greatest degree of freedom, self determination, autonomy, dignity, and integrity of body, mind, and spirit for the individual while he or she participates in treatment or receives services."[14] The therapeutic programs were to be carried out in the least restrictive environment. Bachrach, in a sound analysis of the problem of deinstitutionalization, aptly stated that the quality of restrictiveness per se does not greatly contribute to better patient care. It is, indeed, important to focus the attention on the quality of the program within the chosen setting, whether it be "essentially therapeutic, maintaining or custodial."[15] The idea of the least restrictive environment lacked the necessary foreseeability and flexibility that would have made it patient specific. However, the focus should be not only on adequate programs but also on dealing with people in a humane way. The mentally ill were placed in a situation that was not conducive to mental healing when deinstitutionalization at any cost was set into motion. And the cost was paid by many of the patients, occasional guests of our jails and permanent guests of our streets. "The argument that being inside the hospital is necessarily worse than anything on the outside simply does not hold. There are cases where patients . . . would be better off inside if those conditions cannot be met," stated Bachrach.[16] The proof that deinstitutionalization, born out of a humanitarian philosophy, economic juggling, and therapeutic frustration, was utopian and impractical lies in the presence of thousands of schizophrenics in our streets or in our jails, often chained and crying out as at the time of Pinel and Dix.

At present, it is very difficult for a mentally ill person to be admitted or readmitted to an institution because of the belief that only a limited number of patients should be kept in a psychiatric ward, to avoid overcrowding and provide better quality care. This phenomenon of "treating the census" in order to ensure the quality of care has added a new dimension to the ethical dilemma of caring for the mentally ill. What of those refused admission? Is it not immoral to maintain proper care for a few at the price of depriving a large group of the mentally ill, especially the chronic mentally ill, of almost any care? For example, many patients are discharged from psychiatric hospital units prematurely. It is unethical to discharge a mentally ill patient prior to the complete stabilization of his or her mental illness. It is also nontherapeutic and often leads to decompensation and irrational behavior at home or on the street. The ethical responsibility to dispense care to the "consumer-patient" is put to the test, and the professional dispensers of that care are pulled apart by having to be loyal both to the patient and to the system. In addition, the provision of care is often fragmented and the professional is bound to lose touch with the total patient. Patients often are seen but not admitted to the mental hospitals. It would be worthwhile to find out how they feel about being denied admission, especially whether they find satisfactory the alternative sources of care to which they are referred, assuming that they follow through with the referrals, and also whether the rejection they may feel creates antisocial behavior. Research should delve into "whether use of community resources (coupled with other available social supports) is sufficient to stabilize their problems and deter further applications for hospital admission."[17]

Our moral and ethical dilemmas seem to increase with the passing of time. Together with deinstitutionalization, a policy of noninstitutionalization has also been instituted. "While many patients are discharged from psychiatric hospitals into supportive settings, and the illnesses of other patients are resolved to the point that little support is needed, thousands [of] other patients have been discharged into inadequate settings or into the streets."[18] A great many of them live on sidewalks or in cardboard box shelters. They often are sent to jail for simple misdemeanors, and from jail they are sent to outpatient psychiatric and social services and then sometimes to poorly supervised halfway houses from where their noncompliance with treatment brings them back to the streets.[19] This transinstitutionalization has compounded the problem of city management and created new moral issues. Is it more ethical for a schizophrenic to be in jail than in an asylum? The average citizen looks stupefied as one more wall of the edifice of social morality comes down—the abandonment of and the lack of adequate psychiatric care for the many mentally ill living in our streets or in our jails.

The issue of futility of treatment for the chronic schizophrenics is raised at times. Indeed, in spite of the advent of new psychotropic medication, 25 percent of all schizophrenics will probably not recover from their mental illness or even improve. Nonetheless, one should assume that illness in general, and mental illness in particular, is basically treatable, and chronic mental patients should not be abandoned and/or discarded like unusable objects. Some illnesses, in comparison to half a century ago, now have specific and successful treatment modalities. Others can be made more tolerable while intensive research is actively going on in the hope of finding a definitive cure. At the same time, mental-health professionals should concern themselves more with the ethics of their profession, become more attentive to the welfare of their patients, and not allow uncalled-for interference in the delivery of appropriate care.

It is to be hoped that moral virtues and ethical standards will be upheld in all aspects of psychiatric practice. It is increasingly evident that the legal focus on liberty interests clashes with the treatment needs of the patients. The paternalistic attitude of psychiatry has been questioned. One could argue that the psychiatrist, like other physicians, clings to "that priestly role which since the dawn of history has been so important a component of the identity of the physician."[20] The professional attitude of any psychiatrist should include not only benevolence but also practicality and objectivity. The view that freedom from hospitalization and treatment should be supported at any cost, on the contrary, is founded on utopian ideas mixed with a great deal of emotionalism. Nevertheless, in order to help the schizophrenics who are roaming the streets of the cities, a certain balance between the paternalistic and the libertarian must eventually be reached.

STATISTICAL DATA

The advent of psychopharmacology in the 1960s was marked by one of those surges of optimism characteristic of psychiatry during the past two centuries,[21] and old institutional structures and traditional psychiatric practices were soon viewed as detrimental to patients. Some European countries, notably Finland, Norway, Germany, and Great Britain, had already pioneered social and hospital reforms even prior to the advent of the antidepressants and psychotropic drugs.[22] The schizophrenics, who constitute the predominant population in mental hospitals, responded positively to the new medications. Chlorpromazine was treated as a panacea, as were other psychotropics and antidepressants that followed later. Chronic schizophrenics seemed to return to life—to become self-sufficient, cooperative, and more friendly—and were again able to engage in a moderate degree of interpersonal life. Acute schizophrenics also responded rapidly to treatment. Patients were discharged to those families willing to accept them back home. Halfway houses or community places with minimal supervision were organized. In some cases, discharged patients were allowed to live alone. Deinstitutionalization and noninstitutionalization were well under way.

In the United States, for humanitarian as well as for socioeconomic reasons, this movement took place rapidly. In 1963, Congress, acting on recommendations by the Joint Commission on Mental Illness and Health, passed the Mental Retardation Facilities and the Community Mental Health Centers Acts. Patients were soon transferred from the snake pits to neighborhoods.[23]

There is no doubt that well-coordinated and humanitarian programs for the mentally ill were long overdue and that a new and more dynamic approach was necessary to combat the chronicity of their illness and to replace antiquated and poorly run institutions. However, as previously stated, the implemented programs were frequently a failure. "Often the ideals of deinstitutionalization amount in practice to little more than the shifting of people from one institutional setting to another—from the lunatic asylum to the nursing home, boarding house, or private hospital."[24] The reality is even more bleak. Indeed, many schizophrenics do not comply with their treatments, resist the supervision of social agencies, and are averse to hospitalization, and these individuals often land in the streets and sometimes end up in jails.[25]

According to the National Coalition for Jail Reform (USA), "at times up to one million (roughly 20 percent) of those filing through jails each year are mentally ill or developmentally disabled."[26] Most of the mentally ill in the jail system are chronic schizophrenics or manic-depressives who have often been charged with petty crimes or misdemeanors committed because they are mentally confused.[27] They should be called pseudo-offenders to differentiate them from real criminals. Nevertheless, they are housed in jails or prisons, and both they and their jailers deny their mental illness. The patients often prefer criminalization to psychiatrization, to hospitalization, and to treatment, confident that an overwhelmed and often lenient judicial system will quickly return them to the liberty of their homeless way of life.[28] "Of those offenders assessed mentally ill only 23 percent claimed to be receiving treatment at the time of arrest or incarceration . . . [and] the asylum-like function of the jail makes the job of maintaining incarcerated persons most difficult . . . an emotionally distraught person [mentally ill] may be stripped naked and chained to the floor to prevent a suicide attempt."[29] What a sad cyclical return of the past!

It is, indeed, ironic that in our so-called progressive society, centuries after the emancipatory vision and the efforts of Pinel, Chiarugi, Tuke, and Dix, for whom the asylum was to have become a place where the mad would be treated humanely, the jails and the streets have become repositories of the mentally ill. Comparative statistics show that in 1955 the census in the United States mental hospitals was 634,000 and United States jails housed 185,780 inmates.[30] In 1988, in a reversal of the situation, that jail census rose to 603,928, while the mental hospital census declined to less than 160,862.[31] The nation's 3,493 local jails had become the dumping ground for the mentally ill in our communities.

Many of those not in jail are cluttering the streets of our cities. At the beginning of 1997, there are approximately 1.8 million people in the United States suffering from schizophrenia, and at any given time approximately 150,000 of them are in the streets. Among the 450,000 homeless people, one-third classify as schizophrenics, one-third as suffering from bipolar illness (personal communication: E. Fuller Torrey, M.D., St. Elizabeth Hospital, Washington, D.C.). As early as 1970, by thorough evaluation of the homeless individuals who were admitted to the Manhattan Bowery Project in New York, Goldfarb had established that 33 percent of them were primarily suffering from schizophrenia and had a secondary diagnosis of alcoholism.[32] The typical chronically homeless person in a Philadelphia study emerged as a white individual, over age 40, with a diagnosis of schizophrenia, substance abuse, or both.[33] A study in Baltimore of 298 men and 230 women randomly selected from missions, shelters, and jails found that 91 percent of the men and 80 percent of the women suffered from some form of psychiatric diagnosis. Schizophrenia was diagnosed in 12 percent of the men and 17 percent of the women.[34]

As in the United States, in England and Wales many arrestees are found to be mentally ill. The majority of them are diverted by the police, gatekeepers to the criminal justice system, to psychiatric care when available. However, many psychotic people who are not acutely ill and therefore not easily identifiable are held in custody for weeks or months at a time, because of the bureaucratic procedures involved, without being transferred for treatment to a psychiatric facility. The above, referred to as "decriminalization of the mentally ill," came about after the deinstitutionalization of the 1960s and has made the jail the repository of the mentally ill. Strangely enough, at times the mentally ill themselves attempt to conceal their illness, preferring a possible fast plea bargain, option for bail, or a probationary period instead of going through the lengthy procedures of being transferred to a psychiatric facility and the stigma of mental illness.

Robertson and colleagues assessed the mental condition of 2,721 detainees held in police stations in England/Wales during a period of 18 weeks for observation. They report that in group one 33 detainees (1.2 percent) were regarded by them as "definitely showing signs of a serious mental illness."[35] A second group, comprising four people (0.1 percent), was regarded as being "probably unwell." A third group of 16 people (0.6 percent) was "known to have a history of treatment for psychotic illness" but seemingly doing well while in detention. Lastly, a fourth group of 21 cases (0.8 percent) was thought to be possible mentally ill. Groups one and two combined, for a total number of 37, showed that "2/3 of the group (25) were thought to be suffering from schizophrenia, six (16%) from an affective disorder, five (14%) from brain damage and one from a psychotic state brought about by chronic solvent abuse."[36] The authors, in further assessing 93 cases of a court sample, found that "more than 90% of the court group were recorded as having had previous psychiatric treatment."[37]

The above study supports the usefulness of diversion from the criminal justice facilities to psychiatric treatment centers, obviously in cases of misdemeanor. However, I am quite sure that even in England/Wales there cannot be any assurance that the schizophrenic criminals will consistently report for treatment once diverted, and in those cases, it must be questioned whether treatment would be adequate. The fact that diversion is no assurance for good supervision and treatment of the criminal schizophrenics is supported by the statement of Robertson and collaborators in referral to the treatment they might have received during incarceration: "The grossly psychotic people arrested for persistent begging in central London now stand less chance than they used to of receiving even temporary relief for their symptoms."[38]

Schizophrenia, substance abuse, and personality disorders are the most common psychiatric diagnosis among the homeless. Except in a few cases, the homelessness of the mentally ill is the result of the way deinstitutionalization has been implemented and not deinstitutionalization per se.[39]

> Deinstitutionalization meant granting asylum in the community to a large marginal population, many of whom can cope to only a limited extent with the ordinary demands of life, have strong dependency needs, and are unable to live independently . . . and can survive and have their basic needs met outside of the state hospital only if they have a sufficiently structured community facility or other mechanism that provides support and controls.[40]

About 40 percent of the homeless suffer from a major mental illness. Orr reported that the percentage of the mentally ill offenders in jail ranged from 10 to 50 percent.[41] Briar stated that about 20 percent of the jail population was composed of former or new patients of mental institutions.[42] They are the social misfits mentioned by Reusch and the pseudo-offenders described by Snow. Adler reported an increase in the arrest rate for the mentally ill that was substantially higher than that of the general population.[43] As causes of this rate of increase, she cited improper pharmacotherapeutic management; abuse of, or noncompliance with, medication; the natural progression of mental illnesses; and the new social phenomenological approach to mental illness. She also stated that her previous figure of 10.9 percent of psychiatrically ill inmates was greatly underestimated. Statistics gathered by Petrick revealed that 35 percent of the prisoners in the King County Jail (Washington State) were psychotic.[44] Out of 102 prisoners referred for psychiatric evaluation in the Los Angeles jail in 1982, 75 percent were diagnosed as schizophrenic, 22 percent as having major affective disorders, and only 2 percent having organic brain syndromes and adjustment disorders.[45] Lastly, in a recent analysis of a sample of 272 inmates in a county jail examined for competency to stand trial, the number of schizophrenics was 103 (37.87 percent of the total sample). Of the offenses, 83.5 percent were misdemeanors and 16.5 were felonies, and only 57.28 percent of all the inmates were found to be competent to stand trial.[46]

IN DEFENSE OF PROVIDING A NEW TYPE OF ASYLUM

Daily observation and statistical studies affirm the fact that many mentally ill live in the streets. It seems clear that we need to provide asylum for people whose disadvantages include "social isolation, vocational inadequacy, and exaggerated dependency needs . . . [and inability] to withstand pressure."[47] "While many chronic patients eventually attain high levels of social and vocational functioning, many cannot meet simple demands of living, even with long-term rehabilitative help."[48] They need an asylum, "an inviolable place of refuge . . . [and] a place of retreat and security."[49] There the homeless mentally ill who presently live on the street should find "the network of interrelated programs that meet the varied needs of a very heterogenous population."[50]

The concept of an asylum is still a valid one, despite previous problems in implementing a system of refuge. "Institutional care has historically included a complex and extensive set of functions in the service of psychiatric patients."[51] The patients were receiving substandard care in antiquated institutions, but the therapeutic efforts, even though inadequate, addressed each patient in his or her totality. At present, the fragmentation of care for the mentally ill has created a never-ending carousel from which they are unable to escape.

One reason for the failure of deinstitutionalization is that it is based on the assumption that mental illness is either sociogenic or even nonexistent. Bachrach stated, "Among the many problems plaguing society today is the failure to recognize that a portion of chronic psychiatric patients still require asylum and a failure to offer that asylum even when the need for it is recognized."[52] In England, the 1982 health legislation promoting the idea of entitlement to mental health services was highly criticized as "an empty promise, if it is not accompanied by places in the form of secure accommodations suitable for that patient. The problem may be exacerbated for offender-patients for whom the only alternative may be prison. . . . There is a serious lack of resources for detained mentally disordered patients who need secure conditions. . . ."[53] In Italy, laws were passed to reform the reform—the Mental Health Law 180.[54] In the United States and other Anglo-Saxon countries, the general feeling is that the earlier changes have to be amended.

In 1989, Mosher and Burti, in support of deinstitutionalization, stated that it provided "practical, common sense, flexible, good enough administrative and clinical guidelines to allow the development and implementation of effective psychosocially oriented community mental health systems."[55] Their guidelines, put forth decades after the implementation of the reform of 1958 in the United States, indicate that even they recognize deinstitutionalization has been less than a total success.

CONCLUSION

Assuming that the role of medical ethics is primarily to sensitize people to the moral issues involved in the practice of caring for the sick, one should try, as objectively as possible, to focus attention on the application of those rules that tend to harmonize the goals and desires of all participants in the care process. It is essential not to forget that the medical ethicists should be driven, not by passionate feeling but by the intention of pursuing an objective ethical analysis of the issue at hand through a process of a detailed assessment of the principles and concepts involved. Ethics is more a process than a pronouncement. Ultimately, any decision, as in the case of deinstitutionalization, rests with the leaders of society. It must be remembered, however, that the consequences are experienced by society at large. Because of that, no major ethical decision involving the welfare of others should be taken solely on sociopolitical grounds.

McHugh, in his essay "Psychiatric Misadventures," points out that, at the basis of occasional misdirection in the field of psychiatry, one usually may find, "oversimplification . . . misplaced emphasis . . . [or] pure invention."[56] In acknowledging the vulnerability of the psychiatric field to error, he reported a comment by Szasz, an important leader of the antipsychiatry movement. According to Szasz, psychiatry creates schizophrenia, since an individual is identified as schizophrenic on the basis of an existing system of psychiatry. Szasz's reasoning is worthy of a sophist, but when the well-being of people is at stake, one should be wary of sophistry. People expect and deserve an objective appraisal of what concerns them. Social theories are certainly important tools in the assessment of the human condition, but social factors per se seem to be only contributing factors in the genesis of schizophrenia and manic-depressive disorders, the most common mental illnesses among the homeless mentally ill.

Although one can be sympathetic with Szasz's motive, which is to do away with unnecessary restrictions, it is unethical to avoid treating people who are genuinely ill. The mental health professionals who accept Szasz's sociological approach to mental illness "abandon the role of protecting patients from their symptoms and become little more than technicians working on behalf of a cultural force."[57]

The idea that institutions were essentially oppressive was part of a cultural view of the 1960s. The vision of the alternative life that the chronic schizophrenics supposedly wanted to live was dreamed up by enthusiastic but wrongheaded reformers. "It is now obvious to every citizen of our cities that these patients have impaired capacity to comprehend the world and that they need protective and serious active treatment."[58]

Bachrach aptly stated, "The public policy initiative, which has for several decades dominated service planning for chronic psychiatric patients, may be viewed as a precipitous effort to change an entrenched and established system of care."[59] The absence of the asylum has greatly limited the effectiveness of community-based services for many chronically ill psychiatric patients. Asylums should be places where people may reside and be provided with up-to-date care, where the mentally ill may find temporary comfortable surroundings and humane attention, where freedom from sickness is the main goal along with restoration of autonomy, personal decisional capacity, self-respect, and human dignity.

Serious devastating illness such as schizophrenia should be of central concern in a moral society. The plight of the mentally ill in the streets or in jails is certainly a reflection of the ongoing moral decay of our society. Bachrach nicely summarizes one of the social and moral dilemmas confronting us today:

> Although the original motivation for deinstitutionalization was humane and well-intentioned, its consequences have, at times, been unexpected and harmful to the chronically ill. . . . Chronically ill psychiatric patients are . . . severely disabled and disfranchised populations with few resources . . . economically deprived . . . [and]

> require help in arranging for life's basic necessities, including food, shelter, medical care and social support.[60]

Recently, Scott and Dixon stated that assertive community treatment (ACT) and case management, which provide a multidisciplinary approach to treatment and rehabilitation for schizophrenics, are designed to "enhance continuity and coordination of care."[61] Their review reports that "ACT programs . . . reduce hospitalization and increase the use of community mental health services."[62]

> The following statement indicates why we need to attempt a solution: People with mental problems are our neighbors. They are members of our congregations, members of our families; they are everywhere in this country. If we ignore their cries for help we will be continuing to participate in the anguish from which those cries for help come. A problem of this magnitude will not go away. Because it will not go away, and because of our spiritual commitments, we are compelled to take action.[63]

Further thoughtful programming is needed in order to restore these persons to a humane type of existence and balance again what is good for society with what is good for the individual. Thus far, it seems that both society and mentally ill individuals are getting a short shrift. The conforming society, tired of being importuned and at times displaced from their own places of relaxation and leisure, is changing its attitude toward the homeless. In many cities, schizophrenic and bipolar homeless are being forced from parks and city streets that they had moved into over the past years and made their own. This changing attitude expresses the recognition by the majority of the citizens that these people, homeless and ill, should be dealt with in a different manner that would allow them to receive custodial care and treatment. Such a solution would envision a temporary placement in a mental institution.

The action must be taken by dedicated humanistic professionals who should treat their patients-clients not as objects but as human beings and who are willing to join in a communal attempt to aid the mentally ill to regain their mental health, their autonomy, their self-respect, and their humanity.

NOTES

1. H. C. Solomon, "The American Psychiatric Association in Relation to American Psychiatry—Presidential Address," *American Journal of Psychiatry* 115 (1958): 1–9.
2. P. Chodoff, "Involuntary Hospitalization of the Mentally Ill as a Moral Issue," *American Journal of Psychiatry* 141 (1984): 385.
3. W. Kymlicka, "The Social Contract Tradition," in *Companion to Ethics,* ed. P. Singer (Cambridge, Mass.: Blackwell Reference, 1991), 190.
4. M. Foucault, *Madness and Civilization,* trans. R. Howard (New York: Vintage Books, 1988); R. Porter, *A Social History of Madness* (New York: Dutton, 1989).
5. M. A. Mackenzie, *Plato on Punishment* (Berkeley, Calif., and Los Angeles: University of California Press), 1981.
6. G. Zilboorg, *A History of Medical Psychology* (New York: Norton, 1941).
7. Porter, *Social History of Madness.*
8. Foucault, *Madness and Civilization,* 10.
9. Ibid., 11.
10. Porter, *Social History of Madness.*
11. Foucault, *Madness and Civilization,* 65.
12. *Webster's Ninth New Collegiate Dictionary,* s.v. "responsibility" and "responsible."
13. P. R. McHugh, "Psychiatric Misadventures," *The American Scholar* (Autumn 1992): 498.
14. L. L. Bachrach, "Is the Least Restrictive Environment Always the Best? Sociological and Semantic Implications," *Hospital and Community Psychiatry* 31 (1980): 97.
15. Ibid., 101.
16. Ibid., 99.
17. J. R. Morrissey et al., "Being Seen but Not Admitted. A Note on Some Neglected Aspects of State Hospital Deinstitutionalization," *American Journal of Orthopsychiatry* 49 (1979): 155.

18. R. Peele, "The Ethics of Deinstitutionalization," in *Psychiatric Ethics,* ed. S. Bloch and P. Chodoff (Oxford, New York, and Melbourne: Oxford University Press, 1991), 303.
19. G. B. Palermo et al., "Escape from Psychiatrization: A Statistical Analysis of Referrals to a Forensic Unit," *International Journal of Offender Therapy and Comparative Criminology* 36 (1992): 89–102.
20. Chodoff, "Involuntary Hospitalization of the Mentally Ill as a Moral Issue," 387.
21. A. Scull, "Deinstitutionalization and the Rights of the Deviant," *Journal of Social Issues* 37 (1981): 6–20.
22. G. Klerman, "The Psychiatric Patient's Right to Effective Treatment: Implications of Asheroff vs. Chestnut Lodge." *American Journal of Psychiatry* 147 (1990): 409–18.
23. R. Sommer and A. Osmond, "The Mentally Ill in the Eighties." *Journal of Orthomolecular Psychiatry* 10 (1981): 193–201.
24. K. Jones et al., "The Current Literature: The 1978 Italian Mental Health Law: A Personal Evaluation: A Review," *British Journal of Psychiatry* 159 (1991): 560.
25. G. B. Palermo et al., "Jails Versus Mental Hospitals: A Social Dilemma," *International Journal of Offender Therapy and Comparative Criminology* 35 (1991): 97–104.
26. K. H. Briar, "Jails: Neglected Asylums," *Social Casework* 64 (1983): 388.
27. P. J. Hilts, "Survey Finds Many Jails Holding Mentally Sick on Minor Charges," *New York Times,* 10 September 1992, A12.
28. Palermo et al., "Escape from Psychiatrization," 89–102.
29. Briar, "Jails," 389.
30. U.S. Bureau of the Census, *Historical Statistics of the United States* (Washington, D.C.: U.S. Bureau of the Census, 1960).
31. U.S. Bureau of the Census, *Statistical Abstracts of the United States* (Washington, D.C.: U.S. Bureau of the Census, 1990).
32. C. Goldfarb, "Patients Nobody Wants: Skid Row Alcoholics," *Diseases of Nervous System* 31 (1970): 274–81.
33. A. A. Arce and M. J. Vergare, "Identifying and Characterizing the Mentally Ill among the Homeless," in *The Homeless Mentally Ill,* ed. H. R. Lamb (Washington, D.C.: American Psychiatric Association, 1984), 75–89.
34. F. Kass, "Mental Illness and Homelessness: Majority of Homeless People Found to Be Mentally Ill," *Psychiatric News* 24 (1989): 14.
35. G. Robertson et al., "The Entry of Mentally Disordered People to the Criminal Justice System," *British Journal of Psychiatry* 169 (1996): 173.
36. Ibid., 174.
37. Ibid., 175.
38. Ibid., 178.
39. C. L. M. Caton, *Homeless in America* (New York and Oxford, England: Oxford University Press, 1990).
40. H. R. Lamb, "Deinstitutionalization and the Homeless Mentally Ill," in *The Homeless Mentally Ill: A Task Force Report of the APA,* ed. H. R. Lamb (Washington, D.C.: American Psychiatric Association, 1982), 58.
41. J. H. Orr, "The Imprisonment of Mentally Disordered Offenders," *British Journal of Psychiatry* 133 (1978): 194–99.
42. Briar, "Jails," 387–93.
43. F. Adler, "Jails as Repository for Former Mental Patients," *International Journal of Offender Therapy and Comparative Criminology* 30 (1986): 225–36.
44. J. Petrick, "Rate of Psychiatric Morbidity in a Metropolitan County Jail Population," *American Journal of Psychiatry* 133 (1976): 1439–44.
45. H. R. Lamb and R. Peele, "The Need for Continuing Asylum and Sanctuary," *Hospital and Community Psychiatry* 35 (1984): 798–802.
46. Palermo et al., "Escape from Psychiatrization," 89–102.
47. Lamb and Peele, "Need for Continuing Asylum and Sanctuary," 798.
48. Ibid.
49. *Webster's Ninth New Collegiate Dictionary,* s.v. "asylum."
50. L. L. Bachrach, "Asylum and Chronically Ill Psychiatric Patients," *American Journal of Psychiatry* 141 (1984): 977.
51. Ibid., 975.
52. Bachrach, "Is the Least Restrictive Environment Always the Best?" 977.
53. J. Shapland and T. Williams, "Legalism Revived: New Mental Health Legislation in England," *International Journal of Law Psychiatry* 6 (1983): 366.
54. La Riforma Della Legge 180: Nuove Norme Sulla Tutela Della Salute Mentale, *Psichiatria e Medicina: Attualità in Neuroscienze, Psicogeriatria e Psicologia Medica* (September 1991): 8–11.
55. L. R. Mosher and L. Burti, *Community Mental Health. Principals and Practice* (New York and London: Norton, 1989), 381.
56. McHugh, "Psychiatric Misadventures," 504.
57. Ibid.
58. Ibid., 501.
59. Bachrach, "Asylum and Chronically Ill Psychiatric Patients," 975.
60. Ibid., 976.
61. J. E. Scott and L. Dixon, "Assertive Community Treatment and Case Management for Schizophrenia," *Schizophrenia Bulletin* 21 (1995): 657.
62. Ibid.
63. R. Carter, "A Voice for the Voiceless: The Church and the Mentally Ill," *Second Opinion* 13 (1990): 47.

Chapter 16

Older People and Long-Term Care: Issues of Access

Robert H. Binstock

In the last decades of the twentieth century the goal of improving access to humane and appropriate long-term care services began to be perceived in the United States. Opinion polls indicated that a substantial majority of Americans—in all adult age groups—fear the financial, familial, psychological, and social consequences of dependence on long-term care and favor the general principle of expanding government financing for such care as the principal means of increasing access to it.[1] A number of bills to provide new programs of public funding for long-term care were introduced in Congress in the late 1980s and early 1990s, with estimated annual price tags ranging up to $60 billion in the first year.

Why did long-term care begin to emerge from the dominant shadows cast in the health care arena by the more dramatic treatments and cures offered by acute-care medicine?

One major element is the enormous growth of our older population—aged 65 and over—that doubled from 16 million in 1960 to 32 million in 1990. Persons in this age category are presently 12.5 percent of our population and are expected to constitute 20 percent in the year 2030.[2]

Another element has been a growing constituency of adult children of elderly patients who are perceiving the importance of long-term care services because of their direct contact with the experiences and issues of providing or arranging for the care of their aged parents. Over 13 million adults in the United States who have disabled elderly parents or spouses are potential providers of long-term care, financial assistance, and emotional support; 4.2 million of them provide direct care in home settings.[3] Disabled children, younger disabled adults, and their families, respectively, are additional potential constituencies to the support of greater access to long-term care.

Despite the underlying needs and hopes of these constituencies, enactment of a government program to substantially expand access to long-term care in the immediate future is problematic because of the substantial funds that would be required. Achieving a "balanced budget" is a rhetorical mainstay of contemporary national politics, and containing government expenditures on health care costs is considered to be one of the major means for balancing the federal and state budgets.

The challenges of ensuring adequate access to long-term care for all who need it are substantial. The number of Americans requiring some form of long-term care is already large and will grow significantly over the next few decades. Financing such care is already very difficult for individuals, their families, and governments. Yet, indications are that the prices for services and their aggregate national costs will continue to escalate, while the role of governments in paying for care of an expanded disabled population may be curtailed.

This chapter primarily focuses on issues of access for older people, although it also considers the need for long-term care for younger disabled persons as well as the political role they might play in improving access for persons of all ages. First, it provides an overview of the growing population that needs long-term care. Second, it discusses the issues of access to care. Third, it briefly recounts how proposals to expand public funding for long-term care rose to the national policy agenda in the early 1990s and then abruptly fell from it. And finally, it considers the political and moral prospects for improving access in the years ahead.

THE GROWING POPULATION NEEDING CARE

The U.S. General Accounting Office (1994) reports that there are more than 12 million Americans who need long-term care. Need for long-term care is generally defined in terms of a person's being functionally dependent on a long-term basis due to physical and/or mental limitations. Two broad categories of functional limitations are widely used by clinicians to assess need for care. One category is dependence in basic activities of daily living (ADLs)—getting in and out of bed, toileting, bathing, dressing, and eating. (Persons who have cognitive impairment, who need cueing from someone else to be able to perform their own ADLs, are regarded as ADL dependent.) The other category is limitations in instrumental activities of daily living (IADLs)—taking medications, preparing meals, managing finances, doing light housework and other chores, being able to get in and out of the home, using the telephone, and so on. (Children and people with mental illness are often assessed by other criteria, such as the ability to attend school or problems in behavior.)

The range of services that may be needed by persons who have difficulties in carrying out their ADLs and IADLs, as well as their primary caregivers, is extensive. A list of such services is presented in Table 16–1. Almost all of the services can be provided for individuals regardless of where they reside—at home, in a nursing home, or in residential settings such as retirement communities, board-and-care facilities, adult-foster homes, assisted-living facilities, and various other forms of sheltered-housing arrangements.

Table 16–1 Services That May Be Needed for Disabled Individuals and Their Families

Acute medical care	Homemaker	Physical therapy
Adult day care	Hospice	Protective services
Audiology	Legal services	Recreation/exercise
Autopsy	Medication and elimination of drugs that cause excess disability	Respite care*
Chore services	Mental health services	Shopping
Dental care	Multidimensional assessment	Skilled nursing
Diagnosis	Nutrition counseling	Special equipment (ramps, hospital beds, etc.)
Escort service	Occupational therapy	Speech therapy
Family/caregiver counseling	Ongoing medical supervision	Supervision
Family/caregiver education and training	Paid companion/sitter	Telephone reassurance
Family support groups	Patient counseling	Transportation
Financial/benefits counseling	Personal care	Treatment of coexisting medical conditions
Home-delivered meals	Personal emergency response system	Vision care
Home health aide		

**Respite care* includes any service intended to provide temporary relief for the primary caregiver. When used for that purpose, homemaker, paid companion/sitter, adult day care, temporary nursing-home care, and other services included on the list constitute respite care.

Source: Adapted from *Confused Minds, Burdened Families: Finding Help for People with Alzheimer's and Other Dementias,* p. 16, 1990, Office of Technology Assessment.

Popular perceptions are that most of the long-term care population is elderly and resides in nursing homes. However, as shown in Table 16–2, this is not the case. People aged 65 and older comprise but 55 percent of the long-term care population. Working-age adults account for 42 percent of the total and children the remaining 3 percent. Moreover, only 22 percent of the elderly population needing long-term care, and 19 percent of the total disabled population, reside in nursing homes and other institutions.

Although it seems apparent that the number of people needing long-term care will grow substantially in the future, reasonably precise predictions regarding the size of that population and its composition are difficult because of many factors that are involved. New and improved medical treatments and technological developments could help to prevent, delay, and compensate for various types of functional difficulties. Moreover, health-related lifestyle changes and environmental-protection measures could markedly reduce rates of disabling diseases and injuries. To the contrary, medical advances could increase the need for long-term care. Lower death rates from heart disease and stroke, for example, could mean that more people will live longer with disabling conditions and into the pathway of late-onset illnesses such as Alzheimer's disease. Similarly, improvements in dealing with the complications of acquired immune deficiency syndrome (AIDS) could engender longer periods of care for patients with this condition.

Future needs for providing and financing long-term care at older ages may also be affected by demographic factors. For instance, the cohorts who will reach old age in the next several decades will be better educated than their predecessors, and higher levels of education are associated with lower levels of disability and need for care.[4] Yet the ethnic composition of these same cohorts suggests that the need for care and governmental subsidies for financing it may be even greater in the future than it is today. From 1990 to 2050, the proportion of Americans aged 65 and older that is nonwhite will more than double from 9.8 percent to 21.3 percent. When they reach old age, these racial minorities may be highly dependent on public subsidies for their long-term care if present patterns of economic-resource distribution among racial and ethnic groups persist throughout the first half of the twenty-first century. Among persons aged 65 and older who have the lowest household incomes, nearly 40 percent are racial minorities, and their aggregate net worth is less than one-third that of older white persons.[5]

Even though precise projections are difficult, it is clear that there will be enormous increases in the number of disabled older people in the twenty-first century. When much of the baby boom—a large cohort of 74 million Americans born between 1946 and 1964—reaches the ranks of old age in 2030, the absolute number of people aged 65 and older will have more than doubled from about 31 million in 1990 to about 65 million. Moreover, the number of persons in advanced old-age ranges will also more than double. The number of persons aged 75 and older will grow from 13 million to 30 million

Table 16–2 Number of Persons Needing Long-Term Care, by Age and Residence (in Thousands)

Age Group Population	*In Institutions*	*At Home or in Community Settings*	*Total*
Children	90	330	420
Working-age adults	710	4,380	5,090
Elderly (aged 65+)	1,640	5,690	7,330
Total	2,440	10,400	12,840

Source: Adapted from U.S. General Accounting Office, 1994.

between 1990 and 2030, and those aged 85 and older will have increased from three million to eight million.[6] Rates of disability increase markedly at these advanced old ages. One reflection of this can be found in the present rates of nursing home use in different old-age categories. About 1 percent of Americans aged 65 to 74 years are in nursing homes; this compares with 6.1 percent of persons ages 75 to 84, and 24 percent of persons age 85 and older.[7] Similarly, disability rates increase in older old-age categories among older persons who are not in nursing homes, from nearly 23 percent of those aged 65 to 74 who experience difficulty with ADLs to 45 percent of those aged 85 and older.[8]

The tremendous future growth expected in the older population, in itself, suggests that there will be millions more disabled elderly people in the decades ahead. Whether rates of disability in old age will increase or decline in the future, however, is a matter on which experts disagree, depending on their assumptions and measures.[9] Assuming no changes in age-specific risks of disability, Cassel et al.[10] calculate a 31 percent increase between 1990 and 2010 in the number of persons aged 65 and older experiencing difficulty with ADLs. Using the same assumption, the Congressional Budget Office projects that the nursing home population will increase 50 percent between 1990 and 2010, double by 2030, and triple by 2050.[11] But even those researchers who report a decline in the prevalence of disability at older ages in recent years, emphasize that there will be large absolute increases in the number of older Americans needing long-term care in the decades ahead.[12]

Predicting whether long-term care needs among people under age 65 will increase or decline is more difficult. One of the principal reasons is that reliable databases for making projections are limited as compared with well-developed national and longitudinal sources available regarding the older population. Data collected on a state basis vary widely with respect to state rates for various types of disabilities.[13] Moreover, the numbers involved with respect to various disabling conditions—such as spinal cord injury, cerebral palsy, and mental retardation—are relatively small and much more susceptible to changing conditions.

Yet, experts agree that the number of younger disabled persons has grown in recent years, and this trend may well persist.[14] New technologies and increased access to medical care continue to enable more people to survive injuries and other conditions that were heretofore fatal, and thereby live for many years with ADL limitations. For example, biomedical advances have enabled many more children with developmental disabilities, as well as low birth-weight infants, to survive much longer than in the past and to have extended years in which they need long-term care.

ISSUES OF ACCESS

Whether a long-term care patient is in a nursing home, living at home, or in another type of residential setting, an ideal system of services would be amply available, would be of high quality, would be provided by well-trained personnel, would be easily located and arranged, and would be readily accessible through private and/or public funding. The present system, however, is far from ideal.

The supply of services is insufficient; service providers lack education and training; and the quality of many services is poor.[15] Moreover, the system is so fragmented that even when high-quality services are sufficiently available, many patients and families do not know about them and require help in defining their service needs and in arranging for them to be provided.[16]

Underlying each of these problems, in turn, is the issue of financing. As is the case with most aspects of the U.S. health care delivery system, the characteristics of long-term care services are substantially shaped by the nature and extent of policies for funding it.

The Costs of Care

Aggregate expenditures for long-term care are sizable and very likely to increase in the decades immediately ahead. The total bill in 1995 was $106.5 billion; 73 percent was spent on nursing-home care and 27 percent on home and community-based care.[17] Out-of-pocket payments by individuals and their families account for 32.5 percent of the total. Private insurance benefits pay for 5.5 percent. Other private funds account for 4.6 percent. The remaining 57.4 percent is financed by federal, state, and local governments. Medicaid pays for 85 percent of nursing-home care.

Paying the costs of long-term care out-of-pocket can be a catastrophic financial experience for patients and their families. The annual cost of a year's care in a nursing home averages more than $46,000 but can cost well over $100,000.[18] While the use of a limited number of services in a home or other community-based setting is less expensive, noninstitutional care for patients who would otherwise be appropriately placed in a nursing home is not cheaper.[19]

For a high percentage of older people, the prices of long-term care are simply unaffordable. Among persons aged 65 and older, 40 percent have a pretax income of less than 200 percent of the poverty threshold—under $14,618 for an individual and $18,440 for a married couple in which the man is aged 65 or older.[20]

The costs of care will undoubtedly grow in the future. Price increases in nursing home and home- and community-based care have consistently exceeded the general rate of inflation. Trends in long-term care labor and overhead costs indicate that this pattern will continue.

Dozens of governmental programs are sources of funding for long-term care services, including Medicaid, the Veterans' Administration, Social Security's Title XX for social services, and the Older Americans Act.[21] Yet, each source regulates the availability of funds with rules as to eligibility and breadth of service coverage and changes its rules frequently. Consequently, persons needing long-term care and their caregivers often find themselves ineligible for financial help from these programs and unable to pay out-of-pocket for needed services. In one study, about 75 percent of the informal, unpaid caregivers of dementia patients reported that the patients did not use formal, paid services because the patients were unable to pay for them.[22]

The Caregiving Role of Families

A number of research efforts have documented that about 80 percent of the long-term care provided to older persons outside of nursing homes is presently provided on an in-kind basis by family members—spouses, siblings, adult children, and broader kin networks. About 74 percent of dependent community-based older persons receive all their care from family members or other unpaid sources; about 21 percent receive both formal and informal services; and about 5 percent use just formal services.[23] The vast majority of family caregivers are women.[24] The family also plays an important role in obtaining and managing services from paid service providers.

The capacities and willingness of family members to care for disabled older persons may decline, however, when the baby boom cohort reaches old age, because of a broad social trend. The family, as a fundamental unit of social organization, has been undergoing profound transformations that will become more fully manifest over the next few decades as baby boomers reach old age. The striking growth of single-parent households, the growing participation of women in the labor force, and the high incidence of divorce and remarriage (differentially higher for men) all entail complicated changes in the structure of household and kinship roles and relationships. There will be an increasing number of blended families, reflecting multiple lines of descent through multiple marriages and the birth of children outside of wedlock through other partners. This growth in the incidence of step- and half-relatives will make for a dramatic new turn in family structure in the coming decades. Already, such blended families constitute about half of all households with children.[25]

One possible implication of these changes is that kinship networks in the near future will become more complex, attenuated, and diffuse,[26] perhaps with a weakened sense of filial obligation. If changes in the intensity of kinship relations significantly erode the capacity and sense of obligation to care for older family members when the baby boom cohort is in the ranks of old age and disability, demands for governmental support to pay long-term care may increase accordingly.

The Role of Private Insurance

Private, long-term care insurance, a relatively new product, is very expensive for the majority of older persons, and its benefits are limited in scope and duration. The best-quality policies—providing substantial benefits over a reasonable period of time—charged premiums in 1991 that averaged $2,525 for persons aged 65 and $7,675 for those aged 79.[27] About 4 percent to 5 percent of older persons have any private long-term care insurance, and only about 1 percent of nursing-home costs are paid by private insurance.[28] A number of analyses have suggested that even when the product becomes more refined, no more than 20 percent of older Americans will be able to afford private insurance.[29]

A variation on the private-insurance-policy approach to financing long-term care is continuing care retirement communities (CCRCs) that promise comprehensive health care services—including long-term care—to all members.[30] CCRC customers tend to be middle- and upper-income persons who are relatively healthy when they become residents and pay a substantial entrance charge and monthly fee in return for a promise of "care for life." It has been estimated that about 10 percent of older people could afford to join such communities.[31] Most of the 1,000 CCRCs in the United States, however, do not provide complete benefit coverage in their contracts, and those that do have faced financial difficulties.[32] Because most older people prefer to remain in their own homes rather than join age-segregated communities, an alternative product termed "life care at home" (LCAH) was developed in the late 1980s and marketed to middle-income customers with lower entry and monthly fees than those of CCRCs.[33] There are, however, only about 500 LCAH policies in effect.[34]

A relatively new approach for providing long-term care in residential settings is the assisted-living facility. It has been created for moderately disabled persons—including those with dementia—who are not ready for a nursing home and provides them with limited forms of personal care, supervision of medications and other daily routines, and congregate meal and housekeeping services.[35] Assisted living has yet to be tried with a private-insurance approach. The monthly rent in a first-class nonprofit facility averages about $2,400 for a one-bedroom apartment; the rent is higher in for-profit facilities.

The Role of Medicaid

For those who cannot pay for long-term care out-of-pocket or through various insurance arrangements, and who are not eligible for care through programs of the Department of Veterans Affairs, the available sources of payment are Medicaid and other means-tested government programs funded by the Older Americans Act, Social Service Block Grants (Title XX of the Social Security Act), and state and local governments. The bulk of such financing is through Medicaid, the federal-state program for the poor, which finances the care—at least in part—of about three-fifths of nursing-home patients[36] and 28 percent of home and community-based services.[37] The program does not pay for the full range of home-care services that are needed for most clients who are functionally dependent. Most state Medicaid programs provide reimbursement only for the most "medicalized" services that are necessary to maintain a long-term care patient in a home environment. Rarely reimbursed are essential supports such as chore services, assistance with food shopping and meal preparation, transportation, companionship, periodic monitoring, and respite programs for family and other unpaid caregivers.

Medicaid does include a special waiver program that allows states to offer a wider range of nonmedical home-care services, if limited to those patients whose services will be no more costly than Medicaid-financed nursing-home care. But the volume of services in these waiver programs—which in some states combine Medicaid with funds from the Older Americans Act, the Social Services Block Grant program, and other state and local government sources—is small in relation to the overall demand.[38]

Although many patients are poor enough to qualify for Medicaid when they enter a nursing home, a substantial number become poor after they are institutionalized.[39] Persons in this latter group deplete their assets in order to meet their bills and eventually "spend down" and become poor enough to qualify for Medicaid.

Still others become eligible for Medicaid by sheltering their assets—illegally or legally with the assistance of attorneys who specialize in so-called Medicaid estate planning. Because sheltered assets are not counted in Medicaid eligibility determinations, such persons are able to take advantage of a program for the poor, without being poor. Asset sheltering has become a source of considerable concern to the federal and state governments as Medicaid expenditures on nursing homes and home care have been increasing rapidly—nearly doubling from 1990 to 1995.[40]

An analysis in Virginia estimated that the aggregate of assets sheltered through the use of legal loopholes in 1991 was equal to more than 10 percent of what the state spent on nursing-home care through Medicaid in that year.[41] A study drawing on interviews with state government staff for Medicaid eligibility determination in four states—California, Florida, Massachusetts, and New York—found a strong relationship between a high level of financial wealth in a geographic area and a high level of Medicaid estate-planning activity. Most of these workers estimated that the range of asset sheltering among single applicants for Medicaid was between 5 percent and 10 percent, and for married applicants, between 20 percent and 25 percent.[42]

A law enacted in 1996 made it a federal crime to shelter assets in order to become eligible for Medicaid. But the law is so vague that, practically speaking, it has been unenforceable.

FORCES FOR IMPROVING ACCESS

From the mid-1980s until the mid-1990s a number of national policy makers were sympathetic to these various dilemmas—the inability of individuals and their families to pay for services, the limitations of private insurance, and the anxieties of spending down. Since then, however, the main concern in Washington, D.C., as well as in the states, has been to limit Medicaid expenditures. In this new context, the most likely prospect is that public resources for long-term care will be even less available, in relation to the need, than they have been to date.

Public recognition of a need to improve access to long-term care has been building over the past two decades. The major initial impetus for this increased awareness has been successful advocacy efforts on behalf of older people, particularly the efforts undertaken by a political coalition concerned about Alzheimer's disease (AD) that began to form in the mid-1970s.[43] This coalition was successful in getting Congress to earmark appropriations for AD research at the National Institute on Aging in the 1980s, and the amount of these funds have been increasing ever since.[44]

Advocates for victims of AD formally coalesced in 1988 with the broader constituency concerned for chronically ill and disabled older persons. The Alzheimer's Association, the American Association for Retired Persons (AARP), and the Families U.S.A. Foundation (a small organization originally established to improve the plight of poor older people) allied during the presidential campaign to undertake a lobbying effort organized under the name Long-Term Care '88.[45] The next year an explicit link was forged between advocates for the disabled and the elderly when Congressman Claude Pepper introduced a bill to provide comprehensive long-term home-care coverage for disabled persons *of any age* who are dependent in at least two ADLs.[46] Although this bill was not voted on by Congress, it was a milestone in that it was the first major legislative effort to programmatically combine the long-term care needs of younger disabled adults with those of elderly people.

Following the Pepper bill, several dozen long-term care bills were introduced in Congress. The lobbying efforts for long-term care that were launched in the 1988 presidential campaign have broadened to encompass the needs of younger disabled people and have been carried forward by a coalition named The Long-Term Care Campaign. This Washington-based interest group claims to represent nearly 140 national organizations (with more than 60 million members) including religious denominations, organized labor and business groups, nurses, veterans, youth and women's groups, consumer organizations, and racial and ethnic groups, as well as older and younger disabled persons.[47]

In the early 1990s, advocates for the elderly and younger disabled persons were optimistic that the federal government would establish a new program for funding long-term care that would not be means-tested as is Medicaid. A number of bills introduced from 1989 to 1994 included some version of such a program, including President Clinton's failed proposal for health care reform.[48] None of these proposals became law. The major reason was that any substantial version of such a program would cost tens of billions of dollars each year just at the outset and far more as the baby boomers reach old age.

By the mid-1990s, optimism regarding expanded governmental funding for long-term care was quashed. A new Republican majority in the 104th Congress reversed the focus on long-term care from expansion to retraction. It proposed to limit federal spending on Medicaid. Advocates for long-term care programs switched from offense to defense.

By 1995, Medicaid's expenditures on long-term care had been growing at an annualized rate of 13.2 percent since 1989.[49] As part of its overall effort to achieve a balanced budget, Congress initially proposed in that year to cap the rate of growth in Medicaid expenditures in order to achieve savings of $182 billion by 2002, to eliminate federal requirements for determining individual eligibility for Medicaid (as an entitlement), and to turn over control of the program to state governments through capped block grants. Such changes were vetoed by President Clinton. They resurfaced in 1996 with proposed reductions totaling $72 billion, but no legislation was enacted that year.

This approach remains on the policy agenda, strongly supported by the National Governors Association. According to one analysis[50] the 1995 congressional proposals for limiting Medicaid's growth would have trimmed long-term care funding by as much as 11.4 percent by the year 2000 and meant that 1.74 million Medicaid beneficiaries would have lost or been unable to secure coverage. In addition, this analysis assumed that states would make their initial reductions in home- and community-based care services (because nursing-home residents have nowhere else to go), and concluded that such services would be substantially reduced from their current levels. Five states were projected to completely eliminate home- and community-based services by the end of the century and another 19 to cut services by more than half. Whether or not such specific predictions come true, if provisions to cap and block-grant Medicaid do become law they will almost certainly engender conflict within states regarding the distribution of limited resources for the care of older and younger poor constituencies.

WHAT PROSPECTS FOR IMPROVED ACCESS?

At the turn of the century, prospects for older people having better access to long-term care seem dim. Out-of-pocket payments for care are becoming larger and increasingly unaffordable for many. Only a minority of older persons—now about 5 percent, and perhaps 20 percent in the decades ahead—may be able to afford premiums for private long-term care insurance. Broad societal trends suggest that informal, unpaid care by family members may become less feasible in the future than it is today. Moreover, the safety net that government programs provide by financing long-term care for the poor is seriously threatened by contemporary federal and state budgetary politics.

How might the outlook improve in the future? The most promising seeds for change lie in the enormous projected growth in the number of older persons needing long-term care, outlined at the outset of this chapter. Moreover, leaders of the American Coalition of Citizens with Disabilities, representing eight million disabled persons, have expressed for some years the hope that it might form a powerful political alliance with organizations representing 32 million older people to pursue this issue of mutual concern.[51]

As the demand for long-term care increases, while the means for access remain limited or become more restricted, a widespread and deeply felt popular demand for expanded government funding of long-term care could well emerge. Even as organized advocates for long-term care access brought the issue to the public policy agenda in the late 1980s and early 1990s, the entrance of the baby boomers into the ranks of old age may precipitate a grassroots movement that will revitalize political awareness of the issue as a major problem in American society.

But even if a grassroots movement is able to elevate the principle of expanded government funding for long-term care to the top of the agenda, that general principle masks some basic value questions that, so far, have just begun to surface in public discussion. Widespread debate on and resolution of these questions will be required for a substantial proportion of Americans to understand and support the implications of any law that is to be enacted. Otherwise, even if enacted, such legislation could be quickly repealed as was the poorly understood Medicare Catastrophic Coverage Act of 1988.[52] Yet depending on the identity of the primary constituency seeking support for long-term care—the aged, the disabled, or a broader coalition of the aged, the disabled, and perhaps others—the configurations and primacy of the values involved may be very different, and the likelihood of generating widespread support may vary substantially.

From the perspective of older persons, long-term care has been seen as a problem besetting elderly people, categorically. And the predominant, though not exclusive, element of interest in additional public insurance has been generated by an economic concern. That concern is the possibility of becoming poor through spending down, depleting one's assets to pay for long-term care and then becoming dependent on a welfare program, Medicaid, to pay nursing-home bills. There is a distinct middle-class fear—both economic and psychological—of using savings and selling a home to finance one's own health care. This anxiety reflects a desire to protect estates, as well as the psychological intertwining of personal self-esteem with one's material worth and independence.

The political weight of this type of concern, however, is not substantial in today's climate of public-policy discourse. Since the late 1970s the political era in which categorical old-age entitlement programs were created and sustained with relative ease appears to be over. The aged have become a scapegoat for a variety of America's problems, and many domestic-policy concerns have been framed as issues of intergenerational equity.[53]

If expanded public long-term care insurance is to be enacted as an old-age entitlement, to serve older persons as a buffer against spending down, there are some fundamental moral and political issues that the American public will need to confront and resolve. Among these issues are: Assuming that we can improve laws for protecting spouses of long-term care patients from impoverishment, why shouldn't older people spend their assets and income on their health care? Why should government foot the bill? Why should it be government's responsibility to preserve estates for inheritance? Should government take a more active role than at present in preserving economic-status inequalities, from generation to generation? On what basis should some persons be taxed to preserve the inheritances of others? Should the taxing power of government be used to preserve the psychological sense of self-esteem that for so many persons is bound up in their lifetime accumulation of assets—their material worth? Widespread public debate on such issues may very well fail to resolve them in a fashion that supports a major initiative in long-term care to protect older persons from paying for their care.

Even if such questions are satisfactorily resolved, there would still remain the challenge of bringing together the different perspectives of the elderly and the younger disabled population. In contrast to older persons, younger disabled persons do not perceive long-term care funding as mostly an issue of whether the government or the individual patient and/or family pays for the care. At least as important to them is the issue of whether such funding covers basic access to services, technologies, and environments that will make it feasible to carry forward an active life. They argue that they should have assistance to do much of what they would be able to do if they were not disabled.

The Americans with Disabilities Act of 1990, achieved through vigorous advocacy efforts, has helped to eliminate discriminatory as well as physical barriers to the participation of people with disabilities in employment, public services, public accommodations, transportation, and telecommunications. But it will not provide the elements of long-term care desired by disabled younger adults, such as paid assistance in the home and for getting in and out of the home, peer counseling, semi-independent modes of transportation, and client control or management of services.

Although the disabled have advocated for long-term care services, they have rejected a "medical model" that emphasizes long-term care as an essential component of *health* services. This is understandable, given their strong desires for autonomy, independence, and as much "normalization" of daily life as possible. By the same token, disabled people have traditionally eschewed symbolic and political identification with elderly people, because of traditional stereotypes of older people as frail, chronically ill, declining, and "marginal" to society.

The efforts of disabled people to advocate on their terms for governmental long-term care initiatives, however, have made little progress. Rather, previous success in getting expanded public funding for long-term care on the national policy agenda—for persons of all ages—was due largely to advocates for the elderly, and to broader concerns about the projected health care needs generated by an increasingly larger and, on average, older population of elderly people.

In any grassroots efforts to elevate long-term care funding to the top of the national policy agenda, advocates for the younger disabled would probably be well-advised to suppress their objections to the health care model of long-term care. The challenge of gaining widespread popular support for long-term care funding is to overcome a long-standing cultural perception that long-term care is separate and detached from the arena of health care.

For most of this century, long-term care has been a comparatively neglected backwater in the overall American health care scene. Except for occasional nursing-home scandals and fires—and subsequent ad hoc activities in response to these events—long-term care has received very little attention from the medical profession and society at large. It has been eclipsed by the glamor and prestige of hospital-based medical care that is inherently dramatic because it deals with acute episodes of illnesses and trauma, and their relatively high-tech and quick-fix dimensions of diagnosis and intervention.

In effect, long-term care has not been perceived as part of health care. Long-term care has not even been covered through traditional health insurance mechanisms such as employee benefit plans. When concerns are expressed about the fact that 40 million Americans are not covered by health insurance, coverage for long-term care is not part of the discussion.

Yet, there are good reasons to believe that long-term care will come to be perceived more widely as part of the continuum of health care that is needed by all of us.[54] As the baby boom cohort begins to approach the ranks of old age, the importance of long-term care—a formidable volume of need for it, the difficulties of financing it, and the challenges of delivering it effectively—is likely to become increasingly accepted throughout American society. Such acceptance could bring with it a widespread understanding that long-term care is health care by another name. This perception may enfold long-term care into the shared understanding of justice in health care that dictates that access to long-term care is as much of a fundamental right as is access to other kinds of health care.

NOTES

1. S. McConnell, "Who Cares about Long-Term Care?" *Generations* XIV, no. 2 (1990): 15–18.
2. F. B. Hobbs, *Sixty-Five Plus in the United States: U.S. Bureau of the Census, Current Populations Reports, Special Studies* (Washington, D.C.: U.S. Government Printing Office, 1996), 23–190.
3. R. Stone and P. Kemper, "Spouses and Children of Disabled Elders: How Large a Constituency for Long-Term Care Reform?" *The Milbank Quarterly* 67 (1989): 485–506.
4. U.S. Bureau of the Census, *Sixty-Five Plus in America: Current Populations Reports, Special Studies* (Washington, D.C.: U.S. Government Printing Office, 1992), 23–178.
5. S. Crystal, "Economic Status of the Elderly," in *Handbook of Aging and the Social Sciences,* 4th ed., ed. R. H. Binstock and L. K. George (San Diego, Calif.: Academic Press, 1996), 388–409.
6. U.S. Bureau of the Census, *Sixty-Five Plus in America: Current Populations Reports, Special Studies.*
7. Ibid.
8. C. K. Cassel, M. A. Rudberg, and S. J. Olshansky, "The Price of Success: Health Care in an Aging Society," *Health Affairs* 11, no. 2 (1992): 87–99.
9. J. F. Fries, "The Compression of Morbidity; Near or Far?" *The Milbank Quarterly* 67 (1989): 208–32; K. G. Manton, L. S. Corder, and E. Stallard, "Estimates of Change in Chronic Disability and Institutional Incidence and Prevalence Rates in the U.S. Elderly Population from the 1982, 1984, and 1989 National Long Term Care Survey," *Journal of Gerontology: Social Sciences* 48 (1993): S153–S166; E. L. Schneider and J. M. Guralnik, "The Aging of America: Impact on Health Care Costs," *Journal of the American Medical Association* 263 (1991): 2335–40; L. M. Verbrugge, "Recent, Present, and Future Health of American Adults," in *Annual Review of Public Health,* vol. 10, ed. L. Breslow, J. E. Fielding, and L. B. Lave (Palo Alto, Calif.: Annual Reviews, Inc., 1989): 333–61.
10. Cassel et al., "The Price of Success."
11. U.S. Bureau of the Census, *Sixty-Five Plus in America: Current Populations Reports, Special Studies.*
12. Manton et al., "Estimates of Change in Chronic Disability and Institutional Incidence."
13. M. P. LaPlante, *Disability Statistics Report: State Estimates of Disability in America* (Washington, D.C.: National Institute on Disability and Rehabilitation Research, U.S. Department of Education, Office of Special Education and Rehabilitative Services, 1993).
14. J. L. Ross, *Long-Term Care: Demography, Dollars, and Dissatisfaction Drive Reform.* Testimony before the Special Committee on Aging, U.S. Senate. U.S. GAO/T-HEHS 94-140 (April 12, 1994).
15. U.S. Congress, Office of Technology Assessment, *Losing a Million Minds: Confronting the Tragedy of Alzheimer's Disease and Other Dementias* (Washington, D.C.: U.S. Government Printing Office, 1987).
16. U.S. Congress, Office of Technology Assessment, *Confused Minds, Burdened Families: Finding Help for People with Alzheimer's and Other Dementias* (Washington, D.C.: U.S. Government Printing Office, 1990).
17. K. R. Levit, H. C. Lazenby, B. R. Braden et al., "National Health Expenditures," *Health Care Financing Review* 7, no. 2 (1996): 175–214.
18. Ibid.
19. W. G. Weissert, "Strategies for Reducing Home Care Expenditures," *Generations* 14, no. 2 (1990): 42–44.
20. U.S. Bureau of the Census, *Poverty in the United States: 1995,* Current Population Reports, Consumer Income (Washington, D.C.: U.S. Government Printing Office, 1996), 60–194.
21. U.S. General Accounting Office, *Long-Term Care: Current Issues and Future Directions* (Washington, D.C.: U.S. Government Printing Office, 1995).
22. S. K. Eckert and K. Smyth, *A Case Study of Methods of Locating and Arranging Health and Long-Term Care for Persons with Dementia* (Washington, D.C.: Office of Technology Assessment, Congress of the United States, 1988).
23. K. Liu, K. M. Manton, and B. M. Liu, "Home Care Expenses for the Disabled Elderly," *Health Care Financing Review* 7, no. 2 (1985): 51–58.
24. E. M. Brody, *Women in the Middle: Their Parent-Care Years* (New York: Springer Publishing, 1990); R. Stone, G. L. Cafferta, and J. Sangl, "Caregivers of the Frail Elderly: A National Profile," *Gerontologist* 27 (1989): 616–26.

25. National Academy on Aging, *Old Age in the Twenty-first Century* (Washington, D.C.: Syracuse University, 1994).
26. V. L. Bengston, C. Rosenthal, and L. Burton, "Families and Aging: Diversity and Heterogeneity," in *Handbook of Aging and the Social Sciences,* 3d ed., ed. R. H. Binstock and L. K. George (San Diego, Calif.: Academic Press, 1990), 263–87.
27. J. M. Wiener and L. H. Illston, "Health Care Financing and Organization for the Elderly," in *Handbook of Aging and the Social Sciences,* 4th ed., ed. R. H. Binstock and L. K. George (San Diego, Calif.: Academic Press, 1996).
28. J. M. Wiener, L. H. Illston, and R. J. Hanley, *Sharing the Burden: Strategies for Public and Private Long-Term Care Insurance* (Washington, D.C.: The Brookings Institution, 1994).
29. W. H. Crown, J. Capitman, and W. N. Leutz, "Economic Rationality, the Affordability of Private Long-Term Care Insurance, and the Role for Public Policy," *Gerontologist* 32 (1992): 478–85; R. Friedland, *Facing the Costs of Long-Term Care: An EBRI-ERF Policy Study* (Washington, D.C.: Employee Benefits Research Institute, 1990); A. M. Rivlin and J. M. Wiener, *Caring for the Elderly: Who Will Pay?* (Washington, D.C.: The Brookings Institution, 1988); Wiener et al. *Sharing the Burden.*
30. R. D. Chellis and P. J. Grayson, *Life Care: A Long-Term Solution?* (Lexington, Mass.: Lexington Books, 1990).
31. M. A. Cohen, "Life Care: New Options for Financing and Delivering Long-Term Care," in *Health Care Financing Review, Annual Supplement* (Thousand Oaks, Calif.: Sage Publications, 1988), 139–43.
32. T. F. Williams and H. Temkin-Greener, "Older People, Dependency, and Trends in Supportive Care," in *The Future of Long-Term Care: Social and Policy Issues,* ed. R. H. Binstock, L. E. Cluff, and O. von Mering (Baltimore: Johns Hopkins University Press, 1996), 51–74.
33. E. J. Tell, M. A. Cohen, and S. S. Wallack, "New Directions in Life Care: Industry in Transit," *The Milbank Quarterly* 65 (1987): 551–74.
34. Williams and Temkin-Greener, "Older People."
35. R. A. Kane and K. B. Wilson, *Assisted Living in the United States: A New Paradigm for Residential Care for Older People?* (Washington, D.C.: American Association for Retired Persons, 1993); V. Regnier, J. Hamilton, S. Yatabe, *Assisted Living for the Aged and Frail: Innovations in Design, Management, and Financing* (New York: Columbia University Press, 1995).
36. Wiener and Illston, "Health Care Financing and Organization for the Elderly."
37. American Association of Retired Persons, Public Policy Institute, *The Costs of Long-Term Care* (Washington, D.C.: American Association of Retired Persons, 1994).
38. R. B. Hudson, "Social Protection and Services," in *Handbook of Aging and the Social Sciences,* 4th ed., ed. R. H. Binstock and L. K. George (San Diego, Calif.: Academic Press, 1996), 446–66.
39. E. K. Adams, M. R. Meiners, and B. O. Burwell, "Asset Spend-Down in Nursing Homes: Methods and Insights," *Medical Care* 31 (1993): 1–23.
40. Levit, Lazenby, Braden, et al., "National Health Expenditures."
41. B. Burwell, *State Responses to Medicaid Estate Planning* (Cambridge, Mass.: SysteMetrics, 1993).
42. B. Burwell and W. H. Crown, *Medicaid Estate Planning in the Aftermath of OBRA '93* (Cambridge, Mass.: The MEDSTAT Group, 1995).
43. P. Fox, "From Senility to Alzheimer's Disease: The Rise of the Alzheimer's Disease Movement," *The Milbank Quarterly* 67 (1989): 58–102.
44. G. D. Cohen, "Alzheimer's Disease: Current Policy Initiatives," in *Dementia and Aging: Ethics, Values, and Policy Choices,* ed. R. H. Binstock, S. G. Post, and P. J. Whitehouse (Baltimore: Johns Hopkins University Press, 1992).
45. McConnell, "Who Cares about Long-Term Care?"
46. U.S. House of Representatives, *Long-Term Care Act of 1989,* H.R. 2263, 101st Congress (1989).
47. Long-Term Care Campaign, Pepper Commission Recommendations Released March 2nd, *Insiders Update* (Jan./Feb. 1990): 1.
48. R. H. Binstock, "Older Americans and Health Care Reform in the 1990s," in *Health Care Reform in the Nineties,* ed. P. V. Rosenau (Thousand Oaks, Calif.: Sage Publications, 1994), 213–35.
49. U.S. General Accounting Office, *Long-Term Care: Current Issues and Future Directions.*
50. E. Kassner, *Long-Term Care: Measuring the Impact of a Medicaid Cap* (Washington, D.C.: Public Policy Institute, American Association of Retired Persons, 1995).
51. P. Rubenfeld, "Ageism and Disabilityism: Double Jeopardy," in *Aging and Rehabilitation: Advances in the State of the Art,* ed. S. J. Brody and G. E. Ruff (New York: Springer Publishing, 1986), 323–28.
52. R. Himelfarb, *Catastrophic Politics: The Rise and Fall of the Medicare Catastrophic Coverage Act of 1988* (University Park, Pa.: Pennsylvania State University Press, 1995).
53. R. H. Binstock, "Policies on Aging in the Post-Cold War Era," in *Post-Cold War Policy: The Social and Domestic Context,* ed. W. Crotty (Chicago: Nelson Hall, 1995), 55–90.
54. R. H. Binstock, L. E. Cluff, and O. von Mering (eds.), *The Future of Long-Term Care: Social and Policy Issues* (Baltimore: Johns Hopkins University Press, 1996).

CHAPTER 17

Treating Senility and Dementia: Ethical Challenges and Quality-of-Life Judgments

Stephen G. Post

This chapter focuses on the patient with a progressive dementia, most often of the Alzheimer's type. Although the discussion centers on the elderly, it should be kept in mind that dementia, the loss of mental function from a previous state, can occur in all ages. If Alzheimer's disease is the dementia of the elderly, increasingly AIDS dementia is the dementia of those who are young. Not every issue related to ethics and dementia can be covered here. Instead, I attempt to provide an introduction to some of the concerns that might be considered most pressing.

DIAGNOSTIC DISCLOSURE

Should patients with Alzheimer's disease be told their diagnosis? An article with this question as its title points out that new diagnostic knowledge about Alzheimer's disease is "likely to swing the pendulum even more decisively in favor of truth-telling."[1] Authors Drickamer and Lachs refer to new clinical biologic markers that may increase diagnostic accuracy. So long as clinical diagnosis of Alzheimer's disease is uncertain, some clinicians regard it as ethical to withhold information about diagnosis and prognosis from patients, even those able to comprehend. If diagnosis becomes certain rather than probable, this position will no longer be tenable.

It is remarkable how truth telling in cases of dementia is much rarer than truth telling in cases of cancer and most other disease diagnoses. Some physicians suggest that with cancer they can at least offer some therapeutic hope to the patient, but progressive dementia is currently incurable. Yet the principles of veracity and patient self-determination require in nearly all cases that the truth is told to dementia patients as early as a reasonably certain diagnosis is possible. Patients have a clear legal and ethical right to decide, while still competent, for or against the use of technologies should they become incompetent. They should know the general course of the disease from mild to profound.

Drickamer and Lachs, however, reject this extension of patient autonomy through advance directives because (1) the new self with severe dementia is arguably no longer the old self, and (2) the old self may have overly grim views of progressive dementia that fail to appreciate the unanticipated "contentment" of some patients in the severe stages of decline. Do these authors mean that progressive dementia is ordinarily benign? Contrary to Drickamer and Lachs, in the final analysis the patient does hold the right to make anticipatory choices for the demented self. Respect for autonomy is the moral principle honoring freedom under conditions of competence.

There are some physicians and other health care workers, as well as many family members, who fear that telling the truth will cause distress to the patient, that he or she will feel stigmatized, become depressed even to the point of despair, and become more difficult to manage. So it is suggested by some that the best interests of patients dictates nondisclosure of progressive dementia. However, most health professionals who work closely with demented patients believe that such concerns are unwarranted, that telling the patient the diagnosis only rarely elicits an adverse reaction. Rather, disclosing the diagnosis to the patient allows him or her to participate as far as possible in the development of a plan of action for the future.

There are important reasons to err on the side of disclosing probable diagnosis. Many patients already suspect that they have Alzheimer's disease even if family members want to "protect" them from knowing. There are patients who want to know their diagnosis so that friends and neighbors will understand that they are not being unpleasant or purposefully forgetting names. Foley describes a case in which the patient was relieved to find out his diagnosis and his prognosis; the revelation obviated embarrassment and annoyance at his forgetfulness.[2] Experienced health care professionals have all known situations where the family agonized over whether to tell the patient about a diagnosis, only to have the patient say, "That's what I've thought all along." In a case with which the author is familiar, Murray C. convinced his wife to bring him into the ElderHealth Center after he read an article about Alzheimer's disease in the newspaper. Once diagnosed, he went to his neighbors and old friends to explain that his forgetfulness was beyond his control and that he meant no offense. There is no reason for a conspiracy of silence regarding progressive dementia.

AUTONOMY

Patients are often denied autonomy once the diagnosis of dementia has been made. This approach, less frequent now than in the past, ignores the variability of the clinical state. In the early stages of progressive dementia, or in a mild case, normal exercise of autonomy is possible. Varying degrees of tactful supervision are necessary. When the dementia is more severe, the exercise of autonomy may have to be restricted, but only in the severe and profound stages should it be denied completely. Here advance directives come into play.

When a decision is to be made about a course to be pursued, autonomy may have to be restricted because the person is psychotic or amnesic or because planning ability and judgment are damaged. Such restrictions should be made only after a detailed history has been obtained and the person has been closely observed over a period of time.[3] The capacity to make decisions does not require that all mental functions be working optimally. Patients who have memory disorders or other kinds of disturbed neurological function are not necessarily incapable of understanding ethical import. There may be periods of clarity or of impairment. Even a severely impaired patient may be able to exercise autonomy for certain matters that seem inconsequential to the caregiver but that have acquired great importance for the demented person.

Obviously, all the wishes of the patient with dementia cannot be gratified. The amnesic patient with bad eyesight should not be driving an automobile; the frail, insulin-dependent, diabetic old woman with cardiac failure cannot live alone; the intractably incontinent and unruly patient without a family or friends must have institutional care. Yet even in exceptional cases, patients have the right to have their problems explained in a way they can understand, not just once but as often as necessary.

Advance directives, generally in the form of a living will, are justified as an extension of autonomy. It is too much to expect that people in any numbers will compose advance directives about how they wish to be managed when or if they become demented. Only a small minority of people, generally less than 20 percent, compose advance directives expressing their wishes in regard to dying and death. Yet ideally the patient with dementia should have a living will and a durable power of attorney for health care. In the case of a progressive dementia, arrangements should be made early in the course of the disease, when the patient is still capable of understanding and deciding.

Early after diagnosis is the time to arrive at decisions about cardiopulmonary resuscitation and about levels of treatment to be undertaken when severe illness occurs, when swallowing fails, or when death is imminent. Many patients are incapable of putting together a specific plan, even with help, but patients with moderate dementia are often able to identify people they trust to make later decisions for them. Usually the person chosen will be the next of kin, but there should always be an alternate if for some reason the first nominee becomes unable to act.

QUALITY OF LIFE AND JUST TREATMENT LIMITATIONS

There is much reason to respect the autonomy of the patient who, in knowing his or her diagnosis, is still able to indicate treatment preferences through advance directives relevant to the later stages of dementia when the patient becomes incompetent. While many, if not most, patients will not request lifesaving treatment, there are some who will. This raises the complicated question of how much health care a just society owes those who become severely demented. For patients in the advanced stages of progressive and eventually fatal dementia, the use of life-prolonging medical technologies for reasons other than palliation remains a matter of medical, moral, and societal debate.

The obvious moral basis for treatment limitation is quality of life. But there are valid cautions about appeals to quality of life, because a reliable qualitative measure of a patient's experience is impossible and because the idea of quality of life can be conveniently misused to rid society of unproductive lives. Also, quality of life is at least partly contingent on the extent to which a supportive environment is created to enhance patient well-being. Even with these cautions in mind, however, quality of life can be objectively assessed to a considerable degree. Were quality of life to be given no moral consideration, then it would be necessary to keep every patient alive to the last minute through the use of every technology available. The essential publication in this area is *The Concept and Measurement of Quality of Life in the Frail Elderly.*[4]

A desirable instrument for assessing the complexities of the severity of dementia is the Washington University Clinical Dementia Rating (CDR), which considers memory, orientation, judgment and problem solving, community affairs, home and hobbies, and personal care. In effect, this is a partial quality-of-life indicator that can be used to identify mild, moderate, severe, profound, and terminal phases of progressive dementia. What it does not do is identify the ethically appropriate limits, if any, on the use of lifesaving interventions along this CDR continuum, for this is an ethical problem rather than an empirical one.

At what point in the progression of dementia is prolongation of life ethically unacceptable? There are times when provision of comfort care has the side effect of prolonging life, creating difficult decisions for physicians and family. Should an airway be placed when dyspnea is causing severe distress or should narcotic and sedative medication be used instead? Should a gastrostomy be placed when aspiration follows dysphagia, or should spoon-feeding or withdrawal of food and fluids be the approach? Should acute appendicitis or acute diverticulitis be treated surgically or with antibiotics or analgesics and sedatives? There are no easy answers for individual cases, and the many considerations that must be taken into account include the stage of the disease, the severity of dementia, the suffering of the patient, the ability of the patient to cooperate with things like surgery or endoscopic examination, and the emotional state of the family.

A degenerative disease such as Alzheimer's, if it is the primary diagnosis, can justifiably be looked on as an extended terminal illness. As early as 1976, Robert Katzman wrote, "In focusing attention on the mortality associated with Alzheimer disease, our goal is not to find a way to prolong the life of severely demented persons."[5] However, as was pointed out in 1985, within the medical community and in society as a whole "consensus breaks down when the attempt is made to determine the nature of the therapeutic obligation to the demented patient, particularly with respect to life-sustaining treatment."[6] Perhaps consensus is now more possible. Discussions about the moral justification for medical interventions with respect to quality and quantity of life and about the importance of avoiding "futile" treatment are now more common.[7] Presumably no physician wishes to provide interventions that will be of no value to the patient.

In an international empirical study of physician attitudes toward aggressive treatment interventions in the case of elderly people with advanced dementia, considerable disagreement was evident both across and within countries.[8] The authors were interested in finding out the decisions physicians would make when confronted with a critically ill, demented elderly man. They presented the case of an 82-year-old man brought to an emergency room with life-threatening gastrointestinal bleeding and blood pressure of 70/40. Three years earlier, the man was diagnosed by a neurologist as suffering from probable Alzheimer's disease. He cannot answer a simple question coherently but seems to understand some simple commands. His behavior is agitated; he wanders, does not recognize his daughter, and has urinary incontinence.

Between March 1987 and April 1989, 897 physicians in academic medical centers at family practice, medical, and geriatric rounds were questioned. Countries included Australia, Brazil, Canada, Scotland, Sweden, the United States, and Wales. Physicians were asked to select from among the following four options (assuming there was no directive from patient or family):

1. MICU [medical intensive care unit] (removal to medical intensive care unit if needed, mechanical ventilation if needed, insertion of a central venous catheter)
2. MAX [maximum therapeutic effort] (no transfer to medical intensive care unit, no mechanical ventilation except for surgery if needed)
3. LIM [limited therapeutic effort] (no transfer to medical intensive care unit, no invasive procedures, limited use of antibiotics, intravenous therapy if needed, radiography and blood tests if medically indicated)
4. SUPP [supportive care only] (comfort and palliation, intravenous fluid only if it improves comfort, no radiography, no blood tests, no antibiotics)

The authors conclude that there is wide variation of opinion both within and between countries, that physicians over 40 years of age and those in family medicine are more likely to decide against aggressive interventions, and that Brazilian and American physicians are the most technologically aggressive while Australians are the least aggressive. For example, only 6 percent of Australian physicians chose MICU, whereas 32 percent of U.S. physicians did so. Conversely, 21 percent of Australian physicians chose supportive care compared to only 3 percent of U.S. physicians.

The variation that this study demonstrated is difficult to interpret. No information is provided regarding the reasons for the differences of opinion. For example, the study does not indicate how strong a factor physicians' fear of legal suit for undertreatment might be. Further, level of training was not the same across physicians recruited from various countries, and availability of technology was not taken into account. Two significant factors may be the number of hospices available and the extent to which hospice access for dementia patients who are not approaching death is limited. As an advocate for a hospice approach to treatment of patients with advanced progressive dementia points out, hospices find dementia difficult to handle because it usually involves a more prolonged dying period than, for example, terminal cancer.[9] But whatever the reasons physicians may have for their approach, this study indicates that a consensus on ethical treatment levels still eludes us.

A less relational view of quality of life might assign a higher value to the inner experiences of the self despite the fact of relational loss or suggest that more self-identity may be present in the patient than meets the eye. Patients with severe dementia do demonstrate underlying affective responses, and they may have occasional windows of clarity when some self-identity surfaces, but in the profound and terminal stages, there is no discernible self-identity remaining. It is very unlikely that self-identity is maintained; the appearances of loss cannot be explained as a deterioration in communicative abilities alone.

David C. Thomasma rightly states that we must be circumspect in judging the quality of life for any patient, since there is ultimately a subjective aspect to all qualitative assessments.[10] There is no absolute certainty about how or when deterioration in communication and short-term memory gives way to a loss of internal sense of self-identity. However, as Aristotle argued, some degree of uncertainty is an aspect of most good practical reasoning. When a person is unaware of his or her environment; is mute, bedridden, and incontinent of bladder and bowel; demonstrates no measurable intellectual functions; and faces inevitable death, comfort care is all that medicine should offer. Comfort care means palliation only, that is, it excludes artificial nutrition and hydration, dialysis, antibiotics, and all other medical interventions unless necessary for the control of pain and discomfort.

There is philosophical literature to support this suggestion, although we need not agree with it in all respects. Dan W. Brock asks an essential question: How much health care does justice require for the elderly with severe dementia?[11] Brock concentrates on the effects of dementia such as the erosion of memory and other cognitive functions that "ultimately destroy personal identity."[12] He notes the crucial role played by "memory and other forms of psychological continuity in maintaining the identity of a person through time."[13] Finally, the person is destroyed by dementia. Experience becomes disconnected, disjointed, and incoherent. The patients are "cut off from the self-conscious psychological continuity with their past and future that is the basis for the sense of personal identity through time and which is a necessary condition of personhood."[14] Brock makes a claim that is uncontroversial: Once a person has died, health care is inappropriate. He also argues that patients in the persistent vegetative state (PVS) have no right to health care since they are no longer the subjects of conscious experience. The patient with severe dementia, however, remains the subject of such experience and is capable of suffering pain and enjoying sensuous pleasures. Nevertheless, both memory and self-identity have been ravaged, the links between past and present are broken, and the "temporal glue" of the self is undermined. This loss implies, for Brock, that the severely demented have "claims to palliative, but not life-sustaining" health care.[15] They retain, however, an interest in care and comfort, so that a painful tumor might be removed for palliative reasons. As for patients who still have memory function to a substantial degree, Brock argues that life-saving care should not be denied them if they desire it.

Daniel Callahan constructs a somewhat similar comparison, pointing out that for the patient who is brain dead, no further care of any kind is called for. The patient in the persistent vegetative state retains an interest in "minimal nursing care only," not inclusive of artificial nutrition and hydration. Of the patient who is severely demented, Callahan writes, "On the one hand, he has lost his capacity for reason and usually—but not always—human interaction. On the other hand, there will be no clear ground for believing that the capacity to experience emotions has been lost."[16] Callahan recommends nursing care only, including artificial nutrition and hydration. Whether or not one agrees with this position on nutrition and hydration, Callahan's main point is that death "need not be resisted."[17] Such treatment limitations are based on the quality of life and the underlying disease condition rather than on old age–based cutoffs.[18]

LONG-TERM CARE

Caring is solicitude. It is present to the extent that anxiety is felt about the well-being of another. Modern rescue medicine has often neglected this aspect of care provision. Caregiving as a vocation has been devalued in our society.

The tasks of long-term caring are readily viewed as demeaning. Partial or constant dependence on others is interpreted as an unreasonable and burdensome imposition. Caring is a basic human need that reminds us of a fundamental reality: We are human beings who share social interdependence. In our age of emphasis on autonomy, rights, and freedoms, it is essential to recognize our inherent dependence on others and the reality of human fragility. At the same time, caring often compels advocacy for the autonomy and rights of dependent people.

The lack of support for caregiving is a measure of its devaluation. To do for others what they cannot do for themselves requires, in addition to compassion, great commitment and expenditure of time and resources. But, it has been noted, "as a society, we have created a situation in which we place a higher value on the act of flipping a hamburger than on the act of caring for chronically disabled individuals."[19] Given this reality, some people who are attracted to the vocation of caring are unable to sustain a minimally decent standard of living for themselves and frequently elect to pursue other career paths. Family caregivers in need of training, encouragement, and assistance must frequently go to unusual lengths to locate people in the community who are willing to devote their time and energies to assist with daily caregiver tasks. We neither adequately train nor adequately compensate caregivers; this remarkable omission can blight the lives of vulnerable citizens.

Complicating this devaluation is the dramatic rise in the need for long-term care in all age groups, a rise partly caused by medical progress. Lifesaving interventions allow people to survive but may leave them in need of extended or even lifelong care. Premature infants may be saved through neonatal intensive care and go on to live reasonably independent lives, but some are permanently impaired and become dependent on family members in ways that are frequently unanticipated and that family members are ill-equipped to deal with. As the human life span increased from approximately 50 years at the turn of the century to nearly 80 years now, periods of dependence on caregivers extend far beyond what was usual a few generations ago.

Daughters and daughters-in-law are the ones typically called on to provide emotional support and assistance for those needing long-term care. Over the last few years, national attention has been focused on "women in the middle"—women sandwiched between job and family responsibilities. The extension of the human life span means that "contemporary adult children provide more care and more difficult care to more parents and parents-in-law over much longer periods of time than ever has been the case before."[20] Studies indicate that daughters or daughters-in-law are more than three times as likely as sons to assist an elderly caregiver with a disabled spouse, and women outnumber men as the caregivers for severely disabled parents by a ratio of 4:1.[21] Although results vary somewhat from study to study, about half of these women caregivers experience stress in the form of depression, sleeplessness, anger, and emotional exhaustion.[22]

While women caregivers must be appreciated for all that they do, we are concerned that significant numbers of women are harmed by the social expectation that they embrace caregiving as their exclusive duty in life no matter how severe the threat to their own well-being. In response to this harm, we propose that policy makers, researchers, and male family members give systematic attention to it. Of course, men provide some direct caring and emotional support, but the bulk of the burden falls on women. Caregiving may require a correction of gender inequities and a revision of gender roles in the family such that men do more direct caring.[23]

There is a vital need to support family caregivers. Remarkably, despite the often unanticipated and unplanned-for burdens of caregiving, more than 80 percent of elderly persons with disabilities are cared for at home. The family is a crucial caring resource. At present, social policy often does little more than cheer the family on. Parents of severely disabled children will sometimes succeed against the odds, but there are many who complain about "extending a child's dependence beyond a parent's natural strength."[24] As one mother writes, "All I see is a sleepy life of never-ending diaper changing for us."[25]

First and foremost, society should *never* assume that caregiving obligations, capabilities, and capacities within the family are unlimited. There are instances of caregivers who have sacrificed themselves radically out of love for a family member and genuinely feel that they discovered themselves in the process.[26] But more generally, extremes of self-denial ultimately take a severe toll on caregivers, and they place the recipients of care at risk for neglect and abuse.

Society must recognize limits to caregiving for most people. Before the point of caregiver burnout is reached, it becomes the responsibility of society to provide aid. Family caregiving is a precious moral resource, and for this very reason it merits careful protection. The surest way to weaken and destroy this resource is to overwhelm it.

Precise limits will depend on individual circumstances. But there is no need to argue about or wait for the precise point at which the burden of caring becomes unsustainable. Rather, we must recognize the proportions of the problem and create programs to deal with it. If many intact families provide care that is uniquely beneficial to the recipient, then it is ethically unsound and poor public policy to press them to the point where they will surrender their parent, spouse, or child to an institution in desperation. Everyone loses.

At present, long-term care is underfinanced, especially as compared to available acute care medical services.[27] Respite care, day care, in-home services, and a broad array of community-based programs could make the burden of caregiving more tolerable, but they do not get adequate attention in our society. We must establish a proper balance between preventive, acute, transitory, and long-term care services and facilities. Priority should be placed on developing a full spectrum of care lest caregivers slide beyond the breaking point. We must be satisfied that simply caring for the dying is appropriate, and certainly severe progressive dementia is a terminal condition. The art of dying should involve caring, and dying should in many cases be allowed to occur, as it once did, in the home. It is not so much death as the absence of caring and the denial of reality that may be the enemy.

Those in need of long-term care are often physically dependent. But this dependence on others does not mean that respect for autonomy and integrity should be denied. Recent reforms stress the development and updating of individualized care plans in which nursing home residents participate and give consent to treatment recommendations. It is easy to overlook the importance of choice in the context of routine, everyday matters. Recipients of long-term care are actually most concerned about everyday matters, including meals, sleep schedules, and bathing time. All reasonable choices of residents should be respected.[28]

Access to personal property, telephone use, and visits by friends and relatives are all important. The use of chemical and physical restraints should be kept to the least restrictive level possible and should be regularly reviewed. Use of restraints should always be discussed with residents and their families. Medical treatments and medications can be legitimately refused. Living wills and other advance directives should be encouraged. These and many other choices are appropriate in the nursing home or in the person's own home.

The basic dignity of the recipient of care should also be respected. This includes allowing choices but goes far beyond it, encompassing a respectful attitude on the part of the caregiver. Basic care and comfort in a clean environment is critical to well-being. Respect for privacy, full participation in care planning, giving or withholding consent to treatment, and all other "civil" rights should be routine expectations for all residents of long-term care. Conflicts inevitably arise about the times of rising and retiring, the necessity of getting dressed and undressed, and what to eat and whom to eat with. Interpersonal problems with personnel or with other patients appear. Intimate relations between patients, even sexual activity, are often seen. Restraints, either physical or chemical, are often used as a solution to problems like wandering or noisiness or falling. Most nursing homes are understaffed, and the pressure of work makes one-on-one relationships between staff and patients very difficult. It is easy for patients under such circumstances to lose all autonomy and to be denied all their rights. Patients with dementia are not able to make quick decisions, and their delay results in the decisions being made by institutional caregivers.

All these factors make for conflict of values. The autonomy of the patients in ordinary aspects of daily living is in conflict with the needs of the staff to dress, bathe, toilet, transport, keep order, and record. Patients must get up, get dressed, eat, sit, walk, and retire on an inflexible schedule determined by others.

BEHAVIOR CONTROL

Family caregivers sometimes put tremendous pressure on the psychiatrist to "do something" quickly about behaviors that are offensive or frightening and result in emotional strain. Our society has come to expect prompt control of such behaviors, often through chemical means. The caregivers might already be women in the middle, and an aging parent in a delusional or agitated state can be the straw that breaks the camel's back. For these and other reasons, some of them economic, it is difficult to sustain the commitment to methods that are not destructive of whatever ability to reason the patient with dementia still possesses. Interventions that do not affect the personal identity of patients (insofar as it still exists), are physically less intrusive with respect to the brain, and require active patient participation both cognitively and affectively are certainly costly.[29] In some cases, the respect owed to the mind of an elderly person becomes grist in the mill of medical efficiency.

While there are no absolute guidelines in this area, it is clear that technological shortcuts can make the demented elderly passive recipients rather than active agents. Families know that the human brain is the center of mentation, emotion, and personality and that, ideally speaking, this ultimate perimeter of personhood should not be invaded except as a matter of last resort after less invasive measures have been exhausted. But this ideal forms a dialectic with the realities of cost containment and family caregiver stress. There is reason to worry about excessive use of drugs and electroconvulsive (electroshock) therapy (ECT) in geriatric psychiatry, for our society lives by the quick fix and can easily make scapegoats of the elderly.

Elderly persons, in their inevitable decline, eventually withdraw from some of the interests and pleasures of youth. Whether elderly persons feel more isolated than other age groups is a matter of some debate.[30] However, there are often selected cases in which an elderly person struggles with what Emil Durkheim first called anomie and what sociologists define as "the homelessness of modernity." Isolation, poor communication, removal from the preferred environment, and loss of mobility are problems that can frequently be solved through social rather than chemical means. Yet the basic forms of assistance that such solutions require take resources and willingness to care in the most basic sense of the term. It is unfortunate that chemical custodianship is sometimes the only timely response.

It is valid and beneficent to treat depression and other psychiatric ailments with drugs. But as Salzman emphasizes, not all unhappiness or sense of uselessness in geriatric patients "represents true depression that requires pharmacotherapy."[31] There are many instances in which social isolation or loss of meaning are the root of the problem, and these factors can be mitigated socially or religiously. Salzman recommends ECT only for those patients who do not respond to antidepressant treatment, whose medical condition does not indicate the use of antidepressants, or whose depression is life threatening and/or delusional.

With specific reference to Alzheimer's disease and associated dementias, Martin and Whitehouse argue that "behavioral interventions (i.e., making modifications in the environment) are generally preferable to medications for the treatment of most behavioral problems."[32] These authors point out that use of medication is important in cases of depression, psychosis, anxiety, and sleep disturbances. But they urge a cautious use of psychoactive drugs, offering two basic guidelines: (1) Treatment should be purposeful, with the target symptom well defined, and (2) "employ as few drugs as possible, start with low doses, increase dosages slowly, and monitor carefully for side effects."[33] Polypharmacy and overmedication are particular problems in this patient population.

Mace suggests caution in using drugs to reduce disturbed behaviors (wandering, restlessness, irritability) "at dosages that interfere with remaining cognitive function and at which side effects occur."[34] She also stresses the importance of changing the physical or psychosocial environment first, prior to use of drugs. Spar and La Rue recommend supportive therapy in the early stages of dementia and individual psychotherapy so long as the patient's capacity for insight is preserved. Family intervention is useful at all stages of illness, as are environmental interventions generally (physical and social). Various drugs can be beneficial but ought not to be the first recourse.[35]

Ours is an overmedicated society. In the ethics literature, two general value orientations with respect to drugs and mental health are often alluded to: pharmacological Calvinism and psychotropic hedonism. Psychiatrist Gerald Klerman originally drew this distinction. The first view is one of general distrust of all drugs but especially those that are not clearly therapeutic. It favors verbal insights and self-determination. Psychotropic hedonists, on the other hand, see drugs as the first response to life's unpleasantries.[36] Those holding the first view might deal with a depressed early-onset victim of dementia through psychotherapeutic measures if possible. Effort is made to engage the patient as an active agent of change—as reasonably cognitively intact and capable of basic insights. Drugs are treated as a secondary means, less valued than insight and self-determination and not to be resorted to prematurely. By contrast, the psychotropic hedonist is more likely to resort to drugs immediately, since they are a valuable technology.

No doubt, behavioral problems such as hyperactivity, restlessness, resistiveness, and assaultiveness can be symptomatically managed by modification of the patient's environment, gentle persuasion, and exercise, but in most cases, sooner or later, the patient will require a psychotropic medication. The question is, will recourse to drugs be sooner or later?

There is tremendous pressure to make it sooner. Patients sometimes need to be controlled in less-than-ideal surroundings and with inadequate personal care. Concern for pressures on caregivers (e.g., adult daughters or daughters-in-law) is valid to a degree. Music therapy, art therapy, and group activities may be inaccessible. It will never be possible to create a state-of-the-art Alzheimer's unit in every nursing home. Unfortunately, the pressure to use drugs for custodial rather than therapeutic reasons, so-called chemical straitjacketing, will remain. Drug use for custodial reasons is a serious problem in long-term care facilities for the elderly, particularly in cases of understaffing or other institutional inadequacies.

Long-term care ombudsmen continue to struggle for the full implementation of resident rights: "You have the right to be free from physical and chemical restraint except to the minimum extent necessary to protect you from injury to yourself, to others, or to property."[37] As much as possible, chemical restraints are to be avoided, not just because of what they do to the mental state of the resident but because of their damaging side effects. Antipsychotics can lead to dry mouth and lethargy, and long-term use can lead to tardive dyskinesia; antimanics can lead to nausea, vomiting, and diarrhea. In home care, the possible need to control outbursts that can terrify a caregiver is predicated on the importance of keeping the care system intact, but major tranquilizers can also have negative consequences. It is important to appreciate the variable effects of disease and to understand that surprisingly small doses are often very effective.

OTHER ISSUES

The decision to withhold food and fluids is very difficult but even more difficult is the decision to withdraw them when they have been administered by artificial means over a period of time. The futility of the effort becomes more convincing with the passage of months and even years. Some who accept the morality of withholding life support are unable to accept the morality of withdrawing it once started. Although most ethicists point out that there is no significant moral difference between withholding and withdrawing, some clinicians are unable to regard them as morally equivalent.

Some neurological disorders that produce dementia may impair swallowing very severely at a time when the patient's dementia has not progressed very far. In such instances, gastrostomy would seem indicated. When the dementia has progressed to a more severe stage, with loss of communication and marked reduction in consciousness, the removal of the gastrostomy tube and cessation of food and fluids is regarded by most physicians as a valid moral option. If the decision to withdraw food and fluids is made, it must be with the approval of the family. If the family is in conflict, it is generally better to delay withdrawal until the conflict can be resolved.

Keeping patients with advanced dementia comfortable requires neither causing death by human hand nor striving for prolongation. The author does not advocate active euthanasia (i.e., mercy killing), chiefly because of the possibilities for abuse. Also, many physicians, probably a substantial majority, regard it as a moral imperative that they not actively kill another human being.[38] Four Austrian nursing aides, after all, did kill 49 elderly demented residents in a long-term care setting five years ago.[39] One aide was quoted by police as saying, "The ones who got on my nerves were dispatched directly to a free bed with the Lord."

NOTES

1. M. A. Drickamer and M. S. Lachs, "Should Patients with Alzheimer's Disease Be Told Their Diagnosis?" *New England Journal of Medicine* 326 (1992): 948.
2. J. M. Foley, "The Experience of Being Demented," in *Dementia and Aging: Ethics, Values, and Policy Choices,* ed. B. H. Binstock et al. (Baltimore: Johns Hopkins University Press, 1992), 31–43.
3. M. P. Alexander, "Clinical Determination of Mental Competence: A Theory and Retrospective Study," *Archives of Neurology* 45 (1988): 23–26.
4. J. E. Birren et al., eds., *The Concept and Measurement of the Quality of Life in the Frail Elderly* (New York: Academic Press, 1991).
5. R. Katzman, "The Prevalence and Malignancy of Alzheimer Disease," *Archives of Neurology* 33 (1976): 217–18.
6. N. Rango, "The Nursing Home Resident with Dementia: Clinical Care, Ethics, and Policy Considerations," *Annals of Internal Medicine* 102 (1985): 835–41.
7. R. D. Truog et al., "The Problem with Futility," *New England Journal of Medicine* 326 (1992): 1560–64.
8. E. Alemayehu et al., "Variability in Physicians' Decisions on Caring for Chronically Ill Elderly Patients: An International Study," *Canadian Medical Association Journal* 144 (1991): 1133–38.
9. L. Volicer, "Need for Hospice Approach to Treatment of Patients with Advanced Progressive Dementia," *Journal of the American Geriatrics Society* 34 (1986): 655–58.
10. D. C. Thomasma, "Ethical Judgments of Quality of Life in the Care of the Aged," *Journal of the American Geriatrics Society* 32 (1984): 525–27.
11. D. W. Brock, "Justice and the Severely Demented Elderly," *Journal of Medicine and Philosophy* 13 (1988): 73–99.
12. Ibid., 74.
13. Ibid., 86.
14. Ibid., 88.
15. Ibid., 73.
16. D. Callahan, *Setting Limits: Medical Goals in an Aging Society* (New York: Simon and Schuster, 1987), 183.
17. Ibid., 183.
18. R. H. Binstock and S. G. Post, eds., *Too Old for Health Care? Controversies in Medicine, Laws, Economics, and Ethics* (Baltimore: Johns Hopkins University Press, 1991).

19. R. Applebaum and P. Phillips, "Assuring the Quality of In-Home Care: The 'Other' Challenge for Long-Term Care," *Gerontologist* 30 (1990): 444–48.
20. E. M. Brody, *Women in the Middle: Their Parent-Care Years* (New York: Springer, 1990), 13.
21. Ibid., 35.
22. Ibid., 42.
23. S. M. Okin, *Justice, Gender, and the Family* (New York: Basic Books, 1989).
24. H. Featherstone, *A Difference in the Family* (New York: Basic Books, 1980).
25. Ibid., 35.
26. R. Darling, *Families against Society* (Beverly Hills, Calif.: Sage Library of Social Research, 1979).
27. Brody, *Women in the Middle,* 260.
28. R. B. Rust, *Understanding Your Rights: A Guide to Ohio's Bill of Rights for Residents of Nursing Homes and Rest Homes* (Cleveland, Ohio: Long Term Care Ombudsman, 1990), 17.
29. G. Dworkin, "Autonomy and Behavior Control," *Hastings Center Report* 6, (1976): 23–28.
30. B. Silverstone and S. Miller, "Isolation in the Aged: Individual Dynamics, Community, and Family Involvement," *Journal of Geriatric Psychiatry* 13 (1980): 27–47.
31. C. Salzman, "Clinical Guideline for the Use of Antidepressant Drugs in Geriatric Patients," *Clinical Psychiatry* 46 (1985): 38–43.
32. R. J. Martin and P. J. Whitehouse, "The Clinical Care of Patients with Dementia," in *Dementia Care: Patient, Family, and Community,* ed. N. L. Mace (Baltimore: Johns Hopkins University Press, 1990), 25.
33. Ibid., 25.
34. N. L. Mace, "The Management of Problem Behaviors," in *Dementia Care: Patient, Family, and Community,* ed. N. L. Mace (Baltimore: Johns Hopkins University Press, 1990), 95.
35. J. E. Spar and A. La Rue, *Geriatric Psychiatry* (Washington, D.C.: American Psychiatric Association Press, 1990), 118–21.
36. G. Klerman, "Behavior Control and the Limits of Reform: The Use of New Technologies in Total Institutions," *Hastings Center Report* 5, no. 4 (1975): 40–45.
37. Rust, *Understanding Your Rights,* 12.
38. L. Kass, *Toward a More Natural Science: Biology and Human Affairs* (New York: The Free Press, 1985).
39. F. Protzman, "Killing of 49 Elderly Patients by Nurse Aids Stuns Austria," *New York Times,* 18 April 1989, 1A.

Chapter 18

Respecting the Autonomy of Elders in Nursing Homes

George J. Agich

To respect autonomy is to treat someone as an adult, to expect him or her to act responsibly, and to acknowledge and support his or her capacity for self-determination. Elders who reside in nursing homes often exhibit incapacities that make these usual attributions of autonomy difficult at best. In this chapter, I explore why respecting the autonomy of elders living in nursing homes is so difficult and why a reconceptualization of autonomy is so critical to enhancing their dignity and quality of life. I first discuss the way that autonomy misleads us about what characteristics require protection in elders living in nursing homes. I then discuss the way that actual autonomy is founded on who the elder is and why identity precedes autonomy. I discuss the institutional character of nursing homes and consider the conflict between the nursing home as a protective environment and a place where autonomy can be expressed and consider the implications of identity for establishing a sense of home for elders living in nursing homes. I conclude by arguing that the assumption that an elder lacks autonomy simply because she or he lives in a nursing home is not supported by the reality that everyday autonomy is compatible with considerable degrees and kinds of dependence and incapacity. Hence, respecting the autonomy of elders living in nursing homes requires that we allow ourselves to view them as individuals first. The features of autonomy that are most important line up on the side of dignity and self-expression and not self-determination and independence.

INDEPENDENCE, RIGHTS, AND THE PARADOX OF AUTONOMOUS LIFE IN A NURSING HOME

Respecting individuality is often glossed in terms of respect for individual self-determination or decision making. To respect people's individuality is to allow them to exercise choices about how to live their lives, which often amounts to nothing more than noninterference or forbearance, what political theorists term *negative freedom.*[1] Policies designed to protect autonomy are accordingly structured to afford individuals independence as well as relevant information and the freedom to make choices. Clearly, some individuals who live in nursing homes not only have chosen to do so, but they also retain a voluminous capacity for choice. Other individuals, however, live in nursing homes because they feel they have no other choice. *Having no other choice* does not literally mean that there are no alternatives, but simply that their decision to live in a nursing home was influenced by economic, medical, and social circumstances that make the decision appear to be more a matter of acceptance than free choice. Indeed, coupled with the advice of physicians and family members, the decision to enter a nursing home might appear to be coerced. To be sure, there is no lack of literature addressing the nursing-home experience as a situation in which loss of personal freedom is prominent.[2] Remedial recommendations to deal with these circumstances include protecting patient rights through legal and policy mechanisms. Collectively, these approaches are designed to restore self-determination to elders by correcting various autonomy-subverting features of nursing homes. These approaches, however, do not seem to be able to deal adequately with the reality of compromise that affects the cognitive, communicative, physical, or emotional capacities of the majority of these elders. Whatever their economic, medical, psychological, or social circumstances, these elders are very dependent on others in ways that significantly alter the basic features of autonomy that are assumed in this line of criticism, namely, independence and self-reliance. Imputing a rigorous standard of autonomy to such compromised individuals is not only phenomenologically wrong, but also ethically distracting, because it directs attention from the myriad practical and concrete ways that autonomy can be protected or enhanced in frail elders and channels it instead into the pursuit of the impossible ideal of full self-reliance and independence.

Although many elders living in nursing homes are dependent, they are not entirely dependent. Like competence, dependence is situated and instrumental. One is dependent for some particular reason, dependent on a particular person, or dependent under particular circumstances. Generalizing from dependence in one area to other areas of life leads to serious erosions of autonomy. Elders who cannot ambulate may nonetheless be fully capable of deciding where and when they should be taken, what they want to do, and with whom they want to spend time. Even elders who are cognitively impaired can and do function on their own in many ways. Elders who wander may appear to do so aimlessly, but they are still doing so on their own. That means that many elders retain some capacity for self-initiated action, and it is a mistake to think that they are totally dependent. Viewing the dependence of elders as situated therefore requires caregivers to rethink their approaches to patients and to reevaluate the ways that these approaches do not incorporate the elders' own autonomous strivings.

Although there is a wide variation in the meanings and uses of the term *autonomy* both in public discourse and philosophical discussion, the core meaning of autonomy is usually understood to be related to the literal meaning of self-rule.[3] To be autonomous means to be capable of self-determination and decision making. Furthermore, an autonomous person is characterized by the attributes of independence, self-reliance, absence of restraint on choice and action, and his or her own ability to reflect on preferences or desires as well as to act in accord with them. These features collectively define autonomy as it is understood in the Western, liberal tradition.[4] In this tradition, autonomy points to an individual whose identity is constituted primarily by individual action, belief, and choice. Such an individual is not only independent but also regarded in isolation from others as a very condition of the individual's liberty. These features make discussion of autonomy for elders living in nursing homes extremely problematic. Indeed, the notion of autonomy for such frail and dependent individuals is, if not contradictory, at least paradoxical.

Influenced by the liberal vision of autonomy, one might feel compelled to insist that the contradiction or paradox posed for elders who live in nursing homes is itself a problem that can be remedied only by strict observance of autonomy. Such observance is made possible by insistence on the rights of elders. The motivation for such insistence is, of course, understandable. A long line of criticism of nursing homes views them as what Goffman called *total institutions,* namely, institutions that comprehensively control the daily lives of inmates.[5] As such nursing homes are regarded as oppressive settings in which autonomy can be protected only if rights are affirmed.

There is good reason, however, to believe that simply insisting that elder rights be respected only deals with a limited range of well-recognized but largely superficial concerns. These concerns include rights to information, representation by surrogates or ombudsmen, personal property within the nursing home, privacy, or confidentiality.[6] These rights are undeniably important ways that autonomy can be respected. Such insistence is defensible whenever the conditions for exercising rights are or can be realized by elders. As a reminder to caregivers that elders still deserve respect and deference despite their dependencies is, of course, another important ethical implication of the language of rights. However, not all rights imputed to elders living in nursing homes can actually be exercised by them or, more important, are central to their day-to-day life. Some rights are simply too peripheral or require conditions that elders living in nursing homes seldom possess. For example, a right to full disclosure of nursing-home policies, procedures, and rules is relevant only if the elder is able to understand the information and able to use it in weighing the advantages and disadvantages of one nursing home over another. It adds little in situations where the elder lacks the ability to understand or choose or where there are no other nursing-home alternatives. Taken to an extreme, the insistence on rights leads one to insist that elders living in nursing homes have a right to be free of the shackles of the institution, to be free to live without supervision and without professional health care. Such extreme insistence on liberating elders in nursing homes seems to commit some of the follies that have occurred in the liberation of the mentally ill from institutions. As one commentator put it, they have a right to rot and that right is respected with no further moral claim on our conscience.[7] Such a putative *right to rot* is no more problematic in the case of the seriously mentally ill than is a frail elder's right to deteriorate. Such a right should be defended only if we are prepared to face its actual consequences in the concrete lives of elders, which we (hopefully) are not prepared to do.

Making liberty rights the focus of our effort to respect dependent or incapacitated individuals is as problematic for frail elders living in nursing homes as for seriously ill patients in psychiatric institutions. Many of these elders lack basic capacities to ambulate, to direct themselves according to even a minimal plan of action, or to meet their own daily care needs. Unlike a psychotic individual, who might seem able to act even if he or she does so on the basis of irrational or delusional schemes and plans, elders with cognitive or memory impairments often cannot form or maintain a concept of a plan even if able to bodily enact it. Other elders are simply too frail to execute an action or plan. Although there is no denying that respecting the myriad rights of elders is a common approach to the problem of respecting their autonomy, to restrict our attention to these rights overlooks the everyday struggles of many elders in nursing homes whose autonomy is unaffected by the insistence on rights. The language of ideal autonomy and rights tends to encourage an oversimplified vision of the ethical problems associated with actually respecting autonomy and, in doing so, overlooks the everyday occasions in which autonomy is either advanced, enhanced, or thwarted as dependent elders are cared for in nursing homes. Thus, a rights-dominated account of autonomy is not so much wrong as it is too blunt a tool to deal with the subtle concrete complexities associated with the practical caring of elders in nursing homes. If autonomy is to be a guide to these everyday practical concerns, it will have to be understood in a fashion that is less austere than commonly expressed in the language of patient rights. It will have to connect with the day-to-day experience of elders.

ACTUAL AUTONOMY AND IDENTITY

Viewed in everyday terms, autonomy has to be compatible with dependence of varying sorts and with some kinds and degrees of external influence.[8] In fact, the demands of ideal autonomy are so rigorous that few human agents, and not simply frail elders, would be autonomous for the simple reason that human agents often lack sufficient knowledge and experience to act without reasonable reliance on others. Whenever autonomous individuals rely on the advice of others or defer to experts or authorities, they reveal their own lack of independence and thus, their own interdependence. This commonplace occurrence is, however, a problem only for those who insist that autonomy must be understood in terms of independent, rational decision making. Understandings of autonomy that take seriously how autonomy is revealed in everyday life will have no such difficulties. Such understandings of *actual autonomy* will see autonomy as compatible not only with reliance on others for advice but also on others for actions and services that the individual is not able to perform alone, because to be actually autonomous is to behave in a way that essentially interacts with others.[9]

A concept of actual autonomy recognizes that individuals are not created as adults capable of rational decision making on the basis of their own pregiven beliefs and values but as entities who achieve autonomy in the course of their living with others. Autonomous persons are not found fully formed in the world. They are raised by parents and develop through relationships with others within the family or other important social institutions such as school or work. Autonomy emerges over a lifetime and is shaped in the course of lived interactions with others. As a result, autonomous persons have values and beliefs that are connected with their life experiences. Some of those beliefs are background beliefs and values against which individuals exercise deliberation and rational choice. There is no rational deliberation about beliefs, choices, or values without a taken-for-granted frame of reference. Such a reference existentially defines who the autonomous person is and within which or in terms of which the person realizes himself. *Realizing oneself* is the most pedestrian form of autonomy; it does not involve attainment of ideals of self-actualization but simply points to the processes through which a self actually emerges in the course of a life. Such a self might embody widely shared cultural or ethical ideals just as well as the self might deviate from these ordinary values and beliefs. This means that respecting elders' actual autonomy must involve recognizing and dealing with individuality. Individuality is consistent with constraints and responsibilities that arise because of the communal nature of nursing-home life. Autonomous individuals not only make themselves but also discover and reveal themselves to themselves through their interactions with others. An autonomous elder is thus fully autonomous only in light of her or his identity formed through these interactions. Another way of making this point is to say that an individual is not autonomous unless he or she is a person. Here, the concept of person is used not as an ontological category but as a psychological construct, a framework or scaffolding from which the action, choice, and work that we usually regard as autonomous is conducted. Identity, thus, precedes autonomy.[10]

A person's identity is formed in interaction with others. One's identity always involves degrees of dependence on others, for example, parents or other authority figures. We learn to trust these individuals. From a certain point of view, trust implies that one must yield some degree of liberty to others, but it does not always follow that this surrender diminishes autonomy. Sometimes, this yielding to others enhances our autonomy by linking our individuality with significant others and by allowing us to adapt or cope with anxiety. Respecting actual autonomy thus requires that we respect who the individual is, not simply the individual's abstract or concrete choices. Whenever individuals make choices that are self-destructive or irresponsible, it is not clear that there is a compelling obligation to support their action. Awareness of responsibility introduces an entirely new sphere of ethical analysis that is often overlooked in standard discussions of elder rights.[11] In the context of a nursing home, where individuals live communally and where they suffer from conditions marked by cognitive and other degeneration, this point defines a critical vantage from which to respect their actual autonomy.

Responsibility, after all, is linguistically dependent on the notion of response. All autonomous individuals are responsive. They may, however, not be responsive to language or oral rules, but they can respond to perceptual and other cues. Although the objective behaviors may be the same, the difference is that locked doors and limitations of movement compromise basic expressions of autonomy, whereas a structured environment can provide the cues for elders to responsibly negotiate the difference between permitted and public spaces on the one hand and private or prohibited spaces on the other.[12] Elders are and should be treated as responsible because autonomy is essentially relational. Treating persons as responsible means that they are due respect, not simply that they are expected to follow institutional rules. Rules as such are often not useful because the situations are unique and dynamic. Problems are person dependent or situation dependent, so caregivers need to guard against the tendency to overlook the demands of actual autonomy. This means that administrators and family should be more in tune with the everyday life of elders in the nursing home and the practical caregiving problems. Whenever a gap between the lived experience of elders and that of daily caregivers is allowed to persist, rules proliferate and respect for the fragile and fleeting moments of autonomy is sacrificed.

If identity precedes autonomy, then those things that are important for elders should be respected. Some elders are subjected to all sorts of diagnostic or therapeutic interventions designed to enhance their well-being without seriously considering the effect on their most basic sense of autonomy. Although medical ethics permits surrogate decisions for elders who are not able to make decisions for themselves,[13] this practice is defensible not only when decisions are made on the basis of an understanding of the elders' own preferences or values but also when the decisions reflect who the elder currently is. Because many of us do not have clear preferences or specific values about particular medical treatments, surrogates are not able to make decisions that reflect what patients themselves would decide. Instead, surrogate decision makers are often forced to rely on "best interests" judgments that tend to protect the patient's physical well-being. Physical well-being, however, can be burdensome if it is bought at the price of thwarting the patient's own identity. Here, daily caregivers may be more useful in forming a decision than family surrogates, because they have the clearest and most basic understanding of the patient's present desires and preferences through their day-to-day care. What might be rationally not very burdensome, namely, a hospitalization stay for a diagnostic work-up, may be extremely disconcerting and confusing for a frail elder. The effect of transferring the elder from a familiar and protective environment into that of a medical-care institution should not be undertaken lightly. Too often, these transfers occur without critical discussion with those who most intimately know the patient. Rather, family members are consulted to make decisions when they do not themselves know the patient as intimately as do daily caregivers. If autonomy is to be relevant, then attention to the current identity and quality of experience of the elder is essential.

NURSING HOMES

Respecting the actual autonomy of elders in nursing homes requires that we consider the institutional nature of the nursing home. Some nursing homes exclusively provide skill, that is, care for the most physically dependent individuals who are themselves incapable of performing daily self-care activities or whose medical condition requires skilled nursing care; other nursing homes provide minimal care for individuals who need a sheltered environment including basic services such as laundry, hygiene, food, and some custodial care; and still other institutions provide a mixture. Thus, the notion of a nursing home is a broad one, though for present purposes, I limit discussion to nursing homes that provide skilled levels of care. Even with this limitation, there is a variability in the kinds of institutions. Joining these is a variation in the capacities of the individuals who live in nursing homes. This latter variability, more than any other feature, must be kept in mind because respecting autonomy of elders in nursing homes is first and foremost a matter of acknowledging and respecting their individuality.

Although many elders in nursing homes require highly skilled care, others live in nursing homes because they have no other alternative. In fact, the vast majority of elders in nursing homes are there mainly because they lack family caregivers. Some lack financial resources to extend their living independently. Some are admitted from a hospital after an acute illness for skilled rehabilitative care. Some *frail* elders are admitted for a wide but variable range of incapacities. Although many of these elders have medical problems, their frailty is multidimensional and usually precludes their own self-care. For many, the nursing home is the last stage before death, and some even regard the nursing home as a fate worse than death. Like other so-called total institutions, the nursing home is sometimes regarded as oppressive, but oppression here is as much determined by the vulnerability as by the frailty of the elders who reside there. It does not take much to direct or influence an individual who is fundamentally incapable of daily self-care. Celebrating elder rights, however, involves denying the strikingly dependent and fragile nature of many elders who live in nursing homes. Thus, respect for elder autonomy needs to be based on more commonplace and accessible features of autonomy than rights and must be focused on the peculiar and everyday features of the nursing home that thwart or support autonomy. For present purposes, I focus on two aspects of the nursing home as the environment within which elders live: first, as a place of safety and protection and second, as a place that belongs to the elders as their "home."

SAFETY VERSUS AUTONOMY

Many nursing homes take an overprotective attitude toward elders. For example, believing that injuries from falls are preventable, staff restrain or confine frail elders who have any potential for falling.[14] Some suggest that this tendency is motivated by the nursing home's desire to avoid litigation even though there is no good evidence to support this worry. Insisting on an elder's right to freedom of movement is far too abstract a response to the practice of restraining because the problem of falls and related problems such as wandering are clinically too complex to be so conveniently resolved. Rights simply raise all the wrong kinds of questions. Rights belong to elders, but if they cannot exercise them, then they are thought to transfer to their surrogates. But how can a surrogate exercise an elder's own right to freedom of movement? Often, the surrogate is asked to consent to the imposition of constraints. Thus, patients' safety is juxtaposed with their right to movement, which itself is not understood to be vitally related to their own best interest or autonomy. It is no wonder, then, that restraints are accepted as an easy way out of this dilemma. The right to movement is itself too abstract to be protected whenever the elder's own safety is an issue. If the right to freedom of movement is not an adequate approach, how can actual autonomy help us to address the problems associated with falls and wandering?

Actual autonomy focuses on how individuals experience and interact with the world. As such, autonomy is basically manifested in the spontaneous interaction with the world. As autonomous, individuals make the world and they make their way in the world. Making the world involves a wide range of activities in which individuals give meaning to their experience of the world. As embodied beings, autonomous persons physically make their way in the world; they shape and reshape its meaning through their actions. This means that bodily movement is an important way by which elders enact their autonomy in the world. Because frail elders are prone to falls and the injuries that result therefrom, nursing homes as well as the families of elders are inclined to restrict the opportunities for such accidents. Restriction, however, has two other consequences that are significant. The first consequence is that elders who are restrained are actually prone to greater injury and require greater degrees of attention and care. The second consequence is that restraints not only limit movement but the chance to explore the world and to encounter opportunities to make sense of their experiences. To appreciate this point, we must consider the experience from the point of view of the elder.

Assume that the elder is confused. The elder does not know what she wants. She simply experiences a sense of things amiss, out of order, or lost. She longs for something, something that is missing in her life. As a result, the patient experiences anxiety and concern that naturally manifests itself in motor activity. She sets out to find what is missing. She acts not on the basis of rational thought or deliberation but simply out of a basic need. Her agitation moves her to action. Her action brings her into a wider range of experience outside of her room. Close observation of the movement of elders indicates that it is not correctly described as purposeless. Although we do not explicitly know its intention or purpose for the elder, it does exhibit rational patterns.

Observational studies of institutionalized elders, for example, report that even seriously compromised and cognitively impaired elders actively work and struggle to fill up their time.[15] Indeed, the movement and activities of elders are not continuous or entirely aimless. They change and are divided up, much like the institutional day, into three parts punctuated by meals.[16] One of the effects of movement is to keep the elder attuned to the world and to others. Although cognitive and perceptual abilities may progressively deteriorate, he or she is actively engaged in the world around. Seeing the elder's everyday activities as attempts to make sense of her or his world of experience rather than as problems to be controlled or managed is fundamental to respecting the actual autonomy of elders in nursing homes. Such a change of perspective involves much more than idealistically denying that cognitively impaired elders pose significant challenges to caregivers. Rather it recasts the problems of management in a new and, hopefully, more malleable form.

Uriel Cohen and Gerald D. Weisman argued that interest in the therapeutic potential of the physical environment has grown during the last two decades to the point where it is now possible to place the concept of autonomy in its proper environmental context.[17] They identify three environmental aspects of autonomy—mobility and independence, control and freedom of choice, identity and continuity—that support a set of two dozen principles for the design of environments for people with dementia.[18] It has been reported that the use of color-coordinated doorways or hallways and the use of color-coordinated barriers including Velcro strips across doorways can allow elders freedom of movement within the institution but restrict their movement to areas that are both supervised and safe. Restraints, however, stop movement, or limit it severely, because the movement itself is viewed as a problem. Viewed from the perspective of actual autonomy, movement is not the problem but is an expression of the finite and fragile nature of actual autonomy. Humans are not normally stationary beings. They need opportunities for interacting with the environment around them. Artificially restricting the horizon of perception by significantly limiting movement itself creates agitation. Whenever the range of experiences is restricted, the opportunities for the elder to autonomously impart meaning to experiences is itself limited. Considering actual autonomy thus suggests ways to understand movement that allow movement to be viewed positively while at the same time recognizing that enhancing autonomy through movement is compatible with safety, provided that the environment is structured in ways that prevent or limit the possibility of injury.

The world is always potentially a dangerous place, and it is impossible to rule out all risks. Parents cannot do so for their children, and children cannot do so for their aged parents. Placement in a nursing home, however, gives many family members the sense that the elder is now fully protected. There is round-the-clock supervision, medical and personal care is provided, and so there should be no accidents. However, if autonomy is to be taken seriously and is to be respected, some kinds of risks need to be accepted.[19] Protection that insulates the elder from others, that keeps the elder from "dangerous" activities such as walking, or prevents an elder from visiting a library or church needs to be reexamined. Overprotection can thwart autonomy by nipping it at its most basic level, namely, in the everyday ways that elders express their individual preferences and styles through their *own action* in the world of the nursing home.

IDENTITY AND THE SENSE OF HOME

One is autonomous in terms of the particular values and beliefs that define importantly who one is. However, the beliefs and values that are central to people's autonomy are not necessarily those that they articulate but those that they live or enact in the everyday world. We identify with many things, and our orientation in the world is structured from a primordial identification with our own bodies. As elders deteriorate, their bodies become resistant to them. Frail elders require nursing-home care in large part because of their own inabilities to care for themselves. They can no longer dress themselves, prepare food, or perform bodily cleaning and toilet. As a result, autonomy itself is threatened for these elders because autonomy is linked to the functioning of the body. It would be absurd to think that according these elders substantial rights would make a meaningful difference to their everyday existence. Instead, we need to think about the important role that identification plays in assisting these elders to maintain their own sense of self. The most basic values that define the identity of an elder are not abstract propositions. Rather, they exist in a far more concrete way in everyday experiences. We come to know ourselves in large part through our life in the world.

Through action in the world, personal values are expressed and found by the elder as components of who she or he is. In other words, one does not intellectually decide that one loves one's child, but one responds to the child. Through myriad everyday interactions involving concern and caring the child is valued and given a place within the identity of the parent. To speak here of free choice is to vastly oversimplify the complex, concrete reality of parental regard for children. Parental regard for children is a useful paradigm for understanding how it is that an elder experiences and develops values integral to a sense of self, namely, through basic body awareness, emotional interaction, and caring.

Another component of identification involves not only the individual's body or bodily experience but also the space immediately surrounding the body. That space, namely, the familiar, is a mobile environment in which we are "at home." Home not only has historical and social meaning for individuals but also has a continuous meaning throughout one's life in virtue of the space in which one lives. Insofar as elders are able to personalize their space, they make it their own. For space to belong to someone does not imply a right of ownership as in the case of property but rather a sense of self-definition. Thus, allowing elders and, indeed, encouraging elders and their families to bring various personal items into the nursing home, to decorate the room, and to use their own clothes are important ways that elders can be assisted in maintaining continuity with their identity. Maintaining a continuous sense of self is important for elders because their frailty and incapacities already represent a significant loss not simply of capacity but of who they are. In other words, we need to understand that the incapacities that bring elders into nursing homes are not just physical, cognitive, or communicative inabilities but rather alterations in the elder's own fundamental self-identity. As a result, nursing homes should provide an environment that encourages and permits a rebuilding of the elder's sense of self by allowing ample space for new identities to develop.

The identity of elders is not constituted simply in terms of their "private" space but in terms of the public ways that they comport themselves. Thus, elders need to be accorded considerable latitude in defining relations with others in the nursing home. Too often, families try to secure private space for an elder from the "intrusion" of others. If a nursing home is to be anything like a home, it will develop only as a dynamically defined sense of "yours" and "mine" develops. No matter what the motivation, be it concern for safety or protection of personal property, family members or administrators who insist on defining territory actually violate a fundamental feature of actual autonomy, namely, its prerogative to impart meaning to the world. The elders themselves should be allowed to define the limits and meaning of their worlds. As a consequence, caretakers will need to attune themselves to the elders' own definition and understanding of the environment. After all, the nursing home is the elder's home. The caregivers are only *working* there, whereas elders *live* there. Because meaning cannot simply be read off their behaviors nor consciously defined by impaired elders themselves, caregivers will be challenged to assess the dynamic development of the identity of elders in their everyday actions and interactions.

Along with an identified space, elders should be permitted to reach out and to have visitors within their space. Both allowing and assisting elders to entertain in their own personal space, for example, by providing and maintaining the ability to serve drinks and food, are important ways that elders can maintain links with their past lives. All-too-often, however, nursing nursing-home administrators are motivated by concern to routinize and institutionalize life. As a result, a whole range of spontaneous interactions among (and between) elders, caregiving staff, and family or other visitors becomes strained. Ways need to be found to augment the elder's autonomous use of space if the nursing home is truly to be a *home* rather than an institution. Unfortunately, space is often treated as fungible. An elder is admitted to the hospital for an acute illness and returns only to find herself placed in another room, with another roommate, with a different view out the window. Prohibiting such transfers can, of course, be secured by insisting on elders' rights, but rights alone will not help nursing-home administrators to understand how important space is for respecting the autonomy of elders.

Communal spaces are not always shared equally. Some individuals congregate and form groups that exclude others. Care must be taken, of course, to prevent these natural groups from infringing on the rights of others, but nursing-home administrators should not forget the important role that communal or public space plays in our everyday lives. It is a space in which we feel capable of being ourselves with others. Sharing is an important human experience, but what constitutes *good sharing* cannot be decided abstractly. In nursing homes, a good deal of sharing occurs surrounding a television or before a window with a view. Clearly, not all residents in a nursing home will feel or even be welcomed into this space. Rather than insisting on equal access, multiple spaces amenable to different and creative uses might be provided. Wherever such options are not available, administrators must be careful not to arbitrarily define space by creating rules to regulate its use. Such rules often only result in labeling some elders who cannot comply with the rules as problem residents who must be dealt with, whereas a better approach would involve trying to foster creative and individual accommodation. Admittedly, rules are often created to make it easier for caregivers to carry on their daily care tasks. However, such "bed and body work" ignores the richer reality of elder autonomy and experience. Overregimentation of life within a nursing home curtails communal action just as overrigid urban planning curtails rather than promotes communal or public use of space in cities. Rigidly designated uses for particular spaces can thwart other spontaneous uses. If the actual autonomy of elders matters, then spontaneous definition of space should be cultivated rather than controlled.

If autonomy is to be actually respected for elders in nursing homes, greater attention needs to be paid to the way that elders have access to the private and communal spaces within the facility. One major problem with nursing homes in the United States is their tendency to be isolated from the surrounding community. Because administrators are concerned to prevent wandering and to "protect" confused elders, they tend to keep the elders indoors. With the perception of confinement, however, comes agitation and anxiety.[20] However, enclosed gardens or courtyards can restrict movement but also afford experiential variety so important to many elders. Because our relation with our environment is important, elders should be encouraged and assisted in developing and maintaining the nursing home's space, both in and out of doors. This will be possible in all but the largest cities. Clearly, many elders will not be able, for example, to engage in gardening, but some will be able to give advice regarding plants and make suggestions to custodians or maintenance personnel who care for the grounds. In these ways, elders can be permitted to place their own mark on the "home" in which they live. Indoor space is equally important. It can be a setting for positive experiences only if elders can experience it as theirs. Special attention should be given to the day-to day ways that the nursing home is regimented and made into an institution rather than a home because these routines thwart autonomous expression.

CONCLUSION

Our tacit assumptions about autonomy lead to a number of misconceptions about elders in nursing homes. Because an elder is in a nursing home, even a nursing home delivering skilled care, it does not follow that the individual is decisionally incapacitated. Some elders clearly maintain decisional capacity even though their medical condition can limit their ability to execute or to act on their choices. For example, a patient who is bedridden but otherwise cognitively intact can make decisions about not only her or his own medical care but also about other important life matters. Nonetheless, she might require assistance in carrying out her decisions. It is also important to note that decisional incapacity is seldom global but is more often an incapacity for making a certain kind of decision or for undertaking a certain kind of action in reference to a particular time and circumstance. It is both an instrumental and local concept. It is well to remember that the kinds of inabilities that do not in ordinary life count against one's being regarded as autonomous should not count against an elder just because of his or her dependencies.

Decisional incapacity that is based on lack of information does not mean that patients cannot decide but only that their decisional capacity needs to be supplemented by expert advice and information. In similar fashion, I may want to install a satellite television receiver but not know how to do so. I am not normally regarded as decisionally incapacitated if I rely on a professional installer. In fact, for a whole range of services, it seems prudent that I do rely on specialists because they can usually deliver a quality service or product better than I can provide on my own. Hence, not only should executional incapacity not be mistaken for decisional incapacity but also truly autonomous decisions reflect one's identifications, including beliefs, preferences, habits, and wants that define who the individual is. Thus, elders in nursing homes should not be regarded as nonautonomous simply because their decisional capacity is exercised under conditions of dependence. We are all dependent in a wide variety of ways. Thus, it may be too much to ask of a compromised or frail elder to articulate reasons reflective of deeply held beliefs or values because articulating reasons may be too stringent a demand to make. Ordinarily, we do not impose rigorous decisional standards on everyday decision making. Similarly, it has been argued that informed-consent standards vary depending on the medical circumstances, the nature of the medical intervention, and the degree of risk and benefit.[21] Thus, how decisions are made, what impedes or thwarts self-expression and decision making, and what conditions are in place to augment or enhance it are themselves critically important points for respecting the autonomy of elders in nursing homes. The dependence of elders should not be contrasted with the independence of those living outside nursing homes as if the simple need for nursing care defines a different class of individual—one who is not fully autonomous because he or she is not independent.

Consider adults living outside of nursing homes. Although we consider them independent, most well-functioning adults exist in highly dependent and interdependent relationships. They have spouses, children, parents, families, friends, coworkers, service providers, and others with whom they interact in everyday life and on whom they depend. Commuters rely on transit drivers and others to take them to work. Shoppers rely on supermarket managers, clerks, and others to stock items that they purchase and to assist them, for example, in taking groceries to the car. The need for help is hardly inconsistent with independence. Some kinds of help do conflict with some kinds of independence, but independence is compatible with the need for help. Similarly, dependence is compatible with autonomy. We need to reject the view that autonomy means independence and that dependence is something to be avoided, because such a view obscures the concrete reality of everyday autonomy.

Consider the high level of autonomy that even frail elders might exhibit. They might be able to engage in various kinds of activities, including maintaining social contacts with family or friends by telephone or having visitors. They might enjoy and participate in games or hobbies. Even individuals who seem to wander aimlessly do so in a way that attempts to define a space and to make a world for themselves. Such efforts are not dependent on others, although they require the cooperation of others. Such cooperation is not different in kind from that needed by most adults living outside of nursing homes. In addition, elders in nursing homes are not necessarily dependent perceptually or communicatively. We think that elders in nursing homes exhibit deficient perceptual or communicative capacities only because of our reluctance to spend time in their world. Because individuals or groups exhibit different ways of seeing and experiencing the world, we cannot conclude that they lack perceptual or communicative capacity. In fact, the anthropological and ethnographic evidence suggests the contrary. We simply should not forget the degree to which our own experience is culturally and socially determined. From the inside, our experiences are always full of meaning, but viewed from the outside they might appear to be senseless. In ordinary and everyday experience, the actions and experiences of others are taken for granted as meaningful because we see their actions as typical of those performed by other adults in situations that are similar or analogous to our own. We fail to do so in the case of elders in nursing homes, only because our society has failed to integrate experience of dependent and frail elders into our common social world. In part, this failure is related to the austere concept of autonomy that dominates American social and political discourse. The advantages afforded by the concept of actual autonomy are due largely to our directing our attention away from the ideals of autonomy and back onto the everyday reality of the lives of elders in nursing homes. We can only respect the actual and not some putative ideal of autonomy of elders in nursing homes. Such attention to autonomy importantly turns us away from the abstract language of ethics and to the concrete lives of the elders themselves. Seeing and respecting elders as individuals is thus a fundamental requirement for respecting their autonomy.

NOTES

1. I. Berlin, *Four Essays on Liberty* (Oxford, England: Oxford University Press, 1969), 118–72.
2. J. F. Gubrium, *Living and Dying at Murray Manor* (New York: St. Martin's Press, 1975); C. Laird, *Limbo: A Memoir of Life in a Nursing Home by a Survivor* (Novato, Calif.: Chandler and Sharp, 1979); C. W. Lidz, L. Fischer, and R. M. Arnold, *The Erosion of Autonomy in Long-Term Care* (New York and Oxford, England: Oxford University Press, 1992); M. O'Brien, *Anatomy of a Nursing Home: A New View of Residential Life* (Owings Mills, Md.: National Health Publishing, 1989); J. S. Savishinsky, *The Ends of Time: Life and Work in a Nursing Home* (New York: Bergen & Garvey, 1991); R. R. Shield, *Uneasy Endings: Daily Life in an American Nursing Home* (Ithaca, N.Y., and London: Cornell University Press, 1988); M. Vesperi, "The Reluctant Consumer: Nursing Home Residents in the Post-Bergman Era," in *Growing Old in Different Societies: Cross-Cultural Perspectives,* ed. J. Sokolovsky (Belmont, Calif.: Wadsworth, 1983), 225–37; and W. Watson and R. Maxwell, *Human Aging and Dying: A Study in Sociocultural Gerontology* (New York: St. Martin's Press, 1977).
3. J. Christman, "Constructing the Inner Citadel: Recent Work on the Concept of Autonomy," *Ethics* 99 (October 1988): 109–24.
4. G. J. Agich, *Autonomy and Long-Term Care* (New York

and Oxford, England: Oxford University Press, 1993), 13–36.

5. E. Goffman, "Characteristics of Total Institutions," in *Identity and Anxiety: Survival of the Person in Mass Society,* ed. M. R. Stein, A. J. Vidich, and D. M. White (Glencoe, Ill.: Free Press, 1960), 449–79.
6. B. F. Hofland, "Introduction," *Generations* 14 (Supplement, 1990): 5–8.
7. P. S. Appelbaum and T. G. Gutheil, "Rotting with Their Rights On: Constitutional Theory and Reality in Drug Refusal by Psychiatric Patients," *Bulletin of the American Journal of Psychiatry in the Law* 7 (1979): 308–17; T. G. Gutheil and P. S. Appelbaum, "The Patient Always Pays: Reflections on the Boston State Case and the Right to Rot," *Man and Medicine* 5 (1980): 3–11.
8. Agich, *Autonomy and Long-Term Care,* 76–113.
9. G. J. Agich, "Reassessing Autonomy in Long-Term Care," *Hastings Center Report* 20, no. 6 (1990): 12–17.
10. F. Bergmann, *On Being Free* (Notre Dame, Ind.: University of Notre Dame Press, 1977).
11. A. Jameton, "In the Border Lands of Autonomy: Responsibility in Long-Term Care Facilities," *Gerontologist* 28 (Supplement, June 1988): 18–23.
12. Recent work suggests that the physical activity is correlated with better quality of life in older adults. H. Elderly et al., "A Randomized Trial Comparing Aerobic Exercise and Resistant Exercise with a Health Education Program in Older Adults with Osteoarthritis: The Fitness Arthritis and Seniors Trial (VAST)," *JAMA* 277, no. 1 (January 1977): 25–31; A. C. King et al., "Moderate-Intensity Exercise and Self-Rated Quality of Sleep in Older Adults: A Randomized Control Trial," *JAMA* 277, no. 1 (January 1977): 32–37; D. M. Buchner, "Physical Activity and Quality of Life in Older Adults," *JAMA* 277, no. 1 (January 1977): 64–66.
13. A. E. Buchanan and D. W. Brock, *Deciding for Others: The Ethics of Surrogate Decision Making* (Cambridge, England: Cambridge University Press, 1989).
14. A. Jameton, "Let My Persons Go! Restraints of the Trade: Case Commentary," in *Everyday Ethics: Resolving Dilemmas in a Nursing Home Life,* ed. R. A. Kane and A. L. Caplan (New York: Springer, 1990), 166–77; B. J. Collopy, "Safety and Independence: Rethinking Some Basic Concepts in Long-Term Care," in *Long-Term Care Decisions: Ethical and Conceptual Dimensions,* ed. L. B. McCullough and N. L. Wilson (Baltimore: Johns Hopkins University Press, 1995), 137–52.
15. T. Diamond, "Social Policy and Everyday Life in Nursing Homes: A Critical Ethnography," *Social Science and Medicine* 23 (1986): 1287–95; J. F. Gubrium, *Living and Dying at Murray Manor* (New York: St. Martin's Press, 1975).
16. Gubrium, *Living and Dying at Murray Manor,* 161–68.
17. U. Cohen and G. D. Weisman, "Environmental Design to Maximize Autonomy for Older Adults with Cognitive Impairments," *Generations* 14 (Supplement 1990): 75–78.
18. U. Cohen and G. D. Weisman, *Holding onto Home: Designing Environments for People with Dementia* (Baltimore: Johns Hopkins University Press, 1991).
19. Collopy, "Safety and Independence."
20. J. Cohen-Mansfield and N. Billig, "Agitated Behaviors in the Elderly I: A Conceptual Review," *Journal of the American Geriatric Society* 34 (1986): 711–21; "Agitated Behaviors in the Elderly II: Preliminary Results in the Cognitively Deteriorated," *Journal of the American Geriatric Society* 34 (1986): 722–27.
21. J. Drane, "Competency to Give an Informed Consent," *JAMA* 282 (1984): 925–27.

Chapter 19

The Ethics of Prediction: Genetic Risk and the Physician–Patient Relationship

Eric T. Juengst

Medicine has always been devoted to interpreting signs in order to help patients plan their futures. To that extent, clinicians share an occupational hazard with weather forecasters and fortunetellers: people set great store by the predictions they make, even when they are notoriously inaccurate. Much of that inaccuracy just reflects the limits of technique. Laboratory test results, barometer readings, and palm line lengths are not always precise and reliable indicators of things to come. Even sure signs can yield false predictions when their meanings are misinterpreted, and since false predictions carry the appearance of certainty, they can be dangerous for both professionals and their clients.

How professionals should interpret predictive signs for their clients depends on the nature of their services. Meteorologists predict the circumstances their clients will face as they go about their lives but not how their clients will experience that environment. By contrast fortunetellers are expected to predict the course of their clients' future life experiences. Medical prediction lies somewhere in between, and as its powers grow, so will the medical profession's need to decide just where.

Precise, reliable, long-range predictions about the health of individual patients have always been rare. There are few biologic processes sufficiently inexorable to provide such certainty and fewer techniques for detecting sure signs of those processes in patients. Prognoses with this power have been largely confined to genetically determined conditions and limited by our ability to detect their causal mutations in patients, but that subset of medical problems is growing fast. As the international initiative to map and sequence the human genome makes possible an increasingly wider range of DNA-based health risk assessments, the interpretive challenges that long-range medical predictions entail are becoming an acute professional and social policy problem.

This chapter examines the challenges that will be raised for health professionals and policy makers by the advent of new and more powerful DNA-based prognostic tools. The first section begins with an example, to illustrate the power of medicine's new tools and a metaphor to suggest a thesis regarding their use. The next two sections describe the most urgent ethical and health policy challenges that these tools will raise. Since the issues often appear simply to be new examples of old professional ethical and health policy challenges, the following section steps back to analyze the origins of their unusual grip on the moral imagination, by examining the historical dynamics of the physician–patient relationship in this context. In the closing section,

Source: Reprinted with permission from E. T. Juengst, The Ethics of Prediction: Genetic Risk and the Physician–Patient Relationship, *Genome Science & Technology,* Vol. 1, No. 1, © 1995, Center for Biomedical Ethics, School of Medicine, Case Western Reserve University.

the thesis suggested in the opening section is explicated in light of the intervening analysis, and a new lexicon for genetic diagnostics is proposed to help professionals and the public understand their relationship more clearly.

WEATHER WATCHING, FORTUNETELLING, AND GENETIC TESTING

Consider the situation faced by Jean, a hypothetical young member of a family that displays the pattern of the Li-Fraumeni syndrome. In her family, the distribution of breast cancers, sarcomas, and other neoplasms fits the model of an autosomal dominant genetic trait. Jean has an even chance of inheriting the genetic mutation that causes this trait and, if she has inherited the mutation, faces a 50 percent risk of developing an invasive cancer by age 30 (90 percent by age 70).[1] Until recently, all the members of her family have had to live with these odds. However, with the identification of the molecular basis of Li-Fraumeni syndrome (as a mutation of the tumor suppressor gene named *p53*), molecular diagnostic tests have been developed that can determine with certainty whether or not Jean carries the mutation.[2] Her heightened risk of developing cancer by age 30 can now either be eliminated or doubled through testing.

How should a positive test result be interpreted for Jean? Calling this result a "presymptomatic diagnosis of cancer"[3] would imply that Jean already has the cancer syndrome, albeit in its early stages; that is, that she is already diseased in an important way. Alternatively, her physicians could reassure her that she is now healthy but that her genes may cause her family's syndrome later in life. Conceptually, it is a matter of emphasis, of where one draws the line between a clinical entity and its cause. Practically, however, this emphasis may affect people's ability to use the test effectively in planning their lives.

If Jean understands the test as diagnostic of a life-threatening disease, its prediction will seem to tell her fortune by revealing her to be fatally ill. On that construction, it is not surprising that Jean might sink into depression or hide the bad news from other family members. It is also understandable for others to treat Jean as fatally ill—to place her in the sick role, to begin to say goodbye, to discourage her from demanding such pursuits as medicine, politics, or childbearing—even though her serious health problems may be no closer than their own.

By contrast, Jean's carrier status could be interpreted as something closer to a weather report. It forecasts circumstances that will challenge Jean's life but does not prejudge the outcome of that challenge for her identity as a person. We can predict that, given time, she is likely to face a deadly oncologic storm, but that storm has not yet, and may never, hit and will depend much on other aspects of her genome and her local environment. This interpretation keeps the disease distanced from Jean's identity, to be dealt with as an anticipated problem in her life plans. Since her ability to anticipate her fatal illness does not make her fatally ill, there is no reason, under this interpretation, for the rest of us to treat her as if she were already sick.

Jean's situation suggests a general thesis about the use of DNA-based diagnostics that might be fruitfully explored in more concrete terms. It suggests that modeling genetic prediction after the meteorologist's service rather than the medium's will be fundamental to using the new DNA diagnostic tests to advance the interests of patients.

THE CHALLENGES IN GENETIC PREDICTION

Among the most immediate and recurrent consequences of human genome research will be the localization and identification of medically interesting genes, like *p53,* and their mutations and the subsequent development of DNA-based tests to detect specific alleles in individuals. With the development of the first detailed index and reference marker maps of the human genome, the pace of gene localization and subsequent diagnostic and predictive test development is accelerating dramatically.[4]

The identification of the mutations within the *p53* gene that cause Li-Fraumeni syndrome is a good example of this phenomenon because it suggests both the power and the limits of molecular medicine. Characterizing the *p53* mutations should be an important step toward unraveling the pathophysiology of sporadic as well as inherited forms of cancer, and it enables more precise forms of genetic risk assessment for members of Li-Fraumeni families, like Jean, with known *p53* mutations. It does not, however, immediately lead to a new therapy for the disease. DNA-based tests for the presence of the mutation will be available long before subsequent therapeutic advances are made on the basis of this new knowledge. During the interval, clinicians will be able to offer better risk assessments to their patients, but only against the backdrop of existing preventive and therapeutic prescriptions.

Managing the acquisition and delivery of genetic risk information will involve addressing a cascade of challenges through three social spheres: (1) the individuals and families who seek genetic information, (2) the health care professionals and institutions that provide it, and (3) the public and private institutions that create the social context of that transaction. This chapter focuses on the latter two spheres, but it is important to begin by appreciating the first.

Individual and Familial Challenges

In the absence of effective therapies, the promise of accessible genetic information lies in its ability to allow individuals and their families to identify, understand, and sometimes control their inherited health risks. This promise puts the individuals and families who receive genetic services at the moral fulcrum of the enterprise. If genetic testing and counseling are to be judged a success, it must be from the recipients' point of view, in terms of their ability to use the results to enrich their lives.

For the individuals and families who might avail themselves of these tests, questions will arise about the relative benefits of the knowledge they might gain, given their tolerance for uncertainty and their interpretation of the personal significance of genetic risk information. For individuals at familial risk of carrying recessive genes or genes for late onset disorders, identification of these markers can provide the benefit of increased certainty about their personal carrier status. For those who are found not to carry these genes, this benefit is clearly high. For those who test positive for these genes, the benefit depends on how well they can use the knowledge of their carrier status to prevent or prepare for the ill effects of the gene.

On the other hand, genetic information is almost always about relatives as well as the individual. As a result, genetic testing can also raise fundamental questions about the mutual obligations of kin. Do special obligations flow from the discovery of an inherited health risk to alert extended family members to the risks they may also face?[5] Conversely, do extended kin have an obligation to donate DNA for analysis to assist a relative to clarify a genetic risk when unwanted information about themselves may be generated in the process?[6] How should parents' obligations to protect the interests of their children be interpreted in the face of the expanding range of genetic information available to them in making reproductive decisions?[7] Given that the growing range of genetic risk assessments will be able to be performed prenatally as easily as postnatally, what set of risks should conscientious parents use for a part of their reproductive decision making?

Unfortunately, there is no well-received generic theory of the moral dynamics of family life to draw upon in addressing these questions. This is primarily because there is a rich pluralism of strongly held specific theories on the subject, views that reflect the convictions and experiences of different family histories and traditions.[8] Moreover, in practice, answers to the dilemmas of familial obligation often emerge from the family's interactions with the health professionals providing their care. In this context, there is at least a more explicit moral tradition to appeal to and draw from in considering these policy dilemmas.

Professional Challenges

Many of the patients' challenges, and thus the clinician's, are first encountered during the research that leads to clinical diagnostics.[9] The approaches taken in that setting set precedents for clinical practice. Extrapolating from the challenges that clinical investigators in genetics are already experiencing, several kinds of issues can be anticipated: (1) issues in conveying prognostic information to individuals and families, (2) issues in defining the indications for predictive genetic testing, and (3) issues in limiting the kinds of genetic testing offered individuals and families.

Conveying Prognostic Information. *When to disclose.* The traditional approach in developing a new genetic test has been to condition subjects' participation on the understanding that no individual findings would be disclosed until pilot clinical testing programs determined the protocols that should govern testing, including the extent of pretest education and posttest counseling. This approach was justified, in part, by the slow pace of disease gene isolation, which allowed the clinical community to prepare for the translation of research findings into clinical practice. Thus, the linkage studies localizing markers for the Huntington's disease gene established the policy of withholding preliminary research results from all subjects until the level of scientific confidence in the reliability of the markers justifies the establishment of pilot clinical testing programs.[10]

The increasing pace of gene isolation, however, is putting pressure on this approach. Many investigators now find themselves in possession of information they could use clinically but without a developed program for delivering the information. Increasingly, individuals and families themselves request early results from the researchers. A group at the University of Michigan has reported that a young woman participating in a linkage study of familial breast cancer announced her decision to undergo a prophylactic bilateral mastectomy. The researchers knew that there was little chance that she had inherited any increased risk.[11] Even though the gene in question had not been isolated, the evidence available through flanking markers seemed compelling enough to obligate the team to shift from the research to the clinical mode and disclose their findings to the subject. Their decision is supported by those who argue that subjects should have the right to information about themselves at all stages of the research, particularly when it could have a bearing on clinical decision making.[12] In fact, legal concerns about "look-back liability" on the part of investigators who hold but do not communicate important findings have already been raised.[13]

Intermediate approaches to the question of disclosing early results take two forms. One is to establish decision-making guidelines by suggesting the variables to be considered in each instance. For example, one report recommends that investigators consider (1) the magnitude of the threat posed to the subject, (2) the accuracy with which the data predict that the threat will be realized, and (3) the possibility that action can be taken to avoid or ameliorate the potential injury.[14] The other approach to these issues is procedural: to recommend the creation and use of committees analogous to the data safety and monitoring committees used in clinical trials.[15] These committees are charged with deciding when particular new tests are clinically reliable and useful enough to offer to patients and families. If they involve research subjects or family representatives, these committees hold the potential to offer a useful middle ground between the paternalistic and client-centered views.

These approaches show the difficulty of establishing firm substantive standards for the clinical reliability of new, uncertain genetic information. Moreover, as the Human Genome Project progresses and linkage marker testing gives way to direct clinical testing based on DNA sequence information about the mutations in question, the nature of geneticists' uncertainty problem will change. Increasingly, as tests for genetic factors in more complex diseases become available, the question will become less whether one has the mutation in question but more what that signifies for one's future. To be able to use the results of genomic research intelligently, subjects will need to be able to think in terms of shifting ranges of probabilities, influenced by both other genes and environmental factors. To learn to do so, both the subjects and the investigators will find themselves swimming upstream against our culture's tendency to understand genetic risk factors in a deterministic, even fatalistic fashion.[16]

Quality control. As DNA-based diagnostics and risk assessment tests become applicable to a wider range of cases, the need to develop quality control and quality assurance mechanisms for the laboratories engaged in testing becomes more urgent. Currently, professional organizations and several state governments are experimenting with different systems to monitor and ensure the quality of DNA testing procedures, but no uniform national standards or mechanisms exist. The regulation of commercial genetic test development is a professional issue that is becoming intensified by human genome research. Whereas there are policies to ensure the quality of testing services and accuracy of particular tests, there is no consistent professional oversight for which tests are chosen for development and how they are introduced into clinical practice.[17] Increasingly, there are calls for a mechanism to provide that kind of assessment for new genetic tests.[18]

Informed consent. Compared with more physically invasive forms of clinical intervention, the risks of genetic testing seem minimal. Taking a blood sample is usually the only physical contact the clinician imposes on a patient. As a result, consent forms for genetic testing drafted against standard biomedical templates sometimes cite only the minor physical risks of blood drawing. In the research context, however, investigators are now admonished that genetic studies that generate information about subjects' personal health risks can provoke anxiety and confusion, damage familial relationships, and compromise subjects' insurability and employment opportunities. For many genetic research protocols, these psychosocial risks can be significant enough to warrant careful institutional review board review and discussion. The fact that genetic studies are often limited to the collection of family history information and blood drawing should not, therefore, automatically classify them as "minimal risk" studies qualifying for expedited institutional review board review.[19] Supporting this position is the growing body of literature that documents the range of psychologic responses,[20] stigmatization,[21] and economic discrimination[22] that can attend the disclosure of genetic information about health risks.

One of the more common unanticipated consequences of tracing the inheritance of DNA markers within a family can be the inadvertent disclosure of misidentified paternity. Longstanding recommendations to address that risk prophylactically in the informed consent process[23] are now always followed. In 1992, one research group published a disguised pedigree of a family that disclosed the existence of two children in whom "paternal genotype inconsistencies" were identified.[24] The sequelae of this disclosure within the immediate family were disastrous and led to new guidance to National Institutes of Health (NIH) researchers to include the risks of misidentified paternity in the informed consent process for these studies.

Confidentiality. Deciding how to deal with inadvertent findings of misidentified paternity is a challenge in the clinical setting as well. The most common clients at a genetics clinic are couples who have a child with a genetic disease and desire an assessment of their future risks. Occasionally, these tests reveal that only the mother is a carrier of the child's disease, when two carriers are required to cause it. The obvious deduction from this is that the husband is not the father of the afflicted child. How does the diagnostician live up to his or her obligations to disclose to this couple their reproductive risks?

Here, the geneticist's commitments to patient education and to confidentiality clash. The couple presented themselves as a joint patient, but only the mother actually carries the genetic defect. As an individual patient, she has the need to know her risks in case her course of reproductive decision making continues to diverge from her husband's. On this basis, some geneticists will treat her as their primary client, tell her what they have discovered first, and offer to help her work through the news with her husband if she so desires. Others approach the problem preemptively, by warning all their clients ahead of time that inadvertent findings of nonpaternity are one possible consequence of genetic testing.[25]

If the patient decides not to warn relatives about their common risks, does the professional have an obligation to do so? Occasionally, clients refuse to allow the disclosure of their (positive) genetic test results to the members of their extended family who are also at risk for the disease in question. Once again, the geneticist feels obligations to prevent harm that seem to test the limits of the speciality's client-centered commitments. The question is, how far into the gene pool do the geneticist's professional obligations go? In its report on social issues in genetic screening, the U.S. President's Commission for the Study of Ethical Problems in Medicine gave four strict criteria for breaking confidentiality in clinical genetics: (1) reasonable efforts to elicit voluntary consent to disclosure have failed, (2) there is a high probability both that harm will occur if the information is withheld and that the disclosed information will actually be used to avert harm, (3) the harm that identifiable individuals would suffer would be serious, and (4) appropriate precautions are taken to ensure that only the genetic information needed for diagnosis or treatment of the disease in question is disclosed.[26]

This is a useful set of guidelines, and its restriction of disclosure on behalf of "identifiable individuals" serves to tie it to medicine's traditional patient-centered ethos. Few situations could meet these criteria in genetics, but what about involuntarily disclosing the client's test results to the sperm banks he contributes to, on behalf of the future generations at risk? Here, one starts to feel in earnest the ethical tension that genetics creates between medicine's traditional commitment to the presenting patient and its obligations to the future.

Indications for Testing. The concerns over the risks of linkage research are also important for clinical policy decisions about who should be considered eligible for genetic risk assessment testing. The most prominent example is the debate over involving children in this testing.[27] In situations where little can be done to benefit subjects as a result of a positive marker test, the risks of labeling, stigmatization, and insurability suggest that linkage studies should not involve children, and that has been the traditional position on the issue within medical genetics.[28]

Increasingly, however, the policy of excluding children from linkage testing has come under question.[29] Some argue that the potential benefits of early warning of cancer risk and the benefits of a negative result justify the inclusion of young children in predictive testing programs, even when the risks are acknowledged to be more than minimal.[30] Since the absence of efficient monitoring or preventive interventions in this case still weakens the clinical value of early warning, the weight of this judgment rests on the benefit of a negative test—the relief of anxiety it can give to the children found free of the tested mutations and their parents. Others remain concerned enough about the psychosocial burden of positive tests results [such as the imposition of a "vulnerable child syndrome" on children found to be mutations carriers[31]] to strike the balance the other way, in favor of excluding minors from testing. A third, moderating response is to approach the involvement of minors in a stepwise fashion, in the tradition of beginning research with the least vulnerable population of subjects. For family studies, this means collecting and analyzing DNA samples from adult members of the family first and involving minors only after clinical testing with adults has helped demonstrate the relative medical benefits of presymptomatic testing in that case.[32]

Limits to Testing. Finally, new challenges are being posed for geneticist's interactions with their clients over the uses to which test results might be put. With the advent of sophisticated new procedures (DNA amplification methods such as polymerase chain reaction, and analytic techniques, such as fluorescent in situ hybridization), it has become possible to isolate fetal cells from samples of maternal blood and use them for a limited range of prenatal genetic diagnoses.[33] This technique is viewed as a major advance for prenatal diagnostic technology, primarily because of its ability to improve public access to such testing. By avoiding the invasiveness and physical risks of current techniques, allowing women to undertake testing earlier in their pregnancies, and dramatically lowering the costs of testing, this technique makes it possible to contemplate extending prenatal testing to the entire population, rather than only to those at risk.[34]

The convenience of this test is two-edged, however. One of the easiest fetal traits to identify through this technique, for example, is the sex of a fetus, raising the prospect of using this testing technology to identify and select fetuses of a particular gender. Are there limits to the kinds of testing that responsible practitioners may offer or be willing to provide on request? Increasingly, professional groups are concurring that prenatal testing for gender identification falls beyond the boundaries of medicine.[35] The principal argument is that, as health professionals, genetic diagnosticians should limit their services to providing prospective parents with information about the presence or absence of pathology in the fetus. Since gender is not pathologic, it lies beyond the limits of their service. Of course, drawing a line between normal and pathologic traits will not always be as easy as it is in the case of gender. This argument will be increasingly challenged as the range of human genes and their alleles that can be detected expands beyond the obviously pathologic. Should, for example, responsible geneticists comply with requests for prenatal testing for correctable or minor genetic defects? Is earner status for a recessive genetic disease an appropriate "pathology" to justify prenatal testing? These questions directly affect the commitment of geneticists not to second-guess the reproductive value judgments made by their clients.[36]

PUBLIC POLICY ISSUES

In addition to the questions that geneticists will have to face as clinicians, there are also public policy issues that will be brought to a critical urgency by the availability of more convenient, reliable, and powerful genetic tests. Unlike the health professional's clinical issues, these issues involve weighing the interests of the individuals who learn their genetic health risks against the interests of society or other parties outside the therapeutic relationship who could be affected by the information.

Genetic Services and Public Health

Should genetic services ever be used and evaluated as public health tools to lower the incidence of genetic disease in the population? What role, if any, should public health goals play in implementing techniques designed to expand access to prenatal testing? Unlike the client-centered ethos that generally prevails in genetic services, testing programs evaluated in terms of their ability to reduce the incidence of disease or disability will have an interest in seeking particular reproductive outcomes from their use, which may conflict with the goals of the individuals and families who use them.

Public policies that propose to use carrier screening or prenatal genetic testing as public health tools to reduce the incidence of a particular disease face challenges from three quarters. First, the clinicians whose testing programs would be evaluated under such a policy by the numbers of births avoided would question the pressures placed on their commitment to respect the reproductive autonomy of their clients. Second, their clients, prospective parents, would resist attempts by the state to direct their reproductive choices. Finally, the increasingly articulate organizations and advocates for people with disabilities argue that such a policy is an unjustifiable form of quarantine against patients with those diseases. From their point of view, it is no less discriminatory to exclude persons from society on the basis of their genotype than it would be to do so on the basis of other (genetically determined) single traits, such as gender or color.[37]

Private Control of Genetic Information

The availability of new techniques for acquiring genetic information also has implications for social practices that range far beyond health care policy. Organs and tissues banked for research purposes and blood samples collected during public health screening programs (such as newborn phenylketonuria [PKU] screening) or for personal identification purposes (e.g., by the military or the criminal justice system) all become rich repositories of genetic information about individuals and their families, as a result of DNA amplification techniques, such as the polymerase chain reaction (PCR). Currently, there are no uniform standards governing the management of these de facto DNA databanks[38] or their uses for purposes beyond the intent of their collection, such as clinical diagnoses. Who should have access to and control over this information and for what purposes?

Again, this is a public policy question that has its beginnings in genomic research. Subjects in genetic family studies are routinely assured that they are free to withdraw from the research at any time. Yet their participation consists primarily of their presence on a pedigree and their DNA in a freezer. Does the subjects' right to end their association with a study oblige the investigator to discard their DNA or return it to them for clinical use? Most teams treat DNA samples like other donated human biologic material over which the subjects no longer hold a claim. However, unlike most donated tissue, which can be studied anonymously, DNA samples in a family collection gain their research value precisely to the extent that they continue to identifiably represent their donors. Increasingly, amid concern that intentionally withholding clinically relevant information from subjects may lead to legal liabilities later, investigators are concluding that "the day for informal donations of DNA samples is past" and that explicit "ownership" arrangements must be made with donors to classify questions of subsequent control.[39]

Complicating these arrangements, of course, is the fact that scientists and clinicians themselves are making ownership claims of various sorts to the results of their research and seeking to commercialize the genetic diagnostics that they develop.[40] These claims raise legal and public policy questions that span the spectrum from basic patent and intellectual property law to the regulation of commercial laboratory practices and the conflicts of interest that can be created for the health professionals who operate them. The biotechnology industry's interest in capitalizing on new testing capabilities as they become available by marketing them directly to health professionals and the public makes these questions of professional standards particularly acute.

Genetic Discrimination

Once tests are developed and deployed in clinical practice, another class of public policy questions emerges, questions about how the results of such tests might be used by parties outside the clinical setting. Knowledge of a person's genetic health risks can work to the individual's disadvantage if that information is used to determine his or her access to opportunities provided by social institutions and practices beyond the clinical setting. Should life insurance providers, for example, be allowed to use genetic risks assessments to underwrite prospective clients? Might self-insured employers adopt exclusionary genetic screening programs to avoid potentially high-cost employees? For countries like the United States that depend on private markets in health care coverage, genetic risk information could even be put to use by commercial health insurance providers as part of their underwriting process. For social policy makers, advances in human genome research will increasingly raise the challenge of defining the nature and limits of genetic discrimination as it arises within different institutions and practices.[41]

Most genetic information currently available is of relatively low actuarial value, and it is unlikely that any particular genetic test would be cost-effective enough to use as a routine insurance screen. However, as more people become aware of their genetic risks, commercial insurers will have to decide whether to seek such information from applicants to include in their underwriting process to address increased economic pressure by knowledgeable consumers and competitors who do use such information.[42]

For clinicians, these policy issues also raise practical questions about how to advise their clients and patients. Even if test results are kept scrupulously confidential, patients found to be at genetic risk for serious illness may themselves be asked to disclose any knowledge they have as part of an insurance application. To do so risks being denied coverage for that health problem as a preexisting condition, but to fail to do so risks being charged with fraud and the cancellation of all coverage.[43] Either outcome could be a dire consequence of clinical genetic risk assessment, albeit not a consequence for which the clinicians can be held responsible. Thus, clinical testing programs are now faced with deciding to what degree and at what stage psychosocial risks of participating in genetic studies, such as risks to insurability, should be included in the informed consent process.

In the research setting, investigators and institutional review boards have been discouraged from overemphasizing remote or speculative risks of harms that might occur as a consequence of developing new knowledge.[44] But the risks to insurability have been singled out by several groups as material elements for consent to clinical genetic testing,[45] and the NIH Office of Protection from Research Risk now includes insurability among the social risks that should be disclosed to participants in genetic studies.[46] Critics of this practice point to studies that show little evidence of "genetic underwriting" on the basis of genetic testing,[47] whereas advocates applaud it for its foresight, affirming that "testing of apparently healthy [individuals] for a trait that might stigmatize them for a lifetime requires adequate protections and safeguards, particularly informed consent."[48] Others argue that, given the lack of evidence that economic discrimination is a bona fide risk of genetic testing, it might be better simply to alert patients that if the project succeeds, subjects could eventually obtain information about themselves that they might have to voluntarily divulge to others, such as insurance companies, in the future. This casts the problem as one of recognizing the limits to the clinician's ability to guarantee the confidentiality of the test results rather than as a known risk of genetic testing.[49]

Genetic Literacy

For choices by families, professions, institutions, and governments to be sound in the face of the challenges this complicated context imposes, people at every level need to be as well-informed as possible. Part of the information decision makers need is scientific, and it is the responsibility of the genomics community to help provide that. Indeed, by clarifying the nature and limits of genetic causation and by providing clinical handles on genetic disease processes, scientific research using the genome project's tools may go far to mitigate the concerns about these choices. Sound decision making in this area needs to be well-informed in other ways as well: informed by the experiences of families at risk for genetic disease, by accurate accounts of public perceptions and historical precedents, by well-researched and -articulated policy alternatives, by religious perspectives and ethical considerations. Even the best crafted professional and public policies will not prevent the misuse of genetic information if those who collect and use it do not understand its significance correctly. Ultimately, the best ways to decrease the risks of genetic discrimination are to promote better understanding of human genetics and to involve the public in deliberations over its use.

Several forms of education seem to be needed if we are to become a genetically literate society. First, as genetic technologies become more widely available, the demand for health professionals trained to address the clinical and ethical challenges of managing and interpreting genetic information will quickly outpace the current supply.[50] Second, just as important as improved professional understanding of potentials and limits of genetic information is the appreciation of these parameters by the public. A third important target for educational efforts is those who are in positions to influence the public's response to genetic advances: the news media, the scholarly and scientific community, and public policy makers.

IS GENETICS SPECIAL? THE IDEOLOGIC ARCHEOLOGY OF CLINICAL GENETICS

It has become commonplace to point out that genetic medicine faces a developmental lag between the invention of new genetic tests and the development of the therapeutic interventions that will complement them and that it is during this therapeutic gap that the field faces its professional and public policy challenges in their sharpest form.[51] However, clinicians have coped with similarly lopsided diagnostic challenges in other settings[52] without making a special issue of them. Why should uncomplemented genetic diagnostics merit special attention? In the United States, $5 million a year of the NIH budget for the National Center for Human Genome Research has been devoted for the last four years to the study of ethical, legal, and social issues raised by the clinical application of new genetic information, an unprecedented public investment.[53] The issues of communicating uncertainty, keeping confidentiality, juggling loyalties to multiple family members, insurance discrimination, and personal control over biologics are not unique to genetic medicine. Indeed, some have argued that as DNA-based risk assessments become relevant for a wider spectrum of multifactoral health problems, the distinction between genetic and nongenetic diagnostics is increasingly indefensible for professional and public policy purposes and should be abandoned.[54]

To understand the grip that genetic risk assessments have on the moral imaginations of human geneticists and their public, it is important to put the development of genetic testing in context. Discussions of how best to use DNA-based diagnostics in the absence of therapy do seem to be animated by special concerns that are not as urgent in other settings. But it is not the fact of the therapeutic gap that sets genetic testing issues apart. Rather it is the fact that it is during this therapeutic gap that these tests are most traditionally "genetic." That is, it is during this gap that they behave most like a traditional genetic risk assessment and, as a consequence, pass on to their users the psychosocial burden traditionally associated with genetic explanations of illness. It is not some new set of unanticipated problems that concern people about genetic medicine's new capacities. Rather, faced with the prospect of a burgeoning epidemic of traditional issues, public expectations and professional attitudes both end up cutting against each other, scissors-fashion, to sharpen the issues.

The Social Power of Genetic Information

For patients, three features of what it means to have an illness explained in genetic terms seem particularly strong as sources of concern.

Determinism. Health risk assessments based on information about the presence or absence of genetic mutations have traditionally been limited to the set of health problems classified as genetic disorders. Since relatively few genetic mutations create easily discernible patterns of disease inheritance within a family, the clearest examples of genetic disorders (e.g., Huntington's disease) have been both predictable and intractable. They have appeared in highly penetrant Mendelian patterns in the unfortunate families who inherit them and unfold inexorably in their individual victims. This history still affects the way many people think about genetic risk information, by leading them to assume that genetic diagnostics of any kind have more predictive power than other kinds of health risk assessments. This assumption is corroborated by popular (and academic) accounts of genetic tests as crystal balls, capable of exposing individuals' future diaries.[55] Unfortunately, overly deterministic understandings of genetic test results can foreclose, rather than facilitate, the recipient's ability to make plans for the future by encouraging unnecessary fatalism and exposing the recipient to social stigmatization.

In actuality, of course, genetic risk assessment tests for most multifactorial health problems will have modest predictive power. For example, Jean's *p53* test can clarify whether she has inherited the mutations associated with Li-Fraumeni syndrome and thereby tell her more about her general risks of experiencing cancer. It cannot predict with certainty, however, whether she will experience cancer or, if she does, what her clinical experience will be, that is, which kind of tumor she may experience or how severe it will be or how treatable. In the end, these questions are likely to be more important to her than the bare fact of her increased risk.

Reductionism. Because of the causal power genetic risk factors are often (mistakenly) given, they also tend to play a disproportionate role in the social identification of those who carry them, reducing their identities to their carrier status. Genetic information can identify health risks we inherit from (and often share with) our families and explain those risks at what seems to be a very basic biologic level. Together, the familial and constitutional connotations of genetic information make it easy to interpret genetic health risks as a reflection on the recipient's identity as a person and to label people accordingly.[56] To the extent that genotypic labels are interpreted as indicative of hidden weaknesses within individuals, this reductionistic understanding of genetic test results simply exacerbates any stigmatization that the target disease may carry.[57]

Familial Implications. Overly deterministic and reductionistic interpretations of genetic health risks are cultural perceptions that the facts of genetics do not demand. However, there is one objective feature of genetic risk information that colors almost all genetic testing. When genetic information reveals an individual's risk for disease, it also suggests the possibility that family members are also at risk. This information can bear on reproductive decision making before and after conception and can confront other family members with predictive information that they may not wish to know. In addition, unlike other stigmatizing conditions that affect and label only the individual, genetic conditions can stigmatize families as well. Even if no evidence of the condition exists in other family members, they may be stigmatized by their relationship to an individual who has such a condition.[58]

These three features serve to raise the stakes and animate the discussions of genetic diagnostics because together they give genetic testing a social meaning that other health risk assessments do not share. To the extent that genetic tests are understood to implicate patients' futures, their identities, and their closest relationships, they become centrally important to the patient's lives. It is against this potent psychosocial backdrop that individuals and families, health professionals, and policy makers must consider how best to use new genetic diagnostic tests.

The Professional Ethos of Medical Genetics

At the same time, the other scissor blade in the genetic testing context is the unusual ethos of medical genetics. As in other clinical sciences, the challenge to medical genetics is to explain clinical problems in a way that will help address their patients' concerns. However, the form of these explanations is shaped by the tools that the geneticist brings to bear on the task: the theories of molecular, Mendelian, and population genetics. Until very recently, the explanations that these tools yielded, framed as they were in terms of genes, families, or populations, could not suggest interventions to directly help patients with their own somatic health problems. Instead, geneticists shifted their emphasis from curative interventions to reproductive and preventive planning. This explanatory shift has produced a distinctive and unusual ethos for the specialty that has implications for all aspects of practice.

This perspective gives the clinical geneticist a clear sense of where his or her allegiances lie: The fundamental value of genetic screening and counseling is the ability to enhance the opportunities for individuals to obtain information about their personal health and childbearing risks and to make autonomous and noncoerced choices based on that information.[59]

The specialty's allegiance to the interests of its clients considerably sharpens its general goals of "combatting genetic disease" by focusing on the problems that genetic diseases pose to the patients who present themselves for help. In somatic medicine, this focus is traditional and unproblematic. In genetic medicine, however, the hereditary nature of genetic diseases can suggest other candidates for the practitioner's attention as well: the extended family at risk for the disease, the population carrying its genetic load, or the future generations that the disease may strike. At various times, each of these candidates has been proposed as the proper object of medical genetic practice.[60] However, since 1950, three factors have converged to suggest that the welfare and interests of the presenting patients should take priority over the interests of any other parties their decisions may affect.

The Shadow of Eugenics. In part, the contemporary client-centered ethos in medical genetics is an intentional reaction to the excesses of the eugenics movement in the first half of this century. During that period, the relevance of genetic knowledge to decision making about future generations prompted some to take people's reproductive planning into their own hands, with scandalous consequences.[61] In reaction, the contemporary discipline has deliberately shifted its focus from future generations to prospective parents and taken pains to avoid value judgments about the social consequences of their clients' choices.

Respect for Reproductive Autonomy. Closely related to the discipline's reaction to eugenics has been society's growing conviction that individuals' reproductive choices are intertwined tightly enough with their most important beliefs and values to be given the kind of protection that pluralistic societies give to other important personal freedoms.[62] Medical geneticists thus find themselves working with families on what are usually very private decisions. The client-centered ethos, by reinforcing the confidentiality of the medical genetic exchange and reserving decision-making authority for the clients, represents a professional affirmation of this sphere of privacy.

Prognostic Uncertainty and Therapeutic Impotence. Finally, the ethos of medical genetics also functions as a strategy for coping with uncertainty. Since almost every genetic risk assessment decision will remain a gamble in the absence of effective therapeutic interventions, geneticists claim that the parties who will bear the consequences of those decisions should have the right to make them. This view is usually combined with the claim that, in fact, the patients are in the best position to make the decision because they know their own resources for living with its results.[63] As a result, although medical geneticists still express a general concern to decrease the genetic burden of disease, they are committed to channeling their efforts through the choices of their clients. In the genetics clinic, this client-centered emphasis is most recognizable in the unusual tradition of nondirective communication that distinguishes the practice of genetic counseling. It also underlies the other distinguishing marks of the professional ethics of clinical genetics: the importance given to full, effective disclosure of diagnostic information, to the confidentiality of screening results, and to placing control of subsequent clinical decision making entirely in the client's hands.

In the face of this ethos and its expectations for ethical practice, the prospect of a groundswell of new genetic tests is daunting. Against the pressures created by commercially driven efforts to disseminate convenient and technically accurate multiplex genetic risk assessments to a public that is likely to overinterpret the significance of the test results for themselves and their families, clinical geneticists are faced with deciding how much of their distinctive ethos they can afford to preserve. The fine line between adapting the specialty's ideology to new circumstances and corrupting its professional integrity makes any discussion of these issues a charged one for the field.

CONCLUSION: A NEW LEXICON FOR GENETIC DIAGNOSTICS

There is a common theme to the professional and public policy issues that challenge the development and use of new genetic diagnostics: All are either rooted in or exacerbated by simplistic interpretations of genetic causation and the predictive power of genetic tests. In part, these interpretations are consequences of public and (sometimes) professional misunderstanding of the scientific basis of genetic diagnostics. In part, they are due to the occult imagery that surrounds genetics in the popular press. However, critics also point to the human genetics community itself as a source of the public's confusion about the significance of genetic risk assessments.[64] One way in which this occurs is through the generic use of deterministic adjectives, such as presymptomatic or predictive, to describe the entire range of genetic risk assessment tests. As a consequence, one way in which the clinical community could contribute to resolution of the policy challenges described would be to take more care with its nomenclature by establishing professional conventions to clarify the clinical significance of different categories of genetic risk assessment tests.

As a starting point for such a discussion, and the conclusion to this one, consider the following suggestions for a new genetic testing lexicon.

1. *Diagnostic* genetic tests should be tests that are capable of confirming the diagnosis of an active genetic disease process, such as the use of mutation analysis to diagnose fragile X syndrome in developmentally delayed children.[65]
2. *Prognostic* genetic tests should be tests that are capable of forecasting the emergence of a clinical health problem with a high degree of certainty, such as mutation analysis for Huntington's disease. Such testing is only presymptomatic if one concedes that to carry the mutations is to have Huntington's disease in its earliest stages.[66]
3. *Predictive* genetic tests should be tests that can detect a true genetic predisposition to a clinical health problem, that is, a tendency or inclination to go wrong in a particular way, if not inhibited by other genetic or environmental checks. In these cases, a positive test result would allow us to predict that unless the predisposition is controlled, the clinical problem will result. Newborn testing for PKU fits this model of genetic testing.[67]
4. *Prophylactic* genetic testing, on the other hand, would describe those tests that detect the presence of a genetic susceptibility, that is, a vulnerability to a particular environmental stimulus. For example, alpha$_1$-antitripsin deficiency creates such a susceptibility. In the absence of tobacco smoke, it does no harm, but in those who do smoke, it represents a serious liability.[68] By calling it prophylactic, we would simply be emphasizing that there are interventions to be made, that the problem is not internal or inevitable.
5. *Probabilistic* genetic testing would be a less determined category of genetic risk assessment. Here, one thinks of a test like the test for *p53* mutations in Li-Fraumeni family members, a test that can serve to alert the clients that they are at a statistically higher risk than the population for a particular kind of health problem but cannot make stronger claims about the specific course of the future.
6. *Genetic profiling* would be the category of tests that simply identify a loose empirical association between a particular mutation and an increased incidence of a given health problem. An illustration is the putative association between deletions in the gene for angiotensin-converting enzyme (ACE) and the risk of myocardial infarction.[69]

The point of such a lexicon is not to create watertight categories to which particular genetic tests would be permanently assigned. The categories are clearly overlapping, and one test could fall into several categories depending on the clinical situation. For example, a Huntington's disease mutation test could be diagnostic if it were used to rule out a diagnosis of Huntington's disease in a neurologically impaired patient. The point is to develop some conventions for describing tests in ways that give the public a more nuanced understanding of the epistemic power and their practical significance. In short, what is needed is a way of distinguishing between different kinds of forecasts in the same way meteorologists have a range of predictions to offer based on what their own testing technologies tell them about the imminence, severity, and extent of the weather to come.

Admittedly, this meteorologic approach to genetic diagnostics strains against our modern inclination to invest genes with occult powers to determine the fate of individuals. Just as it is easy to identify Jean as a member of a "cancer family," explaining the presence of other mutations as presymptomatic of multifactoral diseases, such as diabetes, schizophrenia, or heart disease, also can be misread to mean that their carriers are already flawed by these health problems—that they are latent diabetics, schizophrenics, or cardiac patients. These tests, however, need not diagnose personal weakness. If they can be reinterpreted as barometer readings rather than palm lines, their forecasts can strengthen their carriers by giving them the opportunity to prepare for the environmental pressures they will face. If the purpose of medical prediction is to enhance rather than constrain personal autonomy, the weather watcher's perspective may be worth remembering in trying to sort through what genes mean for patients.

If a sense of the true range and limits of different genetic diagnostic tools can be conveyed, professionals and the public can begin to assess and use them in a more realistic manner. The day that DNA testing comes to be seen as simply another kind of biomedical barometer, a large portion of medicine's contemporary challenge will have been overcome.

ACKNOWLEDGMENTS

The Ethical, Legal and Social Implications Program of the NIH/Department of Energy Human Genome Project supported much of the research reviewed here, as well as my own efforts to collect and interpret it. The chapter was facilitated by invitations to develop my views for the U.S. Department of Energy's 1994 Workshop on the Concept of Genetic Predisposition, the Centre for Health Care Ethics at the University of Newcastle, Australia, and the Boehringer Mannheim company's 1995 public education project, "The Diagnostic Challenge."

NOTES

1. D. Malkin et al., "Germ-line p53 Mutations in a Familial Syndrome of Breast Cancer, Sarcomas and Other Neoplasms." *Science* 250 (1992): 1233–38.
2. F. P. Li et al., "Testing for Germ Line p53 Mutation in Cancer Families," *Cancer Epidemiol. Biomarkers Rev.* 1 (1991): 91–94.
3. C. Caskey, "Presymptomatic Diagnosis: A First Step toward Genetic Health Care," *Science* 260 (1993): 48–49.
4. D. N. Cooper and J. Schmidtke, "Molecular Genetic Approaches to the Analysis and Diagnosis of Human Inherited Disease: An Overview," *Ann Med.* 24 (1992): 29–42.
5. M. Huggins et al., "Ethical and Legal Dilemmas Arising during Predictive Testing for Adult-Onset Disease: The Experience of Huntington's Disease," *Am. J. Hum. Genet.* 47 (1990): 4–12.
6. M. Yarborough, "The Role of Beneficence in Clinical Genetics: Nondirective Counseling Reconsidered," *Theor. Med.* 10 (1989): 139–49.
7. K. Rothenberg and E. T. Thompson, *Women and Prenatal Testing: Facing the Challenge of Genetic Technologies* (Columbus, Ohio: Ohio State University Press, 1994).
8. S. Post, *Spheres of Love: Toward a New Ethics of the Family* (Dallas: Southern Methodist University Press, 1994).
9. M. Frankel and A. Teich, *Ethical and Legal Issues in Pedigree Studies* (Washington, D.C.: AAAS, 1993).
10. C. MacKay, "Ethical Issues in Research Design and Conduct: Developing a Test to Detect Carriers of Huntington's Disease," *IRB Rev. Hum. Subjects Res.* 6 (1984): 1–5.
11. B. B. Biesecker et al., "Genetic Counseling for Families with Inherited Susceptibility to Breast and Ovarian Cancer," *JAMA* 269 (1993): 1970–74.
12. D. Wertz and J. Fletcher, "Communicating Genetic Risks," *Science Sci. Technol. Hum. Values* 4 (1987): 60–66.
13. M. Z. Pelias, "Duty to Disclose in Medical Genetics: A Legal Perspective," *Am. J. Med. Genet.* 39 (1991): 347–54.
14. P. R. Reilly, "When Should an Investigator Share Raw Data with the Subjects?" *IRB* 24 (1980): 5, 12.
15. C. MacKay, "Discussion Points to Consider in Research Related to the Human Genome," *Hum. Gene Ther.* 4 (1993): 489.

16. N. A. Holtzman, *Proceed with Caution: Predicting Genetic Risks in the Recombinant DNA Era* (Baltimore: Johns Hopkins University Press, 1989).

17. S. Wilkinson and S. Perry, *Biotechnology and the Diagnosis of Genetic Disease: Technical, Regulatory, and Societal Issues, Program on Technology and Health Care* (Washington, D.C.: Georgetown University Press, 1991).

18. B. S. Wilfond and K. Nolan, "National Policy Development of the Clinical Application of Genetic Diagnostic Technologies: Lessons from Cystic Fibrosis," *JAMA* 270 (1993): 2948–54.

19. U.S. Office for the Protection from Research Risk, *Protecting Human Subjects: Institutional Review Board Guidebook* (Bethesda, Md.: OPRR, 1993).

20. S. Wiggins et al., "The Psychological Consequences of Predictive Testing for Huntington's Disease," *New England Journal of Medicine* 327 (1992): 1401–5.

21. H. Markel, "The Stigma of Disease: Implications of Genetic Screening," *Am. J. Med.* 939 (1992): 209–15.

22. P. Billings et al., "Discrimination as a Consequence of Genetic Screening," *Am. J. Hum. Genet.* 50 (1992): 476–82; M. Rothstein, "Genetic Discrimination in Employment and the Americans with Disabilities Act," *Houston Law Rev.* 29 (1992): 23–85; E. Draper, *Risky Business: Genetic Testing and Exclusionary Practices in the Hazardous Workplace* (New York: Cambridge University Press, 1991).

23. President's Commission for the Study of the Ethical Problems in Medicine and Biomedical and Behavioral Research, *Screening and Counseling for Genetic Conditions* (Washington, D.C.: U.S. Government Printing Office, 1983).

24. J. G. Comptom, "Linkage of Epidermolytic Hyperkeratosis to the Type II Keratin Gene Cluster on Chromosome 12Q," *Nature Genet.* 1 (1992): 301–5.

25. G. J. Annas, "Problems of Informed Consent and Confidentiality in Genetic Counseling," in *Genetics and the Law,* ed. A. Milnunsky and G. J. Annas (New York: Plenum Press, 1976), 111–22.

26. President's Commission, *Screening and Counseling,* 44.

27. D. Wertz et al., "Genetic Testing for Children and Adolescents: Who Decides?" *JAMA* 272 (1994): 875–81; P. S. Harper and A. Clarke, "Should We Test Children for 'Adult' Genetic Diseases?" *The Lancet* 334 (1990): 1205–6.

28. P. Harper, "Research Samples from Families with Genetic Diseases: A Proposed Code of Conduct," *Br. Med. J.* 3061 (1993): 391–93; Huntington's Disease Society of America, *Guidelines for Predictive Testing for Huntington's Disease* (New York: Huntington's Disease Society of America, Inc., 1989).

29. M. Bloch and M. R. Hayden, "Predictive Testing for Huntington's Disease in Childhood: Challenges and Implications," *Am. J. Hum. Genet.* 49 (1990): 1–4.

30. F. P. Li et al., "Recommendations on Predictive Testing for Germ-Line p53 Mutations among Cancer-Prone Individuals," *J. Natl. Cancer Inst.* 84 (1992): 1156–60.

31. M. Green and A. J. Solnit, "Reactions to the Threatened Loss of a Child: A Vulnerable Child Syndrome," *Pediatrics* 34 (1964): 56–77.

32. R. Kodish et al., "Cancer Risk Research: What Should We Tell Subjects?" *Clin. Res.* 42 (1994): 396–402.

33. C. Camaschaella et al., "Prenatal Diagnosis of Fetal Hemoglobin Lepore Boston Disease on Maternal Peripheral Blood," *Blood* 75 (1990): 2101.

34. K. Klinger et al., "Prenatal Detection of Chromosomal Abnormalities Using Fluorescent In Situ Hybridization," *Proc. Miami Bio/Tech* 1 (Winter Symposium 1991): 95–100.

35. L. Andrews et al., *Assessing Genetic Risks: Implications for Health and Social Policy* (Washington, D.C.: National Academy Press, 1993).

36. R. Cowan, "Genetic Technology and Reproductive Choice: An Ethics of Autonomy," in *The Code of Codes,* ed. D. Kevies and L. Hood (Cambridge, Mass.: Harvard University Press, 1992), 244–63.

37. M. Saxton, "Prenatal Screening and Discriminatory Attitudes about Disability," in *Embryos, Ethics and Women's Rights,* ed. E. Baruch et al. (New York: Hayworth Press, 1988), 298–312.

38. L. B. Andrews, "DNA Testing, Banking and Individual Rights," in *Genetic Screening: From Newborns to DNA Typing,* ed. B. M. Knoppers and C. M. Laberge (New York: Elsevier, 1990), 217–42.

39. V. Hannig, "Whose DNA Is It, Anyway? Relationships between Families and Researchers," *Am J. Med. Genet.* 47 (1993): 257–60.

40. W. J. Curran, "Scientific and Commercial Development of Human Cell Lines—Issues of Property, Ethics, and Conflict of Interest," *New England Journal of Medicine* 324 (1991): 998–1000; Eisenberg, "Patenting the Human Genome," *Emory Law Journal* 39 (1990): 721–45.

41. M. Natowitz et al., "Genetic Discrimination and the Law," *Am. J. Hum. Genet.* 50 (1992): 465–75.

42. R. Porkorski, "The Genetic Testing Debate: New Technologies Present Challenges in Risk Selection," *J. Insurance Med.* 20 (1988): 57–61.

43. NIH/DOE, *Task Force Report on Genetic Information and Insurance* (Washington, D.C.: U.S. Government Printing Office, 1992).

44. B. Gay, "Changing Federal Regulations of IRBs," *IRB* 2 (1980): 1–5, 12.

45. Li et al., "Recommendations"; National Institutes of Health, "Workshop on Population Screening for the Cystic Fibrosis Gene: Statement," *New England Journal of Medicine* 323 (1990): 70–71.

46. U.S. Office for the Protection from Research Risk, *Protecting Human Subjects: Institutional Review Board Guidebook.*
47. H. Oster et al., "Insurance and Genetic Testing: Where Are We Now?" *Am. J. Hum. Genet.* 52 (1993): 565–77; J. McEwan et al., "A Survey of Medical Directors of Life Insurance Companies Concerning the Use of Genetic Information," *Am. J. Hum. Genet.* 53 (1993): 33–46.
48. Li et al., "Recommendations," 1159.
49. NIH CF Studies Consortium, "June 1992 Workshop Report" (Unpublished Report, National Center for Human Genome Research, NIH, Bethesda, Md., 1992).
50. Andrews et al., *Assessing Genetic Risks.*
51. F. S. Collins, "Medical and Ethical Consequences of the Human Genome Project," *J. Clin Ethics* 2 (1991): 260–67; J. R. Botkin, "Ethical Issues in Human Genetic Technology," *Pediatrician* 17 (1990): 100–7.
52. G. H. Guyatt et al., "The Role of Before-After Studies of Therapeutic Impact in the Evaluation of Diagnostic Technologies," *J. Chronic Diseases* 39 (1986): 295–304.
53. E. T. Juengst, "Human Genome Research and the Public Interest: Progress Notes from an American Science Policy Experiment," *Am. J. Hum. Genet.* 54 (1994): 121–28.
54. NIH/DOE, *Task Force Report.*
55. G. Annas, "Rules for 'Gene Banks': Protecting Privacy in the Genetic Age," in *Justice and the Human Genome Project,* ed. T. Murphy and M. Lappe (Berkeley, Calif.: University of California Press, 1994), 227–242.
56. D. Brock, "The Human Genome Project and Human Identity," *Houston Law Rev.* 29 (1992): 7–22; E. Fox-Keller, "Genetics, Reductionism and Normative Uses of Biological Information," *Southern California Law Rev.* 65 (1991): 285–91.
57. D. Nelkin and L. Tancredi, *Dangerous Diagnostics: The Social Power of Biological Information* (New York: Basic Books, 1990).
58. R. H. Kenen and R. M. Schmidt, "Stigmatization of Carrier Status: Social Implications of Heterozygote Genetic Screening Programs," *Am. J. Public Health* 49 (1978): 116–20.
59. President's Commission, *Screening and Counseling,* 55.
60. M. Lappe, "Allegiance of Human Geneticists: A Preliminary Typology," *Hastings Center Studies* 1 (1973): 366–74.
61. P. R. Reilly, *The Surgical Solution: A History of Involuntary Sterilization in the United States* (Baltimore: Johns Hopkins University Press, 1991).
62. J. Robertson, "The Potential Impact of the Human Genome Project on Procreative Liberty," in *Gene Mapping: Using Law and Ethics as Guides,* ed. G. Annas and S. Elias (New York: Oxford University Press, 1991), 215–25.
63. J. R. Sorenson, "Biomedical Innovation, Uncertainty, and Doctor-Patient Interaction," *J. Health Soc. Behav.* 15 (1974): 366–74.
64. D. Nelkin, "Promotional Metaphors and Their Popular Appeal," *Public Understanding of Science* 3 (1994): 25–31.
65. F. Roussea et al., "Direct Diagnosis by DNA Analysis of the Fragile X Syndrome of Mental Retardation," *New England Journal of Medicine* 325 (1991): 1673–81.
66. J. Brandt et al., "Presymptomatic Diagnosis of Delayed Onset Diseases with Linked DNA Markers: The Experience of HD." *JAMA* 261 (1989): 3108–14.
67. N. A. Holtzman, "Dietary Treatment of Inborn Errors of Metabolism," *Annu. Rev. Med.* 21 (1970): 115–32.
68. H. D. Stokinger and L. D. Scheel, "Hypersusceptibility and Genetic Problems in Occupational Medicine: A Consensus Report," *J. Occup. Med.* 15 (1973): 564–73.
69. F. Cambien et al., "Deletion Polymorphism in the Gene for Angiotensin Converting Enzyme: A Potent Risk Factor for Myocardial Infarction," *Nature* 359 (1992): 5641–44.

CHAPTER 20

Human Experimentation and Clinical Consent

George J. Agich

Although much has been written about informed consent, there are still uncertainties about the relation of consent and experimentation in research and clinical contexts.[1] In this chapter I first discuss some definitional aspects of informed consent in between research and therapy that are complicated by the place of experimentation in each. In so doing, I contrast the ethics and structure of the physician–patient relationship and the researcher–subject relationship as well as consider the definitions and standards of informed consent in common law and federal regulations governing research with human subjects. Second, I consider some salient practical problems associated with consent to experimentation in clinical settings against this definitional background. I argue that consent requirements vary with the relationship in question—whether it is research or therapy—and with risk-benefit considerations, patient competence, and the actual medical circumstances.

THE DEFINITIONAL PROBLEM

Informed consent is the cornerstone of contemporary medical ethics. At least since the Nuremberg tribunals, it has been widely acknowledged that the voluntary consent of a human subject is ethically required before that subject can participate in experiments.[2] Despite the importance of informed consent in current medical ethics, it has hardly been uniformly respected even in American research.[3] Since 1974, federal regulations have required institutions receiving federal funds to conduct prospective and continuing formal review of all biomedical and behavioral research involving human subjects.[4] These regulations accord informed consent a central place in human subjects research. A doctrine of informed consent has also developed separately in common law that makes it a duty of physicians to disclose relevant information prior to securing patients' permission to undertake diagnostic or therapeutic interventions.[5] It is a matter of scholarly debate whether informed consent in clinical settings is a nineteenth- or twentieth-century phenomenon.[6] What is clear is that while examples of consent in medical practice can be found prior to the twentieth century, the doctrine of *informed* consent came to be recognized generally as a legal obligation of physicians in the relatively recent period between 1957 and 1972.[7]

In response to the Nazi medical experiments, the Nuremberg Code of 1947 was promulgated with an absolute commitment to informed consent: "The voluntary consent of the human subject is absolutely essential."[8] The duty and responsibility for ascertaining the quality of the consent was said to rest "upon each individual who initiates, directs, or engages in the experiment. It is a personal duty and responsibility which may not be delegated to another with

---

impunity."[9] Presumably, this emphasis on the investigator's primary moral responsibility in conducting human experimentation was a response to one of the common defenses made before the Nuremberg tribunals, namely, that the accused was merely following orders or serving a subsidiary role in the research. The Nuremberg Code stresses that moral responsibility is primarily an individual rather than an institutional matter, and the code does not provide a mechanism for ensuring that research with human subjects conforms to its ideals. This approach differs considerably from that taken under federal regulations that require institutional review board (IRB) review of biomedical and behavioral research involving human subjects. Although the regulations also assume that the principal investigator is primarily responsible for designing and conducting the research in a manner consistent with ethical standards and protective of the rights and welfare of subjects, formal review of proposed research is nonetheless focused on institutions that implement the federal research regulations under contract with the Department of Health and Human Services (DHHS). The IRB is the central mechanism through which the regulatory goal of protecting the rights and welfare of subjects of research is carried out.

Federal regulations require that consent forms generally involve the following: (1) the subject's involvement must be identified as research, and a description of the research and its purposes must be provided; (2) the risks must be described; (3) the benefits must be described; (4) if the investigation is clinical, then diagnostic and therapeutic alternatives must be described; (5) a description must be given of the confidentiality of research records and data; (6) an explanation must be given of the availability or unavailability of compensation or treatment for injury; (7) identification must be made of whom to contact for answers regarding the conduct of the research and the subject's rights as well as whom to contact in the event of an injury; (8) an explanation must be given of the subject's rights to refuse participation and to withdraw from the study.[10] Additional elements may be required by the IRB when appropriate, for example, information regarding currently unforeseeable risks, reasons why an investigator might expel a subject from a study, identification of additional costs to the subject incurred as a result of participation in the study, consequences of the subject's withdrawal from the study (e.g., risk of severe side effects if study medication is withdrawn precipitously), information about pertinent new findings, and information about the number of subjects participating in the research project.[11]

These elements of informed consent for human subjects of research point up a significant difference between consent in therapeutic and research settings. Under common law, informed consent is a positive duty of the physician to disclose information regarding the proposed course of treatment, alternatives, and the risks and benefits that are material to patient decision making.[12] As a legal standard, informed consent is imposed retrospectively. That is, courts are involved only after a malpractice suit is filed. Prospective review is not conducted, because such review would be intrusive into the special professional relationship of physician and patient. The physician is thus free from external scrutiny except after the fact and only if a lawsuit is initiated. The researcher, however, is subject to prospective and continuing review requirements, including explicit and detailed standards for the information disclosed.

This difference in the structure of review and the establishment of consent standards reflects an important difference between our therapeutic and research relationships.[13] The physician–patient relationship has traditionally been regarded as a fiduciary relationship in which the physician is obligated to act as the agent of the patient and primarily in the patient's best interest. The research relationship, however, is designed to gather evidence or data for testing a hypothesis with a goal of advancing scientific knowledge rather than benefiting the subject. Of course, in some instances the subjects of research stand to benefit from participating in the study, but such benefit is not the primary goal of the research relationship. In all studies, the subject undertakes risks associated with the research. The expectation is that subjects should be apprised of specific elements of information pertinent to a decision whether or not to participate in the research. In contrast, therapeutic relationships have as their goal patient welfare. The vector of the relationship is toward patient well-being and, so, trust is presumed.

Research is a formal activity supported in large part through public funds, with the aim of advancing scientific knowledge. Therapeutic relationships, however, are fiduciary relationships that primarily aim at enhancing individual patient welfare. The practice of medicine, however, has come to combine research and therapeutic activities—in what Talcott Parsons has termed the *professional complex* of research, service, and teaching[14]—to such an extent that the distinction between research and therapy has proven difficult to apply. Although it is not clear how the term *therapeutic research* entered usage, it has certainly caused difficulty. The concept is at least implicit in the World Medical Association's Declaration of Helsinki, which distinguishes clinical research combined with professional care from "non-therapeutic clinical research."[15] Since it is not conducted for the benefit of the subjects involved, nontherapeutic research is often seen as suspect ethically and as requiring stronger justification than therapeutic research, which, it is often implied, is of benefit to the subject.[16] This assumption, however, is not well-founded, because whether a treatment being researched will benefit a subject is often precisely what is in question. The objective of clinical research usually is to determine the safety or efficacy of a particular therapeutic method or procedure or to gain knowledge of basic physiological processes. Implicit in the need to ask the research question is a basic scientific uncertainty regarding which method or procedure provides the best outcome. This uncertainly means that the question of therapeutic benefit is unresolved and so cannot validly be assumed, even though the question is being investigated in the context of a relationship that aims at providing clinical benefits.

Karen Labacqz and Robert J. Levine, both members of the National Commission for the Protection of Human Subjects of Biomedical and Behavioral Research, have separately criticized the Commission's early definition of "therapeutic research," or "the spurious distinction between therapeutic and non-therapeutic experimentation" in its first report, *Research on the Fetus.*[17] Both argue for a view that was later articulated in the National Commission's *Belmont Report:*

> For the most part, the term "practice" refers to interventions that are designed solely to enhance the well-being of the individual patient or client and that have a reasonable expectation of success. The purpose of medical or behavioral practices is to provide a diagnosis, preventive treatment or therapy to particular individuals. By contrast, the term "research" designates an activity designed to test a hypothesis, permit conclusions to be drawn and thereby to develop or contribute to generalizable knowledge (expressed, for example, in theories, principles, and statements of relationships).[18]

On this view, research and practice (or therapy) are logically distinct activities. The term *research* refers to a class of activities designed to produce generalizable knowledge, whereas *therapy* or *practice* refers to a class of activities that is meant to benefit patients and enhance patient welfare. The distinction is primarily predicated on the intention behind both activities and is reflected in their planning, execution, and the structure of the attendant relationships. While research may be joined with therapy—as in research on the treatment of individuals—the research itself does not thereby become therapeutic.[19] Confusion occurs because research and therapy can occur together in the practice of clinical medicine, for example, research designed to evaluate the safety and efficacy of a therapeutic method or drug, and because notable departures from standard practice are often called experimental when the terms *experimentation* and *research* are not carefully distinguished.[20]

Levine argues that the departures from standard practice, which the *Belmont Report* terms "innovations," should be thought of as a class of activities separate both from research and from those therapies that have been scientifically validated and established. He terms this class "nonvalidated practices." He states, "Novelty is not the attribute that defines this class of practices, rather it is the lack of suitable validation of the safety or ethics of the practice."[21] In the *Belmont Report,* however, the National Commission focused on innovation:

> When a clinician departs in a significant way from a standard or accepted practice, the innovation does not, in and of itself, constitute research. The fact that a procedure is "experimental" in the sense of new, untested or different, does not automatically place it in the category of research. Radically new procedures of this description should, however, be made the object of formal research at an early stage in order to determine whether they are safe and effective.[22]

Requiring that innovations and nonvalidated practices be made the object of research and, hence, subject to formal prospective and continuing review by IRBs raises the important question, What is the proper function of "experimentation" in the practice of medicine and how does this bear on the problem of clinical consent?

An experiment is not simply a formal test of something; it is also a tentative procedure adopted under conditions of uncertainty regarding whether it will achieve the desired purposes or results. On this definition, much of the practice of medicine is experimental in nature. As Herman L. Blumgart has argued,

> Every time a physician administers a drug to a patient, he is in a sense performing an experiment. It is done, however, with therapeutic intent and within the doctor–patient relationship since it involves a judgment that the expected benefit outweighs the risk. . . . We can standardize drugs, but we cannot standardize patients; medical care of the patient demands adjusting the drug to the individual's unique characteristics.[23]

Francis D. Moore has made a similar observation in the context of surgery: Every new operation, for example, is an experiment; indeed every operation of any type contains certain aspects of experimental work."[24] The important point to note is that the experimentation in question is done on the basis of established knowledge and with the primary intention of enhancing the well-being of the patient. Experimentation in this sense is not only compatible with the therapeutic relationship but seems essential to it.

When the treatment is innovative or experimental, things become more complicated ethically. Experimentation (in the sense of novel or new procedures) is a common feature of clinical medicine, especially in emergency or critical care. It is essential that a physician respond quickly and sometimes creatively to unusual presentations of serious illness or trauma. Some responses will be routinized; others will of necessity be novel. Similarly, in the course of surgery, untoward events or unexpected occurrences require modifications of normal procedures. Sometimes, these modifications are due to individual, biological variation or because there is simply not sufficient time for standard approaches. This seems to indicate that such experimentation can be conducted without meeting formal requirements of informed consent when the situation presents no feasible alternatives and when the risk-benefit ratio for the particular subject is acceptable. However, this does not mean that consent can be waived *by the investigator* for experimentation designed to test a hypothesis, to permit conclusions to be drawn, or to develop generalizable knowledge, though IRBs are now permitted to authorize waivers in certain kinds of emergency research.[25]

Any research that asks fundamental questions about the nature of an abnormality and the extent of the human body's response but has no immediate or long-range therapeutic potential for the individual patient would have to be regarded as nontherapeutic. Nontherapeutic clinical research has been regarded as morally suspect in some quarters unless a stringent standard of an informed consent is observed. For example, the Declaration of Helsinki requires that nontherapeutic clinical research meet the following requirements:

> Clinical research on a human being cannot be undertaken without his free consent, after he has been fully informed. . . . The subject of clinical research should be in such a mental, physical, and legal state as to be able to exercise fully his power of choice. Furthermore, the doctor can combine clinical research with professional care, the objective being the acquisition of new medical knowledge, only to the extent that clinical research is justified by its therapeutic value for the patient.[26]

This view would seem to preclude clinical research as we know it, for example, research into basic physiological processes. The thrust of the Declaration of Helsinki is to prevent human subjects from being coerced by the trust they placed in physicians qua physicians. If the physician is also a researcher, the activities of research and practice should be strictly kept distinct. But this approach is problematic because it attempts to force the social role to reflect what is merely a conceptual distinction between research and practice. Modern medicine combines these activities. Rather than proscribe nontherapeutic clinical research, procedures have been developed under federal regulations that require that clinical research protocols be subject to IRB review, a review mandated to protect the welfare and rights of the subjects of research. This provides protection of subjects by institutionalizing the ethical review of consent and thus avoids outright proscription of nontherapeutic clinical research.

The problem of consent to experimentation thus needs to be addressed by examining at least three categories of experimentation. The first includes a wide range of experimentation conducted for the purpose of advancing knowledge, in which case the researcher–subject relationship is in force and strict consent requirements apply. The second category includes experimentation conducted for the purpose of research but involving medical procedures performed on the subject with little or no prospect of immediate benefit to the subject. The third category includes experimentation or innovative therapy for the purpose of benefiting subjects within physician–patient relationships. The experimentation is conducted as part of formal research. Although this categorization melds the distinctions between research and practice, research ethics and clinical ethics, and the intentional and social definitions of these activities, it accurately reflects the ambiguous conceptual background that complicates the ethical problems associated with clinical consent to experimentation.

PRACTICAL ASPECTS

Consent is morally important because it is a significant means for respecting persons. Competent individuals clearly deserve disclosure of relevant information regarding proposed diagnostic and treatment procedures, available alternatives, and risks and benefits reasonably to be expected from a proposed intervention. As Alan Donagan has forcefully expressed it, "A physician is simply not competent if he is unable to describe, in words intelligible to his patients, everything that could matter to them as patients about the character of any course of treatment he proposes."[27] However, even in an alert, communicative adult, there are potential problems of comprehension. The relevant information is often complicated. The patient's own emotional state sometimes makes understanding and assessment of the information difficult. To suffer an illness or disability compromises one's autonomy; hence, consent to experimental procedures in clinical settings is made especially difficult. To address these difficulties, I discuss three related issues concerning consent to experimental procedures or innovative therapies in clinical settings: what constitutes a valid consent, patient competence, and the contribution of cost-benefit considerations.

Informed consent generally involves adequate information, comprehension or understanding of the information, and voluntariness or absence of coercion. Adequate information would include everything that rational persons want to know, including the benefits and costs involved in the various alternatives and the probabilities associated with each. In addition, each individual should know of anything else that might affect his or her personal decision, such as information that might bear on cultural, personal, or religious beliefs or values. Individuals, however, do not need to know the technical details regarding the treatment.[28] Patients, of course, may refuse information. Such waivers of the right to obtain adequate information regarding a particular procedure, however, should never be *inferred* but must be explicitly and unequivocally stated by the individual.

Ideally, comprehension of the information disclosed should allow the individual's personal beliefs and values to be reflected in any decision. That is, the highest level of comprehension will include a reflective consideration of the proposed course of treatment, available alternatives, and risks and benefits in light of an individual's personal beliefs.[29] Various tests for patient competence have been proposed in the literature. These tests focus on the evidence that a choice has been made, the reasonableness or rational basis of the choice, and the ability to understand or the actual understanding of the information provided. However, as Loren H. Roth et al. argue,

> In effect, the test as actually applied combines elements of all the tests described above. However, the circumstances in which competency becomes an issue determine which elements of which tests are underplayed. Although in theory competency is an independent variable that determines whether or not the patient's decision to accept or refuse treatment is to be honored, in practice it seems to be dependent on the interplay of two other variables: the risk/benefit ratio of treatment and the valence of the patient's decision, i.e., whether he or she consents to or refuses treatment.[30]

Common law and medical ethics recognize situations in which a patient is unable to grant consent. Obvious examples are patients who are obtunded or comatose. Other, more troublesome examples involve patients who are confused or simply too physically ill to comprehend the information and implications of the decision they are being asked to make. In such circumstances, the patient's representative or proxy, usually a spouse or family member, is permitted to grant consent on the patient's behalf. Proxy consent is permitted, because the overriding value in situations of acute illness is patient welfare. The principle of respect for persons involves two essential components: that individuals should be treated as autonomous agents and that persons with diminished autonomy are entitled to protection.[31] Proxy consent is intended to satisfy the latter. However, in a situation of acute illness such as cardiac arrest, it is naive to believe that a spouse or family member is able to grant a fully *informed* consent for the patient. Even if the surrogate were immediately available, it is unlikely that many individuals could resist the natural urge to "do something" or be able to evaluate the subtler aspects of the therapeutic alternatives in a purely rational and objective fashion. For these reasons, emergency treatment relies on a concept of *presumed* or *implied* consent because of the strength obligation of the beneficence that requires that actions be taken to ensure patient welfare.

Underlying this discussion is the belief that the requirements of consent vary not only with patient competence but with the degree and kind of risks and benefits associated with the procedure for which consent is sought. This is clearest in the therapeutic relationship. The physician is not obligated to inform a patient of *all* aspects of treatment but only of those aspects that are material to the patient's informed choice. Another way of expressing this point is that the physician is obligated to obtain patient consent for the proposed *course of treatment,* but not for every component of the actual treatment as it proceeds. As Donagan expresses it, "Advancing a claim to decide a course of treatment that one is to undergo in no way encroaches upon the physician's authority over how that course of treatment is to be carried out."[32]

Risk and benefit considerations and actual clinical circumstances are also relevant in the researcher–subject relationship, but they serve to constrain investigator authority rather than to enhance it. Because advancing scientific knowledge is the primary goal of the research relationship, research ethics (as expressly stated in federal regulations) constrain the investigator to describe in detail the purposes of the research and the details of the subject's involvement. Even in cases where IRBs do not require that the consent forms include detailed discussion of every single aspect of the investigational procedure, the IRB is required to evaluate them in making an assessment of the risk-benefit ratio. Thus, the principal investigator is required to provide sufficient information in the protocol to permit the IRB to estimate the risk-benefit ratio even though the IRB may permit this information to be summarized and explained in lay language to prospective subjects in the consent form.

Unless subjects stand to benefit from the research in a substantial way—as is the case in some clinical research—the principle of respect for persons requires that autonomy be respected by according the individual maximal free choice. When free choice is problematic (e.g., with so-called vulnerable subjects, namely, prisoners or children), specific regulations apply that either proscribe or limit the involvement by placing burdens on the principal investigator to justify involving these subjects and to develop additional methods for ensuring that autonomy is respected. For example, in the case of the institutionalized mentally ill, an ombudsman or consent monitor might be used to ensure that subjects are uncoerced by the principal investigator in securing consent. In the case of children, assent or agreement of a child to an experimental procedure is required in addition to informed consent from parents or guardians. These requirements indicate that consent is balanced by risk-benefit considerations and concern for subject welfare in such a way that the authority is located primarily in the IRB rather than in the investigator. It is the IRB that has the authority to make the final judgment regarding the application of the required and additional elements of consent given the risk-benefit considerations of the particular protocol. In the therapeutic relationship, however, it is the physician who bears final responsibility for modifying consent requirements. In both situations, however, the underlying principles are the same: respecting patient autonomy and protecting patient welfare. These goals serve as the touchstone for judging the ethical acceptability of a consent process, though their application can vary with the conditions just discussed.

In the case of clinical research, the standards of clinical medical ethics and research ethics overlay the problem of consent. Not surprisingly, then, consent in clinical experimentation or innovative therapy is complex. One factor contributing to this complexity is that subjects are often under stress and naturally suffer from anxiety or other emotional reactions to illness. Imposing a high standard might overlook the subtleties associated with the actual competence of patients in clinical settings. In point of fact, there are degrees and qualities of consent that need to be distinguished. As discussed earlier, consent itself must be seen in terms of patient competence, risk-benefit considerations, and the actual clinical circumstances surrounding the consent. Along these lines, James F. Drane has proposed a "sliding-scale model" for determining competence.[33] The model involves three standards of consent that apply to different objective medical decisions. The first standard proposes the minimal requirements of *awareness* (orientation to one's medical situation) and *assent* (explicit or implicit acceptance or refusal). Such a standard would be appropriate for refusing, for example, an effective treatment or for consenting to effective treatment for acute illness or procedures involving high benefit and low risk where the alternatives are limited and where there is diagnostic certainty. Generally, emergency situations would meet these requirements.

The second standard involves the median requirements of *understanding* the medical situation and the proposed treatment and of *choice* based on medical outcomes. This standard would apply, for example, in the case of a chronic condition with a doubtful diagnosis or the case where the outcome of therapy for acute illness is uncertain, where risks and benefits of proposed interventions are balanced, or where a proposed treatment is possibly effective but burdensome.

The final standard involves the maximum requirements of *appreciation* (critical and reflective understanding of the illness and treatment) and *rational decision making* (making choices that reflect one's own articulated beliefs and values). This highest standard of competency is necessary for consent to ineffective treatment, i.e., experimental and unproven treatment, or for refusal of effective treatment for acute illness either where diagnostic certainty and benefit are high, risk is low, and there are limited alternatives or where the disorder is immediately life threatening. This approach is of particular interest because the standard of competency for *refusing* ineffective treatment is the minimal requirement of awareness and assent, whereas the competency standard for *consent* to ineffective treatment, including experimental treatment with a high risk to benefit ratio, is the maximum requirement of appreciation and rational decision making.

The threat of coercion is always present in clinical settings where patients suffer the stress of illness and disability and exhibit anxiety, grief, or psychological defense mechanisms.[34] There is a spectrum of cases to be sure. On the one side is the situation in which the physician is commonly perceived as "my doctor," who has "my interest" foremost; in such a case, a physician can often get a patient to agree to almost any procedure. The use of experimental procedures under such circumstances is problematic because the possibility of subtle coercion is always present. However, if the procedure has minimal or low risk and the benefit is potentially great and no standard treatments are available, then consent that relies simply on patient assent and awareness might be justified. Alternatively, a device or drug might be justified for use if there is scientific evidence for its effectiveness but the drug or device has not yet received Food and Drug Administration (FDA) approval. A minimal standard of consent could be justified because the primary obligation of the physician in the clinical setting is the care of the patient. When experimental procedures have a relatively high degree of probability of enhancing patient welfare, consent that meets the minimal requirements set forth by Drane is adequate.

What might be an example of such a procedure or intervention? Consider the use of cimetidine for duodenal ulcer. The drug was widely used abroad, with clinical results reported a number of years prior to its approval for use under FDA regulations. To be sure, the drug could not be used without conforming to FDA and IRB consent requirements, including the use of a detailed consent form. However, if a patient were to listen distractedly to the information, read the consent form perfunctorily, and sign it without evidence of complete understanding, would it be ethical for the physician to proceed to administer the medication? Here, the patient is compliant to such an extent that he or she would accept a *treatment* even if not fully informed. It does not seem that the physician is obligated to ensure that the highest standard of comprehension is met in this circumstance if there are valid clinical and ethical reasons for the patient's less-than-full understanding because the investigational drug is so far along in the approval process that the therapy is more like a standard than an experimental one. The prospect of benefit to the patient outweighs the demand for a high standard of consent in this case.

At the other end of the spectrum, patient defense mechanisms such as denial or regression, which might hinder a patient in assuming the necessary active role in therapy (consider the so-called cardiac cripple, who avoids even usual and desirable activities such as sexual relations for fear of inducing another attack), can lead to a patient's refusing the procedure. If the patient meets only the lowest standard of competence as described above, should the physician desist from offering an innovative therapy? In this case, the obligation of the physician is to benefit the patient. The physician should work with the patient and family to attain a higher level of understanding. Of course, unless the situation is life threatening, the physician has to respect the patient's decision in the end, no matter how minimal the standard of competence. The important point is that the initial refusal (based solely on the standard of assent and awareness) does not ethically justify the physician's accepting the patient's refusal.

If a patient manifests denial of his illness, yet mistakenly believes that his or her participation in the research protocol would benefit others because it would provide normal control required by the experimental design, what standard of consent would need to be met? On the face of it, such a patient does not manifest sufficient understanding of her or his medical situation and the proposed experimental intervention to meet even median standards. Therefore, he or she could not validly consent to any experimental procedure that involved more than minimal risk. But would a minimal level of awareness and assent be adequate for experimentation involving minimal risk? If one analyzes the situation from the point of view of the ethics of the physician–patient relationship, the answer must be that consent is not valid unless the patient were to benefit. Otherwise, one would simply *use* the patient for one's own end. Such an action would pervert the fiduciary character of the physician–patient relationship. A researcher, however, is under no similar direct and overriding obligation to the subject. Therefore, the focus shifts from enhancing the patient's welfare in physician–patient relationships to respecting the subject's autonomy by providing full disclosure of information and by avoiding coercion in the process of recruitment.

In cases of experimentation with no or low benefits, meeting the highest standards of consent may not be achievable. For such cases, the authority for modifying consent requirements shifts from the investigator to the IRB, which is charged with balancing requirements of consent with considerations of risk and benefit in light of clinical circumstances. For example, the regulations governing human subjects research permit the waiver or alteration of informed consent requirements in cases in which the research involves minimal or no risk to the subject and in which the knowledge to be gained is significant. Specifically, federal regulations permit an IRB to approve a consent procedure that does not include, or that alters, some or all of the elements of informed consent or even to waive the requirements to obtain informed consent provided that the IRB finds and documents the following: (1) that the research involves no more than minimum risk to the patient; (2) that the waiver or alteration will not adversely affect the rights and welfare of the patient; (3) that the research could not practicably be carried out without the waiver or alteration; and (4) that the patient will be provided, whenever appropriate, with additional patient information after participation.[35] The authority for determining whether these conditions apply in particular protocols rests with the IRB, not with the principal investigator. If the social good of advancing scientific knowledge is to compromise in any way the principle of informed consent, it is only the IRB, removed from the research itself, that can make such a determination.

The ethical justification of consent to experimentation in clinical settings involves consideration of the clinical circumstances, patient competence, and the risk-benefit ratio in the light of the intentions behind and the social objectives of the research and therapy. Underlying and justifying informed consent is the principle of respect for persons, which also requires that persons be protected, sometimes from their own choices. The solution to the problem of consent, thus, inevitability depends on how one addresses the issue of paternalism and the wider problem of the degrees and kinds of influence that are compatible with respect for patient autonomy. This latter question has not been addressed directly in this chapter, but an answer is implicit in the ways that consent requirements actually vary in therapeutic and research relationships. Whether these answers are ultimately paternalistic and whether they can be justified is another matter, one that requires further discussion.

NOTES

1. Two good recent summary discussions are T. L. Beauchamp, "Informed Consent," in *Medical Ethics,* 2d ed., ed. R. M. Veatch (Boston: Jones & Bartlett, 1996), 185–208 and A. M. Capron, "Human Experimentation," in *Medical Ethics,* 2d ed., ed. R. M. Veatch (Boston: Jones & Bartlett, 1996), 135–84.
2. Nuremberg Code, *Trials of War Criminals before the Nuremberg Military Tribunal under Control Council Law No. 10* (vol. 2) (Washington, D.C.: U.S. Government Printing Office, 1949).
3. Final Report of the Advisory Committee on Human Radiation Experiments, *Human Radiation Experiments* (New York and Oxford, England: Oxford University Press, 1996).
4. "Protection of Human Subjects," *Code of Federal Regulations* 45 CFR 46, revised March 8, 1983.
5. Three 1972 court decisions are informed-consent landmarks: *Canterbury v. Spence,* 464 F.2d 772 (D.C. Cir. 1972); *Cobbs v. Grant,* 104 Cal. Rptr. 505, 502, P.2d 1 (1972); and *Wilkinson v. Vesey,* 295 A.2d 676 (R.I. 1972).
6. M. S. Pernick, "The Patient's Role in Medical Decisionmaking: A Social History of Informed Consent in Medical Therapy," in *Making Health Care Decisions,* vol. 3, President's Commission for the Study of Ethical Problems in Medicine and Biomedical and Behavioral Research (Washington, D.C.: U.S. Government Printing Office, 1982), 1–35; Jay Katz, *The Silent World of Doctor and Patient* (New York: Free Press, 1986).
7. R. R. Faden and T. L. Beauchamp, *A History and Theory of Informed Consent* (New York: Oxford University Press, 1986), 125–32.
8. *Trials of War Criminals before the Nuremberg Military Tribunals,* 2.
9. Ibid.
10. "Protection of Human Subjects," sec. 46, 116.
11. Ibid.
12. Faden and Beauchamp, *History and Theory,* 23–49, 114–50; Jay Katz, *Experimentation with Human Subjects* (New York: Russell Sage Foundation, 1972).
13. L. R. Churchill, "Physician-Investigator/Patient-Subject: Exploring the Logic and Tension," *Journal of Medicine and Philosophy* 5 (1980): 215–24.
14. T. Parsons, "Research with Human Subjects and the 'Professional Complex,'" in *Experimentation with Human Subjects,* ed. P. A. Freund (New York: George Braziller, 1970), 116–51.
15. World Medical Association, "Declaration of Helsinki," adopted by the 18th World Medical Assembly, Helsinki, Finland, 1964, and revised by the 29th World Medical Assembly, Tokyo, Japan, 1975.
16. A proposed but never implemented policy of the Department of Health, Education and Welfare involved prohibiting entire categories of "non-beneficial research" without regard to consideration of risk involved. See Department of Health, Education and Welfare, "Proposed Policy," *Federal Register* 39 (August 23, 1974): 30648–57.
17. K. Labacqz, "Reflections on the Report and Recommendations of the National Commission: Research on the Fetus," *Villanova Law Review* 22 (1977): 367–83; Robert J. Levine, "Clarifying the Concepts of Research Ethics," *Hastings Center Report* 9 (1979): 22; National Commission for the Protection of Human Subjects of Biomedical and Behavioral Research, *Report and Recommendations: Research on the Fetus,* DHEW Publication no. (OS) 76-127 (Washington, D.C.: U.S. Government Printing Office, 1975).
18. National Commission for the Protection of Human Subjects of Biomedical and Behavioral Research, *The Belmont Report: Ethical Principles and Guidelines for the Protection of Human Subjects of Research,* DHEW Publication no. (OS) 78-0012 (Washington, D.C.: U.S. Government Printing Office, 1975).
19. Lebacqz, "Reflections," 362.
20. National Commission, *Belmont Report,* 2.
21. Levine, "Clarifying the Concepts," 22.
22. National Commission, *Belmont Report,* 3.
23. H. L. Blumgart, "The Medical Framework for Viewing the Problem of Human Experimentation," in *Experimentation with Human Subjects,* ed. P. A. Freund (New York: George Braziller, 1970), 44.
24. F. D. Moore, "Therapeutic Innovations: Ethical Boundaries in the Initial Clinical Trial of New Drugs and Surgical Procedures," in *Experimentation with Human Subjects,* ed. P. A. Freund (New York: George Braziller, 1970), 358.

25. Department of Health and Human Services, "Protection of Human Subjects: Informed Consent and Waiver of Informed Consent Requirements in Certain Emergency Research: Final Rules," *Federal Register* 61 (October 2, 1996): 51531–33.
26. World Medical Association, "Declaration of Helsinki."
27. A. Donagan, "Informed Consent in Therapy and Experimentation," *Journal of Medicine and Philosophy* 2 (1977): 315.
28. The view of the adequacy of information in consent is developed by C. M. Culver and B. Gert, *Philosophy in Medicine* (New York: Oxford University Press, 1982), 43–50.
29. H. Morreim, "Three Concepts of Patient Competence," *Theoretical Medicine* 4 (1983): 239–46.
30. L. H. Roth et al., "Tests of Competency to Consent to Treatment," *American Journal of Psychiatry* 134 (1977): 274.
31. National Commission, *Belmont Report,* 4.
32. Donagan, "Informed Consent," 313.
33. J. F. Drane, "Competency to Give an Informed Consent," *JAMA* 252 (1984): 925–27 and "The Many Faces of Competency," *Hastings Center Report* 15 (1985): 17–21.
34. For discussion of related concerns, see S. D. Mallary et al., "Family Coercion and Valid Consent," *Theoretical Medicine* 7 (1986): 123–26; T. Tomlinson, "The Physician's Influence on Patients' Choices," *Theoretical Medicine* 7 (1986): 105–21.
35. "Protection of Human Subjects," sec. 46, 116–46, 117.

BIBLIOGRAPHY

Advisory Committee on Human Radiation Experiments, *Final Report of the Advisory Committee on Human Radiation Experiments.* New York and Oxford, England: Oxford University Press, 1996. Complete report of the Advisory Committee on Human Radiation Experiments that reviews radiation experiments conducted by the United States government and critically discusses these experiments in their historical context and in light of prevailing ethical and legal norms.

Faden, Ruth R., and Tom L. Beauchamp, *A History and Theory of Informed Consent.* New York: Oxford University Press, 1986. A comprehensive historical and theoretical discussion and analysis of informed consent in practice and research settings.

Katz, Jay. *Experimentation with Human Beings.* New York: Russell Sage Foundation, 1972. A comprehensive casebook with edited coverage of the principal documents pertaining to human subjects research and relevant secondary material; somewhat dated, but nonetheless an important work for consultation.

———. *The Silent World of Doctor and Patient.* New York: The Free Press, 1986. Katz argues that disclosure and consent requirements, except the most rudimentary, are obligations that are alien to medical thinking and practice.

Levine, Robert J. *Ethics and Regulations of Clinical Research,* 2d ed. Baltimore: Urban, 1986. An overview of problems and present solutions regarding the ethics and regulation of clinical research; it is strongly oriented toward federal research guidelines.

National Commission for the Protection of Human Subjects of Biomedical and Behavioral Research. *The Belmont Report.* DHEW Publication no. (OS) 78-0012. Washington, D.C.: U.S. Government Printing Office, 1975. A summary of the ethical principles that guided the work of the National Commission. Importantly, this report came after the majority of the Commission's work was completed and is basically a reflection on the principles that guided its decision making rather than a justification of them.

CHAPTER 21

The Ethics of Research on the Mentally Disabled

Adil E. Shamoo and Joan L. O'Sullivan

HISTORY OF THE MEDICAL ABUSE OF THE MENTALLY DISABLED[1]

Prior to Second World War

Since colonial times, persons with mental disabilities have been treated as less than equal to the rest of the population. Governments have been more concerned with securing the local population from imagined threats by the mentally disabled than with the health and well-being of persons suffering from mental illness. This attitude is reflected in the lack of treatment for persons with mental illness until the 1950s.[2] Inadequate health care for persons with mental illness compared to those with other illnesses is one example of the historical deprivation of human rights for persons with mental illness.[3] The use and abuse of persons with mental illness as human subjects in research is an extension of such an attitude.

The notion that all evil thoughts and acts are the result of a few monsters such as Attila the Hun, Genghis Khan, or Hitler is mythical. Those three individuals stand out in history; nevertheless their monstrous acts could not have been carried out without tens of thousands of other human beings who shared their views, objectives, and methods. Caplan, writing about the Nazi concentration camps, points out that "Those physicians and public health officials who staffed the camps, murdered the demented, and advanced theories of racial hygiene were, according to this myth, simply lunatics, charlatans, and quacks."[4] But the unethical behaviors of such individuals and societies have intellectual underpinnings that were respected in their times. It is important to the question of research subjects to recognize the dangers of these ideas.[5]

The eugenic movement in the first half of this century provided the basis for government-approved sterilization of thousands of persons with mental illness. Eugenics is a science that deals with all influences that improve the inborn qualities of a race. In an attempt to eradicate "negative factors" in the early 1900s, 28 U.S. states and 1 Canadian province enacted legislation to allow sterilization not only for those who were criminally insane but also for those who were mentally ill.[6] By 1939, about 30,000 persons had been sterilized in the United States. Close to 13,000 sterilizations were conducted in California alone.[7] These sterilizations are not the moral equivalent to the genocide that occurred in Germany in 1930s and early 1940s but nevertheless illustrate a discriminatory government policy that is based on a questionable moral theory. In addition to sterilization, the German medical researchers conducted numerous medical experiments on unsuspecting, unconsenting, or coerced human beings. Some of these experiments subjected human beings to severe hypothermia, high-altitude decompression, drinking sea water, irradiation to cause sterility, and stress and starvation.[8]

The Nazi racial hygienists emphasized the importance of genetics in the development of human characteristics and downplayed the importance of environment. They argued that the mentally ill were not only a burden to society economically but also that their sterilization or euthanasia would purify the race, producing one that was physically and mentally healthy.[9] German scholars experimented with trait transmissions of diseases and studied family trees in order to buttress their theories. Adolf Hilter in his *Mein Kampf* said, "Whoever is not bodily and spiritually healthy and worthy, shall not have the right to pass on his suffering in the body of his children."[10]

Germany enacted its law on sterilization in 1933. It authorized the genetic health court to order sterilization for "feeblemindedness, schizophrenia, manic-depressive insanity, genetic epilepsy, Huntington's Chorea, genetic blindness or deafness, or severe alcoholism."[11] Twelve other European nations followed suit and enacted sterilization laws. The sterilization laws were based largely on the false premise that these traits are passed on as single-locus Mendelian genetic transmissions. This has been disproved, and it is well-accepted that these illnesses are multifactorial, involving both genetic predisposition and environmental factors. The genetic and environmental causes of mental illnesses are similar to most physical illnesses, such as diabetes and cardiovascular diseases.[12]

Hitler was the leader of the Nazi Party Congress when he proposed "the murder of the mentally ill" in Nuremburg in 1935[13] to purify the German race. The prevalence of Nazi racial thinking was so dominant in Germany then that it became the accepted paradigm among research circles, publications, journals, scientific leaders, and students. Lack of criticism of that paradigm illustrates the strength behind the movement.

Post-Second World War

The civilized world was disgusted by the atrocities committed by Nazi doctors and scientists on hundreds of thousands of German citizens, including the mentally ill. After the Nuremburg war-crimes trials, during which these experiments came to light, the American Medical Association[14] (AMA) quickly adopted three requirements for experiments using human subjects: (1) voluntary consent, (2) prior animal experimentation, and (3) proper medical protection. The judges at the Nuremburg trials drafted their own code of ethics, known as the Nuremburg Code. The first principle of the Nuremburg Code is that no one should be forced to take part in medical research. "The voluntary consent of the human subject is absolutely essential," they wrote.[15] The Nuremburg Code further requires that the subject should have sufficient understanding to give consent, and that there should be no coercion or duress.[16]

A second important document, the Declaration of Helsinki, augments and refines protections for human subjects enrolled in research. The Declaration of Helsinki was a product of the World Medical Association meeting in 1964. The Helsinki Declaration binds the researcher to the concept of "direct therapeutic benefit." If the patient is not legally competent to consent to participate in a research protocol, a surrogate decision maker can give consent to only research that will deliver a direct therapeutic benefit to the patient. The Declaration ensures that the interest of science and society will never take precedence over the interest of the patient.[17]

The Helsinki Declaration was signed at a time when the press had recently reported cases of patient abuse in research studies in the United States. In 1963, in the Jewish Chronic Disease Case in Brooklyn, New York, it was discovered that researchers had injected foreign live cancer cells into 22 patients without informing patients or attaining informed consent.[18] Later, in 1966, Henry K. Beecher listed numerous cases in which patients were exposed to risks in research protocols without their knowledge or consent.[19] In 1972, Jay Katz published an anthology of cases culled from court files, medical literature, and the media, detailing dubious and unethical research protocols conducted on uninformed subjects.[20]

The most notorious case was the Tuskegee syphilis study conducted from the 1930s to

1973. In this study 600 African-American men (400 experimental subjects and 200 control subjects) were enrolled to study the natural course of syphilis disease.[21] In the 1940s it was clear that those infected with the disease were dying at twice the rate of the control group. More important, penicillin had been proven to be effective in eradicating syphilis. However, none of the subjects received penicillin, and the experiment went on until 1973.

In all of these cases, there was a violation of one or more of the three pillars of informed consent—sufficient knowledge, lack of duress and coercion, and comprehension.

CURRENT PRACTICES

Federal Action

The first federal law in the United States to protect human subjects in research was established in 1974 by the National Research Act.[22] The act and subsequent regulations[23] established local institutional review boards (IRBs) to judge the appropriateness of research protocols. The federal law defines research as "a systematic investigation, including research development, testing and evaluation, designed to develop or contribute to generalizable knowledge."[24]

A key report on the issue of using the mentally ill as research subjects was the *Belmont Report*[25] of the National Commission for the Protection of Human Subjects of Biomedical and Behavioral Research. The *Belmont Report* confirms the need for the three elements of informed consent, especially for those with "mental disability," who should be considered vulnerable and in need of greater protections.

The report of the President's Commission for the study of Ethical Problems in Medicine and Biomedical and Behavioral Research[26] that followed the *Belmont Report* again emphasized the vulnerable status of persons who are "mentally disabled."[27] But despite the fact that both of those two national commissions recommended that special status be accorded to those with mental disability, the final federal regulations did not give this status to the mentally disabled. Instead, the regulations awarded "vulnerable status" only to children, prisoners, and pregnant women who are subjects in research studies.

The recent Office for Protection from Research Risk (OPRR) guidebook[28] offers new language based on the federal regulations in order to give greater protections for the mentally disabled. For example the OPRR guidebook states, "Persons who are institutionalized, particularly if disabled, should not be chosen for studies that bear no relation to their situation just because it would be convenient for the researcher."[29] The OPRR guidebook further states, "Persons who are totally dependent on an institution may be vulnerable to perceived or actual pressure to conform to institutional wishes for fear of being denied services or privileges."[30]

In 1991, the federal government adopted the "Common Rule" that codifies the acceptance by 15 federal agencies and the Central Intelligence Agency (CIA) of a uniform set of rules governing research using human subjects.[31] The Common Rule is basically identical to the policy in 45 CFR 46, Subpart A, which has been in effect since 1974 and has been revised several times since.

The current OPRR guidebook interpretations of the federal regulations regarding research using mentally disabled subjects are covered under the heading "Cognitively Impaired Persons."[32] The federal regulations use several terms to describe this group, such as "cognitively impaired" and "mentally disabled."

The OPRR guidelines on IRBs are based closely on the federal regulations and state that "IRBs that regularly review research involving vulnerable subjects (such as the mentally disabled) are required by DHHS and FDA regulations to consider including among their members one or more individuals who are knowledgeable about and experienced in working with those subjects. In addition, the IRB must be sure that additional safeguards are in place to protect the rights and welfare of these subjects."[33]

The federal regulation clearly indicates that if an IRB regularly deals with another vulnerable group not specifically mentioned in the regulation, it should be treated as a vulnerable group[34] and a member of that group who is knowledgeable about the vulnerable group (i.e., mentally disabled) should be a member of the IRB.[35] Certainly, those IRBs that regularly review washout/relapse studies (removal of patient from all medications for a few weeks or up to a year to test return of symptoms of the illness, or a relapse) or other research protocols with the mentally disabled fall in this category. However, there are no specific regulations governing the mentally disabled. The mentally disabled were never declared by a specific language as a vulnerable subject despite the recommendations of the two national commissions.[36]

IRBs

Federal regulations require that IRBs be established in order to review and approve or disapprove research proposals that use human subjects.[37] The primary objective is to protect the rights and welfare of human subjects participating in research. Therefore, IRB approval is a prerequisite to proceeding in any research protocol involving human subjects.

IRBs must have one member from the community outside the research institution. The minimum number of IRB members is five,[38] but usually membership varies between 15 and 25 persons representing diverse aspects of the research institution.

IRBs use a risk-benefit analysis in order to judge research proposals. The IRBs, therefore, must identify probable benefits from the research as well as probable risks. IRBs are to ensure that subjects are informed of risks, benefits, and available alternative treatments.[39] Research risks usually are those over and above those risks associated with therapies the subject may be undergoing. The OPRR is in charge of overseeing compliance with regulations concerning human subjects enrolled in research experiments.[40]

Regarding the mentally disabled, the OPRR guidebook cites the National Commission for the Protection of Human Subjects:

> For such subjects, the Commission recommended that minimal risk be defined in terms of the risks normally encountered in the daily lives or the routine medical and psychological examination of healthy subjects. IRBs should therefore determine whether the proposed subject population would be more sensitive or vulnerable to the risks posed by the research as a result of their general condition or disabilities. If so, the procedures would constitute more than minimal risk for those subjects.[41]

The Department of Health and Human Services (DHHS), the follow-up agency to the Department of Health, Education and Welfare (DHEW), revised its regulations in 1981, 1983, 1986, 1991, and 1996. The final revision as interpreted by the OPRR[42] addresses the issue of the cognitively impaired and their participation in research. OPRR in its latest modification does consider the mentally disabled as vulnerable subjects.[43] The OPRR's guidebook on IRBs states that "IRB's . . . regularly review research involving vulnerable subjects (such as the mentally disabled)."[44]

ABUSES OF THE MENTALLY DISABLED

Modern-day medical research is big business for drug and medical equipment companies, with billions of dollars at stake. Therefore, research is often intertwined with personal concerns for financial gains, glory, fame, ego, and extreme competition.[45] Securing research grants is essential for scientists to survive professionally and personally. This pressure translates into an urgent need to sign large numbers of human subjects into research protocols and to produce quick results to satisfy research sponsors.[46] Persons with mental illness are vulnerable to researchers pressured to enroll research subjects.

As we mentioned earlier, there are many reports of abuses of the mentally disabled in research settings. However, until recently, there have been no systematic studies of the past experimental protocols that used mentally disabled subjects including the most controversial research protocol, washout/relapse. Washout/relapse protocols involve the complete, sudden withdrawal of medication from patients (washout) before the subject is enrolled in new experimental research in order to test a new drug. The subject most likely will suffer a relapse, a return of symptoms such as psychosis and delusions either during the washout period or during the testing of the new drug, due to the ineffectiveness of the drug or a placebo. The absence of a critical examination of such studies was recognized by Wyatt, a noted psychiatric researcher, who said, "Surprisingly, there has been little investigation into these areas despite the large number of withdrawal studies."[47] None of the regulatory agencies (the Food and Drug Administration [FDA] or OPRR) have conducted such a study.

Because of the dearth of information, we undertook to survey the past 30 years of literature on washout/relapse studies of patients with schizophrenia.[48] A group of psychiatric researchers[49] published a similar survey but with greatly different questions and parameters. A commentary on the Gilbert study noted that, "This review comes at a time of increased public and professional concern about the ethics of research concerning neuroleptic withdrawal in schizophrenia, stimulated in part by national attention to complaints from the families of patients who participated in a neuroleptic withdrawal study at the University of California—Los Angeles."[50] In that study, a patient named Craig Aller suffered permanent damage after his medication for schizophrenia was suddenly withdrawn. Another patient, it is claimed, committed suicide due to the withdrawal of medication.[51]

The key finding of both studies is that the sudden washout/withdrawal experiments resulted in a relapse rate of 39 percent[52] to 53 percent of patients.[53] This high rate of recurring symptoms is compared to a relapse rate of 16 percent when patients remain on medication.[54]

In our survey of U.S. studies[55] we found that 32 percent of patients signed informed consent. The reports make no mention of informed consent in 56 percent of the patients studied. In 39 out of 41 studies, the reports make no mention of the patient's competence to give informed consent, despite the fact that subjects were diagnosed with schizophrenia, a diagnosis that severely affects cognition, and despite the fact that federal regulations require that those signing informed-consent forms comprehend what they have signed.

We found that 10.5 percent of patients dropped out of the studies and that there was no follow-up on those patients. More disturbing is the fact that in 36 of 41 studies, the reports did not specify the number of dropouts.[56]

In addition to the ethical concerns about the conduct of washout/withdrawal experiments, there is the question of physical harm to patients when full-blown symptoms of an illness go untreated for a considerable period of time while the research is going on (up to one year and sometimes longer). It is potentially harmful to the brain to allow symptoms of a brain disorder to go unchecked, just as it would be for diseases such as diabetes and cardiovascular diseases to go untreated. Concerns about the safety of such research were raised as early as 1986, by Crow et al., and by Wyatt in 1991 and Loebel in 1992.[57] The risks of washout/withdrawal cited were (1) seven times more criminal activities, (2) increased bizarre behaviors that stigmatize the patient further, (3) increased morbidity, (4) psychosis that by itself may be toxic, and (5) delayed intervention resulting in poor long-term outcome.[58]

The sudden washout/withdrawal of medication is known to be harmful in numerous drug treatment studies including those studies with patients with schizophrenia. Gilbert et al.[59] and Jeste et al.[60] have cited that rapid reduction of medication resulted in a 50 percent relapse rate, whereas slow reduction (tapering off) over six months resulted in an 8 percent relapse rate. Baldessarini and Viguera, leading psychiatric researchers, state: "The sudden removal of much or all of a maintenance psychopharmacologic treatment carries an excess risk for severe symptomatic exacerbation or relapse within several months."[61] Baldessarini and Viguera estimate the ratio of relapse risk in schizophrenia after continued versus discontinued neuroleptic treatment is 2 to 13, a very significant increase in risk.

Our survey indicates that the UCLA incident, covered extensively by the media, is not an isolated case.[62] The survey reveals that, in part, the design and conduct of the washout/withdrawal research plans were inadequate, raising ethical[63] and legal concerns about compliance with various federal regulations.[64]

We found that in two cases, one in Texas and one in New York, psychiatric researchers for years used incompetent institutionalized mentally disabled patients as subjects in research.[65] In both cases, the researchers' consent forms were signed by patients who had been declared incompetent or by their inappropriately chosen surrogates. Court challenges in both cases have halted the research until there is further resolution of the problem, either by the courts or by new regulations.[66] In the New York case, the New York State Supreme Court, Appelate Division, in a landmark unanimous ruling declared that nonconsensual, nontherapeutic experimental studies on mentally disabled adult patients and children that offer them no direct benefit "violate the state and federal constitutional rights to due process, as well as the common law right to personal autonomy of the patients. . . ."[67] These two cases clearly demonstrate how seriously mentally disabled patients are used as guinea pigs, fitting Katz's description: "Consent is tantamount to conscripting citizen-patients for participation in research."[68]

The cavalier attitude of some researchers toward the rights of the mentally disabled is most dangerous. Some justify these experiments by saying they are for the good of science, for the public interest, or to advance knowledge, albeit at the expense of the civil liberties of the disabled.

Thomasma argued well against this position when he stated,

> "Recent revelations about our own government and scientific community conducting radiation research without consent on the retarded and pregnant women in the 1950s and 1960s demonstrates that the Nazis did not have a lock on the cavalier treatment of vulnerable populations. Boundaries must be established on the power of the state and on the power of science over individuals in our society."[69]

INFORMED CONSENT AND THE MENTALLY DISABLED

The three cornerstones of informed consent are derived from the Nuremberg Code, the AMA code, and the Helsinki Declaration. Federal regulations require that the patient have sufficient knowledge, that there is no duress or coercion, and that the patient comprehend the issue.[70] Protections of the mentally disabled in research have entered the international arena, as well. The International Covenant on Civil and Political Rights (ICCPR), ratified by United States in 1992, provides further protection of informed consent as part of international human rights.[71] It is noteworthy to remember that

> "informed consent is only a minimal way to protect individuals and honor their personhood. Essentially it defines the borders beyond which we cannot go without the participation of the individual. Without consent we cannot reduce a person to an object for any purpose. This is not the same as honoring and promoting individual worth, no matter what the circumstance of their neurological condition."[72]

Levine supports having a "federal policy for the ethical conduct of research on persons who by reason of mental or behavioral disorders are vulnerable in that they are not capable of giving adequately informed consent."[73]

The three pillars of informed consent are crucial when obtaining informed consent from persons with neurobiological impairment such as mental illness and Alzheimer's disease. The neurobiologically impaired are susceptible to persuasion and may strive to please the caretaker by signing an informed consent that is legally and ethically invalid. There is evidence that when a physician/investigator's role is combined, the patient is not really "volunteering" to be a subject of research.[74] The investigator has a high legal and ethical standard to meet when obtaining informed consent from seriously mentally ill patients.[75] The more serious and chronic the patients' mental illness, the more difficult it becomes to obtain a valid informed consent.

This is especially true when the patient has schizophrenia, the severest form of mental illness that affects cognition and volition. Large numbers of schizophrenic patients have impaired cognition and volition.[76] The early DSM-III clearly states that schizophrenia disturbs "content of thought," "perception," and "volition."[77] Psychiatric textbooks in the past 30 years emphasize these symptoms. In patients with schizophrenia, impaired comprehension is one of the major symptoms. Thus, for many schizophrenic patients, it would be impossible to give valid informed consent. Recent data[78] confirms that at a minimum 50 percent of schizophrenic patients lack "adequate" range of decision making.

A researcher seeking informed consent should disclose honestly the nature of research and how it differs from therapy. This is especially important for those cognitively impaired patients enrolled in risk-laden research. Katz[79] suggests seven points that all relate to informing the subject that he/she is agreeing to be a research subject and, as such, that his or her best interests may not be served.

GUIDELINES FOR FUTURE RESEARCH USING THE MENTALLY DISABLED

There has been a recent flurry of suggested guidelines for allowing mentally disabled subjects into research studies.[80] Important documents are the position paper of the American College of Physicians[81], the Code of Federal Regulations[82], and National Alliance for the Mentally Ill (NAMI) Standards for Protection of Individuals with Severe Mental Illnesses Who Participate as Human Subjects in Research.[83] Keyserlinck et al.[84] have proposed guidelines primarily for subjects with Alzheimer's disease. His article emphasizes the progressive nature of the illness and that an advance medical directive (i.e., health care power of attorney), if properly executed when the patient is still competent, can serve as the basis for a surrogate to enroll the patient in research.[85]

Therapeutic vs. Nontherapeutic Research

It is important to note that the term *therapeutic research* means that the research carries a potential direct therapeutic benefit to the patient. OPRR recognizes the fact that research differs from treatment: "Research itself is not therapeutic; for ill patients, research interventions may or may not be identical."[86] Nontherapeutic research by design has no potential for direct benefit. This is a crucial distinction. As Katz recognizes,

> in therapy physicians are expected to attend solely to the welfare of the individual patient before them, while in research patient-subjects also serve as means for the ends of science and therefore their individual needs have to yield to the dictates of the research question and protocol.[87]

Berg's article recognizes the historical abuses of human subjects in research, and it calls for the "greatest protection" for "research that involves high risk and little or no potential direct therapeutic benefit."[88]

Legal Competence

The term *competence* has been taken to mean legal competence. An adult is presumed to be competent until a court finds him or her incompetent. Informed-consent laws refer to comprehension, not competence, in testing the validity of informed consent. Comprehension means the ability to understand the ramifications of the research, the risks and benefits of participating, and any available alternative treatment. A person who cannot understand these things may be incompetent to sign an informed-consent form although no court has ruled him or her incompetent.

Comprehension

The *Belmont Report*[89] addressed the issue of comprehension as an important item. The *Belmont Report* stresses not only that the information be sufficient, but also that it be presented in an understandable manner. The *Belmont Report* then specifically addresses the issue of comprehension and mental disability.

Comprehending Subjects. Most individuals fall into this category. These patients can be asked to sign informed consents, provided that the informed-consent process has followed all of the required standards.

Questionably Comprehending Subjects. The patients in this category are perhaps the most difficult to assess. The investigator should be cognizant of red flags that require him or her to assess comprehension, such as:

1. The patient is diagnosed with serious mental illness such as schizophrenia, major depression, manic-depression, anxiety disorder, or personality disorder.
2. The patient is currently institutionalized or has been in the recent past (within five years), whether in a mental-health facility or in jail.
3. The patient or any member of his family reports to the physician that the subject has or has had a psychiatric disorder.
4. The staff on the research team perceive that the subject may not be comprehending the content or the process of informed consent.

The position paper of the American College of Physicians emphasizes that "Cognitive impairment renders persons incompetent to make their own decisions to participate in research if it eliminates the person's ability to understand, make choices about, or communicate a decision regarding particular research."[90]

We proposed not only that the mental status of the subject should be evaluated but also that the evaluator should be an independent psychiatrist not involved in any way with the research project.[91] NAMI later adopted this position as part of NAMI ethics standards that strongly emphasize comprehension:

> Research participants should be carefully evaluated before and throughout the research for their capacity to comprehend information and their capacity to consent to continued participation in the research. The determination of competence shall be made by someone other than the principal investigator or others involved in the research. Except for research protocols approved by the Institutional Review Board (IRB) as minimal risk, whenever it is determined that the subject is not able to continue to provide consent, consent to continue participation in the research shall be sought from families or others legally entrusted to act in the participant's best interest.[92]

Uncomprehending Subjects. If the subject cannot comprehend the impact of participating in research, then it may be possible to obtain consent from a surrogate.

If the patient has signed an advance directive for health care and has appointed an agent, then the health care agent may be able to authorize the person's participation in research. This will depend on state laws governing surrogate consent to medical treatment. However, one could argue that the health care agent should not authorize a subject's participation in greater than minimal-risk research unless the research has a direct therapeutic medical benefit to the patient. Contrarily, one could also advance the argument that in unique medical circumstances and with the approval of the IRB or hospital ethics committee or its equivalent, the health care agent may authorize nontherapeutic research that falls below high risk (i.e., a small increment above minimal risk).

When the court appoints a guardian for an incompetent subject, the guardian, subject to court approval, may be able to authorize the enrollment of the patient into minimal-risk research. Again, this would be subject to local statutes. However, one may argue that the guardian should not be authorized to enroll the subject in *any* nontherapeutic research. This position would be consistent with the best-interest philosophy conveyed by the American College of Physicians' position paper[93] and the Helsinki Declaration.[94]

Many states have statutes that authorize family members or close friends to make health care decisions for incompetent patients. Whether consent to participate in research studies is included in the term *health care* would have to be determined on a state-by-state basis. The federal guidelines refer to informed consent given by a "legally authorized representative."[95] This may mean only a court-appointed guardian, or may include surrogates, depending on the law in each state.

Morally Justified Experiments. Tom L. Beauchamp,[96] in his article analyzing the final report of the Advisory Committee on Human Radiation Experiments (ACHRE), uses the committee's enunciated six Universal Moral Principles to judge past practices of those who conducted research. The six principles are (1) One ought not to treat people as mere means to the ends of others, (2) One ought not to deceive others, (3) One ought not to inflict harm or risk of harm, (4) One ought to promote welfare and prevent harm, (5) One ought to treat people fairly and with equal respect, and (6) One ought to respect the self-determination of others. Beauchamp concludes, "A hundred years or a thousand years ago would not alter their [the six principles] moral force,"[97] a statement consistent with the committee's report. Beauchamp cites Elizabeth Zitrin, a lawyer and ACHRE committee member: "If the experiments [here they were referring to human radiation experiments, but for our purpose they could be any experimental research study with humans] were consistent with accepted medical practices at the time, it does not make them ethical. And they were not consistent with the highest standards of the time articulated by the government, the profession or the public."[98]

The survey we have conducted on the use of the mentally ill in research for over 30 years clearly shows a greater abuse of these patients than in the radiation studies. The human radiation experiments stopped over 30 years ago, but tens of thousands of mentally disabled people are still subjected to experiments with adverse consequences. The use of the mentally ill in high-risk nontherapeutic research violates all of the six ethical standards enunciated by ACHRE. This is especially true regarding the first principle, "One ought not to treat people as mere means to the ends of others." The most recent Statement of Principles of Ethical Conduct by the American College of Neuropsychopharmacology (ACNP), the largest and most powerful organization of psychiatric researchers, in response to the recent revelations says: "All persons living in society have a moral responsibility to participate in efforts to promote and contribute to the present and future welfare of that society. Research is one of these obligations."[99] It is an unfortunate and dangerous idea to demand by "moral obligation" that the mentally ill "volunteer" for research. Even if these experiments are the accepted norms of psychiatric research, "it does not make them ethical," as Zitrin stated.[100] Beauchamp's rebuke to the human radiation experiments applies equally to the ACNP's expectation that the mentally disabled participate as research subjects: "Never in the history of civil medicine has it been permissible to exploit patients by using them to the end of science in non-therapeutic research that carries risk of harm."[101]

CONCLUSIONS

Persons with mental illness have been and continue to be used in high-risk, nontherapeutic research. Persons with mental illness and especially those diagnosed with the severest form of mental illness such as schizophrenia may lack the capacity to comprehend the risks associated with their participation in research. Patients who have comprehension and who have a valid surrogate or a health care agent to give informed consent should be able to participate in research protocols only if they impose minimal risk to the patient. If the research protocol represents a greater-than-minimal risk to the patient, the surrogate or health care agent may allow the participation of the patient only if there is direct medical benefit to the patient. Only in unique and highly unusual and compelling circumstances should patients lacking comprehension be allowed to participate in riskier experiments without direct medical benefits to them.

NOTES

1. *Neurobiologically impaired* or *neurologically disordered* (NBDs) or *brain disordered* are less stigmatizing terms. We will use the term *mentally disabled.* However, all documents and literature refer to the mentally ill. We will use the terms *mental illness* and *mentally ill* whenever they are necessary to accurately reflect the literature.
2. H. A. Foley and S. S. Sharfstein, *Madness and Government: Who Cares for the Mentally Ill?* (Washington, D.C.: American Psychiatric Press, 1983).
3. A. E. Shamoo, "Human Rights in Reference to Persons with Mental Illness," *Accountability in Research* 4 (1996): 207–16; id., "Ethical Considerations in Medication-Free Research on the Mentally Ill," in *First National Conference on Ethics: Ethics in Neurobiological Research with Human Subjects,* ed. A. E. Shamoo (New York: Gordon and Breach Science Publishers, 1996), 197–202; id., "The Inhumane Use of Persons with Mental Illness in Biomedical Experimental Research" (Testimony to the Committee on Governmental Affairs, United States Senate, March 1996).
4. A. L. Caplin, "How Did Medicine Go So Wrong?" in *When Medicine Went Mad,* ed. A. L. Caplan (Totowa, N.J.: Humana Press, 1992), 56.
5. Caplan, "How Did Medicine Go So Wrong?" 53–94; ed. B. Muller-Hill, *Murderous Science* (Oxford: Oxford University Press, 1988).
6. R. Proctor, *Racial Hygiene-Medicine under the Nazis* (Cambridge: Harvard University Press, 1988), 97.
7. Ibid.
8. Caplan, "How Did Medicine Go So Wrong?" 64; J. Katz and R. S. Pozos, "The Dachau Hypothermia Study," in *When Medicine Went Mad,* ed. A. L. Caplan (Totowa, N.J.: Humana Press, 1992), 135.
9. Proctor, *Racial Hygiene-Medicine*; Muller-Hill, *Murderous Science*; Caplan, "How Did Medicine Go So Wrong?"
10. Proctor, *Racial Hygiene-Medicine,* 95, quoting A. Hitler, *Mein Kampf.*
11. Proctor, *Racial Hygiene-Medicine,* 96.
12. A. E. Shamoo, "Brain Disorders: Scientific Facts, Media, and Public Perception," *Accountability in Research* 5 (1996): 161–73.
13. Proctor, *Racial Hygiene-Medicine,* 195.
14. Advisory Committee on Human Radiation Experiments (ACHRE), *Final Report* (Washington, D.C.: U.S. Government Printing Office, 1995), 135, quoting the AMA, 1946; AMA Board of Trustees, minutes of the 19 September 1946 meeting, AMA Archive, Chicago, Ill. (ACHRE No. IND-072595-A).
15. The Nuremberg Code, 1947, quoted in ACHRE, *Final Report,* 103.
16. Ibid.
17. World Medical Association, *Declaration of Helsinki: Recommendations Guiding Physicians in Biomedical Research Involving Human Subjects* (Helsinki, Finland: World Medical Association, 1964), quoted in R. E. Bulger and H. E. Riser, eds., *The Ethical Dimensions of the Biological Sciences* (Cambridge, Mass.: Cambridge University Press, 1993).
18. World Medical Association, *Declaration of Helsinki,* quoted in R. R. Faden and T. L. Beauchamp, *A History and Theory of Informed Consent* (New York: Oxford University Press, 1986), 161.
19. H. K. Beecher, "Ethics and Clinical Research," *New England Journal of Medicine* 274 (1966): 1354–60.
20. J. Katz, *Experimentation with Human Beings* (New York: Russell Sage Foundation, 1972).
21. ACHRE, *Final Report,* 178; J. H. Jones, *Bad Blood* (New York: Free Press, 1993), 114.
22. ACHRE, *Final Report,* 676.
23. 45 Code of Federal Regulations (CFR), part 46 (1996).
24. 45 CFR, part 46 (1996), 102(d).
25. National Commission for the Protection of Human Subjects of Biomedical and Behavioral Research, *The Belmont Report* (Washington, D.C.: U.S. Department of Health, Education, and Welfare, 1978).
26. President's Commission for the Study of Ethical Problems in Medicine and Biomedical and Behavioral Research, Summing Up (Washington, D.C.: U.S. Government Printing Office, 1983).
27. A. E. Shamoo and D. N. Irving, "Accountability in Research Using Persons with Mental Illness," *Accountability in Research* 3 (1993); 1–17.
28. Office for Protection from Research Risk (OPRR), *Protecting Human Research Subjects: Institutional*

Review Board Guidebook (Washington, D.C.: U.S. Government Printing Office, 1993).

29. OPRR, *Protecting Human Research Subjects,* 6.27.
30. Ibid.
31. ACHRE, *Final Report,* 677.
32. OPRR, *Protecting Human Research Subjects,* 6.26.
33. Ibid., 6. 27. 45 CFR, part 46, 107.
34. Shamoo and Irving, "Accountability in Research."
35. J. T. Puglisi and G. B. Ellis, "Neurobiological Research Involving Human Subjects: Perspectives from the Office for Protection from Research Risks," 4 (1996): 264.
36. Shamoo and Irving, "Accountability in Research."
37. 45 CFR, part 46, 103.
38. Ibid., 107(a).
39. S. Hoppe, "Institutional Review Boards and Research on Individuals with Mental Disorders," *Accountability in Research* 3 (1996): 187–95.
40. 45 CFR, part 46.
41. OPRR, *Protecting Human Research Subjects,* 3.6.
42. 45 CFR, part 46; OPRR, *Protecting Human Research Subjects.*
43. Shamoo and Irving, "Accountability in Research"; OPRR, *Protecting Human Research Subjects.*
44. OPRR, *Protecting Human Research Subjects,* 6.27.
45. A. E. Shamoo and Z. Annau, "Ensuring Scientific Integrity," *Nature* 327 (1987): 550; A. E. Shamoo, "Organizational Structure and Function of Research and Development," in *Principles of Research Data Audit,* ed. A. E. Shamoo (New York: Gordon and Breach Science Publishers, 1989), 39–63; id., "Role of Conflict of Interest in Scientific Objectivity: A Case of a Nobel Prize Work," *Accountability in Research* 2 (1992): 55–75; id., "Role of Conflict of Interest in Public Advisory Councils," in *Ethical Issues in Research,* ed. D. Cheney (Frederick, Md.: University Publishing Group, 1993), 159–74; V. H. Sharav, "Independent Family Advocates Challenge the Fraternity of Silence," in *First National Conference on Ethics: Ethics in Neurobiological Research with Human Subjects,* ed. A. E. Shamoo (New York: Gordon and Breach Science Publishers, 1996), 177–83; J. Katz, "Ethics in Neurobiological Research with Human Subjects: Final Reflections," *Accountability in Research* 4 (1996): 277–83.
46. Shamoo, "Role of Conflict of Interest"; D. N. Irving and A. E. Shamoo, "Which Ethics for Science and Public Policy," *Accountability in Research* 3 (1993): 77–100.
47. R. J. Wyatt, "Risks of Withdrawing Antipsychotic Medication," *Arch. Gen. Psychiatry* 52 (1995): 206.
48. A. E. Shamoo and T. J. Keay, "Ethical Concerns about Relapse Studies," *Cambridge Quarterly on Health Care Ethics* 5 (1996): 373–86.
49. P. L. Gilbert et al., "Neuroleptic Withdrawal in Schizophrenic Patients: A Review of the Literature," *Arch. Gen. Psychiatry* 52 (1995): 173–88.
50. H. Y. Meltzer, "Neuroleptic Withdrawal in Schizophrenic Patients: An Idea Whose Time Has Come," *Arch. Gen. Psychiatry* 52 (1995): 200.
51. R. Aller and G. Aller, *First National Conference on Ethics: Ethics in Neurobiological Research with Human Subjects* (Langhorne, PA: Gordon and Breach Scientific Publishers, 1997).
52. Shamoo and Keay, "Ethical Concerns about Relapse Studies."
53. Gilbert et al., "Neuroleptic Withdrawal in Schizophrenic Patients: A Review."
54. Ibid.
55. Shamoo and Keay, "Ethical Concerns about Relapse Studies."
56. Ibid.
57. Wyatt, "Risks of Withdrawing Antipsychotic Medication," 206; T. J. Crow, J. F. MacMillan, A. L. Johnson, and B. C. Johnstone, "A Randomized Controlled Trial of Prophylactic Neuroleptic Treatment," *British Journal of Psychiatry* 148 (1986): 120–27; R. J. Wyatt, "Neuroleptics and the Natural Course of Schizophrenia," *Schizophrenia Bulletin* 17 (1991): 325–51; A. D. Loebel, J. A. Lieberman, J. M. Alvir, D. I. Mayerhoff, S. H. Geister, and S. R. Symanski, "Duration of Psychosis and Outcome in First-Episode Schizophrenia," *American Journal of Psychiatry* 149 (1992): 1183–88.
58. Wyatt, "Risks of Withdrawing Antipsychotic Medication."
59. Gilbert et al., "Neuroleptic Withdrawal in Schizophrenic Patients: A Review."
60. D. V. Jeste, "Considering Neuroleptic Maintenance and Taper on a Continuum: Need for Individual Rather Than Dogmatic Approach," *Arch. Gen. Psychiatry* 52 (1995): 209–12.
61. R. J. Baldessarini and A. C. Viguera, "Neuroleptic Withdrawal in Schizophrenic Patients," *Arch. Gen. Psychiatry* 52 (1995): 189–91.
62. Aller and Aller, *First National Conference on Ethics*; Shamoo and Keay, "Ethical Concerns about Relapse Studies."
63. A. E. Shamoo, "Policies and Quality Assurance in the Pharmaceutical Industry," *Accountability in Research* 1 (1991): 273–84.
64. A. E. Shamoo, "Executive Summary," in *First National Conference on Ethics: Ethics in Neurobiological Research with Human Subjects,* ed. A. E. Shamoo (New York: Gordon and Breach Science Publishers, 1996), 5–27.
65. P. Hilts, "Judge Tells Health Department to Stop Experiments on Patients," *The New York Times,* 26

March 1995; L. Beil, "Psychiatric Research Raises Legal Red Flags," *The Dallas Morning News,* 29 April 1996, sec. H.

66. Ibid.
67. *T. D. et al. v New York State Office of Mental Health et al.,* (N.Y./App. Div. Lexis 12293 1996).
68. Katz, "Ethics in Neurobiological Research with Human Subjects," 282.
69. D. C. Thomasma, "A Communal Model for Presumed Consent for Research on the Neurologically Vulnerable," *Accountability in Research* 4 (1996): 227–39.
70. OPRR, *Protecting Human Research Subjects.*
71. E. Rosenthal and L. Rubenstein, "International Human Rights Advocacy under the 'Principles for the Protection of Persons with Mental Illness,'" *International Journal of Law and Psychiatry* 16 (1993): 257–300; Shamoo, "Human Rights in Reference to Persons with Mental Illness"; E. Rosenthal, "The International Covenant on Civil and Political Rights and the Rights of Research Subjects," *Accountability in Research* 4 (1996): 253–60.
72. Thomasma, "A Communal Model for Presumed Consent for Research on the Neurologically Vulnerable," 237.
73. R. J. Levine, "Proposed Regulations for Research Involving Those Institutionalized as Mentally Infirm: A Consideration of Their Relevance in 1995," *Accountability in Research* 4 (1996): 177–86.
74. A. Meisel and L. H. Roth, "Toward an Informed Discussion of Informed Consent: A Review and Critique of the Empirical Studies," *Arizona Law Review* 25 (1983): 265–346; L. H. Roth et al., "Informed Consent in Psychiatric Research," *Rutgers Law Review* 39 (1987): 425–41; Katz, "Ethics in Neurobiologial Research with Human Subjects."
75. Shamoo and Irving, "Accountability in Research."
76. American Psychiatric Association, *American Psychiatric Association: Diagnostic and Statistical Manual of Mental Disorders,* DSM III (Washington, D.C.: American Psychiatric Association, 1980).
77. Ibid.
78. T. Grisso and P. S. Appelbaum, "The MacArthur Treatment Competence Study, III: Abilities of Patients to Consent to Psychiatric and Medical Treatments," *Law and Human Behavior* 19 (1995): 149–74; P. S. Appelbaum, "Patients' Competence to Consent to Neurobiological Research," *Accountability in Research* 4 (1996): 241–51.
79. Katz, "Ethics in Neurobiological Research with Human Subjects," 280.
80. E. W. Keyserlink et al., "Proposed Guidelines for the Participation of Persons with Dementia as Research Subjects," *Perspectives in Biology and Medicine* 38 (1995): 319–62; J. W. Berg, "Legal and Ethical Complexities of Consent with Cognitively Impaired Research Subjects: Proposed Guidelines," *Journal of Law, Medicine, and Ethics* 24 (1996): 18–35; R. Dresser, "Mentally Disabled Research Subjects: The Enduring Policy Issue," *JAMA* 276 (1996): 67–72.
81. American College of Physicians, "Cognitively Impaired Subjects," *Annals of Internal Medicine* 3 (1989): 842–48.
82. 45 CFR, part 46.
83. A. E. Shamoo et al. "NAMI's Standards for Protection of Individuals with Severe Mental Illness Who Participate as Human Subjects in Research," in *The First National Conference on Ethics: Ethics in Neurobiological Research with Human Subjects,* ed. A. E. Shamoo (New York: Gordon and Breach Science Publishers, 1996), 327–29.
84. Keyserlinck et al., "Proposed Guidelines for the Participation of Persons with Dementia as Research Subjects."
85. T. Sunderland and R. Dukoff, "Informed Consent with Cognitively Impaired Patients: An NIMH Perspective on the Durable Power of Attorney," *Accountability in Research* 4 (1996): 217–26.
86. OPRR, *Protecting Human Research Subjects,* 1–2.
87. Katz, "Ethics in Neurobiological Research with Human Subjects," 278.
88. Berg, "Legal and Ethical Complexities of Consent with Cognitively Impaired Research Subjects," 29.
89. National Commission, *The Belmont Report.*
90. American College of Physicians, "Cognitively Impaired Subjects," 843.
91. A. E. Shamoo, "Our Responsibilities toward Persons with Mental Illness as Human Subjects in Research," *The Journal* 5 (1994); 14–16.
92. A. E. Shamoo et al., "NAMI's Standards," 327–29.
93. American College of Physicians, "Cognitively Impaired Subjects."
94. World Medical Association, *Declaration of Helsinki.*
95. 45 CFR, part 46, 117(2).
96. T. L. Beauchamp, "Looking Back and Judging our Predecessors," *Kennedy Institute of Ethics Journal* 6 (1996): 251–70.
97. Ibid., 253.
98. Ibid., 256.
99. American College of Neuropsychopharmacology (ACNP), "A Statement of Principles of Ethical Conduct for Neuropharmacologic Research in Human Subjects" (1996): 1–14.
100. Beauchamp, "Looking Back," 256.
101. Ibid., 264.

Chapter 22

AIDS Activists and Their Legacy for Research Policy

Loretta M. Kopelman

Advances in medical research have brought new and successful treatments for human immunodeficiency virus (HIV) and acquired immunodeficiency syndrome (AIDS). These treatments became available to patients in 1996, giving new hope to those with these conditions. Those who are HIV-positive now often find that their "viral loads" drop sharply and those with AIDS that their apparent death sentence is transformed to life with a chronic illness.[1] Hope, however, should be tempered with the knowledge that this pandemic remains out of control in many parts of the world, and not everyone can tolerate or afford these therapies. Many of the 22.6 million persons with HIV or AIDS do not have the $15,000 or more price tag for these "drug cocktails."[2]

Even if treatments offered cures for all and were widely available at low cost, the AIDS epidemic would have left its legacy upon research policy and politics. AIDS activists and patients helped change how research is conducted, altering the balance of power between investigators and subjects. Activists and investigators have clashed over who should control the testing and use of promising new treatments for those with HIV infection and AIDS. AIDS activists believe that people's interests are sometimes needlessly sacrificed to rigid and overdemanding research procedures. For example, they decried the slow pace of testing by the Food and Drug Administration (FDA) and its tight control over who can receive untested or experimental therapies. Typically, only those enrolled in clinical trials (CTs) of investigational new drugs can receive them; women, children, and those with serious complications are often excluded from these studies. Activists find such rules misguided since they prevent many people from receiving treatment for a rapidly progressing fatal illness. They want access to promising new drugs (whether or not they are being tested) as well as to preliminary information about the efficacy and safety of those drugs currently being tested. Activists contend that patients should have more choice about whether they are willing to undergo risky, experimental, or even untested therapies.

For example, in 1994, the Centers for Disease Control and Prevention (CDC) found that if women with HIV infection were given zidovudine (ZDV) during pregnancy, there was a 67.5 percent reduction in the risk for HIV transmission to their progeny.[3] Consequently, all pregnant women were urged to get testing for HIV infection, and to be treated to help prevent vertical transmission of HIV infection to their fetus. Up until that publication, however, many clinicians did not inform, let alone offer, pregnant women the only available treatment for AIDS or HIV because it had not been tested on pregnant women. Clinicians feared harm would come to the fetus and subsequent liability if they prescribed treatments that had not been tested and approved for pregnant women. Yet withholding this information constituted a violation of informed-consent policy, which requires that people be told of alternative treatments available.[4] The mother is decision maker for herself and her fetus, and clinicians manipulated her decision by withholding pertinent information. Rather than adopt the paternalistic position of deciding what is best for her to know, clinicians and investigators could have given her the best available information and admitted that they are uncertain about the effects of this treatment on the fetus, thereby letting the woman decide. One could adopt the policy that if an otherwise successful intervention has not been tested on a certain population, competent patients will be able to decide if they should take it. This example illustrates why many patients and activists want less paternalism from clinicians and investigators and more information and choices. People resent automatic exclusion from studies because they are pregnant, or of a certain age, gender, or ethnic or racial group. Participation not only benefits individuals but the group to which they belong.

Many clinicians and investigators fear that giving up more control could harm patients and undermine proven research methods. Modifications in the testing and availability of new treatments might help a few, investigators argue, but will hurt many in the long run if untested or poorly tested therapies become widely available. They argue that the government has a duty to protect the public from dangerous and ineffective "therapies." They also point to the remarkable gains that have been made in many diseases in a relatively short time because new treatments were systematically evaluated. The best way to improve treatments and protect the public, some argue, is to give investigators the freedom to set the goals, priorities, and methods for testing promising new treatments.[5]

In contrast, activists continue to reject such protectionism, seeking a more active role in setting priorities and in saying how studies are conducted. They have drawn attention to the evaluative and ethical nature of many issues regarding the testing and use of promising new treatments. These evaluative and ethical judgments concern decisions about the initiation of trials, the use of placebos, randomization, the selection of subjects, the ending of trials, and how best to protect the general public with respect to promising new treatments. These are not matters that can be settled entirely by science, and activists want a say in resolving them.

In what follows, I argue that the conflicts between investigators and activists should be resolved by acknowledging that research needs to be a cooperative venture in which investigators accommodate patients' views of what is in their interests, and patients accommodate proven research methods. Cooperation can take many forms including mutual respect for each other's point of view, values, and goals. For example, the investigators' primary interests may be pursuing studies to measurable "hard" endpoints such as death, opportunistic infections, or survival over five years. Patients are generally most interested in their overall quality-of-life and the likelihood of increased pain, costs, and dementia. When people believe that their views of rights, harms, and benefits shape the review process of protocols and evaluation of new treatments, they are more trusting and feel a greater sense of control over their lives. Research cannot be a cooperative venture, however, if potential patient-subjects cannot understand enough to be partners. There is a line between what constitutes too much and too little protection of the public, and the dispute between AIDS activists and many investigators concerns where to draw that line and who should draw it. After discussing how research methods are beginning to change, I will examine critics' charges that, in general, patients do not know enough about medical research to be regarded as genuine partners in a cooperative venture.

TRADITIONAL METHODS UNDER ATTACK

In the last 50 years, investigators developed techniques to protect the public from untested and dangerous drugs. These methods now usually involve several different stages of testing and so-called hard endpoints to evaluate the effectiveness of treatments. In AIDS research, these hard endpoints are usually death or opportunistic infections.

The FDA has a fourfold classification of drug studies, and traditionally one phase is completed before the next begins. *Phase I* studies focus on the safety of the investigational new drugs and are usually conducted with small numbers of people. The subjects, often normal volunteers or selected patients, are typically not randomized. *Phase II* testing usually continues with a small number of patients, carefully monitored to determine the efficacy as well as the safety of the new treatment. *Phase III* clinical trials are often expanded so that efficacy and safety can be studied in many patients. Investigators prefer Phase III studies to be double-blind (neither doctors nor their patients know which treatment they receive) and randomized (the assignment to treatment arms is made by a chance mechanism). If there is a drug currently being used, investigators will test it against the new treatment. If there is not, they prefer to test the investigational new drug against a placebo (an inert preparation such as a sugar pill or saline injection). Hundreds, and sometimes thousands, of patients participate to allow well-grounded comparison between the experimental treatment and the standard treatment. If there is no standard treatment, investigators generally test the new treatment against a placebo.

Patients may have to meet strict eligibility requirements to be enrolled in Phase III trials. The more similar, or "homogeneous," the subjects, the more assurance that the results reflect differences among the treatments studied. Often women of childbearing years, older people, children, and those with severe complications are excluded. While such restrictions enhance the trial's internal validity by making subjects more homogeneous, they raise problems about generalization of the results to other groups. If the therapies are tested only on adult men, for example, one does not know how the therapies affect women or children. If pregnant women are routinely excluded, no information can be calculated about how treatments affect them or their fetuses. Results of studies are not usually made public until Phase III trials have been completed and published.

Phase IV studies are used to collect additional information after the new therapy has been released for marketing. Once a drug has been marketed, investigators continue to compile information by monitoring physicians' use of the new therapy. They often use it in ways other than those for which it has been tested and may also find rare reactions. In this way, investigators gather data about new uses or previously excluded populations such as children, women, and those individuals with complications. This, however, constitutes an "off-label" use of these drugs, since the drugs have not been tested for use on these groups. Some clinicians are reluctant to prescribe under such circumstances, especially for pregnant women.

This way of conducting clinical trials often takes many years to complete, keeping promising new drugs away from the public and in the control of investigators. Activists charged that the strict eligibility criteria slowed the pace of testing and were unfair to those excluded.[6] In addition, when testing takes so long, newer studies often show that the ongoing protocol no longer provides optimal care for all its patient-subjects. Hence, activists demanded more flexibility and some changes have resulted.

First, the medical establishment responded to criticisms that studies unfairly excluded certain groups such as women and people of color. The National Institutes of Health (NIH) in 1986 adopted a policy of inclusiveness. Investigators and reviewers were directed to go case by case and decide when it was reasonable to include more women or racial or ethnic minorities in studies. The Women's Congressional Caucus, alarmed by continuing criticism, commissioned the General Accounting Office (GAO) to study the inclusion of women and minorities in studies, especially with reference to clinical trials.[7] It took a year to complete the study, and in 1990, the GAO reported that it had found no real changes since 1986. The NIH policy of going case by case had apparently failed.

The members of Congress, especially the 29 members of the women's caucus, decided that legislative action was needed. They argued that the U.S. taxpayers were supporting the NIH, and half of them were women. Yet women's conditions, disorders, and maladies were not receiving proportional attention, and they were excluded from studies that provided benefits to the subjects and the groups they represented. Louise M. Slaughter (D-NY)[8] wrote, "Women [are] still excluded from the bulk of government-sponsored medical research. . . . It has been almost three decades since the Civil Rights Act of 1964 began tearing at the notion that women could not hold certain jobs because, surely, we were handicapped by our hormones and menstrual periods. But medical science did not follow suit. Menstrual cycles and irregular hormone levels were blamed for data too difficult to analyze, becoming a convenient excuse to ignore female subjects in many cases."

Consequently, in 1993, Congress passed The NIH Revitalization Act[9] requiring that studies supported by the NIH must include representative populations, particularly women and various racial and ethnic groups, and that cost cannot excuse noncompliance. Members of Congress thought participation in research was a benefit that, out of fairness, should be made available to all. It seemed unjust to exclude women, children, and others from studies representing their only or best chance for good treatment. Moreover, if studies are not conducted using these groups as subjects, then it is less clear how to generalize findings to them, especially given environmental, or gender, differences that exist between these and other groups.[10] Without testing on the populations for whom the interventions are intended, it is uncertain if the best means are being used to treat their HIV infection, depression, stroke, diabetes, vascular, or other diseases.

A second change concerned replacing hard endpoints in ending trials, such as death or opportunistic infection with so-called soft endpoints that are markers for these hard endpoints.[11] For example, soft endpoints were used in approving dideoxyinosine (DDI) for marketing. Investigators did not know how DDI affected the hard endpoints of death or opportunistic infections, but they did know it increased lymphocyte levels. The use of soft or surrogate endpoints to end trials satisfied those who wanted to speed up trials but brought criticism from those who questioned whether we understood enough about the relationship between the hard and soft endpoints.[12]

Third, the Public Health Service (PHS) expanded the availability of investigational new drugs by means of a parallel track.[13] Patients with HIV-related diseases can obtain experimental drugs even though they are not enrolled as subjects in the clinical trials of the drug. These regulations require that there are no therapeutic alternatives, the drugs are being tested, there is some evidence of their efficacy, there are no unreasonable risks for the patient, and the patient cannot participate in the clinical trials.

Byar et al. favor this and other ways of modifying the traditional manner of doing trials.[14] Many more doctors could include their patients in trials if investigators streamlined data sets by asking fewer but more pertinent questions. In addition, investigators can sometimes speed up testing by using factorial designs that compare two or more drugs simultaneously. The use of more flexible entry criteria and streamlining of data sets also encourages more collaboration with physicians around the country. This would have the consequence of enabling more patients to enroll, making results more generalizable. It would also make treatments available to more patients and minimize the use of parallel treatment tracks. Byar et al., however, spell out a proposal for parallel track or uncontrolled Phase III trials to meet the following requirements:

> (1) There must be no other treatment *appropriate* to use as a control; (2) there must be sufficient experience to ensure that the patients not receiving therapy will have a uniformly poor prognosis; (3) the therapy must not be expected to have substantial side effects that would compromise the potential *benefit* to the

> patient; (4) there must be *a justifiable expectation* that the potential *benefit* to the patient will be sufficiently large to make interpretation of the results of a non-randomized trial unambiguous; and (5) the scientific rationale of the treatment must be sufficiently strong that a positive result would be widely *accepted.*[15]

I added emphasis to certain words in this quotation because they are highly evaluative: "appropriate," "justifiable expectation," "benefit," and "accepted." Appropriate for what? Expected by whom? Acceptable or beneficial in what way? Answering these questions involves more than scientific judgments. Careful answers also require evaluative and moral judgments about risks and benefits in relation to some goal, and the patients' perspectives on these issues are often different from investigators' views. Investigators are interested in improving care for future patients. Patients may be more interested in how the treatment will affect them personally. For example, an investigator's primary interest may be assessing differences in group survival over five years, while a patient may be more interested in such quality-of-life aspects as potential cost, hospital stays, nausea, confusion, or dementia.

Thus, the concept of a clinical trial as a cooperative venture could be undermined by having investigators alone determine when flexibility is acceptable or appropriate, and when expectations are justifiable for some goal. For example, why should this proposal be limited to life-threatening diseases? How poor must the prognosis be to qualify? These are not questions that science alone can answer. AIDS activists want to help make key judgments about what sort of testing and priorities are *appropriate.*

Certain studies illustrate these new approaches. For example, in May 1992, a promising new antiviral agent, D4T (Stavudine), began Phase II and III testing. Unlike the past, Phase II testing was not completed before Phase III began, and physicians could obtain D4T for their HIV patients on a parallel track free from the manufacturer. The manufacturer distributed DDI (trade name didanosine) to over 23,000 patients on expanded-access programs. Still excluded, however, were children under 13 years of age and women who were pregnant or breastfeeding their infants.[16]

Some believe these changes reduce public safety by undercutting proven methods and scientific standards. The general public may not understand that drugs available on a parallel track are largely untested or why insurance companies refuse to pay for untested therapies. Moreover, critics fear members of the public may not participate in clinical trials once they realize the promising new drug is available outside the study. As we shall see, these critics typically believe that research cannot be a cooperative venture between investigators and subjects or activists.

CRITICS OF RESEARCH AS A COOPERATIVE VENTURE

Some contend that viewing research as a cooperative venture, where patient-subjects are seen as partners in the clinical trials, rests upon a "shaky foundation."[17] Such critics doubt whether so-called informed consent is really informed or whether patients can understand enough about risks or potential benefits of alternative treatments, randomization, interim data, probabilities, or the scientifically vigorous methodology used in testing to make them anything like partners.[18] Some assert that the problem is that patients, families, and their advocates tend to rely upon anecdotal information and "common sense" rather than aggregate data.[19]

Critics who doubt if research can be a cooperative venture generally fall into two distinct groups. Their disagreements are over whether to defend or reject the traditional clinical trial methodologies.

Defenders of Traditional Clinical Trial Methods

Some critics believe that we must defend investigators' freedom to design what they regard as the best studies, and to do this they want to restrict patients' "rights." These critics argue that patients have a right to optimal treatment but not to pick their treatment.[20] The current understanding of patients' rights is unreasonable, they hold, and disrupts clinical trials. If investigators give up more control, they claim, we would further slow medical progress and muddy the waters with generalizations based on poor methodology. These critics conclude that for the sake of public utility we should support the investigators' freedom to design the best clinical trials and modify patients' rights.

It seems unlikely, however, that AIDS activists will be satisfied with *fewer* rights and less control, even given these critics' assurances that future patients will benefit from better clinical trials. These activists do not agree that investigators are making choices that are most socially useful. Granting investigators more control to design trials without interference is a shallow victory for them, especially if patients will not enroll in the studies or comply with directions.

Critics of Traditional Clinical Trial Methods

Other critics who deny that research can be a cooperative venture with patient subjects because patients do not understand enough to be partners, reach a different conclusion about what policies should be adopted. These critics maintain that investigators do not help patients to understand the central point that as the information comes in, it will be increasingly apparent that some groups are getting suboptimal care.[21] Without genuine understanding and informed consent on this point, traditional methods put medical advances ahead of patients' rights and welfare. The patient should come first, and doctors should not enroll their patients in studies where they do not come first. Traditional research methods, they hold, typically violate physicians' duties to their patients.[22]

These critics understand the physicians' duty, or what some call the *therapeutic obligation,* as the duty to provide patients with what their doctors believe is the best available care. These critics view traditional clinical trial methodology as entailing that some patients will receive suboptimal care, and they conclude that such methods are incompatible with the traditional duties of health care professionals. This understanding of the therapeutic obligation, however, presumes that there is a best treatment and that it is up to physicians to determine what is best for their patients. Both assumptions are often false.

First, this understanding of the therapeutic obligation is problematic because many times it is uncertain which treatments are best. A moral requirement for justifying clinical trials is that the different treatment arms must be in clinical equipoise. This is usually understood to mean that the community of investigators and physicians are uncertain about which treatment being tested is best, so there is no known therapeutic advantage to a patient's assignment to any one of the various treatment arms.[23] If physicians must provide what they believe is the best treatment available for their patients, then we must assume they believe there is a best treatment. Yet, this is incompatible with the assumption underlying clinical trials—that the best treatment is recognized to be unknown. It is not surprising, therefore, that these critics reject traditional methods of testing. They assume that treatments cannot be in clinical equipoise.

Second, this formulation of the therapeutic obligation (that physicians must provide patients with what they believe is the best available care) is paternalistic because it assumes that physicians know what is best for patients. Yet, AIDS activists have demonstrated that they are unwilling to let clinicians or investigators simply decide what is best for them. They want themselves or their surrogates to be part of these decisions. Many patients want to consider treatments in light of their goals, values, and principles to determine how alternative treatments affect the quality of their lives. Activists support this. If patients do not think the treatment arms of the trial are in equipoise from their perspective, they will refuse to participate. This led Lo to conclude, "Thus, the concept of equipoise should include the potential volunteers of the clinical trial, as well as the community of investigators."[24]

What links both kinds of critics of research as a cooperative venture is their belief that patients cannot understand enough to be genuine partners, and that as a result we have to make some hard choices between the investigators' freedom to design what they consider the best trials and the patients' rights or welfare. In what follows, I want to question their common assumption that patient-subjects cannot participate as partners because they lack sufficient knowledge and understanding.

UNDERSTANDING OR CONTROL?

If we suppose, as some critics believe, that the difficulties about viewing research as a cooperative venture centered around the patients' lack of understanding, then these disagreements would evaporate where there exists a competent and informed subject population. Quite the reverse has happened with the AIDS epidemic, even though many of the patients are highly educated and informed. While individual patients are sometimes ignorant and uncertain, as a group these patients and their families or advocates grow increasingly more informed and more vocal. There are a large number of newsletters, home pages on the Internet, media, and government reports about HIV infections (and other chronic diseases) that many patients, families, and advocates carefully follow.

It is also doubtful to say that the primary problem is just an information gap. Consider how investigators and clinicians react when results seem counterintuitive or when they or their family members are sick. In the January 1991 issue of the *Journal of Clinical Oncology,* an article by Belanger et al. shows that physicians and nurses may accept the results of large randomized trials theoretically but reject them in practice when the results are inconsistent with their own intuitions.[25] In addition, they found that oncologists and oncology nurses were reluctant to agree to participate in clinical investigations when they viewed themselves as the patients. In an editorial in the same issue, Hayes writes, "First, we must be certain that our recommendations to patients are no different than those we would make for ourselves or our families. . . . Moreover, when possible, we should base our treatment recommendations on properly generated data. To do so requires that we not be too quick to accept results of studies that support our biases."[26]

When faced with insufficient data, oncologists and oncology nurses ought to conclude that this is an ideal time to conduct and enroll as patients in a clinical trial. When making decisions for themselves or their families, however, they tended to break the tie with hunches or intuitions. The explanation for their reaction cannot be a lack of understanding. It is possible that this study shows some oncologists recommend clinical trials for others but not for themselves, or that they are suspicious of how clinical trials are conducted.

Another important explanation is that when the decision is *personal* and *risky,* we are reluctant to admit there is genuine uncertainty. When patients enroll in a randomized, controlled, double-blind clinical trial, they do not select their treatment options. When the stakes are high, clinical trials and randomization force us to confront uncertainty and our lack of power. We have to admit that we may do badly when depending upon a chance assignment. Our uncertainty may give rise to images of alternative ways our lives may go, and it makes most of us very uncomfortable.

When the people are asked to enroll in randomized clinical trials, they have to admit uncertainty and a lack of control. This is very hard when the stakes are high. Like the oncologists in the Belanger survey, or patients who demand greater access, we prefer to think our intuitions are reliable. I believe that this has less to do with ignorance and more to do with a very human response to uncertainty, risk, and loss of control. People do not want to admit to themselves that they lack understanding about what to do.

Critics might object that this tendency to operate by intuitions when we are personally involved shows why investigators—not subjects or activists—should be in charge, and thus why research should not be a cooperative venture.

Potential subjects, critics argue, either lack the impartiality, or do not know enough to be partners in the designing, testing, or use of promising new treatments.

This response, however, ignores subject-patients' power to defeat trials they dislike, distrust, or do not see as being in their best interest. If a study does not seem to be in their best interest (assuming that they are properly informed of the risks and benefits), they will not enroll or if they do enroll, they may refuse to follow the investigators' directions. Thus, one practical reason for agreeing that patients should be regarded as partners is that they have the power to undercut trials. Achievement of the freedom to design and execute studies as investigators wish, without interference from patients, families, or advocates, will be an empty victory if few patients will participate in them or cooperate if they do enroll.

One way that patients can defeat trials is by not following the investigators' instructions. For example, Merigan, in a recent issue of the *New England Journal of Medicine,* revealed that the clinical trial of zidovudine (AZT) against a placebo was jeopardized by the fact that 9 percent of the patients who were given a placebo were taking AZT on their own. As Merigan writes, "If these irregularities had been more widespread, the useful effects of the drug could have been obscured in the trial, to the detriment of future patients infected with human immunodeficiency virus (HIV). Specifically, the early initiation of zidovudine therapy in asymptomatic patients would not have become standard practice."[27]

Another way that patients can defeat trials is by refusing to enroll in them. For example, the National Surgical Adjuvant Project for breast and bowel cancers set out to conduct randomized clinical trials on the survival rates of women with breast cancer. Women were asked to give consent before randomization to lumpectomy versus simple mastectomy with or without radiation. Women were asked to go into surgery not knowing if they had cancer, and if they had it, not knowing which treatments they would receive. Because of this uncertainty many physicians were reluctant to ask their patients to participate in these studies, other doctors found many women unwilling to accept such conditions.[28] In response to the slow accrual rate, investigators switched to a prerandomized schema. Subjects were informed of their proposed group assignment, treatment options, and the nature and purpose of the study at the time consent was sought. The accrual rate increased sixfold. Several authors found this suspicious and questioned if physicians, perhaps unconsciously, were enthusiastic about whatever assignment the women got since they knew the assigned treatment in advance of seeking consent.[29]

This bias may exist in some cases, but consider another explanation. Patients may find the prerandomization design more acceptable because they know which treatment they will receive. It is not that most patients lack the capacity to understand randomization; it is no harder to understand than the flip of a coin. The problem with chance assignments is related, I believe, to how we react to uncertainty when we are very apprehensive. When there is great potential for loss or gain, agreeing to randomization forces us to confront uncertainty. We cannot rationalize that we have control or that there is some reasonable way to break the tie. The issue is not merely about information but also involves our difficulty in admitting that we have little control. Randomization forces us to admit that we have no defenses against uncertainty, risk, and loss of control. Thus, critics of research as a cooperative venture need to consider how they can enroll and keep subjects in studies if they do not build their trust and cooperation. As the potential harms and benefits of studies increase, people increasingly want to understand why some trials are started or finished, when placebos are used, what information is available, and how unjustifiable biases are eliminated. People's desire to participate stems from rights of self-determination, our need to protect our own well-being, and a variety of social interests in the use of tax dollars and the enhancements of civil rights.

MORAL AND VALUE JUDGMENTS IN RESEARCH

AIDS activists have drawn attention to long-standing debates over how new therapies should be tested and used. Many of these are evaluative and ethical, not just scientific disputes, and informed people of goodwill can legitimately disagree about the issues involved.

Beginning Trials

Activists sometimes disagree with investigations about when to begin systematic study. One such disagreement was over compound Q, a substance derived from Chinese cucumber roots. AIDS activists were eager to have compound Q tested because of evidence from laboratory tests that it could combat the HIV virus. Frustrated by what they took to be a slow reaction to a promising new drug, members of Project Inform organized trials on their own. They obtained compound Q illegally. Their trial had no institutional review and no independent data safety monitoring committee; some subjects suffered serious complications and death. Critics argue that people rushed to conduct a trial before safe dosages had been established.[30] Sadly, some people died because of the lack of agreement and cooperation about when to begin a trial.

Using Placebos

There are many methodological advantages to using placebos. A placebo control trial can show a treatment's efficacy uncontaminated by the patient's expectations (the placebo effect) and can also unequivocally establish one drug as a standard therapy. This happened for AZT and aerosol pentamidine for treatment of HIV and opportunistic infections. Such conclusive tests have important practical consequences. For example, if insurance companies are shown that these therapies work, they will pay for them.

To use a placebo in clinical trials, however, it should be uncertain at the beginning whether the patients are better off with the placebo or the experimental treatment. If a reasonable and informed person would want the promising treatment, it may be wrong to use a placebo.[31] Moreover, the subjects in clinical trials are patients, and their health care professionals have a duty to provide optimal treatment for all their patients. If the placebo arm is not offering good care, the health care professionals are not fulfilling their moral commitment to their patients, and investigators are violating research codes.[32]

There are, of course, genuine disagreements about what we really know or what the reasonable person would want. For example, when AZT was first being tested, some objected that it was wrong to use a placebo. They maintained that under the circumstances, a reasonable person would want AZT because the drug *might* help them. They knew that the placebo would not help them fight the virus. Others argued that until the testing was completed, we did not really know if the treatment was better or worse with a placebo. Since informed people of goodwill can disagree about these matters, it is important to have their various views represented at the table where decisions are made.

Selecting Subjects

Participation in research is increasingly seen as a benefit to oneself or one's group. Many people with life-threatening illnesses want to enroll in trials as a way to gain access to promising investigational new drugs. For example, some people may see participating in a clinical trial as their only way of receiving state-of-the-art medical care. Excluding large groups, such as women of childbearing years, older people, or children, also raises issues of fairness. It is harder to generalize findings to groups that have not been tested. In short, people have come to see participating in research as a potential benefit to themselves and their group and, all things being equal, view restrictions based on age, gender, or race or ethnic group as creating problems about fairness and generalizability. For example, Pizzo argued that a variety of regulatory obstacles kept children with AIDS from getting the only drugs that could help them.[33] Federal and state rules then restricted the use of untested drugs such as AZT on children to "protect" these vulnerable subjects.

Women also claimed that rules allegedly designed to protect them from untested drugs actually harmed them. One reason that women were excluded was that they might become pregnant and the fetus could be harmed by an experimental drug. Barring women from participating in trials just because they are or might become pregnant denies them the same access to new and promising therapies as men. It assumes that there will be a conflict of interest between the needs of the mother and fetus and that the welfare of the fetus should come first as a matter of policy. Also troubling is that if drugs are only tested on men, the effect on women will be unclear. This seems unjust since women's tax dollars support these studies, yet women do not get the same benefit from them as men. The NIH, under the leadership of Bernadine Healy, sought to address this problem, but the progress so far has been discouraging.[34]

The 1993 NIH Revitalization Act requires that studies supported by the NIH must include representative populations, particularly women, and various racial and ethnic groups. Cost cannot be a consideration for noncompliance. People no longer think of all research as a risky burden they want to avoid. Consequently, the rule "women, children, and the sickest last" no longer seems gallant; it seems unfair.

Randomization

The gold standard for clinical trials is double-blind, placebo-control methodology. Randomization eliminates nuisance variables, such as age, nutritional habits, or living styles that might confound the results by distributing people randomly throughout the arms of the studies. This helps ensure that the results of the study are due to the different treatment modalities that patients receive.

When the treatments are equally good, randomization is justifiable. It is unethical to assign patients randomly to clinical trials when the arms are not in clinical equipoise, especially when a disease is fatal or rapidly progressing. The view of investigators and patients about what is *equally good,* however, may be different. Investigators may view what they regard as insufficiently tested treatment as no better than a placebo. Patients may see the treatment as their only hope because there are no others and their disease is progressing rapidly. Thus, they do not want to be in a randomized, controlled trial. For example, ganciclovir is an antiviral drug. Investigators wanted to use it to treat cytomegalovirus retinitis, which is an opportunistic infection causing blindness. A randomized, placebo-control trial was planned that would exclude patients taking AZT, but critics objected that such a randomized clinical trial would be unethical.[35] The views of the critics won the day, but others objected that this drug was released without rigorous testing. Investigators argue for the utility of randomization to counteract unintended bias.

Bias

Another reason for regarding research to be a cooperative venture is that, by including many points of view, we minimize a variety of biases and conduct better scientific studies. Investigators, like the rest of us, tend to ignore their own ingrained biases or regard themselves as more immune from unjustified biases than others. It is hard to assess how much bias exists among medical investigators, but studies document disturbing patterns of unjustified bias by clinicians against certain groups of patients, including those who are female, poor, elderly, Latino, and African American. These are the very groups targeted by the 1993 NIH Revitalization Act for greater *inclusion.*[36] If we do not study and compare populations, we do not expose biases, prejudices, or misconceptions. Investigators who want unilateral control may minimize how difficult it is to recognize and deal with their unjustified biases. Their particular point of view will dominate all others if they control what and whom to study, when to begin and end trials, and what studies are funded or published.

By including more diverse groups with different perspectives in the designing, review, and implementation of studies, we increase the likelihood of recognizing important interests and unjustified biases. Clinicians, investigators, and institutional review boards (IRBs) can learn from groups that have often felt excluded, such as women, African Americans, and other minorities and ethnic groups.

Ending Trials

When AZT was first shown to help some AIDS patients, a double-blind, placebo-controlled, randomized clinical trial was begun. Some patients received AZT; others, a sugar pill placebo. After several months of testing the AZT against a placebo, 16 of the 137 patients on the placebo arm died while only 1 of the 145 patients receiving AZT died. The trial was ended, and those having gotten the placebo then received AZT.[37] Arguments about whether this trial should have ended earlier or later are moral arguments about how to balance two important values: the safety of individual patients and the social utility of reliable research. The controversy was not just about what we know and when but about who controls the decision when to end studies or use placebos.

Investigators, patients, and health care professionals may have different perspectives. Investigators typically focus on helping future patients and are reluctant to end a study unless they believe that the results are conclusive. Doctors and nurses, however, are committed to providing their individual patients good care. Many wanted their patients to get AZT and not the placebo.

To justify the clinical trials, it should be uncertain whether the patients are better off with the placebo or with the experimental treatment. If thalidomide (at one time given for nausea in pregnancy but later found to cause severe birth defects) had been tested against a placebo, those in the placebo group would have performed far better. After the thalidomide tragedy, when many of the FDA's regulations were put in place, a dominant concern was to protect the public from untested and potentially dangerous new treatments. If AZT had been not clearly useful but harmful, this attitude might have persisted. But AZT was very successful compared to the placebo and appeared to be so from the beginning. Although a double-blind format was used in the study, rumors persisted that physicians and nurses knew which patients were getting the AZT and opposed giving placebos to their patients.

THE CASE FOR RESEARCH AS A COOPERATIVE VENTURE

AIDS activists have focused attention on some long-standing moral disputes over how to conduct trials. They have helped to change how clinical trials are done by speeding up the approval of drugs, getting patients access to therapies being tested, obtaining some information about preliminary trends, and changing how patients are selected for trials. AIDS activists want more of a say in making moral and evaluative choices about when to begin trials, end studies, randomize, use placebos, and select subjects from different groups. Advocates for other diseases also have newsletters, follow promising new treatments, and demand more control. In the late 1980s and 1990s, these disputes became political. For example, the 1993 NIH Revitalization Act makes it clear that excluding women and various racial and ethnic groups from studies is often unfair. Without this testing, it is uncertain how the new procedures would affect them.

Even if activists were justified in bringing to light certain problems, this does not show that research should be a cooperative venture. Critics argue that activists and potential subjects are either too ignorant or too partial to be genuine partners. In contrast I have argued here and elsewhere that research should be viewed as a cooperative venture between patient-subjects and investigators.[38]

The first reason why research needs to be a cooperative venture is that subjects or their surrogates have rights of self-determination regarding research participation that are a part of a web of important civil rights. In addition, they have interests in protecting their own well-being and advancing as best they can their own life plan. The broad powers that some investigators want are discordant with other values of our country. We live in a country where people can do dangerous and foolish things. They can swim in shark-infested waters and camp near active volcanoes if they wish. Accordingly, patients may object when they are prohibited from taking promising new treatments that they believe are their only hope for improved health. If they can assume risks for themselves for sport, why can they not take risks for health? Since neither patients, investigators, nor clinicians can succeed in achieving the goal of fighting disease without the others, the best policy is to foster cooperation, mutual trust, and a spirit of compromise. Trust is built through the process of informed consent and by having individuals similar to the subject population or their advocates have a role in planning for the testing and use of promising new therapies.

Second, if investigators do not acknowledge research as a cooperative venture and learn to build trust, they will find that fewer subjects will enroll in studies or follow directions. Moreover, studies that clearly violate people's rights that come to the attention of the public make it more difficult for other investigators to enroll subjects.

Third, patients or their advocates should acknowledge the common goal of medical advances and concede the importance of and rapid progress that has been made as a result of proven research methods. This common goal should build trust and a spirit of research as a cooperative venture. Investigators should acknowledge that public funding creates responsibilities to benefit the entire public. Policies excluding women, some ethnic groups, and other minorities give the perception that the interests are insufficiently represented. In addition, a policy of inclusion helps combat unjustified bias that plague us all in the pursuit of knowledge.

Finally, there are difficult social and moral choices to be made about the degree of protection or access we want regarding new drugs or medical procedures. Deciding how much testing we as a society consider appropriate for establishing the safety and efficacy of promising new treatments before allowing them to be made available is like determining how much screening we desire in airports or how much safety inspection of buildings we want. It is only natural that when we think about the drugs that caused great harm, such as thalidomide, we want a lot of protection. But when we think about drugs that turned out to be beneficial, such as AZT, we want to have early access to them and are impatient with long trials. We cannot have it both ways, and it is best to make these decisions cooperatively with investigators.

Thus, research needs to be a cooperative venture where patients or their advocates acknowledge proven research methods and investigators acknowledge patients' views of what is in their interest. Representatives from affected groups should have a role in planning for the testing and use of promising new therapies. The degree of protection we want in testing the safety and efficacy of promising new treatments is a social and moral decision, not just a scientific matter.

NOTES

1. A. S. Fauci, "AIDS in 1996: Much Accomplished, Much to Do," *The Journal of the American Medical Association* 276 (1996): 155–56.
2. The Associated Press, "AIDS cocktail offers hope at Duke Medical," *Daily Reflector* 2 December 1996, 1, 7.
3. U.S. Centers for Disease Control and Prevention, "Zidovudine for the Prevention of HIV Transmission from Mother to Infant," *Morbidity and Mortality Weekly Report* 4 (29/94) vol. 43, no. 16 (1994): 285–87.
4. L. M. Kopelman, "Informed Consent and Anonymous Tissue Samples: The Case of HIV Seroprevalence Studies," *The Journal of Medicine and Philosophy* 19 (1994): 525–52.
5. M. Zelen, "A New Design for Randomized Clinical

Trials," *New England Journal of Medicine* 300 (1979): 1242–45; J. S. Tobias, "Informed Consent and Controlled Trials," *Lancet* 2 (1988): 1194.

6. R. Dresser, "Wanted: Single, White Males for Medical Research," *Hastings Center Report* 22, no. 1 (1991): 24–29; B. Healy, "The Yentl Syndrome," *New England Journal of Medicine* 325 (1991): 275; P. A. Pizzo, "Pediatric AIDS: Problems within Problems," *Journal of Infectious Diseases* 161 (1990): 316–25.
7. Institute of Medicine, "Inclusion of Women in Clinical Trials: Policies for Population Subgroups," *Women and Health Research: Ethical and Legal Issues of Including Women in Clinical Studies,* vol. 1, ed. A. C. Mastoianni, R. Faden, and D. Federman (Washington, D.C: National Academy Press, 1994).
8. L. M. Slaughter, "Recruitment and Retention of Women in Clinical Studies," Office of Research on Women's Health, U.S. Department of Health and Human Services, NIH Publication No. 95-3756 (1994): vii–x, vii.
9. U.S. Congress, "NIH Revitalization Act" (June 10, 1993). For reprint see *Institute of Medicine* (1994): 233–36.
10. L. M. Kopelman, "Research Policy/II. Risk and Vulnerable Groups," in *Encyclopedia of Bioethics,* rev. ed., vol. 4 (New York: Simon & Schuster, 1995), 2291–96; L. M. Kopelman, "Children/III: Health Care and Research," in *Encyclopedia of Bioethics,* rev. ed., vol. 4 (New York: Simon & Schuster, 1995): 357–68.
11. D. P. Byar et al., "Design Considerations for AIDS Trials," *New England Journal of Medicine* 323 (1990): 1343–48; U.S. Public Health Service, "Expanded Availability of Investigational New Drugs through a Parallel Track Mechanism for People with AIDS and HIV-Related Disease," *Federal Register,* 21 May 1990, 20856–60.
12. B. Lo, "Ethical Dilemmas in HIV Infection: What Have We Learned?" *Law, Medicine and Health Care* 20 (1992): 92–103.
13. U.S. Public Health Service, "Expanded Availability of Investigational New Drugs through a Parallel Track Mechanism for People with AIDS and HIV-related Disease."
14. Byar et al., "Design Considerations for AIDS Trials."
15. Ibid., 1344.
16. S. Staver, "New Antiviral Agent, D4T, Now Available to Treat HIV," *American Medical News,* 19 October 1992, 4.
17. K. Schaffner, "Ethical Problems in Clinical Trials," *Journal of Medicine and Philosophy* 11 (1986): 297–315.
18. G. J. Annas, "AIDS, Compassion and Drugs," *Hastings Center Report* 21, no. 4 (1991): 44–45; J. B. Kadane, "Progress toward a More Ethical Method for Clinical Trials," *Journal of Medicine and Philosophy* 11 (1986): 385–404; M. J. Lacher, "Physicians and Patients as Obstacles to a Randomized Trial," *Clinical Research* 26 (1978): 375–79; J. Waldenstrom, "The Ethics of Randomization," in *Research Ethics* (New York: Alan R. Liss, 1983), 243–49; M. Zelen, "A New Design for Randomized Clinical Trials"; J. S. Tobias, "Informed Consent and Controlled Trials."
19. G. J. Annas, "AIDS, Compassion and Drugs."
20. M. Zelen, "A New Design for Randomized Clinical Trials."
21. D. Wikler, "Ethical Considerations in Randomized Clinical Trials," *Seminars in Oncology,* 8 December 1981, 437–41.
22. C. Fried, "Medical Experimentation: Personal Integrity and Social Policy," in *Clinical Studies,* vol. 5, eds. A. B. Bearn et al. (New York: Elsevier Press, 1974); F. Gifford, "The Conflict between Randomized Clinical Trials and the Therapeutic Obligation," *Journal of Medicine and Philosophy* 11 (1986): 347–66; J. B. Kadane, *Journal of Medicine and Philosophy*; D. Marquis, "An Argument That All Prerandomized Clinical Trials Are Unethical," *Journal of Medicine and Philosophy* 11 (1986): 367–84; D. Wikler, "Ethical Consideration in Randomized Clinical Trials."
23. B. Freedman, "Equipoise and the Ethics of Clinical Research," *New England Journal of Medicine* 317 (1987): 141–45.
24. B. Lo, "Ethical Dilemmas in HIV Infection: What Have We Learned?" 94.
25. D. Belanger et al. "How American Oncologists Treat Breast Cancer, An Assessment of the Influence of Clinical Trials," *Journal of Clinical Oncology* 9 (1991): 7–16.
26. D. F. Hayes, (editorial) "What Would You Do If This Were Your . . . Wife, Sister, Mother, Self?" *Journal of Clinical Oncology* 9 (1991): 1–3.
27. T. C. Merigan, "You Can Teach an Old Dog New Tricks. How AIDS Trials Are Pioneering New Strategies," *New England Journal of Medicine* 323 (1990): 1341–42.
28. S. S. Ellenberg, "Randomization Designs in Comparative Clinical Trials," *New England Journal of Medicine* 310 (1984): 1404–8; B. Fisher, "The National Surgical Adjuvant Project for Breast and Bowel Cancer," NSABP Protocol B-06, distributed in 1980 to surgeons; K. M. Taylor et al., "Physician's Reasons for Not Entering Eligible Patients in a Randomized Clinical Trial of Surgery for Breast Cancer," *New England Journal of Medicine* 310 (1984): 1363–67.
29. T. L. Beauchamp and J. L. Childress, *Principles of Biomedical Ethics,* 4th ed. (New York: Oxford University Press, 1994); S. S. Ellenberg, *New England Journal of Medicine*; D. Marquis, *Journal of Medicine and Philosophy.*

30. B. Lo, "Ethical Dilemmas in HIV Infection: What Have We Learned?"

31. L. M. Kopelman, "Consent and Randomized Clinical Trials: Are There Moral or Design Problems?" *Journal of Medicine and Philosophy* 11 (1986): 317–45.

32. World Medical Association, Declaration of Helsinki. [1964]: 1989. "Recommendations Guiding Medical Doctors and Biomedical Research Involving Human Subjects," adopted by the 18th World Medical Assembly, Helsinki, Finland, and amended in 1975, 1983, and 1989; Germany (Territory Under Allied Occupation, 1945–1955: U.S. Zone) Military Tribunals, "Permissible Medical Experiments," *Trials of War Criminals before the Nuremberg Tribunals under Control Law No. 10* 2 (Washington, D.C.: U.S. Government Printing Office, 1947), 181–83.

33. P. A. Pizzo, "Pediatric AIDS: Problems within Problems."

34. R. Dresser, "Wanted: Single, White Males for Medical Research"; B. Healy, "The Yentl Syndrome."

35. B. Lo, "Ethical Dilemmas in HIV Infection: What Have We Learned?"

36. K. H. Todd, N. Samaroo, and J. R. Hoffman, "Ethnicity as a Risk Factor for Inadequate Emergency Department Analgesia," *JAMA* 269 (1993): 12 (March 24–31): 1537–39; K. H. Todd, T. Lee, and J. R. Hoffman, "The Effect of Ethnicity on Physician Estimates of Pain Severity in Patients with Isolated Extremity Trauma," *JAMA* 271 (1994): 12 (March 23–30): 925–28; I. S. Udvarhelyi, C. Gatsonis, A. M. Epstein, C. L. Pashos, J. P. Newhouse, and B. J. McNeil, "Acute Myocardial Infarction in the Medicare Population: Process of Care and Clinical Outcomes," *JAMA* 268 (1992): 18 (November 11): 2530–36; N. K. Wenger, L. Speroff, and B. Packard, "Cardiovascular Health and Disease in Women," *New England Journal of Medicine* 329 (1993): 247–56; M. Angell, "Caring for Women's Health—What Is the Problem," *New England Journal of Medicine* 329 (1993): 4 (July 22): 271–72; J. Z. Ayanian, I. S. Udvarhelyi, C. A. Gatsonis, C. L. Pashos, and A. M. Epstein, "Racial Differences in the Use of Revascularization Procedures after Coronary Angiography," *JAMA* 269 (1993): 20 (May 26): 2642–46; J. Z. Ayanian, and A. M. Epstein, "Differences in the Use of Procedures between Women and Men Hospitalized for Coronary Heart Disease," *New England Journal of Medicine* 325 (1991): 221–25; M. E. Gornick, P. W. Edgers, T. W. Reilly, R. M. Mentnech, L. K. Fitterman, L. E. Kucken, and B. C. Vladeck, "Effects of Race and Income on Mortality and Use of Service Among Medicare Beneficiaries," *New England Journal of Medicine* 335: 11 (1996): 791–799; E. D. Peterson, L. K. Shaw, E. R. DeLong, D. B. Pryor, R. M. Califf, and D. B. Mark, "Racial Variation in the Use of Coronary-Revascularization Procedures," *New England Journal of Medicine,* 336: 7 (1997): 480–486.

37. T. L. Beauchamp and J. L. Childress, *Principles of Biomedical Ethics.*

38. L. M. Kopelman, "Informed Consent and Anonymous Tissue Samples: The Case of HIV Seroprevalence Studies"; L. M. Kopelman, "Consent and Randomized Clinical Trials: Are There Moral or Design Problems?"; L. M. Kopelman, "Research Methodology/II. Controlled Clinical Trials," in *Encyclopedia of Bioethics,* rev. ed., vol. 4 (New York: Simon & Schuster, 1995), 2270–85.

CHAPTER 23

The IRB: Current and Future Challenges

Kenneth C. Micetich

Advances in medicine are made only through the process of clinical research. Clinical research is the involvement of humans in carefully designed, performed, completed, and analyzed clinical trials with the intention of publishing the results so that the scientific and medical communities can evaluate the results and the conclusions. It is only with the consensus of the medical and scientific communities after review and replication of the published results that a claim of an advance in medicine is authenticated.

Clinical research cannot be done without human involvement. At the present time nonhuman models that mimic or predict the human response to disease and treatments do not exist. Persons participating in the clinical research process are informed of the aims of the research project, the procedures, and the potential risks and benefits of the research project. A person who consents to participate in a clinical trial agrees to voluntarily assume the risk that is associated with the participation. Obviously, the consenting individual performs an individual risk-benefit analysis and decides that the risks are proportional to the potential benefits.

The individually determined risk-benefit analysis is variable from person to person. Factors influential in making a decision about participation in research include personal values and beliefs, life experiences, goals, and expectations. An individual may assign different weights to these factors depending on personal circumstances. Thus, a person who is faced with the threat of a fatal illness may opt for participation in a therapeutic research project while the same person in a healthy state may opt out of participation in a nontherapeutic research project.

Before human participation in any research, institutional review boards (IRBs) must review and approve all clinical research plans. The federal regulations mandate IRB review and approval of all research involving humans. IRB approval of a project, in part, means: (1) that procedures are used that are consistent with sound research design and that do not expose the participant to excess risk, thereby minimizing the risk of participation; (2) risks to humans are reasonable in relation to benefits; (3) prior informed consent will be sought and documented.[1] In practice, IRBs review the protocol, any supporting information, and the consent document.

IRBs have been in existence since 1974. The federal regulations that govern the conduct of human research are deeply rooted in accepted, fundamental, ethical principles.[2] While the federal regulations establish a set of minimum expectations that must be met, local IRBs are free to, and are expected to, establish local expectations consistent with the values of the institution, its constituency, and its research participants. Institutional values, goals, and resources may also determine whether the project is done after IRB approval, but an institution may never implement a project after a negative finding by the IRB.[3]

An examination of the federal regulations and the ethical principles that govern research clearly state that IRBs will be responsible for reviewing the scientific aspects of a clinical research project, the risks and the potential benefits and the adequacy of the informed-consent document.[4] It is likely that most IRBs meet the letter of the regulations and thus the minimum expectations. IRBs can show that they meet, deliberate, keep minutes, and issue approval letters. They can also show that the approved consent document states that the individual is participating in a research project and that risks and benefits are stated in the consent document. IRBs, in the first 25 years of their existence, have been successful in making certain that research is identified as such to an individual and that an individual receives mandated information prior to participation. This is the IRB process, and this process is now firmly established.

It is easy to verify that IRBs follow correct process. It is simply a matter of reviewing files, minutes, and documents. The determination of whether an IRB is meeting the spirit or substance of the regulations is more important. Assessment is difficult if not impossible at the present time. Quality control of the IRB decisions and findings would be ideal, but the IRB findings cannot be objectively measured as can the sodium concentration in a vial of blood that a regulatory agency sends as an unknown to clinical laboratories around the country to assess accuracy of the laboratory. A tremendous amount of faith and trust is placed in local IRBs.

There are forces present in the research environment today that were not present 25 years ago. First, new technology and knowledge yield complex protocols to test even newer and more complicated concepts. Second, the last 25 years have witnessed the birth and rapid growth of the medical industrial establishment. There are now many different for-profit companies making new products that must be tested and approved so that the product can be sold and a profit perhaps made. Third, in the past, patient care revenue supported important research at academic medical centers. However, health care reimbursement has changed, depleting research and education funds at academic medical centers. Now academic medical centers and other institutions compete with each other to be performance sites for the clinical testing of products of the medical industrial establishment. A successful center in the high stakes competition gains not only money and favorable press but also patients. Billions of dollars are at stake. Money is the engine that drives the research machine. It is now imperative that clinical research be done as quickly and efficiently as possible.

The forces that shape the research environment today impact the IRB. The protocols are more numerous and more complex than they were 25 years ago. The medical industrial research community expects quick review of complicated projects. Participant enrollment must be brisk and results collected and analyzed quickly. Informed-consent documents can be written in such a way as to favor participation.

The danger is that it is possible, in this new and complicated research environment, that an IRB can be procedurally correct but not meet the spirit of the regulations. IRBs must directly confront the new research environment. The challenge for IRBs now and into the twenty-first century is to establish substance. IRBs must more fully examine protocols in the context of the definition of clinical research, and they must more carefully examine the quantity and the quality of the information given to prospective participants.

CLINICAL RESEARCH—THE PROTOCOL

Clinical research is the involvement of humans in carefully designed, performed, completed, and analyzed clinical trials with the intention of publishing the results so that the scientific and medical communities can evaluate and put into proper perspective the results and the conclusions. The IRB can and must review all components of clinical research in reviewing a protocol.[5]

Rationale, objectives, procedures, outcomes of interest, experimental design, provisions that minimize risk, and methods of analysis must be clearly stated in the IRB reviewed protocol. In addition, there must be well-defined starting and stopping points as well as a provision for monitoring and reporting adverse events. It is important that the IRB ascertain the qualifications of the investigator and ensure that selection of subjects is equitable and without coercion. Most pharmaceutical company protocols and cooperative group protocols do a reasonable job in presenting these details in a protocol. However, local protocols developed "in-house" may be lacking in one or more of these important protocol features.

The following areas merit the careful attention of the IRB: (1) justification of number of participants; (2) the method of analysis; (3) the experimental design; (4) selection of participants; (5) qualifications of the investigator to perform the research; (6) investigator, institutional, and company commitment to the research; (7) the worth of the research; (8) the dynamic nature of the approval process.

Participant Number

The investigator must justify the participant number. If a larger number of patients than the number needed to accept or reject the null hypothesis is enrolled in the research project, then excess participants will be needlessly exposed to risk. If too few participants are enrolled in the project so that a statistically credible answer will never be obtained, then all the participants in the project will have assumed risk for no reason, since the stated objectives of the protocol will never be met. The responsibility for justification of the participant number must rest with the principal investigator of the research project, usually in consultation with a biostatistician, and it is the responsibility of the institution to provide the investigator with the support necessary to conduct clinical research.

Method of Analysis

The investigator must present a proposed method of analysis of the results in the protocol. Without the analysis of the results, the findings of the clinical trial will not be meaningful and will never be published. Participants will have assumed risk for no good reason. Again, the responsibility for the analysis rests with the investigator, and the institution or department must provide the investigator with the necessary support for the proper conduct of clinical research.

Experimental Design

IRBs must pay particular attention to the use of a placebo in a research study.[6] A placebo-controlled clinical trial is justified when no satisfactory treatment exists for the disease that is being investigated in the research project. If the scientific and medical literature support the efficacy of a treatment for a disease process, then the use of a placebo control in the research project is neither warranted nor ethical and should be disapproved by the IRB.

A problematic experimental design is the randomized, double-blind, placebo-controlled clinical study (RDBS) that is immediately followed by participation in an open-label extension study (OLES).[7] This study design compares a placebo to the active medication. To achieve balance in the two treatment groups, participants are randomly assigned to receive either placebo or active medication. To avoid reporting bias, participants and investigator do not know the identity of the treatment assignment (double-blinded). After the participant receives study medicine for the prescribed time, he or she may take active medicine for an additional length of time. This is called an open-label extension study because all participants in this study take the active medicine and not the placebo and participation in the OLES immediately follows participation in the RDBS.

The RDBS and the OLES are accepted experimental designs. The problem is the relationship of the OLES to the RDBS. Participation in the OLES requires prior participation in the RDBS. All participants in the OLES take open-label active study medication without knowing the identity of the treatment assignment in the RDBS.

We have taken the position that such a design is not ethical because the existence of the OLES after the parent RDBS, if known to the research subject at time of consent for the randomized trial, serves as an inducement to participate in the parent randomized trial.[8] Moreover, since the blind of the parent trial is not broken, some patients will continue to receive active medication when it was not helping them during the randomized trial. This violates a well-known principle of medical therapeutics; namely, a medicine that is not helping should be stopped since a therapeutic benefit does not balance the risks of continued treatment. Such experimental designs do not serve the interest of the participant and society and serve only the financial interest of the company that is developing the study medication because this experimental design may save time and money.

Selection of Participants

The IRB must ascertain that selection of participants is equitable and that inducements are not offered that would lead participants to enroll in a study in which they might otherwise decline to participate were it not for the inducement.[9] Most clinical studies do not offer payment to the participants, although free study medication and some free medical care may be offered. This is generally felt to be appropriate. Some normal volunteer studies offer money for participation. The IRB must find that the amount of money offered is not coercive and that the schedule of payments must not be such that the patient is forced to complete the study in order to be paid. No guidelines exist, and each IRB must decide what is fair compensation in relation to the study procedures. The absolute amount of money paid is not the only determining factor, however. The monies offered must be judged in relation to the socioeconomic status of the potential participants.

Recently, *The Wall Street Journal* reported that the Eli Lilly Company paid homeless people to participate in some of their phase 1 clinical trials of new investigational drugs.[10] The amount of money and other inducements (temporary housing) was not huge but was large relative to the average income of a homeless person. The other problem with this payment schema is that a disadvantaged segment of society shouldered a disproportionately large share of the research burden. This violates the principle of justice.[11]

IRBs must realize that money is not the only inducement that can be associated with participation in a research project. There are some research projects that use normal volunteers. Normal volunteers can be research laboratory technicians, medical students, graduate students, secretaries, or any other convenient institutional personnel. If one of these individuals enrolls in a research project that a superior is conducting, he or she may, on the one hand, reason that failure to participate will displease a superior and may affect future career opportunities. On the other hand, participants may feel that enrolling in the research project may lead to a better evaluation or career opportunity in the future. Also, there may be pressure to participate when someone else within a group of workers enrolls in the study because the nonparticipant may feel that the participant will be treated more favorably by the supervisor or chief in the future.

The IRB cannot judge motives, but the IRB can deal with perceptions. Therefore, it is within the scope of authority of the IRB to prevent this situation from ever developing. The IRB should give strong consideration to insisting that participants for whom the investigator has direct or indirect supervisory responsibility be prohibited from participating in the research project. In addition, many people would find it hard to decline participation when the supervisor directly solicits the employee. General solicitation, rather than face-to-face solicitation, should be the only means of recruiting normal-volunteer research participants.

We recently had the opportunity to review a normal-volunteer research study in which anesthesia residents would be asked to undergo three spinal anesthetics to determine the effect of different anesthetic agents on the sympathetic nervous system. The IRB reasoned that the job market is so poor for anesthesia residents finishing training that the participant might feel that he or she would get a better letter of recommendation from the chair of the anesthesia department if the individual participated. To be fair to all and to prevent people from participating based on a wrong perception, the IRB determined that a condition of approval of the project would be that only department of anesthesia faculty members could participate in the research project. The other advantage of this solution to our problem was that the participants would be truly informed!

Qualifications of the Investigator

The IRB must be certain that the investigator is qualified to carry out the proposed research and that the institution has the necessary facilities to support the research. There are three questions to ask. Is the investigator trained to perform the procedures the protocol requires? Does the institution support the procedures that the protocol requires? Is the investigator trained in the conduct of clinical research?

The IRB should not approve protocols when the investigator or his or her designee is not trained in the performance of a specific procedure. Many times this question can be answered by examining the curriculum vitae. Training and board certification will usually provide the answer. On occasion it will be necessary to verify that the hospital has credentialed the investigator to perform a particular procedure. It is also important that a particular hospital or research institution of any type support the research-required procedures.

The investigator must be qualified to conduct clinical research in general. The investigator must be willing to follow the details of the protocol and must not commit protocol violations without justification. Failure in this regard could lead to the exclusion of one or more participants from the data analysis, and these participants would have assumed risk for no good reason. In fact, poor recordkeeping and numerous protocol violations can render the whole study invalid. This would be a serious situation, since the entire participant population assumed risk for no good cause. IRBs must remember that very few physicians have taken formal courses in clinical research. Most of the time the training is "on the job," even though some clinical research was probably a requirement of a clinical training program. IRBs would do well to consider the past experience of the investigator in the performance of clinical research, the track record of the investigator in completing previously approved projects, any reports of patients enrolled on the research protocol who are later found to be ineligible for participation, and the presence or absence of a data management team in the investigator's department.

Commitment to Research

There must be evidence of commitment to the protocol. The IRB should have every reason to believe that the protocol will be completed, once approved. This is becoming a problem lately. Recent changes in the health care reimbursement system have decreased research budgets of medical-center departments, leading to less research support. This is particularly true for locally developed protocols. IRBs should insist as a condition for review that departmental resources exist to support the protocol to its completion.

A different sort of problem is noted in multicenter company protocols. The investigator can ensure that the company pays for data collection and data management. However, companies make financial decisions concerning drug development. We have seen protocols started, patients enrolled, and projects terminated when the company made a financial decision that further development of the treatment was no longer in the best interest of the company. Patients have assumed risk for no good reason when the protocol is not completed for marketing reasons.

Worth of the Research

IRBs must determine that the project has worth. Projects can be designed perfectly and be statistically valid but the information may not be that important. Projects of minimal or no value cannot be associated with any risk inasmuch as there is no benefit to balance a risk.

The merit or worth of a project is extremely difficult to judge. There are several lines of evidence of worth on which the IRB can validly rely. First, the IRB can examine the rationale for the protocol. Information concerning the importance of the findings must be present in the protocol. If not, then the IRB should ask for further information. Second, external agency funding of the research project can be taken as evidence of worth, since funding is competitive and a group of experts judged the importance of the information. Third, the commitment of the institution to the research may be taken as evidence of worth. Generally, if the institution or department commits financial and personnel resources to the project, the project appears to have merit. Fourth, the sense of the IRB can be an indicator of the worth of a project. If the nonscientific members of the IRB are not convinced of the worth of the project, it is either because the investigator has not explained it well or worth does not exist.

A caveat is in order. The investigator's department support of a research project without making a financial commitment to the project cannot necessarily be taken as evidence of worth of a project. Changes in health care reimbursement have depleted hospital and academic department research and education funds. More and more departments are looking to company-sponsored clinical research activities to fund departmental activities and staff salaries. Thus, departmental support of a project without concomitant commitment of institutional funds should be considered a potential conflict of interest because the department may have something to lose if it is not a performance site for the project. It is not beyond comprehension that a department could support a project even if it is not totally convinced of the worth of the project.

The Dynamic Nature of the Approval Process

Once the IRB grants approval to a research project, the review process does not stop. At any time, the IRB must be willing to reevaluate the risk-benefit ratio of a project if new information becomes available. The researcher may not voluntarily bring new information to the IRB, for two reasons. First, the researcher may not realize that the new information impacts on the study. Second, the researcher may have a vested interest (a perceived conflict of interest) in seeing the project to completion. While it is good that projects are completed, it is not good if the researcher supports the project when new information becomes available that negatively impacts on the risk-benefit analysis. Thus, any board member aware of information from any area is duty-bound to bring the material to the attention of the full board and insist that the project be reevaluated. Examples of information include unreported adverse protocol reactions, reports of irregularities in the conduct of the study and/or the consent process, reports in the press, the medical literature, and scientific meetings as well as participant reports of problems.

Federal regulations reasonably require that projects be reviewed no less frequently than every 12 months.[12] The period of re-review can be less frequent, and the level of risk determines the frequency of review. The IRB determines the frequency of review. Periodic review of research activity must be as substantive and meaningful as the initial review. Researchers should take this opportunity to report any recent advances and adverse protocol reactions that may have an impact on the risk-benefit analysis of the project. At any time during the conduct of the project, the IRB has the authority to close the project to further participant enrollment, pending clarification and analysis of new information. The IRB must also be willing to revise the consent document as new information becomes available. Additionally, investigators must submit changes to the protocol and reports of adverse protocol reactions as they are noted for timely board review. Any of these changes and adverse reactions can prompt a more thorough reevaluation of the study even if the study is not due for re-review.

CLINICAL RESEARCH INFORMED CONSENT

Having determined that the risks of participation are proportional to the potential benefits and having found that it is appropriate that the participant can voluntarily assume the risk of participation, the IRB must examine the consent document. There are eight required elements of consent:[13] (1) a statement that the study involves research along with an explanation of the purposes and procedures, duration of participation, and identification of experimental elements; (2) a description of risks; (3) a statement of benefits to the individual or to others that may reasonably be expected from the research; (4) alternatives to participation; (5) provisions for confidentiality; (6) medical treatments and compensations available in the event of research-related injury; (7) an explanation of whom to contact for answers to questions about the research, for information about a research-related injury, and for information about the rights of research subjects; (8) a statement that participation is voluntary and that the participant may discontinue participation at any time without loss of benefits or penalty.

Most IRBs insist that all of the required elements of consent are present, thus meeting the letter of the regulations. However, federal regulations and common sense mandate that the information given to the potential participant shall be in language that is understandable to the person giving consent. To give informed consent, you must understand what you read and what is told to you.

The following areas concerning informed consent merit careful consideration by the IRB: (1) the language of the consent; (2) the time and place of the consent; (3) the purpose, procedures, risks, and alternatives section of the consent; (4) consent and the cognitively impaired.

Consent Language

Proper consent requires that participants understand the potential benefits, risks, and procedures associated with participation. The IRB never knows who actually wrote the consent document. Most investigators copy the company or the cooperative-group consent document and add required local information. The role of the companies, the cooperative groups, and the investigators in writing the consent document represent a real conflict of interest. These parties have the most to gain from brisk participant enrollment in the research project.

The consent document is the most important document that the IRB reviews, and we never know the credentials of the person who wrote the consent. Consents are long (averaging six to seven pages), contain technical language, require a twelfth-grade education or higher to comprehend, and are frequently exhaustive lists of any and all known complications of the treatment under investigation.[14] This is very disappointing given the financial resources of the cooperative groups and the pharmaceutical industry. The tendency to include every single adverse event, no matter how rare, is particularly reprehensible, especially when there is no attempt to rank the order of the side effects and their likelihood, and suggests a purely legalistic approach to consent. For the above reasons, many consent documents are unacceptable and require considerable revision even though they contain the required elements of consent. It would be ideal if a disinterested third party reviewed the protocol and relevant supporting information and then wrote the consent document. IRBs review many informed consents and should consider themselves experts on consent and consent documents.

Inadequate and overly enthusiastic consent documents are not easy problems to solve and require huge amounts of time to revise. Consent documents should be written for a sixth-to-eighth-grade reading comprehension level. The consents can be shortened and simple declarative sentences used. One possible solution is for an IRB to consult with a journalist who has experience in creating popular works. If the consent documents can be written with the above in mind, it is likely that we will have a more informed participant population. I emphasize that consent documents that contain all of the required elements of consent are frequently inadequate from the comprehension standpoint, even though they might be judged as adequate for the information contained, and they constitute a serious problem.

Time and Place of Consent

Ethical considerations and the federal regulations require that the prospective participant have ample opportunity to consider participation. A patient who is told of the project and has only a brief time to make a decision about participation is not giving truly informed consent. The emotional and physical state of the participant must also be considered. Participants in acute emotional distress and pain are not likely to comprehend the nature of the research project. There are some protocols involving interventions during cardiac catheterization in which the investigator will not know until halfway through the procedure if the patient is eligible to participate. It is not appropriate to present the study to the participant during the cardiac catheterization. For studies such as this, the IRB must specifically discuss and mandate when consent can be obtained. In this case, the consent must be obtained prior to the cardiac catheterization.

Specific Consent Issues

There are two levels of decision making that a potential participant in the research process uses in deciding about participation in a clinical trial. The first level is a generic screen. The second level is detailed. Some human subjects refuse participation based on generic issues of clinical research. For example, some people will never participate in research and state that they do want to be "guinea pigs." Others will object to the concept of randomization (assignment by lottery) to a treatment. Still others will not want to participate in a clinical research project because they have a defined chance of receiving a placebo or the research project is double-blinded (neither researcher nor participant will know the identity of the treatment). This is not unusual. All of us when deciding about participating in certain activities have a set of internal screening issues that are critical for us as individuals and determine whether we will consider the activity any further.

The IRB must require that consent documents allow the participants to understand that the project before them is research (experimental), and if applicable, explain the assignment of treatment and other generic aspects of the experimental design. For example, we find the following wording useful in the consent for a randomized, double-blind placebo-controlled trial:

> If you agree to participate in this research project you will receive either one of three doses of [the study medicine] or a placebo (a harmless, inactive substance). Which you receive will be determined by lottery. Neither you nor your doctor will know which you are receiving, but this information can be learned in the event of an emergency. In this study, one out of every four patients will receive a placebo and three out of every four patients will receive the active medicine.

If a project passes the generic screen of the individual, then the potential participant requires further details to make a final decision. The details of the procedures, risks, and alternatives are most important for the person who is deciding about participation in clinical research and provide the information necessary to make an individual risk-benefit assessment.

It is critical that the consent document contain truthful information. IRBs will find it most useful to compare the objectives stated in the protocol with the purpose of the study in the consent. A consent document cannot state that a purpose of the study is to determine the efficacy of a new medicine when the study is a phase 1 dose-finding study and efficacy is either not being assessed or is not a stated objective. A consent for a phase 1 oncology study[15] might include the following:

> The purpose of this research is to determine the maximum amount of medicine that we can safely give to people. The first three patients will receive a low dose of the study medicine. If they do not experience severe side effects, the next three patients will receive a higher dose of the drug. The dose of drug will be raised after every three patients as long as the patients have not had serious or troublesome side effects. The study

> is completed when we find a dose of study medicine that causes serious problems.
>
> The dose of study medicine that you receive in this research project will be determined by how many patients have been treated before you and what side effects they have had. Your doctor can tell you what dose level of study medicine you will receive and what side effects patients treated before you have had.

While the above wording may seem harsh, it does accurately reflect the purpose of a phase 1 study.

The risks section of the consent document for a phase 1 study will also have specific requirements. On the one hand, the patient enrolling late in the study may experience more side effects since the dose has been escalated, but the antitumor effect may be better. On the other hand, patients enrolling early in the study will receive a low dose of the study medication and may have few side effects, but the antitumor effect of the drug may be low.

It is also important that participants understand the alternatives to participation. Sometimes the alternative is only nonparticipation. However, in the case of therapies, it is vital that the investigator list any standard treatments. It is also necessary to state that the doctor will discuss the risks and the benefits of the standard treatments with the participant.

IRBs must carefully review the benefits section of the consent document and broaden the beneficiaries. Benefits cannot be promised or implied because the participant is enrolling in a research project and the purpose of that research project may be to determine efficacy. However, other groups may benefit. The drug companies may benefit if the Food and Drug Administration allows them to sell the drug for treatment. The institution and the investigator's department may benefit from the budgeted indirect costs of the research project that may allow hiring of additional staff to perform other duties. A graduate nursing student collecting data for a Ph.D. dissertation will clearly benefit. Thus, others may benefit from the participant's enrollment in the research project. It is the truth and should be so stated. A benefits section might state:

> "We cannot predict the effect of a treatment on your disease. The purpose of this research is to determine if the research treatment can help people with your condition. Therefore, we do not know if you will personally benefit from participating in this research project. The information we learn may benefit future patients with your condition.
>
> The [company] may benefit financially if, based on the results of research, the Food and Drug Administration allows the [company] to sell the new medicine for the treatment of patients with your condition. Your doctor and the Department of Medicine of University Medical Center may also benefit from your participation in this research project.

Lastly, it is important to remember that research participants do not understand the process of clinical research. Participants are generally not aware that information on how they do will be collected and sent somewhere, usually to a company or a clinical-data management firm. This should be explicitly stated. We have generally included the following information in our consents:

> Information on how you do will be sent to [sponsor]. At a later time the results will be studied. The group of patients who received the inactive medicine will be compared to the group of patients who received the study medicine. In this way we will learn about the safety and the usefulness of [investigational treatment] in the treatment of patients with your condition.

The IRB should strive to guarantee that patients and the clinical research process and personnel work together as a team. Truthful and understandable consent documents, easy access to study personnel, and informing past participants about the study results at the completion of the project enhance the team concept. Informing participants about the results of the study is rarely done. The investigators and the IRB should consider possible mechanisms for informing past participants of the results of the clinical trial.

Consent and the Cognitively Impaired

The cognitively impaired are a heterogeneous group of patients that includes those mentally disabled from birth, those with an acquired dementia (Alzheimer's disease), and those with an acute problem that renders them impaired (stroke, cerebral hemorrhage, head trauma, and so forth). The cognitively impaired cannot give consent since their problem limits the capacity to understand, and they cannot weigh the risks and benefits of the research project. This does not mean, however, that research involving this class of participants is prohibited. A distinction must be made between therapeutic and nontherapeutic research. Thus, research with therapeutic intent after obtaining surrogate consent is appropriate.

Research without direct therapeutic intent in this class of people has no chance of direct individual benefit, and the appropriateness of enrolling these people in research projects after obtaining surrogate informed consent is less clear.[16] If the project is of minimal risk (defined as no greater risk than the risk associated with everyday life or the risk associated with performance of a routine physical examination or routine tests), then surrogate consent may be appropriate, but the worth of the study should be examined carefully. In projects of greater-than-minimal risk, surrogate consent may be relied upon, but all should agree that the results of the project will provide generalizable information of vital importance for the understanding of the problem that may enhance therapeutic development for this class of affected individuals. IRB review of nontherapeutic research using cognitively impaired participants must not be hasty. Where judged necessary, the IRB must seek the opinions of experts, caregivers, and specialty societies in determining the worth of the project. The surrogate, however, must provide consent before the person is enrolled in the research project.

Several years ago, the government of the United States admitted that it gave radioactive iron to mentally disabled persons in a research project designed to learn more about the effects of radioactivity. No consent was obtained from anyone. This was clearly wrong. IRBs today would not approve such research because the project is without individual benefit, and the information learned is not important to an understanding of the disease process. The government determined that the outcome of the research was of vital national interest, but this argument would be rejected today as well.

IRBs will soon confront a new challenge. Recently, the Food and Drug Administration and the Department of Health and Human Services announced a change in policy that would allow the cognitively impaired to participate in research without prior consent. This policy change applies to research in emergency situations when consent is not possible.[17] The pharmaceutical industry and experts in critical-care medicine argued that unless the requirement for consent is relaxed in certain patients, research cannot be done in emergency situations.[18] Additionally, there are some disorders (stroke, cerebral hemorrhage) in which there may be a narrow critical window of opportunity to act to prevent further damage. Due to the acute onset and the life-threatening nature of the illness as well as the inability to find a consenting surrogate within the critical time interval, regulations now allow enrolling these patients in clinical trials (including those that are double-blinded and placebo-controlled) without prior consent.

The policy change is dramatic. Proponents have introduced the concept of relative risk.

IRBs in approving this type of research must find that the risk of participation in the research project is low compared to the threat to life posed by the illness. The new policy requires that a mechanism be in place to advertise the existence of the study to the community prior to commencing the study. It is not clear how this should be done or what useful purpose it serves.

There are problems with the new policy. First, it is true that sooner or later there will be a treatment given under the new policy that will be shown to be deleterious to survival. In this case, patients will have involuntarily assumed the risk of having a poorer outcome than if they had not participated in the study. Second, the policy assumes that even if the participant does not personally benefit, there may be greater good to society that participation achieves. Note that there is no moral or ethical mandate that requires participation in research because it may help others. The problem is that patients rarely enter clinical trials based totally on altruism. The priority for the participant is that the project may help the participant directly. Third, the policy represents a substitution of society's values for the values of the cognitively impaired participant. Society views this research as potentially good and, therefore, so should the cognitively impaired patient. Fourth, it is very difficult to justify enrollment without consent of a cognitively impaired individual in a research trial in which there is a chance that he or she will receive a placebo in a life-threatening situation.

The issue is not research involving the cognitively impaired but research involving the cognitively impaired without consent. This research can be done without waiver of consent but it will just take longer. At the present time, there is no apparent justification for the waiver of consent in the emergency situation. One can make a case for the waiver in the face of 100 percent mortality, but it is still not clear what constitutes a life-threatening situation that would trigger the implementation of the policy. So far, statements and explanations have not given concrete examples of the types of studies that may invoke the new policy. It is expected to be used sparingly. Although the policy has gone into effect, individual IRBs and institutions can decline to review and approve emergency research. IRBs should consult the responsible institutional officials and other members of the lay and scientific communities that it serves for guidance. To date, a national debate on this policy has not taken place, and the changes have not been widely publicized. Companies have much to gain if the study drug or procedure is eventually approved by the Food and Drug Administration. Institutions will be paid some money to enroll the participants. Institutional performance sites for these types of studies must thoroughly and vigorously debate the policy. The critical question remains: Under what circumstances, if any, is it ever justified to enroll a cognitively impaired person in a research study without prospective consent from a surrogate?

SUMMARY

Since 1974 IRBs have reviewed and approved clinical research and consent documents. The challenges that the IRB faces today are the challenges it will face in the twenty-first century. Review of protocols must become more detailed and IRBs must strive to ensure that the consent process permits the person time to make an informed decision and that the consent document is not only accurate and tells the truth but also is understandable and free of coercion.

Clinical research is complex. The clinical trials done today are more complicated than those done 20 years ago. The reporting requirements to and of the IRB are voluminous.[19] Chairing the IRB is rapidly becoming a full-time occupation. While it is expected that all IRBs will obey the letter of the regulations, we have a long way to go to ensure that the IRB will obey the spirit of the regulations and its ethical roots. There are numerous issues that need debate and resolution. Many IRB chairs and committee members have no training in ethics or understanding and appreciation of the historical events and the codes that bolster ethical clinical research. Perhaps they should. IRBs would do well to remember that they exist to protect the research participant. However, it is possible to merge the sometimes-perceived competing interests and motives of the research establishment, the institution, and the research participant. This is possible only if each of these three components of clinical research understands and respects the others and they work together as a team in the clinical research process. The forging of this alliance for the mutual benefit of all is the real challenge for IRBs in the twenty-first century.

NOTES

1. Department of Health and Human Services, Protection of Human Subjects, Title 45, Code of Federal Regulation, Part 46: 46.111.
2. Department of Health and Human Services, Protection of Human Subjects, Title 45, Code of Federal Regulation, Part 46: Revised June 18, 1991: 46; The Belmont Report, *Ethical Principles and Guidelines for the Protection of Human Subjects of Research* (Washington, DC: US Government Printing Office, 1978), DHEW Publication No. (OS) 78-0012; World Medical Association, "Declaration of Helsinki," as amended by the 41st World Medical Assembly, Hong Kong, September 1989, reprinted in *Law, Medicine and Health Care* 19, no. 3–4 (Fall/Winter 1991): 264–65.
3. Department of Health and Human Services, Protection of Human Subjects, 46.112.
4. Office for Protection from Research Risk, *Protecting Human Research Subjects: Institutional Review Board Guidebook* (Washington, DC: US Government Printing Office, 1993), sec. 3 and 4.
5. K. C. Micetich, "Reflections of an IRB Chair," *Cambridge Quarterly of Healthcare Ethics* 3 (1994): 506–9.
6. Office for Protection from Research Risk, *Protecting Human Research Subjects,* 4–16.
7. K. C. Micetich, "The Ethical Problems of the Open-Label Extension Study," *Cambridge Quarterly of Healthcare Ethics* 5 (1996): 410–14.
8. Ibid.
9. Office for Protection from Research Risk, *Protecting Human Research Subjects,* 3–44.
10. "To Screen New Drugs for Safety, Lilly Pays Homeless Alcoholics," *The Wall Street Journal,* 14 November 1996.
11. C. Weijer, "Evolving Ethical Issues in Selection of Subjects for Clinical Research," *Cambridge Quarterly of Healthcare Ethics* 5 (1996): 334–45.
12. Department of Health and Human Services, Protection of Human Subjects, 46.109(e).
13. Ibid., 46.116.
14. S. A. Grossman et al., "Are Informed Consent Documents That Describe Clinical Oncology Research Protocols Readable by Most Patients and Their Families?" *Journal of Clinical Oncology* 12 (1994): 2211–15.
15. The purpose of a phase 1 oncology study is to determine the maximal tolerated dose of a new chemotherapeutic agent. In contrast, the purpose of a phase 2 oncology study is to determine the activity of the agent against a particular cancer.
16. E. DeRenzo, "Surrogate Decision Making for Severely Cognitively Impaired Research Subjects: The Continuing Debate," *Cambridge Quarterly of Healthcare Ethics* 3 (1994): 539–48.
17. Department of Health and Human Services, Food and Drug Administration, Title 21, Code of Federal Regulation, Part 50: 50.24.
18. M. H. Biros et al., "Informed Consent in Emergency Research: Consensus Statement from the Coalition Conference of Acute Resuscitation and Critical Care Researchers," *JAMA* 273 (1995): 1283–87.
19. D. F. Phillips, "Institutional Review Boards under Stress: Will They Explode or Change?" *JAMA* 276 (1996): 1623–26.

Part III

Critically Ill and Dying Patients

Chapter 24

Ethical Issues in the Use of Fluids and Nutrition: When Can They Be Withdrawn?

T. Patrick Hill

The issue of withholding and withdrawing artificial nutrition and hydration from dying and permanently unconscious patients has become a serious ethical problem in the last 10 years. It helps to measure the gravity of the problem when we remember that between 10,000 and 60,000 dying or permanently unconscious patients are actually maintained on sustenance supplied artificially by tubes.

In the case of one million recovering patients who annually receive artificial nutrition and hydration, no one doubts that artificial sustenance is a boon. But for those patients who, with or without artificially provided sustenance, have no hope of recovering from their illness, supplying nutrition and hydration may be as inappropriate as maintaining a brain-dead body on a ventilator. "Yet, perhaps because of the uniquely symbolic significance of nourishment in the minds of many, artificial feeding appears to be more difficult to discontinue than any other treatment. And this applies both to patients who are expected to die in a relatively short time, and to permanently unconscious and other patients whose death may not occur for months or years unless sustenance by tube is stopped."[1]

Is there something intuitively sound about this symbolism? If so, does it justify the difficulty we feel when we consider discontinuing artificial feeding? Or is it possible on the basis of rational analysis to come to the conclusion that there are indeed sound ethical reasons why we should withhold or withdraw artificial nutrition and hydration? This chapter will attempt to show that in the case of dying and permanently unconscious patients, our intuitive sensitivity to the symbolism of nourishment notwithstanding, there are solid ethical grounds for discontinuing artificial sustenance and permitting death from natural causes to occur.

The ethical questions surrounding the withdrawal of fluids and nutrition from a dying patient are more complicated in one significant respect than the withdrawal of any other life-sustaining treatment, such as antibiotics or cardiopulmonary resuscitation. The basic medical justification for the withdrawal of antibiotics, for example, is that under a particular set of clinical circumstances, they can no longer achieve their clinical purpose. When that happens, the basic ethical justification for withdrawal would come from the absence of any inherent value, again under these particular circumstances, in continuing to provide antibiotics. The ensuing death of the patient is medically acceptable on the grounds that it results from an underlying pathology now no longer considered treatable. The death is ethically acceptable as something that has happened in the natural course of events, in this case, the inevitable progress of a fatal illness over which there is now no human control and for which there is no human responsibility.

Fluids and nutrition used in the care of a dying patient do not fit quite as readily into this line of medical and ethical reasoning. For one thing, they embody the natural instinct to care for the most vulnerable, the dying, when all hope of cure is gone. But they can also serve to draw the distinction between cure and care in the medical setting. There may be a point in the course of illness beyond which medical treatment is useless and can, as a result, be stopped or withheld; it appears counterintuitive to say the same of care. There is no medical justification for ceasing to provide care to a dying patient, and since there is always inherent value in providing care, there is no ethical justification for withholding it either. According to this line of reasoning, as long as fluids and nutrition are seen only as being a means of caring for, not curing, a dying patient, there would be no medical or ethical justification for withholding them in some form or another or in some degree or another.

Consequently, it is of paramount importance to determine if and when fluids and nutrition can be regarded as having a medical purpose in addition to that of providing human care and, beyond that, to determine if and when the provision of fluids and nutrition to a dying patient serves no medical purpose and does not constitute the provision of human care to that patient.

In order to do this, it is necessary to acknowledge the difference between food and drink, on the one hand, and artificial nutrition and hydration, on the other. "The common forms of eating and drinking are not at issue; this is not a matter of denying a person a lunch. At issue here is a range of medical technologies that vary in complexity, sophistication and, at times, danger. Total parenteral feeding is a world apart from dining on fried chicken, and the difference between them is obvious."[2] There is a universal need for food and drink to sustain life. There is no such need for artificial nutrition and hydration to sustain life.

As a universal need, food and drink might best be seen as a means of human care. Artificial nutrition and hydration, however, since they are designed to address a medical condition, such as a temporary or permanent inability to swallow, are better seen as a form of clinical treatment. Consequently, their use and purposes will be determined by the patient's diagnosis and prognosis. Understood this way, according to Devine, artificial nutrition and hydration are an integral part of a larger medical effort to restore someone to health or maintain that person at a certain level of human functioning. But when that effort ceases overall to have a medical purpose, nutrition and hydration, as a constitutive part of the effort, also cease to have any purpose.[3] In other words, just as the purposes of the medical treatment plan for the patient justify the decision to provide nutrition and hydration, so any eventual purposelessness of the same medical treatment plan can justify the cessation of treatment, including nutrition and hydration.

If one is not prepared to accept the clean distinction, as suggested here, between food and drink and nutrition and hydration, one can at least admit that nutrition and hydration may oscillate between being administered for purposes of care and purposes of cure. In that sense, nutrition and hydration can be seen as positioned somewhere on a spectrum that is defined at one end as only a means of curing and at the other end as only a means of caring. As a means of curing, nutrition and hydration are morally neutral in themselves; as a means of caring, they become morally positive in themselves. Consequently, the more they move on this spectrum away from being means of care and toward being means of cure, the more legitimate it can become to withdraw nutrition and hydration when the overall medical plan, of which nutrition and hydration are a part, is suspended on the grounds of medical futility. At that point, alternatives for the purposes of care to deal with the patient's hunger and thirst can be used.

The difference between food and water and nutrition and hydration is then an important consideration when making an ethical decision to withhold the latter. So also is the difference between hunger and thirst and malnutrition and dehydration. A 1987 report by the Hastings Center draws the distinction by describing hunger and thirst as a need felt by the patient and defining malnutrition and dehydration as a chemical condition of the patient's body. "Medical procedures for supplying nutrition and hydration treat malnutrition and dehydration; they may or may not relieve hunger and thirst. Conversely, hunger and thirst can be treated without necessarily using medical nutrition and hydration techniques, and without necessarily correcting dehydration or malnourishment."[4] To support the validity of this distinction, the report observes that dehydrated patients, for example, can find relief from thirst by having their lips and mouths moistened with ice chips or a lubricant.[5] This observation gives additional weight to the argument that hunger and thirst are more appropriately the object of interventions to provide care whereas malnutrition and dehydration are more appropriately the object of interventions to achieve cure.

Once the case has been made for nutrition and hydration as a medical intervention, one can make the assumption that the ethical criteria used in deciding to withdraw other medical life-sustaining treatments are applicable in deciding when to withdraw nutrition and hydration.

The core criterion around which all the others will congregate is the integrity of the patient as a person. Modern medicine operates by isolating symptoms and treating them accordingly. While this discriminating methodology, which undeniably reflects the sophistication of contemporary medical practice, is highly effective, it runs the serious risk of atomizing the patient organ by organ, system by system, particularly as a terminal illness runs its course and the body decompensates as a result. Under these circumstances, it is all too easy to lose sight of the person who is the patient and discount the personal control over treatment decisions without which it will be impossible for these decisions to be ethical.

This entails, on the part of those providing medical treatment, the utmost respect for the physical integrity of the body on which the patient has a fundamental claim. And central to any recognition of the physical integrity of the body as a necessary condition for ethical medical interventions is the patient's informed consent. Hence the need for the patient's consent to be treated and the need to respect the patient's refusal to begin or continue treatment. In other words, it must be a basic working assumption on the part of those responsible for treatment, in this case nutrition and hydration, that they may not withdraw them without the consent of the patient. Even more important, they must recognize that the only source of final authority in the patient-physician relationship is the patient. "Although physicians must often be authoritative about the options available to patients, all involved must recognize that the actual authority over the patient never resides with the physician. Patients alone, or their legal surrogates, have the right to control what happens to them."[6]

All the requirements for an ethically satisfactory decision to withdraw or withhold nutrition and hydration will not be found in the patient's subjective preferences alone, significant as they are. Without direct reference to the clinical context, namely, the actual medical condition of the patient and its projected course, it would be ethically unacceptable to withhold life-sustaining treatment such as nutrition and hydration. Although it is true that ethical decisions are guided by principles, they are also rooted in the actual circumstances that suggest those particular principles and provide the justification for their use in a given case.

This observation is important for the way it illustrates an essential feature of ethical analysis, which, according to one ethicist, "is an exchange between the moral meaning found in the empirical context and the moral meaning found in the several principles contending for application in this concrete case."[7] The moral meaning of the empirical context will be measured in terms of bodily integrity and the extent to which withholding life-sustaining treatment will enhance or diminish that integrity. And as we have already seen, bodily integrity is something to which the patient has a claim and something that the physician must respect.

The next question then is, what is the strength of this claim? How forcefully can the claim to bodily integrity and its corollary, informed consent, be made to justify the decision to withhold or withdraw nutrition and hydration? In responding to this question, ethicists have resorted to the language of rights, saying that bodily integrity is so central to the patient that it can be claimed as a right.

Rights, according to philosophers like Richard Wasserstrom, are "moral commodities" that automatically create obligations and duties.[8] "In other words, a right is a claim, the force of which derives, not from the physical strength or socioeconomic standing of the right holder but the inherent reasonableness of the right being claimed relative to the circumstances under which it is being claimed."[9] Relative to bodily integrity, that would mean a patient's claim to discretion over his or her body. In the context of deciding to withhold or withdraw nutrition and hydration, the implications of such a claim are troublesome because they create obligations and duties for treatment providers. That could and does result in an adversarial situation as the patient or the physician seeks to control the outcome. In turn, that threatens the moral relationship between the patient and the physician presupposed by the patient's claim and the corresponding responsibilities of the physician.

But this problem has less to do with the concept of rights than it has to do with how we understand their function. Understood as a prerogative of the patient alone to be exercised against the physician, the right to bodily integrity can make it very difficult to achieve "the kind of joint decision-making of all the concerned parties that is required by a full theory of moral responsibility."[10] For this reason, philosophers like John Ladd prefer to understand rights as claims to something rather than claims against somebody. A distinct advantage of this interpretation is that it presupposes cooperation rather than competition. Another is that rather than requiring particular obligations of particular individuals, rights entail collective responsibilities on the part of society at large. Ladd therefore refers to rights as ideal and argues that they "relate to things that a society ought to provide for its members so that they will be able to live a good life, that is, a moral life constituted by moral relationships of responsibility and caring."[11]

If we understand the right to bodily integrity as an ideal right on which the decision to withhold nutrition and hydration can be based, thereby permitting the patient to control the circumstances of his or her death, then the manner of the patient's dying becomes a moral enterprise in the same way that the manner of the patient's life has been a moral enterprise. In which case, the decision to withhold or withdraw life-sustaining treatment, such as nutrition and hydration, may constitute the patient's most profound moral need at that stage in life. "As such it will be a necessary means to pursue whatever moral goals have been directing his life up to this point and should now be directing the circumstances and time of his death, if the two are to be consonant."[12]

But rights have a habit of conflicting with other rights, and it is particularly important to understand what this might mean in the present context. The patient's claim to bodily integrity and its corollary, informed consent, in relation to the withdrawal of nutrition and hydration can and does, for example, conflict with society's right to preserve life as an interest central to the integrity of society itself. This conflict lies in one form or another at the heart of the decision to withdraw nutrition and hydration from the patient. As a decision taken in the interests of bodily integrity and informed consent on the part of one individual that leads inevitably to death, it is, potentially at least, a threat to the communal interests society has in the preservation of life in general.

At the same time, both claims can be justified. As a result, neither claim presumably is absolute. It follows then that one or the other claim can only be made legitimately when in doing so the individual does not essentially compromise society and society does not essentially violate the individual. Therefore, any decision on the part of a patient to withdraw nutrition and hydration, if it is to be ethically acceptable, must not constitute a threat to society's legitimate interests in the preservation of life.

The task then becomes one of establishing a working tension between the two claims so that when they do indeed conflict, there is a way to avoid paralysis and achieve a mutually acceptable way of determining which claim, the individual's or society's, should prevail in a given set of circumstances.

In its seminal decision in the case of Karen Ann Quinlan, the New Jersey Supreme Court was acutely conscious of the conflicting claims and of the need to provide a formula by which to resolve the conflict in a way that does justice to both individual and society at the same time. "We think that the State's interests [in the preservation of life] weakens and the individual's right to privacy grows as the degree of bodily invasion increases and the prognosis dims. Ultimately, there comes a point at which the individual's rights overcome the State interest."[13]

In discussing the ethical criteria to be used in withholding nutrition and hydration, this statement is significant in the way it advances self-determination (or privacy, as the court called it) by protecting the bodily integrity from futile medical treatment in the face of an increasingly dim prognosis. Where there is less and less hope that medical interventions will do anything for the well-being of the patient, there is a greater justification, should the patient wish it, to withhold life-sustaining treatment like nutrition and hydration.

So far, this discussion has attempted to lay the ethical foundation for decisions to withhold or withdraw nutrition and hydration from a patient. When either decision is made, the patient will die eventually, raising the question whether such an outcome is, on the face of it, ethically acceptable. In other words, the assumption is that it is not. Thus, if death has occurred as a result of the decision to withhold or withdraw nutrition and hydration, it becomes necessary to show that someone has the right to make that decision. If someone does, what is the basis of that right? And assuming there is some basis for such a right, what circumstances and outcomes would justify its exercise?

The discussion, up to this point, has attempted to show that the individual with the rights to bodily integrity and self-determination would logically be able to exercise those rights by making decisions, for example, to withhold or withdraw medical treatment in general and nutrition and hydration in particular. In drawing the distinction between care and cure in order to show that nutrition and hydration have more to do with the latter, it becomes possible to see that under appropriate circumstances nutrition and hydration, like any other medical treatment, could be the object of such a decision. In other words, the individual is vested with moral authority to make decisions of this kind, and nutrition and hydration fall within the legitimate range of this authority. And even though this moral authority or right is not absolute, conflicting with a state interest in the preservation of life, there are circumstances in which the individual right to self-determination can take precedence over the state interest.

It remains now to look at those circumstances as they appear in the clinical setting. Since nutrition and hydration are to be considered as a medical treatment, the decision to withdraw or withhold them will depend in some measure on whether, given the patient's condition, they can provide sufficient benefit without imposing at the same time a burden disproportionate to that benefit. Too frequently in this context, the discussion of benefits and burdens is conducted in relation to clinical outcomes. Accordingly, the argument goes, when benefits to the patient's well-being are less than the burdens he or she has to suffer to obtain those benefits, decisions to forgo such treatment are ethically acceptable, even when they hasten death as a result. This is a cogent argument as presented in terms of outcomes. But the real strength of the argument is derived from the individual's right to bodily integrity and self-determination. Otherwise, what would justify ethically the opposite decision to start or continue treatment even though its burdens outweigh the benefits?

This is a critical point because on it rests the principle of self-determination and the correct relationship between the patient and the physician and the responsibility of the physician to provide for informed consent or refusal on the part of the patient. Independently of the patient, the physician can determine that, given his or her patient's diagnosis and prognosis, all treatment options entail greater burden than benefit. On the face of it then, withholding or withdrawing treatment can medically be the right thing to do. But this would not be the ethically acceptable thing, at least minus any consideration given to the principle of patient bodily integrity and the principle of self-determination. Neither of these principles can be secure in the absence of consent or refusal from the patient, who realistically can only provide one or the other on the basis of an awareness of the treatment options and a clear grasp of their respective benefits and harms. Therefore, what gives ethical sanction to the outcomes of a decision, in this instance to withdraw nutrition and hydration, is not solely the objective calculation that the burdens of treatment outweigh any benefits. However necessary that calculation is, for ethical purposes it is not sufficient to meet the demands of the bodily integrity and self-determination of the patient. That will come from the patient's consent to or refusal of treatment informed by a calculation of its burden proportionate to the benefits.

We have seen that in this question of withdrawing nutrition and hydration there is a real and legitimate tension between the rights of the individual and the communal interests of the state. There is also a parallel tension between the rights of the patient and the legitimate claims to professional integrity on the part of the treating physician. Arguably, this tension is never as clearly drawn as when decisions to withdraw nutrition and hydration are being considered. The fundamental ethical question is whether physicians should be involved at all? What in the patient-physician relationship could justify such a decision? Is there anything in the nature of this relationship that would sanction, for example, an obligation on the part of physicians to accede to a patient's request to withdraw nutrition and hydration over their better professional judgment?

At stake, from their point of view, are professional obligations to treat the patient in order to further his or her well-being and to avoid doing harm. In this situation, the question for the physician is how, clinically, does withdrawing nutrition and hydration benefit a patient and also avoid doing harm?

Far from being an oxymoron, the question is reasonable in itself and has been made answerable in part as a result of the argument that nutrition and hydration can be considered a medical treatment. As such, they are morally neither good nor bad in themselves so that there can be no presumption that they should or should not be administered. Like the withdrawal of other treatments then, such as chemotherapy in the case of a patient in the terminal stages of cancer, the withdrawal of nutrition and hydration should be subjected, as we have already said, to a calculation of its benefits proportionate to its burdens in order to provide objective medical reasons why withdrawal not only benefits the patient but also does not harm him or her.

Is that possible? One answer to this question is empirical and will tell us what physiologically happens to a patient from whom nutrition and hydration have been withdrawn. The other is ethical and tells us what becomes of the moral standing of the patient from whom this treatment has been withdrawn. Let us consider the empirical answer first. According to Paul C. Rousseau, artificial hydration has long been thought to ease the discomfort of terminal illness.[14] He points out, however, that recent studies suggest something very different:

> As death approaches, dehydration occurs naturally from inadequate oral intake, gastrointestinal and renal losses, and the loss of secretions from the skin and lungs. Transitory thirst, dry mouth and changes in mental status have been found to develop—but the headache, nausea, vomiting or cramps frequently associated with water deprivation rarely occur. The mental changes—while upsetting to relatives—bring relief to patients by lessening their awareness of suffering.[15]

Rousseau adds that while the administration of intravenous fluids may produce a feeling of well-being, that feeling can be of short duration. "In time, artificial hydration is likely to heighten the discomfort of a terminally ill patient, and often exacerbates underlying symptoms."[16]

There is additional clinical evidence in support of the assertion that nutrition and hydration can be harmful to the dying patient. "Tube feeding itself may produce pain; erosions or hemorrhage of the nasal septum, oesophagus, and gastral mucosa have been reported; and nasogastric feeding as well as gastrostomy feeding has been associated with aspiration pneumonia."[17]

With clinical evidence like this, it is reasonable to conclude that "withholding or withdrawing artificial feeding and hydration from debilitated patients does not result in gruesome, cruel, or violent death."[18] Indeed, Rousseau would go further on the basis of his clinical evidence. "Accompanied by comfort measures and emotional support, dehydration is a humane therapeutic response to terminal illness."[19] The Hastings Center guidelines arrive at a similar conclusion: "Patients in their last days before death may spontaneously reduce their intake of nutrition and hydration without experiencing hunger or thirst."[20] As a result, decisions to withhold such treatment can meet the physician's twin obligation to do what is in the patient's best interests and to do no harm to the patient.

As persuasive as this clinical evidence is, are there ethical reasons as persuasive that would justify a physician withdrawing or withholding nutrition and hydration in order to do what is in the patient's best interests and to do no harm to the patient? Essentially, this question is asking what effect the withdrawal of nutrition and hydration has on the moral standing of the patient. If, as some assert, "life is 'the first right of the human person' and 'the condition of all the others,'"[21] what circumstances would justify a decision that would inevitably lead to the death of the patient?

Kevin O'Rourke, a medical ethicist, is addressing the same issue when he asserts that "one of the basic ethical assumptions upon which medicine and efforts to nurse and feed people are based is that life should be prolonged and because living enables us to pursue the purpose of life."[22] Included in the purpose of life are happiness, fulfillment, and human relationships, which, O'Rourke observes, "imply some ability to function at the cognitive-affective, or spiritual, level."[23]

Despite the theological orientation of these two particular assertions, there is nothing in either of them that is not reaffirmed in the traditional presumption in clinical practice, which is to favor life. But implicit in the question under consideration in this chapter is the possibility that now there are clinical circumstances in which the presumption in favor of life is no longer ethically acceptable.

To rephrase the question for purposes of ethical analysis, what becomes of the obligation to prolong life when, despite the continuation of treatment, the patient will remain alive but will not recover sufficiently to be him- or herself physically, mentally, and psychologically? Recover, that is, to resume the central purposes of his or her life knowingly, willingly, and emotionally. That implies at least that, before the obligation to prolong life ceases, there is a level of purposefulness to which the patient ought to be able to lay claim and to obtain which the physician can reasonably continue to treat. But if no such level can be hoped for given the patient's prognosis, we place an impossible burden on the patient by continuing to treat: the expectation of life without, however, the means to appropriate it in any personal sense through mental, volitional, or emotional behavior.

Considered in those terms, there seems ample justification to agree with O'Rourke when he concludes that "if efforts to prolong life are useless or result in a severe burden for the patient insofar as pursuing the purpose of life is concerned, then the ethical obligation to prolong life is no longer present."[24]

This is an ethical argument for withholding or withdrawing nutrition and hydration from the patient and should not be confused with the clinical argument for withholding or withdrawing nutrition and hydration from the patient on the grounds that their use imposes burdens disproportionate to any benefits. But the basis for making this particular ethical argument rests in part on the clinical calculation that the burdens of treatment will outweigh its benefits. The clinical calculation is necessary but not sufficient to make the ethical argument. It is important to draw this distinction if we are to see the real limitations of the arguments based on clinical data alone and at the same time to see how unsatisfactory it is to make principled ethical arguments that are not informed by clinical data.

The distinction illustrates another critical point. Too frequently we consider treatments like nutrition and hydration as though they possessed some moral quotient of their own. It would be more accurate, as suggested earlier, to view them as essentially amoral or ethically neutral. And so, to be realistic, any ethical analysis of nutrition and hydration begins with the consequences of their use rather than with nutrition and hydration themselves. Here, the important point is that modern medical practice, in sustaining life, can and does overreach itself with consequences for which it is directly responsible but concerning which it has no professional ability to determine to be ethically acceptable or unacceptable. Accordingly, from the perspective of the patient receiving such treatment, we can no longer presume that medicine, whatever the intentions of physicians, is a benign exercise, at least as far as its outcomes are concerned. As one commentator has put it, "Doctors now choose from a vast array of interventions that, when combined with effective therapies for underlying conditions, often greatly prolong survival."[25] However, as the evidence of one intensive care unit after another will verify, "the quality of life so skillfully sought can range from marginally tolerable to positively miserable."[26] In other words, the distinction between clinical and ethical reasons for withholding life-sustaining treatment shows that there is a difference between judging a clinical intervention like nutrition and hydration to be medically successful in the quantitative, technical sense and judging it to be personally acceptable in relation to the qualitative needs and preferences of the patient. And because of this difference, it is necessary, when making an ethical argument for withholding nutrition and hydration, to acknowledge that the patient's preferences and underlying values will take precedence.

Any decision, therefore, to withhold life-sustaining treatment, like nutrition and hydration, should be made only after the most careful consideration of the patients' best interests as reflected in their preferences and apart from the clinical outcomes as such (since they do not necessarily coincide, they must always be viewed separately). The natural hesitation we feel in making a decision to withdraw or withhold life-sustaining treatment cannot, however, justify holding the patient hostage to our hesitation on the grounds that its initiation or continuation will be medically successful. Rather, armed with the principles laid out above, we can conclude not only that it is ethically acceptable to withhold or withdraw nutrition and hydration but that it may be the only ethical thing to do in the circumstances examined here.

NOTES

1. "Choice in Dying, Background Paper on Artificial Nutrition and Hydration" (Choice in Dying, New York, September 1990), 1.
2. R. J. Devine, "The Amicus Curiae Brief: Public Policy versus Personal Freedom," *America* (April 8, 1989): 323–34.
3. Ibid., 324.
4. *Guidelines on the Termination of Life-sustaining Treatment and the Care of the Dying* (Briar Cliff Manor, N.Y.: Hastings Center, 1987), 59–60.
5. Ibid., 60.
6. J. E. Ruark, et al., "Initiating and Withdrawing Life Support," *New England Journal of Medicine* 318 (1988): 25–30.
7. D. C. Maquire, *Death by Choice* (Garden City, N.Y.: Image Books, 1984), 82.
8. R. Wasserstrom, "Rights, Human Rights, and Racial Discrimination," in *Human Rights,* ed. A. I. Melden (Belmont, Calif.: Wadsworth, 1970), 99.

9. T. P. Hill, "The Right to Die: Legal and Ethical Consideration," *Southern Medical Journal* 85, no. 8 (1992): 25–57.
10. J. Ladd, "The Definition of Death and the Right to Die," in *Ethical Issues Relating to Life and Death,* ed. J. Ladd (New York: Oxford University Press, 1979), 135.
11. Ibid., 139.
12. Hill, "The Right to Die."
13. In re Quinlan, 70 N.J., 10, 355 A2d 647, at 37.
14. P. C. Rousseau, "How Fluid Deprivation Affects the Terminally Ill," *R.N.* (January 1991): 73–76.
15. Ibid., 73.
16. Ibid., 74.
17. J. C. Ahronheim and M. R. Gasner, "The Sloganism of Starvation," *Lancet* 335 (1990): 279.
18. Ibid.
19. Rousseau, "How Fluid Deprivation Affects the Terminally Ill," 76.
20. *Guidelines on the Termination of Life-Sustaining Treatment,* 60.
21. U.S. Bishops' Committee for Pro-Life Activities, "Nutrition and Hydration: Moral and Pastoral Reflections," *Origins* 21, no. 44 (1992): 705–12.
22. K. O'Rourke, "The AMA Statement on Tube Feeding: An Ethical Analysis," *America* (November 22, 1986): 322.
23. Ibid.
24. Ibid.
25. Ruark et al., "Initiating and Withdrawing Life Support," 25.
26. Ibid.

Chapter 25

Death, Medicine, and the Moral Significance of Family Decision Making

James Lindemann Nelson

It is one of the best known pieces in literature, a staple of undergraduate curricula: *The Death of Ivan Ilych.*[1] Having access to the title, readers know what's going to happen right from the start: As though to eliminate any possible doubt, we watch the unfolding of Ivan's life, character, and relationships in flashback from his obsequies. Ivan himself, of course, is not so advantageously positioned. A good part of the story's drama consists precisely of his coming to understand that his illness is fatal. This task turns out to be complex and difficult, marked by ambivalence, insight, and denial.

Ivan's story offers us a powerful and particular image of what is involved in coming to grips with dying. It stresses the importance of the jobs we have to do as our lives come to a close, and the value of the insights we can then gain. It also offers an equally forceful and vivid image of the place of the family at the end of life, one that highlights the falsity that permeates relationships, and the unreliability of those who are closest to us.

Tolstoy wrote *Ivan Ilych* in 1886. We die differently now, many of us in hospitals, many in the aftermath of some deliberation and choice about using, withholding, or withdrawing therapies. Should a very low birthweight, brain-damaged baby be removed from her ventilator, a step that will end her suffering, but also any chance she has at life? Should an elderly man with "multiple-organ failure" undergo the violence of cardiopulmonary resuscitation if his heart stops, trading a peaceful death for a tiny chance at staying alive long enough to leave the hospital? Contemporary medicine has introduced new complexities into dying, complexities that often force patients and their families into making choices of a sort Ivan did not face. Yet current clinical practice and legal and ethical policy concerning those decisions reflect a very Tolstoyan construction of what's at stake and what's in danger.

The response of Ivan's family to his dying was not notable for its moral insight. This fact is most marked by the translucent curtain of deceit with which his family veils Ivan's descent to death. Ivan is dying, but his dying is a forbidden subject; Ivan in particular must not acknowledge or even allude to it. The terrible consequence is that he must suffer his dying without familial recognition.

> What tormented Ivan Ilych most was the deception, the lie, which for some reason they all accepted, that he was not dying but was simply ill, and that he only need keep quiet and undergo a treatment and then something very good would result . . . this deception tortured him—their not wishing to admit what they all knew and what he

---

Source: Reprinted with permission from J. L. Nelson, Death, Medicine, and the Moral Significance of Family Decision Making, *Michigan Family Review,* Vol. 1, © 1995.

> knew, but wanting to lie to him concerning his terrible condition and wishing and forcing him to participate in that lie.[2]

In this chapter, I pose a counterimage to Tolstoy, in two parts. My leading idea will be that our most intimate connections—which is what I will take "family" to mean here—will often have very important constructive roles to play in the tasks we face as our lives come to a close. But I will also underscore the fact that families are often deeply involved in those tasks and significantly affected by how they are discharged. Accordingly I will argue that families ought to have some say in how pertinent choices are made. Both these considerations should enrich and help direct our policy concerning end-of-life decision making.

THE STANDARD APPROACH: ROMANTICIZING DEATH, DEMONIZING FAMILIES

We enjoy a considerable measure of social consensus that treatment too burdensome for the benefits it promises may be withheld or withdrawn—even if rejection of treatment is tantamount to acceptance of death. This consensus was perhaps most clearly flagged by the Supreme Court's decision in Cruzan vs. Missouri Department of Health,[3] which upheld a patient's right to decide against life-sustaining therapy. There has also been wide agreement that such decisions are solely authorized by the principle of patient autonomy; that is, the moral claim that people enjoy a certain kind of sovereignty over what interventions in their bodies are consistent with their values, and which are not.[4]

This consensus has a certain instability packed in it. Economic pressures and a reassertion of the autonomy of health care professionals have led some to think that life-prolonging health care can in principle be withheld despite patient/family desires, if it is expensive enough,[5] or withdrawn over patient/family objection, if the odds of it working are low enough.[6] But the major practical problem with the patient sovereignty view has been that when people are sick enough to require decision making of this kind, they are often too sick to make any decisions at all. For the past few decades, states have been experimenting with different means of extending a person's decision-making authority regarding health care, a movement culminating in the federal Patient Self-determination Act of 1990, which mandates that all patients be informed of the procedures approved by their state for directing their health care even if they should become incapacitated.

Practically speaking, what this boils down to is allowing other people to convey a patient's treatment preferences if the patient cannot exercise this authority in his or her own voice at the time a decision is required. Others might assist in the interpretation of "living wills," or more generally, written treatment directives, which are often both vague and ambiguous. They may simply make a decision as the patient's proxy, trying to judge as the patient would have judged. But in either case, the interpreter or proxy decision maker enjoys the position by virtue of relationship to the will of the patient: either because the proxy had been explicitly delegated to fill these roles, or in the absence of an explicit declaration made by the patient, because he or she is assumed to be able to transmit or reproduce the patient's preferences better than anyone else.

The natural assumption is that close relatives will typically be in the best position to decide. But there is an equally natural objection: Family members hardly count as disinterested parties. Because of their very closeness, relatives often have a sizable stake in how treatment decisions go, and if their interests influence the decision making, the orthodoxy regards the process as morally contaminated.

This "standard approach" to end-of-life decision making shares the suspicion about intimates found in Tolstoy's depiction of Ivan's decidedly nasty family, in which those who have some kind of relationship to the dying man—his wife and adult daughter—don't love him, and those who do—which is to say, his young son—seem to be permitted no relationship to him. Our thinking about end-of-life decision making, particularly concerning patients who cannot make decisions on their own behalf, seems to be haunted by specters closely resembling Ivan's wife and daughter, who saw him largely as a means to fulfilling their own desires. Therefore, judgments about starting or stopping life-sustaining therapy are carefully guarded to prevent such manipulation of vulnerable people.

Family members, then, have no standing simply as family members, but only as conduits to the preferences that the patient actually had, or would have had. If their interests influence whether medical treatment of various kinds continues or not, then the patient is at great risk of abuse: either suffering the continual burdens of invasive care for an inadequate goal, or forgoing desired care and with it the chance to extend life.

In fact, the picture for families is even darker. Not only are their motives suspect; it turns out that even their readings of the patient's desires are questionable. Recent studies of proxy decision making have indicated that families are, as it turns out, not very good at guessing the preferences of their relatives when it comes to the end of life.[7] In the standard view, then, their main claim to decision-making authority is undermined, while the main caution against them seems as strong as ever.

The picture for incompetent patients also appears grimmer than has yet been suggested. What they have at stake is not simply the possibility of undergoing extended discomfort or premature death because their families are either mistaken about their preferences or malignantly indifferent to them. Equally significant is the loss of the ability to invest their deaths with the kind of meaning that best comports with their sense of their life overall. Ivan Ilych provides us with a hint of this theme. Recall his painful examination of his life, his insight into how misdirected and trivial he had allowed his life to become, and how his final task is to accept himself, and his suffering, and hence to achieve salvation.

The idea that there is often a "terminal perspective" on life, from which we can get an especially accurate view of our lives, and the idea that how we end our lives is crucial to the success or failure of those lives overall, strike me as at least loosely linked. Together they make up what might be called a romantic view of death, clearly present in Tolstoy, and not at all foreign to contemporary sensibilities. Consider this passage from *Life's Dominion,* the most recent book of the influential philosopher and legal scholar, Ronald Dworkin:

> There is no doubt that most people treat the manner of their deaths as of special, symbolic importance: they want their deaths, if possible, to express and in that way vividly to confirm the values they believe most important to their lives.[8]

Whether or not Dworkin is right about "most people" on this point, he is, I think, surely right about what most ethical and legal theorists think when they take up the issue of how choices should be made at the end of life. We find here another significant reason why our evolving policy on this matter has, since the 1970s, been directed toward empowering patients. It isn't simply to defend them from assaults on what Dworkin would call their "experiential"[9] interests, or how things feel to them: It is also to protect their ability to live and die in accordance with their "critical" interests; that is, with their reflective sense of what is truly significant and characteristic about their lives. How we die is of particular significance to whether or not our critical interest in having lived a good life is achieved, and it is crucial to our achieving such a life that our deaths be as much as possible orchestrated according to our own ideas.

A REVISED ACCOUNT: DYING IN INTIMACY

The contemporary context of decision making in the face of death, then, is in very important respects much the same as it was in the late nineteenth century. We are cynical about families, romantic about death. What's wrong with this standard "Tolstoyan" concept of the significance of death and the suspicious character of families? In my view, pretty much everything.

This is not to say that there are no abusive and otherwise untrustworthy families out there. Nor is it to deny that for some people the process of dying is transformative, offering new and deep insights. Finally, I am not implacably hostile to the idea that the way we die can be crucial to the success or otherwise of our lives overall. Rather, my attitude toward all these claims is that they are all overstated; they ought not to be taken as the predominating feature of either families or death. Many have families who are not decidedly nasty; many die without gaining deep insights into the nature of things; many can have bad deaths who had quite acceptable lives overall; many have good deaths that are not good because they, personally or through carefully directed proxies, have orchestrated every step. And the worst of the overstatement is what might be regarded as its cumulative implication: We face death alone most often as "vulnerable adults" whose chief need is protection from rapacious relatives.

General practice, as opposed to policy and theory, indicates that my misgivings about this tableau are not idiosyncratic. Relatively few people avail themselves of formal advance directives, despite the publicity given to the importance of advance health-care planning; the few who do draw up such directives tend to be disproportionately white, well-off, and well-educated. While there are many possible explanations here, one plausible suggestion is that different subcultures within our nation have different views about how important it is to take a direct hand in end-of-life decision making.

Part of the problem may be that medical practice and legal policy regarding death correctly assume that most people want to die well, but that both practice and policy are confused about what dying well means to many of us. Doing something "well" does not necessarily mean doing it according to our own self-regarding desires; it may mean acting in accord with what strikes us as right, seemly, meet—where these notions guide us in ways that we believe to be good in themselves, and not simply because we happen to accept them. More particularly, many of us may believe that our deaths should cohere with a life lived in important connection with other people. The course of our dying should express concern about their burdens, not because doing so is the crucial task of our lives, nor because death has vouchsafed to us some special moral insight at the end, but because such concern is consistent with long-held views about how to live well, views that need not be abandoned when the job at hand is how to die well.

Not simply speculation, data, drawn largely from the work of High[10] show that many people feel no need to file a formal document because they think of their families as their advance directives. The Harvard-based medical ethicists Linda and Ezekiel Emanuel[11] have wondered whether High's results don't simply reflect most people's uncritical acceptance of the view that families know best what we ourselves would want, and that this enthusiasm for relatives would not survive the growing evidence to the contrary. But their critique makes two crucial assumptions. First, it assumes that the kind of medical choices that are open to us as we die are typically such that we have considered preferences about them, preferences expressing something that matters to us deeply. It also assumes, perhaps even more significantly, that our choices rule the day, however they might affect the interests of those with whom we have been intimate.

But both these assumptions seem unwarranted. The Michigan law professor Patricia White, drawing on her experience in the presumably less emotionally charged area of estate planning, has pointed out that "people find it difficult to predict accurately how they would react to some hypothetical future crisis."[12] The idea, then, that the job of a proxy decision maker is to somehow elicit just what the patient would have wanted if the patient could speak in the present situation assumes that there is some one thing he or she would have wanted, and this assumption may well be false.

One of course could simply make determinations about one's future care, rather than predictions. That is, the decision maker would be exerting her autonomy now, reflecting her current preferences, rather than making a guess about what she would want in a future in which she is incapacitated, if, contrary to fact, she could make a considered decision at that time. But if we are to understand advance decision making as a determination rather than as a prediction, then it isn't clear that decision making at the end of life retains the kind of special moral significance the romantic perspective gave it. Dying "romantically"—i.e., in a way that reflects something crucially important about your life—might well require, not a blunt determination now of how a future event should be handled, but fine-grained sensitivity to the details of that future time. How much pain or discomfort is at issue? What are the chances that a medical intervention will achieve its end, at what cost to the patient or to others the patient cares about? It is not implausible that making decisions of this kind could, in principle, allow the decision maker an opportunity to express and even develop her moral character. But, if so, what would allow her this opportunity is the ability to fit her decision precisely to the circumstances.

The result is that it is far from clear that all, or even many, of the preferences healthy self-aware people have about hypothetical future crises really count as considered or authoritative in any event. And we have yet to consider the point that, even if we assume incompetent patients typically have well-considered and well-ordered preferences that others might put into practice, the interests of their families remain morally relevant to decision making even if those interests run counter to patient preferences.

As John Hardwig[13] has powerfully argued, there is no good reason to think that the ill are totally excused from their moral obligations to their intimates simply because of their illness. Nor is it appropriate to think that family members are required to bear any imaginable burden to further any interest of a relative if that interest happens to be medical. Not a plea to endorse selfishness, the standard approach to decision making at the end of life proceeds as though selfishness were the appropriate standard: The patient's needs must be served, and the only way to assure they are met is to forbid family members to think of anything other than what the patient would. But families quite often have a different way of organizing the distribution of caring work that goes on within them. Sometimes that organization may be open to moral criticism—as when women are assigned an unequal share of caring labor simply because they are women—but the very fact that they distribute the family's resources in a way that is sensitive to many needs ought not to be regarded as beyond the moral pale simply on its face. Maintaining that proxy decision making by family members is to be censured is particularly ironic in the present context of health care delivery, in which the medical interests of patients are sometimes subordinated to the needs of the health maintenance organization in which they are enrolled, or the resources their state is willing to make available for Medicaid.

It is on the basis of considerations of this sort that I think that Ivan Ilych's sort of death ought to be seen as unusual—fit to be the subject of an immortal short story—rather than as a good guide to what challenges and choices will regularly face people as they die. We needn't construct a policy that assumes families are to be carefully controlled, suspected of guilt until proven innocent. We needn't think that putting our own stamp on the precise character of our death is a crucial determinant of the quality of our lives. Therefore, we needn't be so enamored of systems that rely primarily on explicit advance directives, seeing their authority as stemming solely from the patient and, in effect, disadvantaging the many patients and families without advance directives to whom death will come. It seems to me both more realistic, as well as quite defensible morally, to reverse the burden of proof here: We ought to recognize that families have a certain kind of moral authority to serve as proxies, unless perhaps the patient has made an explicit declaration to the contrary, or unless that authority is misused to a point that constitutes abuse.

But this strategy is only part of what should be an overall rethinking of the contexts in which we die, and the assumptions that are prevalent in those contexts—assumptions that tend to undermine the kind of closeness that very ill patients can have with their families. Health care institutions should be set up to be as transparent as possible to these connections, not now the case. Hospitals, for example, remain places in which certain value commitments are evident and powerful: They are hierarchical, unfamiliar places that separate you from daily routines and common sources of identity affirmation, running all the way from your own clothes to your most intimate connections. Hospitals have their own, clear agenda, to which patients are strongly invited to subscribe. The notion that patients need to be empowered in such settings is exactly right; the mistake is in thinking this is likely to happen if patients are allowed to be alienated from their own sources of personal affirmation and authority in the name of giving such authority formal protection.

CONCLUSION: AN OBJECTION AND A REPLY

It might be alleged that, the institutional structure of health care systems apart, the system of deciding currently in place for incapacitated people is actually very well suited to accommodate just the values sketched out here. Many people have families in which there are people whom they trust. Many people don't think it essential that their death reflect precisely what their own decisions would have been, had they been able to make them directly. Such people can easily execute advance directives that say, in effect, "My spouse gets to decide any feature of my medical care, if I am not able to do so." For those people who either do not trust their families, or do not wish to burden them with the task of making end-of-life decisions, appointing nonfamily proxies will be possible. For people who think that it is crucial that the circumstances of their deaths as closely as possible fit some overriding concept of the integrity of their lives, more specific treatment directives are possible. What really gets left out of the standard view?

This very reasonable question has a pragmatic answer, to which I have already alluded, and a rather deeper answer. The pragmatic response is simply that the majority of people will, for the foreseeable future, die without a formal advance directive. At the very least, this fact suggests that we pay more attention to how to make health care decisions for this group of people, and the most reasonable response would seem to be a system of proxies arranged in descending order of priority: spouse, adult children, parents, siblings, and so on. This system would certainly not be without problems—for instance, understanding what "spouse" means in a society where people often live together without formal marriage—but it would at least have the right scope and the right slant. Individuals who felt uncomfortable with the ordering or wanted to leave specific instructions to their proxies would be within their rights to execute specific directives to change it.

The deeper reason is that the standard approach is not neutral among different views of what a person owes to his or her family, or more broadly, of the nature of intimate connections. It contains a certain expressive force suggesting that our intimate ties are insignificant unless formalized by an explicit exercise of our own sovereign authority. This view is neither self-evidently true, nor altogether innocuous with regard to its impact on how we think about family ties generally in this society. Rereading *Ivan Ilych* reminds us that skepticism about the family is not a new phenomenon, but should not distract us from the distinct possibility that new forms of defensiveness about intimate connections can make things worse, as well as better.

NOTES

1. L. Tolstoy, *The Death of Ivan Ilych and Other Stories,* trans. Alymer Maude (1866; reprint, New York: New American Library, 1960).
2. Ibid., 137.
3. *Cruzan v. Director,* Missouri Department of Health, (1990) 110 Ct. 2841.
4. R. Faden and T. Beauchamp, *A History and Theory of Informed Consent* (New York: Oxford University Press, 1986); A. Buchanan and D. Brock, *Deciding for Others* (Cambridge: Cambridge University Press, 1989).
5. L. Fleck, "Just Health Care Rationing: A Democratic Decision Making Approach," *University of Pennsylvania Law Review* 140 (1992): 1597–1636.
6. T. Tomlinson and H. Brody, "Futility and the Ethics of Resuscitation," *JAMA* 264 (1990): 849–60.
7. A. Seckler et al., "Substituted Judgment: How Accurate Are Proxy Predictions?" *Annals of Internal Medicine* 151 (1991): 1276–80; E. Emanuel and L. Emanuel, "Proxy Decision Making: An Ethical and Empirical Analysis," *JAMA* 267 (1992): 2067–71.
8. R. Dworkin, *Life's Dominion* (New York: Knopf, 1993), 211.
9. Ibid.
10. D. High, "All in the Family: Extended Autonomy and Expectations in Surrogate Health Care Decision Making," *Gerontologist* 28 (1988): 46–51; *id.,* "Why Are Elderly People Not Using Advance Directives?" *Journal of Aging and Health* 5 (1993): 497–515; *id.,* "Families' Roles in Advance Directives," *Hastings Center Report* 24 (Special suppl. 1994): 516–18.
11. Emanuel and Emanuel, "Proxy Decision Making."
12. P. White, "Appointing a Proxy under the Best of Circumstances," *Utah Law Review* (1992): 849–60.
13. J. Hardwig, "What about the Family?" *Hastings Center Report* 20 (1990): 5–10.

Chapter 26

Care of the Hopelessly Ill: Proposed Clinical Criteria for Physician-Assisted Suicide

Timothy E. Quill, Christine K. Cassel, and Diane E. Meier

One of medicine's most important purposes is to allow hopelessly ill persons to die with as much comfort, control, and dignity as possible. The philosophy and techniques of comfort care provide a humane alternative to more traditional, curative medical approaches in helping patients achieve this end.[1] Yet there remain instances in which incurably ill patients suffer intolerably before death despite comprehensive efforts to provide comfort. Some of these patients would rather die than continue to live under the conditions imposed by their illness, and a few request assistance from their physicians.

The patients who ask us to face such predicaments do not fall into simple diagnostic categories. Until recently, their problems have been relatively unacknowledged and unexplored by the medical profession, so little is objectively known about the spectrum and prevalence of such requests or about the range of physicians' responses.[2] Yet each request can be compelling. Consider the following patients: a former athlete, weighing 80 lb (36 kg) after an eight-year struggle with acquired immune deficiency syndrome (AIDS), who is losing his sight and his memory and is terrified of AIDS dementia; a mother of seven children, continually exhausted and bed-bound at home with a gaping, foul-smelling, open wound in her abdomen, who can no longer eat and who no longer wants to fight ovarian cancer; a fiercely independent retired factory worker, quadriplegic from amyotrophic lateral sclerosis, who no longer wants to linger in a helpless, dependent state waiting and hoping for death; a writer with extensive bone metastases from lung cancer that has not responded to chemotherapy or radiation, who cannot accept the daily choice he must make between sedation and severe pain; and a physician colleague, dying of respiratory failure from progressive pulmonary fibrosis, who does not want to be maintained on a ventilator but is equally terrified of suffocation. Like the story of "Diane," which has been told in more detail,[3] there are personal stories of courage and grief for each of these patients that force us to take very seriously their requests for a physician's assistance in dying.

Our purpose is to propose clinical criteria that would allow physicians to respond to requests for assisted suicide from their competent, incurably ill patients. We support the legalization of such suicide, but not of active euthanasia. We believe this position permits the best balance between a humane response to the requests of patients like those described above and the need to protect other vulnerable people. We strongly advocate intensive, unrestrained care intended to provide comfort for all incurably ill persons.[4] When properly applied, such comfort care should result in a tolerable death, with symptoms relatively well controlled, for most

Source: Reprinted from *The New England Journal of Medicine*, Vol. 327, No. 19, pp. 1380–1384, Copyright 1992, Massachusetts Medical Society. All rights reserved.

patients. Physician-assisted suicide should never be contemplated as a substitute for comprehensive comfort care or for working with patients to resolve the physical, personal, and social challenges posed by the process of dying.[5] Yet it is not idiosyncratic, selfish, or indicative of a psychiatric disorder for people with an incurable illness to want some control over how they die. The idea of a noble, dignified death, with a meaning that is deeply personal and unique, is exalted in great literature, poetry, art, and music.[6] When an incurably ill patient asks for help in achieving such a death, we believe physicians have an obligation to explore the request fully and, under specified circumstances, carefully to consider making an exception to the prohibition against assisting with a suicide.

PHYSICIAN-ASSISTED SUICIDE

For a physician, assisting with suicide entails making a means of suicide (such as a prescription for barbiturates) available to a patient who is otherwise physically capable of suicide and who subsequently acts on his or her own. Physician-assisted suicide is distinguished from voluntary euthanasia, in which the physician not only makes the means available but, at the patient's request, also serves as the actual agent of death. Whereas active euthanasia is illegal throughout the United States, only 36 states have laws explicitly prohibiting assisted suicide.[7] In every situation in which a physician has compassionately helped a terminally ill person to commit suicide, criminal charges have been dismissed or a verdict of not guilty has been brought[8] (and L. Gostin, personal communication). Although the prospect of successful prosecution may be remote, the risk of an expensive, publicized professional and legal inquiry would be prohibitive for most physicians and would certainly keep the practice covert among those who participate.

It is not known how widespread physician-assisted suicide currently is in the United States, or how frequently patients' requests are turned down by physicians. Approximately 6,000 deaths per day in the United States are said to be in some way planned or indirectly assisted,[9] probably through the "double effect" of pain-relieving medications that may at the same time hasten death[10] or the discontinuation of or failure to start potentially life-prolonging treatments. From 3 to 37 percent of physicians responding to anonymous surveys reported secretly taking active steps to hasten a patient's death, but these survey data were flawed by low response rates and poor design.[11] Every public-opinion survey taken over the past 40 years has shown support by a majority of Americans for the idea of physician-assisted death for the terminally ill.[12] A referendum with loosely defined safeguards that would have legalized both voluntary euthanasia and assisted suicide was narrowly defeated in Washington State in 1991,[13] and more conservatively drawn initiatives are currently on the ballot in California, before the legislature in New Hampshire, and under consideration in Florida and Oregon.

A POLICY PROPOSAL

Although physician-assisted suicide and voluntary euthanasia both involve the active facilitation of a wished-for death, there are several important distinctions between them.[14] In assisted suicide, the final act is solely the patient's, and the risk of subtle coercion from doctors, family members, institutions, or other social forces is greatly reduced.[15] The balance of power between doctor and patient is more nearly equal in physician-assisted suicide than in euthanasia. The physician is counselor and witness and makes the means available, but ultimately the patient must be the one to act or not act. In voluntary euthanasia, the physician both provides the means and carries out the final act, with greatly amplified power over the patient and an increased risk of error, coercion, or abuse.

In view of these distinctions, we conclude that legalization of physician-assisted suicide, but not of voluntary euthanasia, is the policy best able to respond to patients' needs and to protect vulnerable people. From this perspective, physician-assisted suicide forms part of the continuum of options for comfort care, beginning with the forgoing of life-sustaining therapy, including more aggressive symptom-relieving measures, and permitting physician-assisted suicide only if all other alternatives have failed and all criteria have been met. Active voluntary euthanasia is excluded from this continuum because of the risk of abuse it presents. We recognize that this exclusion is made at a cost to competent, incurably ill patients who cannot swallow or move and who therefore cannot be helped to die by assisted suicide. Such persons, who meet agreed-on criteria in other respects, must not be abandoned to their suffering; a combination of decisions to forgo life-sustaining treatments (including food and fluids) with aggressive comfort measures (such as analgesics and sedatives) could be offered, along with a commitment to search for creative alternatives. We acknowledge that this solution is less than ideal, but we also recognize that in the United States access to medical care is currently too inequitable, and many doctor-patient relationships too impersonal, for us to tolerate the risks of permitting active voluntary euthanasia. We must monitor any change in public policy in this domain to evaluate both its benefits and its burdens.

We propose the following clinical guidelines to contribute to serious discussion about physician-assisted suicide. Although we favor a reconsideration of the legal and professional prohibitions in the case of patients who meet carefully defined criteria, we do not wish to promote an easy or impersonal process.[16] If we are to consider allowing incurably ill patients more control over their deaths, it must be as an expression of our compassion and concern about their ultimate fate after all other alternatives have been exhausted. Such patients should not be held hostage to our reluctance or inability to forge policies in this difficult area.

PROPOSED CLINICAL CRITERIA FOR PHYSICIAN-ASSISTED SUICIDE

Because assisted suicide is extraordinary and irreversible treatment, the patient's primary physician must ensure that the following conditions are clearly satisfied before proceeding. First, the patient must have a condition that is incurable and associated with severe, unrelenting suffering. The patient must understand the condition, the prognosis, and the types of comfort care available as alternatives. Although most patients making this request will be near death, we acknowledge the inexactness of such prognostications[17] and do not want to exclude arbitrarily persons with incurable, but not imminently terminal, progressive illnesses, such as amyotrophic lateral sclerosis or multiple sclerosis. When there is considerable uncertainty about the patient's medical condition or prognosis, a second opinion or opinions should be sought and the uncertainty clarified as much as possible before a final decision about the patient's request is made.

Second, the physician must ensure that the patient's suffering and the request are not the result of inadequate comfort care. All reasonable comfort-oriented measures must at least have been considered, and preferably have been tried, before the means for a physician-assisted suicide are provided. Physician-assisted suicide must never be used to circumvent the struggle to provide comprehensive care or find acceptable alternatives. The physician's prospective willingness to provide assisted suicide is a legitimate and important subject to discuss if the patient raises the question, since many patients will probably find the possibility of an escape from suffering more important than the reality.

Third, the patient must clearly and repeatedly, of his or her own free will and initiative, request to die rather than continue suffering. The physician should understand thoroughly what continued life means to the patient and why death appears preferable. A physician's too-ready acceptance of a patient's request could be perceived as encouragement to commit suicide, yet it is important not to force the patient to "beg" for assistance. Understanding the patient's desire to die and being certain that the request is serious are critical steps to evaluating the patient's rationality and ensuring that all alternative means of relieving suffering have been adequately explored. Any sign of ambivalence or uncertainty on the part of the patient should abort the process, because a clear, convincing, and continuous desire for an end of suffering through death is a strict requirement to proceed. Requests for assisted suicide made in an advance directive or by a health care surrogate should not be honored.

Fourth, the physician must be sure that the patient's judgment is not distorted. The patient must be capable of understanding the decision and its implications. The presence of depression is relevant if it is distorting rational decision making and is reversible in a way that would substantially alter the situation. Expert psychiatric evaluation should be sought when the primary physician is inexperienced in the diagnosis and treatment of depression, or when there is uncertainty about the rationality of the request or the presence of a reversible mental disorder the treatment of which would substantially change the patient's perception of his or her condition.[18]

Fifth, physician-assisted suicide should be carried out only in the context of a meaningful doctor-patient relationship. Ideally, the physician should have witnessed the patient's previous illness and suffering. There may not always be a pre–existing relationship, but the physician must get to know the patient personally in order to understand fully the reasons for the request. The physician must understand why the patient considers death to be the best of a limited number of very unfortunate options. The primary physician must personally confirm that each of the criteria has been met. The patient should have no doubt that the physician is committed to finding alternative solutions if at any moment the patient's mind changes. Rather than create a new subspecialty focused on death,[19] assistance in suicide should be given by the same physician who has been struggling with the patient to provide comfort care, and who will stand by the patient and provide care until the time of death, no matter what path is taken.[20]

No physician should be forced to assist a patient in suicide if it violates the physician's fundamental values, although the patient's personal physician should think seriously before turning down such a request. Should a transfer of care be necessary, the personal physician should help the patient find another, more receptive primary physician.

Sixth, consultation with another experienced physician is required to ensure that the patient's request is voluntary and rational, the diagnosis and prognosis accurate, and the exploration of comfort-oriented alternatives thorough. The consulting physician should review the supporting materials and should interview and examine the patient.

Finally, clear documentation to support each condition is required. A system must be developed for reporting, reviewing, and studying such deaths and clearly distinguishing them from other forms of suicide. The patient, the primary physician, and the consultant must each sign a consent form. A physician-assisted suicide must neither invalidate insurance policies nor lead to an investigation by the medical examiner or an unwanted autopsy. The primary physician, the medical consultant, and the family must be assured that if the conditions agreed on are satisfied in good faith, they will be free from criminal prosecution for having assisted the patient to die.

Informing family members is strongly recommended, but whom to involve and inform should be left to the discretion and control of the patient. Similarly, spiritual counseling should be offered, depending on the patient's background and beliefs. Ideally, close family members should be an integral part of the decision-making process and should understand and support the patient's decision. If there is a major dispute between the family and the patient about how to proceed, it may require the involvement of an ethics committee or even of the courts. It is to be hoped, however, that most of these painful decisions can be worked through directly by the patient, the family, and health care providers. Under no circumstances should the family's wishes and requests override those of a competent patient.

THE METHOD

In physician-assisted suicide, a lethal amount of medication is usually prescribed that the patient then ingests. Since this process has been largely covert and unstudied, little is known about which methods are the most humane and effective. If there is a change in policy, there must be an open sharing of information within the profession, and a careful analysis of effectiveness. The methods selected should be reliable and should not add to the patient's suffering. We must also provide support and careful monitoring for the patients, physicians, and families affected, since the emotional and social effects are largely unknown but are undoubtedly far-reaching.

Assistance with suicide is one of the most profound and meaningful requests a patient can make of a physician. If the patient and the physician agree that there are no acceptable alternatives and that all the required conditions have been met, the lethal medication should ideally be taken in the physician's presence. Unless the patient specifically requests it, he or she should not be left alone at the time of death. In addition to the personal physician, other health care providers and family members should be encouraged to be present, as the patient wishes. It is of the utmost importance not to abandon the patient at this critical moment. The time before a controlled death can provide an opportunity for a rich and meaningful goodbye among family members, health care providers, and the patient. For this reason, we must be sure that any policies and laws enacted to allow assisted suicide do not require that the patient be left alone at the moment of death in order for the assisters to be safe from prosecution.

BALANCING RISKS AND BENEFITS

There is an intensifying debate within and outside the medical profession about the physician's appropriate role in assisting dying.[21] Although most agree that there are exceptional circumstances in which death is preferable to intolerable suffering, the case against both physician-assisted suicide and voluntary euthanasia is based mainly on the implications for public policy and the potential effect on the moral integrity of the medical profession.[22] The "slippery slope" argument asserts that permissive policies would inevitably lead to subtle coercion of the powerless to choose death rather than become burdens to society or their families. Access to health care in the United States is extraordinarily variable, often impersonal, and subject to intense pressures for cost containment. It may be dangerous to license physicians to take life in this unstable environment. It is also suggested that comfort care, skillfully applied, could provide a tolerable and dignified death for most persons and that physicians would have less incentive to become more proficient at providing such care if the option of a quick, controlled death were too readily available. Finally, some believe that physician-assisted death, no matter how noble and pure its intentions, could destroy the identity of the medical profession and its central ethos, protecting the sanctity of life. The question before policy makers, physicians, and voters is whether criteria such as those we have outlined here safeguard patients adequately against these risks.

The risks and burdens of continuing with the current prohibitions have been less clearly articulated in the literature.[23] The most pressing problem is the potential abandonment of competent, incurably ill patients who yearn for death despite comprehensive comfort care. These patients may be disintegrating physically and emotionally, but death is not imminent. They have often fought heroic medical battles only to find themselves in this final condition. Those who have witnessed difficult deaths in hospice programs are not reassured by the glib assertion that we can always make death tolerable, and patients fear that physicians will abandon them if their course becomes difficult or overwhelming in the face of comfort care. In fact, there is no empirical evidence that all physical suffering associated with incurable illness can be effectively relieved. In addition, the most frightening aspect of death for many is not physical pain, but the prospect of losing control and independence and of dying in an undignified, unesthetic, absurd, and existentially unacceptable condition.

Physicians who respond to requests for assisted suicide from such patients do so at substantial professional and legal peril, often acting in secret without the benefit of consultation or support from colleagues. This covert practice discourages open and honest communication among physicians, their colleagues, and their dying patients. Decisions often depend more on the physician's values and willingness to take risks than on the compelling nature of the patient's request. There may be more risk of abuse and idiosyncratic decision making with such secret practices than with a more open, carefully defined practice. Finally, terminally ill patients who do choose to take their lives often die alone so as not to place their families or caregivers in legal jeopardy.[24]

CONCLUSION

Given current professional and legal prohibitions, physicians find themselves in a difficult position when they receive requests for assisted suicide from suffering patients who have exhausted the usefulness of measures for comfort care. To adhere to the letter of the law, they must turn down their patients' requests even if they find them reasonable and personally acceptable. If they accede to their patients' requests, they must risk violating legal and professional standards, and therefore they act in isolation and in secret collaboration with their patients. We believe that there is more risk for vulnerable patients and for the integrity of the profession in such hidden practices, however well intended, than there would be in a more open process restricted to competent patients who met carefully defined criteria. The medical and legal professions must collaborate if we are to create public policy that fully acknowledges irreversible suffering and offers dying patients a broader range of options to explore with their physicians.

NOTES

1. S. H. Wanzer et al., "The Physician's Responsibility toward Hopelessly Ill Patients," *New England Journal of Medicine* 310 (1984): 955–59; S. H. Wanzer et al., "The Physician's Responsibility toward Hopelessly Ill Patients: A Second Look," *New England Journal of Medicine* 320 (1989): 844–49; American Medical Association, Council on Ethical and Judicial Affairs, "Decisions near the End of Life," *JAMA* 267 (1992): 369–72; J. Rhymes, "Hospice Care in America," *JAMA* 264 (1990): 369–72; L. Broadfield, "Evaluation of Palliative Care: Current Status and Future Directions," *Journal of Palliative Care* 4, no. 3 (1988): 21–28; K. A. Wallston et al., "Comparing the Quality of Death for Hospice and Non-hospice Cancer Patients," *Medical Care* 26 (1988): 177–82.
2. National Hemlock Society, *1987 Survey of California Physicians Regarding Voluntary Active Euthanasia for the Terminally Ill* (Los Angeles: Hemlock Society, 1988); Center for Health Ethics and Policy, *Withholding and Withdrawing Life-sustaining Treatment: A Survey of Opinions and Experiences of Colorado Physicians* (Denver: University of Colorado Graduate School of Public Affairs, 1988); S. Helig, "The SFMS Euthanasia Survey: Results and Analysis," *San Francisco Medicine* (May 1988): 24–26, 34; M. Overmyer, "National Survey: Physicians' Views on the Right to Die," *Physicians Manage* 31, no. 7 (1991): 40–45.
3. T. E. Quill, "Death and Dignity: A Case of Individualized Decision Making," *New England Journal of Medicine* 324 (1991): 691–94.
4. Wanzer et al., "The Physician's Responsibility toward Hopelessly Ill Patients"; Wanzer et al., "The Physician's Responsibility toward Hopelessly Ill Patients: A Second Look"; American Medical Association, Council on Ethical and Judicial Affairs, "Decisions near the End of Life"; Rhymes, "Hospice Care in America"; Broadfield, "Evaluation of Palliative Care"; Wallston et al., "Comparing the Quality of Death for Hospice and Non-hospice Cancer Patients."
5. D. E. Meier and C. K. Cassel, "Euthanasia in Old Age: A Case Study of Ethical Analysis," *Journal of the American Geriatric Society* 31 (1983): 294–98.
6. P. Aries, *The Hour of Our Death* (New York: Vintage, 1982).
7. S. A. Newman, "Euthanasia Orchestrating 'the Last Syllable of . . . Time,' " *University of Pittsburgh Law Review* 53 (1991): 153–91; L. H. Glantz, "Withholding and Withdrawing Treatment: The Role of the Criminal Law," *Law, Medicine and Health Care* 15 (1987–1988): 231–41.
8. Newman, "Euthanasia Orchestrating 'the Last Syllable of . . . Time' "; Glantz, "Withholding and Withdrawing Treatment."
9. A. Malcolm, "Giving Death a Hand: Rending Issue," *New York Times*, 14 June 1990, A6.
10. American Medical Association, Council on Ethical and Judicial Affairs, "Decisions near the End of Life"; Meier and Cassel, "Euthanasia in Old Age."

11. National Hemlock Society, *1987 Survey of California Physicians Regarding Voluntary Active Euthanasia for the Terminally Ill*; Center for Health Ethics and Policy, *Withholding and Withdrawing Life-sustaining Treatment;* Helig, "The SFMS Euthanasia Survey"; Overmyer, "National Survey."
12. Malcolm, "Giving Death a Hand"; T. Gest, "Changing the Rules on Dying," *U.S. News and World Report*, 9 July 1990, 22–24; Hemlock Society, *1990 Roper Poll on Physician Aid-in-Dying, Allowing Nancy Cruzan to Die, and Physicians Obeying the Living Will* (New York: Roper Organization, 1991); Hemlock Society, *1991 Roper Poll of the West Coast on Euthanasia* (New York: Roper Organization, 1991).
13. R. I. Misbin, "Physicians' Aid in Dying," *New England Journal of Medicine* 325 (1991): 1307–11.
14. R. F. Weir, "The Morality of Physician-assisted Suicide," *Law, Medicine and Health Care* 20 (1992): 116–26.
15. J. Glover, *Causing Death and Saving Lives* (New York: Penguin, 1977), 182–89.
16. N. S. Jecker, "Giving Death a Hand: When the Dying and the Doctor Stand in a Special Relationship," *Journal of the American Geriatric Society* 39 (1991): 831–35.
17. R. M. Poses et al., "The Answer to 'What Are My Chances, Doctor?' Depend on Whom Is Asked: Prognostic Disagreement and Inaccuracy for Critically Ill Patients," *Critical Care Medicine* 17 (1989): 827–33; M. E. Charlson, "Studies of Prognosis: Progress and Pitfalls," *Journal of General Internal Medicine* 2 (1987): 359–61; R. S. Schonwetter et al., "Estimation of Survival Time in Terminal Cancer Patients: An Impedance to Hospital Admissions?" *Hospice Journal* 6 (1990): 65–79.
18. Y. Conwell and E. D. Caine, "Rational Suicide and the Right to Die: Reality and Myth," *New England Journal of Medicine* 325 (1991): 1100–03.
19. G. I. Benrubi, "Euthanasia: The Need for Procedural Safeguards," *New England Journal of Medicine* 326 (1992): 197–99.
20. Jecker, "Giving Death a Hand."
21. American Medical Association, Council on Ethical and Judicial Affairs, "Decisions near the End of Life"; Weir, "The Morality of Physician-assisted Suicide"; C. K. Cassel and D. E. Meier, "Morals and Moralism in the Debate over Euthanasia and Assisted Suicide," *New England Journal of Medicine* 323 (1990): 750–52; W. Reichel and A. J. Dyck, "Euthanasia: A Contemporary Moral Quandary," *Lancet* 2 (1989), 1321–23; M. Angell, "Euthanasia," *New England Journal of Medicine* 319 (1988): 1348–50; J. Rachels, "Active and Passive Euthanasia," *New England Journal of Medicine* 292 (1975): 78–80; J. Lachs, "Humane Treatment and the Treatment of Humans," *New England Journal of Medicine* 294 (1976): 838–40; P. J. van der Maas, "Euthanasia and Other Medical Decisions Concerning the End of Life," *Lancet* 338 (1991): 669–74; P. A. Singer and M. Siegler, "Euthanasia: A Critique," *New England Journal of Medicine* 322 (1990): 1881–83; D. Orentlicher, "Physician Participation in Assisted Suicide," *JAMA* 262 (1989): 1844–45; S. M. Wolf, "Holding the Line on Euthanasia," *Hastings Center Report* 19, no. 1, suppl. (1989): 13–15; W. Gaylin et al., "Doctors Must Not Kill," *JAMA* 259 (1988): 2139–40; K. L. Vaux, "Debbie's Dying: Mercy Killing and the Good Death," *JAMA* 259 (1988): 2140–41; C. F. Gomez, *Regulating Death: Euthanasia and the Case of the Netherlands* (New York: The Free Press, 1991); D. Brahams, "Euthanasia in the Netherlands," *Lancet* 335 (1990): 591–92; H. J. J. Leenen, "Coma Patients in the Netherlands," *British Medical Journal* 300 (1990): 69.
22. Singer and Siegler, "Euthanasia"; Orentlicher, "Physician Participation in Assisted Suicide"; Wolf, "Holding the Line on Euthanasia"; Gaylin et al., "Doctors Must Not Kill"; Vaux, "Debbie's Dying"; Gomez, *Regulating Death*; Brahams, "Euthanasia in the Netherlands"; Leenen, "Coma Patients in the Netherlands."
23. Weir, "The Morality of Physician-assisted Suicide"; Cassel and Meier, "Morals and Moralism in the Debate over Euthanasia and Assisted Suicide"; Reichel and Dyck, "Euthanasia"; Angell, "Euthanasia"; Rachels, "Active and Passive Euthanasia"; Lachs, "Humane Treatment and the Treatment of Humans"; van der Maas, "Euthanasia and Other Medical Decisions Concerning the End of Life."
24. Quill, "Death and Dignity."

CHAPTER 27

Ethical Issues Concerning Physician-Assisted Death

Barbara Supanich and Howard Brody

INTRODUCTION AND KEY DEFINITIONS

Physician-assisted death is a very challenging issue for United States society, which is in many ways ambivalent about death and the process of dying. Movies, TV serials about doctors, the evening news showing us film footage of wars and famines as we eat our evening meal—all sterilize the death experience and at times make it surreal and unreal. In contrast are the poignant experiences of our own personal and professional lives that teach us the realities of death and dying—patients, relatives, and friends who have died from acquired immune deficiency syndrome (AIDS), heart disease, cancer, or traumatic injuries. It is in this societal, professional, and personal milieu that we ask questions about *how* people die and *how they decide* the context of their dying process.

Although various faith traditions and other ethical guidelines, including the American Medical Association Council on Ethical and Judicial Affairs, prohibit assisted suicide and active euthanasia, public-opinion polls show that United States society is sharply divided on these topics. It is important that physicians and health care providers understand the issues and the surrounding controversies. In this chapter, we will review some of the major ethical arguments, propose clinical strategies for responding to a patient's request for death assistance, and finally discuss the broader context necessary for a deeper understanding of the challenge of assisted death.

Before proceeding, we need to clarify some basic definitions and distinctions.

Assisted suicide refers to the patient's intentionally and willfully ending his or her own life, with the assistance of a third party. This assistance may include different levels of involvement—merely providing information about how to commit suicide; providing the means to commit suicide, such as a lethal quantity of pills; or actively participating in the suicide, such as being present at the scene and inserting an intravenous line through which the patient may then administer a lethal dose.[1] The widely publicized actions of Drs. Timothy Quill[2] and Jack Kevorkian[3] provide examples of the second and third levels of involvement respectively.

In **voluntary active euthanasia,** patients freely choose to have a lethal agent directly administered to them by another individual, with a merciful intent. As practiced in the Netherlands, this might involve the physician's injecting intravenously a quick-acting sedative followed by a paralytic agent to halt respiration.

Assisted death is the term we will use in the remainder of the chapter to refer jointly to the practices of voluntary active euthanasia and assisted suicide. Most of the ethics literature has focused on the special problems of the physician's role; and so we will most commonly refer to **physician-assisted death.** However, in intensive care units (ICUs), in hospice settings, and in nursing homes, as well as in the homes of people who choose to die in their own homes, the roles of other health care professionals and the family are extremely important. In many of these settings, patients may actually request assistance in dying from one or more of these individuals as well as (or instead of) from the physician.

It is also important to be clear about what is *not* assisted death. It is *not* an assisted death if a competent person decides not to initiate a specific therapy (e.g., antibiotics for a pneumonia or other septic process, artificial nutrition and hydration, further cardiac medications); nor is it assisted death to withdraw any of these options from a patient. The use of high doses of opioids, where the intent is to relieve pain and not to hasten death, is *not* physician-assisted death. While many still believe that high-dose opioids pose a serious risk of fatal respiratory depression, palliative specialists know that this very seldom occurs with proper titration of analgesic doses, even when very large doses of opioids are administered in terminal illness.[4] Even in the rare case in which respiratory depression is a foreseen (but unintended) consequence of adequate analgesia, administering the analgesics is not considered physician-assisted death. (If, however, the true intent is to cause or hasten death, and analgesia is merely a ruse or a rationalization, then we would classify the case as assisted death.)[5]

Withholding and withdrawing life-sustaining treatment is widely accepted today both in ethics and law as appropriate and compassionate care, provided that the competent patient is fully informed and freely chooses that management option. There are some philosophers, notably Rachels,[6] who have argued that there is no morally relevant difference between this practice and the practice of assisted death. In this chapter, without giving detailed arguments, we will dissent from this view. That is, we will leave open the question of whether assisted death is morally justifiable and will discuss the arguments on both sides of the issue. But we will assume that if assisted death can be justified, it must be justified on its own merits, and not merely because it shares some of the same moral features with the relatively uncontroversial practice of withdrawing and withholding life-sustaining treatment.[7]

ETHICAL ARGUMENTS

Patient Integrity and Autonomy

When patients with terminal illnesses come to see their primary physicians, there are multiple issues on their minds—personal image, ability to maintain control over treatment decisions (including pain management and other treatment issues), family dynamics, personal values and potential conflicts with family and/or physician(s), deeper reflections about their life goals and how they want to continue living life. Patients want to be able to have conversations about life and the effects that the illness is having on it with their physicians in an open and supportive atmosphere. It is in this type of an atmosphere that patients will be more apt to discuss their concerns and fears about their dying process and options for management of that process, including assisted death.[8]

Those supporting assisted death claim that they are honoring patient integrity by being willing to have conversations with their patients that are open to discussing *all* treatment options with the patient (and his or her family members, if so desired by the patient) including assisted death. In support of patient integrity and autonomy, proponents argue that only the patient knows what constitutes a harm, and so may decide that continued life with severe interminable suffering is a greater harm than assisted death.[9]

Opponents claim that patient autonomy is not the supreme moral value and is insufficient to justify choosing assisted death. They understand autonomy as a valid moral value in treatment decisions regarding the withdrawal or withholding of life-sustaining treatments, because in those situations we are respecting personal bodily integrity. But they do not extend the justification to include a right to demand that others take specific actions to end one's life.

Compassionate Response to Suffering

Proponents of assisted death are supportive of efforts to improve pain control and symptom management by physicians and other health care professionals; however, they argue that there still remain cases in which the best palliative care measures are insufficient to relieve these patients' suffering. They argue along with Quill and others[10] that a willingness to discuss the option of assisted death with the patient may often act as a suicide preventive because, during this open conversation, the physician may be able to alleviate the patient's fears and misunderstandings and propose other viable alternatives.[11] Alternatively, if patients do not feel that such a conversation is an option with the physician, they may choose to commit suicide in a manner that is more traumatic for themselves and their families and friends.

In contrast, opponents remind us that suffering is a multifaceted dimension of human existence. Suffering, in their view, is intimately tied to the individual's values, belief system, and sense of meaning. Therefore, at the end of life, suffering is related to one's unique sense of who one is as a person, and how one experiences an illness in the overall context of one's life journey and personal expectations for the future.[12] To relieve suffering, then, by eliminating the sufferer is always unacceptable. Opponents would argue for physicians and others to more competently attend to issues of loneliness, fear of death, depression, forgiveness, unresolved family and personal conflicts, and anger and hopelessness. This is challenging work for the health care professional but ultimately will allow for a richer personal resolution. Attending to these issues is important for another reason—a person may make an assisted death request when the physician or family member is suffering from similar inner turmoil. Rather than actively listen to the reasons and concerns behind the patient's request, the physician or family member may project his or her own suffering onto the patient's request and wrongly conclude that a premature death is a merciful choice for this patient.[13]

Safeguards and the Slippery Slope

Persons on both sides of this issue agree that a policy of assisted death would pose a danger to patients and to society and that some physicians might abuse this option at the end of life.[14] Table 27–1 lists some safeguards and guidelines commonly proposed by supporters of assisted death.[15]

Proponents argue that these safeguards and guidelines create the structure needed for the appropriate conversations between the patient and the physician regarding treatment plans for control of the patient's pain and suffering. These conversations create the rapport and trust necessary for a truly healing relationship. Proponents strongly support recommendations for a consultation from another physician and that there be clear and accurate documentation that all of the guidelines have been followed. Adherence to these guidelines, proponents argue, would

Table 27–1 Safeguards and Guidelines for a Policy of Assisted Death

- The patient must have a condition that is incurable (not necessarily terminal) and is associated with severe suffering without hope of relief.
- All reasonable comfort-oriented measures must have been considered or tried.
- The patient must express a clear and repeated request to die that is not coerced (e.g., emotionally or financially).
- The physician must ensure that the patient's judgment is not "distorted," that is, the patient is competent to make rational treatment choices.
- Physician-assisted death must be carried out only in the context of a meaningful physician-patient relationship.
- Consultation must be obtained from another physician to ensure that the patient's request is rational and voluntary.
- There must be clear documentation that the previous six steps have been taken, and a system of reporting, reviewing, and studying such deaths must be established.

adequately guard against the slippery slope that opponents fear.

Opponents believe that the slippery slope is a much more serious concern. Once the legal protections against physician-assisted death are weakened or dissolved, society will lose interest in protecting the vulnerable against physicians' making inappropriate decisions to hasten death. Given the pressures of cost containment and biases toward vulnerable populations such as individuals who test positive for the human immunodeficiency virus (HIV), minorities, and the disabled, there is also concern that once the legal constraints are lifted, physicians may feel *obligated* to provide assisted death.[16]

Opponents view guidelines and safeguards as, at best, a well-intentioned but inadequate protection against these powerful social forces leading to inevitable abuse; and at worst, a hypocritical facade erected by proponents to win over public opinion. They are concerned that when doctors start providing the means of death for their patients that this will erode the patient-physician relationship. Since physicians would be tempted to choose a like-minded physician to serve as a consultant, second opinions provide dubious safety; nor could any documentation system ensure that physicians would be consistent and compassionate and that patients would be truly safeguarded.[17]

The debate over safeguards and the slippery slope is brought into sharp focus by differing interpretations of the Dutch experience. Proponents point to the Netherlands' history of legally permitted assisted death to support their claim that abuses are minimal and are identified and contained when they occur.[18] Opponents view the Dutch experience as confirming our worst fears of the slippery slope.[19]

Professional Integrity

Opponents of physician-assisted death equate professional integrity with the physician's role as a healer and so view physician-assisted death as antithetical to the basic role and moral integrity of a physician. Physicians, in their view, are to use their knowledge and skills for healing, restoring, and relieving suffering when possible and to offer comfort always, but never to kill.[20] Similar arguments of integrity have been made in the literature for other health care professionals, including nurses and pharmacists.[21]

Many proponents would argue that opponents have narrowly restricted the definition of physician integrity to a very traditional understanding of "healing." They would argue for an expanded understanding of professional integrity to include relief of suffering, respect for the patient's voluntary choices, and aiding patients to achieve a peaceful and dignified death. For proponents, an exception to the general prohibition against physician-assisted death would be a patient who despite excellent palliative care measures is still having unremitting suffering and has made repeated voluntary requests to his or her physician for death assistance. In such a narrowly defined case, a physician of integrity could respond affirmatively to the patient's request, if such an action was not in conflict with the physician's personal moral or religious convictions.[22]

Substituted Judgment

The slippery slope argument also raises concerns about extending physician-assisted death to incompetent patients. At the present time, proposals for physician-assisted death specifically exclude the option of choosing physician-assisted death by an advance directive. Opponents, however, fear that if a legal right to assisted death is ever accepted, death assistance for now-incompetent patients by advance directive would be a logical and unavoidable extension of any such right.[23] A 1996 United States Court of Appeals ruling stated that patients have a constitutional right to physician-assisted death, and left open the possibility that such a right might be exercised by a surrogate on behalf of an incompetent patient. The final decision by the United States Supreme Court has been made: a patient does not have a "right to die."[24]

CLINICAL MANAGEMENT OF REQUESTS FOR ASSISTED DEATH

As outlined above, the ethical debate over assisted death seems as intractable as the abortion debate. One might conclude that proponents and opponents would therefore disagree radically about actual management of individual patients and could not possibly work cooperatively in team settings.

We contend, however, that the irresolvability of the theoretical debate masks a broad area of practical convergence. Note, after all, that opponents do not favor merely abandoning the terminally ill to whatever pain and suffering befalls them. Nor do proponents favor assisted death as the *first* choice for any terminally ill patient. Both share a strong commitment to trying as hard as possible to relieve the patient's distress to the extent that the patient no longer wishes to die—proponents, so that they can be sure that assisted death is truly a last resort; and opponents, because they believe that such efforts will ultimately remove any serious demands for assisted death. Moreover, neither believe that health professionals should be required to participate in any activity that is against their personal moral or religious convictions.

Table 27–2 outlines suggested steps for the clinical management of a request for assisted death. Some scrutiny of these steps will show that most can be followed equally by physicians who support and who oppose the assisted-death option.

Table 27–2 Suggested Steps for the Clinical Management of a Request for Assisted Death

- The provider should listen to the request for assisted death in an open and sympathetic manner and evaluate the issues underlying the request.
- Providers should share their personal stance with patients in an open and professional manner, always assuring patients that they will be supported throughout this personal decision-making process.
- All providers should take appropriate steps to process their personal emotional reactions to the patient's request, e.g., hospice-team meetings.
- The provider should have a continuing dialogue with the patient and appropriate family members or support persons concerning the development and implementation of the therapeutic treatment plans, including a request for assisted death, in a manner that is consistent with the provider's moral values and belief system.

Listen Openly and Evaluate Underlying Issues

Patients demonstrate both courage and trust when they verbalize a request for assisted death to the primary physician. The physician may have strong personal feelings triggered by such a request but should not allow those feelings to derail the necessary conversations with the patient over the ensuing days, weeks, or months. The physician should avoid imposing personal values, but through multiple supportive conversations with the patient should determine the crucial issues. It is important to let the patient know that he or she is not alone, among those facing terminal illness, to consider assisted death as a personal option. It is also important for the physician to convey to the patient that he or she is honored that the patient is confiding in him or her and is prepared for honest discussions with the patient about the option of assisted death.

Both the physician and the patient need to seek out support for themselves as they ponder such a significant decision. The patient may want to discuss the request with other family members, other members of the health care team, clergy, or a close friend. Physicians should not isolate themselves when they are presented with such a request and also should seek out supportive persons in their personal and professional lives to assist them as they reflect on the implications of such requests.

Physicians need to make every effort to understand the reasons that motivate such a request from the patient and respond appropriately with the information and support that the patient needs. For some patients, this may mean addressing issues of loss of dignity, depression, and feelings of intense loneliness; psychological counseling would be an appropriate intervention. Others may have a desire for more information about their disease or specific issues related to the "how" of their dying process. Some patients may have concerns about how their illness affects their family and friends; a social-worker consult might be helpful. Still others may have deep spiritual issues that this illness has brought into sharper focus for them; an appropriate referral to their religious or spiritual mentor would be a critical next step. As one can see from these brief examples, an initial request for assisted death, when approached with active listening and sensitivity to the patient's underlying issues, is always more complex than one initially anticipates and requires repeated conversations to ensure that the request is both enduring and consistent with the patient's life values and goals.

Share Personal Stance with the Patient

It is premature to allow the physician's personal stance on assisted death to derail the deep and careful inquiry into the patient's issues and needs. But physicians are obliged to be truthful and honest with patients regarding *all* aspects of their treatment options, and therefore the next step is to let the patient know what the physician's stance is on the issue of assisted death.

Physicians who morally oppose physician-assisted death should couple refusal to provide this with an assurance that they will stand with the patient until the moment of death and will exhaustively search out all appropriate treatment options to ameliorate the patient's suffering. The physician should stress the importance of continuing the dialogue about the patient's perceptions of his or her suffering, so that they can explore mutually acceptable solutions. Finally, it is important to let the patient know that although the idea of assisted death is morally objectionable to the physician, the person making the request is not.

The physician who is morally willing to be actively involved in assisted death needs to inform the patient of the required procedure for confirming that the patient is making a voluntary and thoughtful choice and that the patient's suffering cannot be relieved by other accepted means. The actual amount of time to make such determinations varies and needs to be negotiated with the patient. The physician should also inform the patient that in most cases of this sort, other interventions can improve the quality of life and remove the need for death assistance and that he or she will try hard to identify such interventions.

At this stage, an occasional patient will break off the dialogue—either because the patient demands assisted death and the physician is not willing to provide it, or because he or she feels entitled to this assistance without going through a long process of exploring alternatives. A few such patients may end up committing suicide without the physician's assistance, perhaps in a way that causes great suffering for both the patient and the survivors. While such outcomes are tragic, they do not, in our view, count as an argument against the stepwise approach. Safeguards will count for nothing if patients are allowed, in effect, to use a threat of suicide by other means as emotional blackmail to get the physician to circumvent the process. In such cases, the physician's obligation to act out of professional integrity takes priority over any rights or wishes of the patient.

Assure Adequate Comfort Care

There are several reports in the literature that document physicians' and other health care providers' poor knowledge about pain control[25] and other comfort measures at the end of life. When a patient makes a request for death assistance, therefore, it behooves the physician to ensure that all reasonable comfort measures have been discussed with the patient and given a trial.

Most patients have concerns and fears about suffering—primarily the fear that they will have unremitting pain and no hope for relief. Frequent discussions with the patient about the multiple techniques available for increasing comfort will help to alleviate such fears. Patients also have concerns about loneliness, abandonment, unresolved family or other personal conflicts, and changed body image and/or personal-identity issues. Spiritual counseling can help to restore a sense of meaning and hope for patients in the context of their life's values and beliefs. Many persons have found that the use of narrative, oral or written, is very comforting and can facilitate restoring meaning and hope for the patient at this point in the life journey. We encourage patients to engage in telling or writing stories about their illness, about their hopes for survival, and about the life events and encounters that have deepened their sense of meaning and core life values.

Assure Voluntariness and Reasonableness of Request

Physicians need to understand the nature of the patient's request and ensure that it is a clear, uncoerced, patient-initiated decision. It is important for the physician to be certain that the patient's request is a serious one, that the patient has seriously considered alternatives and has rejected them for rational reasons, and that the patient has not made the decision for death assistance during a despondent period of the illness. Quill et al.[26] appropriately emphasize that any sign of ambivalence or uncertainty on the part of the patient should abort the process, and that the patient's desire for death must be strong, continuous, clear, and convincing.

Just as important, the physician must be assured that the patient's judgment is based on a clear and accurate understanding of the facts of his or her case and that the patient understands the implications of his or her decision for assisted death. Frequent and compassionate discussions with the patient will facilitate a better understanding of the reasons for the request and ascertain the perseverance of the request by the physician. The physician must be especially alert for signs of depression, which could interfere with judgment as well as add to the patient's suffering. Consultation with a skilled psychiatrist may be essential if there is any suspicion of depression; and in some cases a trial of antidepressant therapy with a rapidly acting drug might be essential before acceding to a request for death assistance.

We agree with Quill and others that patients should be strongly encouraged to share the decision with their family members. Of course, this decision should never be forced on the patients, and they should be able to choose whom to involve and inform as well as when to share the decision with the family. The primary physician can often function as a facilitator in the discussions between the patient and family members when there are conflicting concerns and opinions.

PLACING THE DEBATE IN CONTEXT

The apparent intractability of the assisted-death debate has done more than obscure the broad area of consensus around optimal patient care. By reducing the debate to the fairly technical level of "should we or shouldn't we?" it has tended to distract us from broader social and spiritual questions. Unless we address those questions, we will be unable to comprehend why our society and our health care system is having this particular debate now and why it has assumed the apparently intractable character that it has.

A critical question is whether physicians view their professional obligation to be primarily biomedical or whether they include in that obligation the importance of understanding the life journey and story of their patients. If they choose the latter, then they will probably describe their profession as one of promoting health and wellness and of sojourning with their patients through all of life, including the final journey of the dying process. Persons who have this viewpoint do not describe death as the enemy but rather, as a part of life. Medicine would once and for all accept death as a limit that cannot be overcome and use that limit as an indispensable focal point in thinking about illness and disease.[27] Medicine would change its focus from fighting death at all costs to helping each person live life to its fullest potential.

A key issue often lost in the current intellectual and legal debate is the critical need to improve the quality of care and support for dying patients throughout our health care system. Our own estimate from the current debate is that only about 3 percent of patients who might request assisted death have symptoms that are not remediable by current therapeutic options. This means that proponents and opponents of assisted death agree fully on what should be done to help 97 percent of all patients; and yet the best available evidence is that far too many of that 97 percent are poorly served by our present system. Health care professionals in particular have an obligation to provide leadership in reforming the culture of the health system to be more responsive to the needs of terminally ill patients and their families, including better pain management and better coordination of care.

Many see the assisted-death debate as rooted in unrealistic expectations of what technology can offer in the management of disease and the belief that there is a technological cure available for everyone somewhere in the United States. It is a moral obligation of health care providers to help all of our patients seek a balance between the technological imperative and the "pursuit of a peaceful death" as described by Daniel Callahan.[28] It is Callahan's observation that the technological imperative for some patients and their physicians becomes oppressive and serves "to make our dying all the more problematic: harder to predict, more difficult to manage, the source of more moral dilemmas and nasty choices, and spiritually more productive of anguish, ambivalence and uncertainty."[29]

Merely saying that we accept the inevitability of death does not necessarily free us from the seductive power of the technological solution. For some, the "technical fix" might be the "suicide machine"; for some, it is the hope that ideal hospice care will allay all suffering and put an end to all requests for death assistance. Both positions, in our view, represent failures to grapple with the meaning of suffering and death at the deeper cultural and spiritual level.

Because physician-assisted death is an issue with serious personal and societal implications, we strongly encourage continuing dialogue on this issue in as many societal arenas as possible. Within this dialogue, the physician-patient conversation is primary but not exclusive. Since we are communal by our very nature, discussions about life and death demand that we go beyond the individual context and force us to contemplate what it means to live together as a compassionate society.

NOTES

1. D. T. Watts and T. Howell, "Assisted Suicide Is Not Voluntary Active Euthanasia," *J. Am. Geriat. Soc.* 40 (1992): 1043.
2. T. Quill, "Death and Dignity: A Case of Individualized Decision Making," *NEJM* 324 (1991): 691.
3. J. Kevorkian, *Prescription: Medicide: The Goodness of Planned Death* (Buffalo, N.Y.: Prometheus Books, 1991); G. Annas, "Physician-Assisted Suicide: Michigan's Temporary Solution," *NEJM* 328 (1993): 1573.
4. W. C. Wilson et al., "Ordering and Administration of Sedatives and Analgesics during the Withholding and Withdrawal of Life Support from Critically Ill Patients," *JAMA* 267 (1992): 949.
5. H. Brody, "Commentary on Billings and Block's 'Slow Euthanasia,' " *J. Palliat. Care* 12 (1996): 38–41.
6. J. Rachels, *The End of Life: Euthanasia and Morality* (New York: Oxford University Press, 1986).
7. G. Annas, "Death by Prescription: The Oregon Initiative," *NEJM* 331 (1994): 1240; D. Callahan, "Pursuing a Peaceful Death," *Hastings Center Report* (July/August 1993): 33; Euthanasia: California Proposition 161; New York: Commonweal Foundation (September 1992; Special Supplement): 1–16; E. J. Emanuel, "The History of Euthanasia Debates in the United States and Britain," *Ann. Intern. Med.* 121 (1994): 793.
8. J. Peteet, "Treating Patients Who Request Assisted Suicide," *Arc. Fam. Med.* 3 (1994): 723; B. Ferrel and M. Rhiner, "High-Tech Comfort: Ethical Issues in Cancer Pain Management for the 1990s," *J. of Clinical Ethics* (Summer 1991): 108; D. Steinmetz et al., "Family Physician's Involvement with Dying Patients and Their Families," *Arch. Fam. Med.* 2 (1993): 753.
9. M. Battin, "Voluntary Euthanasia and the Risks of Abuse: Can We Learn Anything from the Netherlands?" *Law. Med. Health Care* 20, no. 1–2 (Spring–Summer 1992): 133; J. Davies, "Altruism towards the End of Life," *J. Med. Ethics* 19 (1993): 111.
10. T. Quill et al., "Care of the Hopelessly Ill: Proposed Clinical Criteria for Physician-Assisted Suicide," (Sounding Board), *NEJM* 327 (1992): 1380; H. Brody, "Assisted Death: A Compassionate Response to a

Medical Failure," *NEJM* 327 (1992): 1384; T. E. Quill, *Death and Dignity: Making Choices and Taking Charge* (New York: W.W. Norton, 1993).

11. T. Quill, "Doctor, I Want to Die, Will You Help Me?" *JAMA* 270 (1993): 870.
12. E. J. Cassell, "The Nature of Suffering and the Goals of Medicine," *NEJM* 306 (1982): 639; *id., The Nature of Suffering and the Goals of Medicine* (New York: Oxford University Press, 1991).
13. S. Miles, "Physicians and Their Patients' Suicides." *JAMA* 27 (1994): 1786.
14. Battin, "Voluntary Euthanasia and the Risks of Abuse"; Quill et al., "Care of the Hopelessly Ill"; F. Miller et al. "Regulating Physician-Assisted Death," *NEJM* 31 (1994): 119; R. F. Weir, "The Morality of Physician-Assisted Suicide," *Law. Med. Health Care* 20 (Spring–Summer 1992): 116.
15. Quill et al., "Care of the Hopelessly Ill"; Miller et al., "Regulating Physician-Assisted Death."
16. C. S. Campbell, "'Aid-in-Dying' and the Taking of Human Life," *J. Med. Ethics* 18 (1992): 128.
17. D. Callahan and M. White, "The Legalization of Physician-Assisted Suicide: Creating a Regulatory Potemkin Village," *University of Richmond Law Review* 30 (1996): 1–83.
18. G. Van de Wal et al., "Euthanasia and Assisted Suicide, 1: How Often Is It Practised by Family Doctors in the Netherlands?" *Fam. Pract.* 9 (1992): 130–34; G. Van der Wal et al., "Euthanasia and Assisted Suicide, 2: Do Dutch Family Doctors Act Prudently?" *Fam. Pract.* 9 (1992): 135–40; *Position Statement* (Gainesville, Fl.: Academy of Hospice Physicians, 1988); *Statement Opposing the Legalization of Euthanasia and Assisted Suicide* (Arlington, Va.: National Hospice Organization, 1989).
19. Quill et al., "Care of the Hopelessly Ill"; Miller et al., "Regulating Physician-Assisted Death"; G. Van der Wal, and R. J. Dillmann, "Euthanasia in the Netherlands," *BMJ* 308 (May 1994): 1346; Van der Wal et al., "Euthanasia and Assisted Suicide, 1"; *id.,* "Euthanasia and Assisted Suicide, 2."
20. W. Gaylin et al., "Doctors Must Not Kill," *JAMA* 259 (1988): 2139; L. R. Kass, "Neither for Love nor Money: Why Doctors Must Not Kill," *The Public Interest* 94 (Winter 1989): 25.
21. C. S. Campbell et al., "Conflicts of Conscience: Hospice and Assisted Suicide," *Hastings Center Report* 25 (1995): 36; A. Haddad, "Physician-Assisted Suicide: The Impact on Nursing and Pharmacy," *Of Value* (Society for Health and Human Values Newsletter) (December 1994); M. T. Rupp and H. L. Isenhower, "Pharmacists' Attitudes toward Physician-Assisted Suicide," *Am. J. Hosp. Pharm.* 51 (1994): 69; A. Young and D. Volker, "Oncology Nurses' Attitudes Regarding Voluntary, Physician-Assisted Dying for Competent, Terminally Ill Patients," *Oncol. Nurse Forum* 20 (1993): 445; S. Kowalski, "Assisted Suicide: Where Do Nurses Draw the Line?" *Nurse Health Care* 14 (1993): 70.
22. F. G. Miller and H. Brody, "Professional Integrity and Physician-Assisted Death," *Hastings Center Report* 25 (1995): 8.
23. Euthanasia: California Proposition 161; New York: Commonweal Foundation; D. Callahan, "'Aid in Dying': The Social Dimensions," *Commonweal* (Supplement, 9 August 1991): 12.
24. Supreme Court, June 1997.
25. "Pain Management: Theological and Ethical Principles Governing the Use of Pain Relief for Dying Patients." *Health Progress* (January/February 1993): 30; Ferrel and Rhiner, "High-Tech Comfort"; Management of Cancer Pain Guidelines Panel, *Management of Cancer Pain,* Clinical Practice Guidelines no. 9 (Rockville, Md.: Agency for Health Care Policy and Research, 1994).
26. Quill et al., "Care of the Hopelessly Ill."
27. Callahan, "Pursuing a Peaceful Death."
28. Ibid.
29. Ibid., 33.

CHAPTER 28

Euthanasia: The Way We Do It, the Way They Do It

Margaret P. Battin

INTRODUCTION

Because we tend to be rather myopic in our discussions of death and dying, especially about the issues of active euthanasia and assisted suicide, it is valuable to place the question of how we go about dying in an international context. We do not always see that our own cultural norms may be quite different from those of other nations and that our background assumptions and actual practices differ dramatically. Thus, I would like to examine the perspectives on end-of-life dilemmas in three countries: The Netherlands, Germany, and the United States.

The Netherlands, Germany, and the United States are all advanced industrial democracies. They all have sophisticated medical establishments and life expectancies over 70 years of age; their populations are all characterized by an increasing proportion of older persons. They are all in what has been called the fourth stage of the epidemiologic transition[1]—that stage of societal development in which it is no longer the case that most people die of acute parasitic or infectious diseases. In this stage, most people do not die of diseases with rapid, unpredictable onsets and sharp fatality curves; rather, the majority of the population—as much as perhaps 70–80 percent—die of degenerative diseases, especially delayed-degenerative diseases that are characterized by late, slow onset and extended decline. Most people in highly industrialized countries die from cancer; atherosclerosis; heart disease (by no means always suddenly fatal); chronic obstructive pulmonary disease; liver, kidney, or other organ disease; or degenerative neurological disorders; they die not so much from attack by outside diseases but from gradual disintegration. Thus, all three of these countries are alike in facing a common problem: how to deal with the characteristic new ways in which we die.

DEALING WITH DYING IN THE UNITED STATES

In the United States, we have come to recognize that the maximal extension of life-prolonging treatment in these late-life degenerative conditions is often inappropriate. Although we could keep the machines and tubes—the respirators, intravenous lines, feeding tubes—hooked up for extended periods, we recognize that this is inhumane, pointless, and financially impossible. Instead, as a society we have developed a number of mechanisms for dealing with these hopeless situations, all of which involve withholding or withdrawing various forms of treatment.

Some mechanisms for withholding or withdrawing treatments are exercised by the patient who is confronted by such a situation or who anticipates it: These include refusal of treatment, the patient-executed do not resuscitate (DNR) order, the living will, and the durable power of attorney. Others are mechanisms for decision by second parties about a patient who is no longer competent or never was competent. The latter are reflected in a long series of court cases, including Quinlan; Saikewicz; Spring; Eichner; Barber; Bartling; Conroy; Brophy; the trio Farrell, Peter, and Jobes; and Cruzan. These are cases that attempt to delineate the precise circumstances under which it is appropriate to withhold or withdraw various forms of therapy, including respiratory support, chemotherapy, antibiotics in intercurrent infections, and artificial nutrition and hydration. Thus, during the past 20 years or so, roughly since Quinlan (1976), we have developed an impressive body of case law and state statutes that protects, permits, and facilitates our characteristic American strategy of dealing with end-of-life situations. These cases provide a framework for withholding or withdrawing treatment when we believe there is no medical or moral point in going on. This is sometimes termed *passive euthanasia;* more often, it is simply called *allowing to die,* and it is ubiquitous in the United States.

For example, a study by Miles and Gomez indicates that some 85 percent of deaths in the United States occur in health care institutions, including hospitals, nursing homes, and other facilities, and of these, about 70 percent involve electively withholding some form of life-sustaining treatment.[2] A 1989 study cited in the *Journal of the American Medical Association* claims that 85–90 percent of critical care professionals state that they are withholding and withdrawing life-sustaining treatments from patients who are "deemed to have irreversible disease and are terminally ill."[3] Still another study identified some 115 patients from whom care was withheld or withdrawn in two intensive-care units; 110 were already incompetent by the time the decision to limit care was made. The 89 who died while still in the intensive-care unit accounted for 45 percent of all deaths there.[4] It is estimated that 1.3 million American deaths a year follow decisions to withhold life support;[5] this is a majority of the just over 2 million American deaths per year.

In recent years, the legitimate practice of withholding and withdrawing treatment has increasingly been understood to include highly specific forms certain to result in death, such as withholding or withdrawing artificial or ordinary nutrition and hydration. The administration of escalating doses of morphine, which, though it will depress respiration and so hasten death, is accepted under the (Catholic) principle of double effect, "foreseen but not intended" to result in death; it is thus said to be distinguished from killing. At least in theory, withholding and withdrawing treatment is the way we in the United States go about dealing with dying. This is the only currently legally protected alternative to maximal treatment recognized in the United States.

In November 1994, however, voters in Oregon passed a ballot measure that would permit a physician to prescribe a lethal medication for a terminally ill patient who requested it, subject to a number of safeguards, though as of this writing the initiative remains tied up in court. In the spring of 1996, two federal circuit courts ruled that state laws prohibiting physician-assisted suicide are unconstitutional; and the United States Supreme Court subsequently announced that it would hear these cases during the spring term of 1997, and decided in June 1997 that a person does not have "a constitutional right to die."

A number of studies have shown that many physicians do receive requests for assistance in suicide or active euthanasia, and that a substantial number of these physicians have complied with one or more such requests, though out of sight of the law. Although reliance on "allowing to die" is currently American medicine's official posture in the face of death, the legal situation in individual states could change quite rapidly. At the moment, we do not legally permit ourselves to actively and intentionally cause death.

DEALING WITH DYING IN THE NETHERLANDS

In the Netherlands, although the practice of withholding and withdrawing treatment is similar to that in the United States, voluntary active euthanasia and physician assistance in suicide are also available responses to end-of-life situations. Although active euthanasia and assistance in suicide remain prohibited by statutory law, they are protected by a series of lower and supreme court decisions and are widely regarded as legal, or, more precisely, *gedoogd,* legally "tolerated." Euthanasia is the more frequent form of assistance in dying and most discussion has concerned euthanasia rather than assistance in suicide, though the conceptual difference is not always regarded as great: Many cases of what the Dutch term *voluntary active euthanasia* involve self-administration of the lethal dose by the patient and so would count for Americans as physician-assisted suicide. In either case, the physician is prepared to be present and to assist in preventing any unwanted side effects. The Dutch court decisions have the effect of protecting the physician who performs euthanasia or provides assistance in suicide from prosecution, provided the physician meets a rigorous set of guidelines.

These guidelines, variously stated, contain five central provisions:

1. that the patient's request be voluntary
2. that the patient be undergoing intolerable suffering
3. that all alternatives acceptable to the patient for relieving the suffering have been tried
4. that the patient have full information
5. that the physician consult with a second physician whose judgment can be expected to be independent

Of these criteria, it is the first that is central: Euthanasia may be performed only at the voluntary request of the patient. This criterion is also understood to require that the patient's request be a stable, enduring, reflective one—not the product of a transitory impulse. Every attempt is to be made to rule out depression, psychopathology, pressures from family members, unrealistic fears, and other factors compromising voluntariness.

In 1990, a comprehensive, nationwide study requested by the Dutch government, popularly known as the Remmelink Commission report, provided the first objective data about the incidence of euthanasia.[6] This study also provided information about other medical decisions at the end of life: withholding or withdrawal of treatment; the use of life-shortening doses of opioids for the control of pain; and direct termination, including not only voluntary active euthanasia but physician-assisted suicide and life-ending procedures not termed euthanasia. This study was supplemented by a second empirical examination, focusing particularly carefully on the characteristics of patients and the nature of their euthanasia requests.[7] Five years later, the researchers from these two studies jointly conducted a major new nationwide study replicating much of the previous Remmelink inquiry, providing empirical data both about current practice in the Netherlands and change over a five-year period.[8]

About 130,000 people die in the Netherlands every year, and of these deaths, about 30 percent are acute and unexpected and 70 percent are predictable and foreseen, usually the result of degenerative illnesses comparatively late in life. Of the total deaths in the Netherlands, the first Remmelink Commission study (data from the death certificate sections) found about 17.9 percent involved decisions to withhold or withdraw treatment in situations where continuing treatment would probably have prolonged life; five years later, this proportion had risen to 20.2 percent. In the 1990 study, another 18.8 percent of decisions at the end of life involved the use of opioids to relieve pain but in dosages probably sufficient to shorten life; this had risen to 19.1 percent by 1995.

The 1990 study revealed that about 2,300 people, 1.8 percent of the total deaths in the Netherlands, died by euthanasia—understood as the termination of the life of the patient at the patient's explicit and persistent request; another 400 people, 0.3 percent of the total, chose physician-assisted suicide. However, another 0.8 percent of patients who died did so as the result of life-terminating procedures not technically called euthanasia. These cases, known as "the 1000 cases," unleashed highly exaggerated claims that patients were being killed against their wills. In fact, in about half of these cases, euthanasia had been previously discussed with the patient or the patient had expressed in a previous phase of the disease a wish for euthanasia if his or her suffering became unbearable; and in the other half, the patient was no longer competent and was near death, clearly suffering grievously although verbal contact had become impossible. In 91 percent of these cases without explicit, current request, life was shortened by less than a week, and in 33 percent by less than a day.

By 1995, although the proportion of cases of assisted suicide had remained about the same, the proportion of cases of euthanasia had risen to about 2.4 percent (associated, the authors conjectured, with the aging of the population and the increase in the proportion of deaths due to cancer). However, the proportion of cases of life termination without current explicit request had declined slightly to 0.7 percent. In 1990, a total of 2.9 percent of all deaths had involved euthanasia and related practices; by 1995 this total was 3.3 percent. Only about 41 percent of cases are reported to the coroner, as required, but there were no major differences between reported and unreported cases in terms of the patient's characteristics, clinical conditions, or reasons for the action.[9]

Although euthanasia is thus not frequent—a small fraction of the total annual mortality—it is nevertheless a conspicuous option in terminal illness, well-known to both physicians and the general public. There has been very widespread public discussion of the issues that arise with respect to euthanasia during the last two decades, and surveys of public opinion show that public support for a liberal euthanasia policy has been growing: from 40 percent in 1966 to 81 percent in 1988.[10] Doctors, too, support the practice, and although there is a vocal opposition group, the opposition is in the clear minority. Some 53 percent of Dutch physicians said that they had performed euthanasia or provided assistance in suicide, including 62 percent of *huisarts* (general practitioners). An additional 35 percent of all physicians said that although they had not actually done so, they could conceive of situations in which they would be prepared to do so. Thus, although many who had practiced euthanasia mentioned that they would be most reluctant to do so again and that "only in the face of unbearable suffering and with no alternatives would they be prepared to take such action,"[11] some 88 percent of Dutch physicians appear to accept the practice in some cases. As the 1995 report commented, "as in 1990, a large majority of Dutch physicians consider euthanasia an exceptional but accepted part of medical practice."[12] The study authors also commented that the data do not support claims of a slippery slope.

In general, pain alone is not the basis for deciding upon euthanasia, since pain can, in most cases, be effectively treated. Rather, the "intolerable suffering" mentioned in the second criterion is understood to mean suffering that is intolerable in the patient's (rather than the physician's) view and can include a fear of or unwillingness to endure *entluistering,* that gradual effacement and loss of personal identity that characterizes the end stages of many terminal illnesses. In a year, almost 35,000 patients seek reassurance from their physicians that they will be granted euthanasia if their suffering becomes severe; there are about 9,700 explicit requests, and more than two-thirds of these are turned down, usually on the grounds that there is some other way of treating the patient's suffering. In 14 percent of cases in 1990, the denial was based on the presence of depression or psychiatric illness.

In the Netherlands, many hospitals now have protocols for the performance of euthanasia; these serve to ensure that the court-established guidelines have been met. However, euthanasia is often practiced in the patient's home, typically by the general practitioner who is the patient's long-term family physician. Euthanasia is usually performed after aggressive hospital treatment has failed to arrest the patient's terminal illness; the patient has come home to die, and the family physician is prepared to ease this passing. Whether practiced at home or in the hospital, it is believed that euthanasia usually takes place in the presence of the family members, perhaps the visiting nurse, and often the patient's pastor or priest. Many doctors say that performing euthanasia is never easy but that it is something they believe a doctor ought to do for his or her patient when nothing else can help.

Thus, in the Netherlands a patient who is facing the end of life has an option not openly practiced in the United States: to ask the physician to bring his or her life to an end. Although not everyone does so—indeed, about 97 percent of people who die in a given year do not do so—it is a choice widely understood as available.

FACING DEATH IN GERMANY

In part because of its very painful history of Nazism, Germany appears to believe that doctors should have no role in causing death. Although societal generalizations are always risky, it is fair, I think, to say that there is vigorous and nearly universal opposition in Germany to the notion of active euthanasia. Euthanasia—usually not understood in the Dutch sense, based on the Greek root *eu-thanatos,* or "good death," but in the horrific sense associated with Nazism—is viewed as always wrong, and the Germans view the Dutch as stepping out on a dangerously slippery slope.

However, it is an artifact of German law that, whereas killing on request (including voluntary euthanasia) is prohibited, assisting suicide is not a violation of the law, provided the person is *tatherrschaftsfähig,* capable of exercising control over his or her actions, and also acting out of *freiverantwortliche Wille,* freely responsible choice. In response to this situation, a private organization, the *Deutsche Gesellschaft für Humanes Sterben* (DGHS), or German Society for Humane Dying, provides support to its very extensive membership in choosing suicide as an alternative to terminal illness.

Although for legal reasons the DGHS no longer publishes its own book of drug dosages for ending life, a person who has been a member of the DGHS for at least a year, provided he or she had not received medical or psychotherapeutic treatment for depression or other psychiatric illness during the last two years, can request a copy of *Departing Drugs* (German title, *Selbsterlösung durch Medikamente*). This booklet, published in Scotland by an international working group, provides a list of prescription drugs, together with the specific dosages necessary for producing a certain, painless death. DGHS has recommended that the member approach a physician for a prescription for the drug desired, asking, for example, for a barbiturate to help with sleep. If necessary, the DGHS would also arrange for someone to obtain drugs from neighboring countries, including France, Italy, Spain, Portugal, and Greece, where they may be available without prescription. In unusual cases, the DGHS may also provide what it calls *Sterbebegleitung* (accompaniment in dying), which involves arranging for a companion to remain with the person during the often extended period that is required for the lethal drug to take full effect. However, the *Sterbebegleiter* is typically a layperson, not someone medically trained, and physicians play no role in assisting in these cases of suicide. To preclude suspicion by providing evidence of the person's intentions, the DGHS also provides a form—printed on a single sheet of distinctive purple paper—to be signed once when joining the organization, expressing the intention to determine the time of one's own death, and signed again at the time of the suicide and left beside the body as evidence that the act is not an impetuous one, and to request that, if the person is discovered before the suicide is complete, no rescue measures be undertaken. Because assisting suicide is not illegal in Germany, provided the person is competent and in control of his or her own will, there is no legal risk for family members, the *Sterbebegleiter,* or others in reporting information about the methods and effectiveness of suicide attempts, and the DGHS encourages its network of regional bureaus, located in major cities throughout the country, to facilitate feedback. On this basis, it has regularly updated and revised the drug information it provides to the international consortium that publishes *Departing Drugs.*

In the wake of the 1992 scandal that engulfed the founder and president of the DGHS, Hans

Henning Atrott, who was convicted for violations of drug laws and tax evasion for selling some members cyanide for exorbitant sums, the DGHS has gone through a period of considerable introspection and reassessment. It has turned much of its attention to the development of other measures for protecting the rights of the terminally ill. It now also distributes newly legalized advance directives, including the living will and the durable power of attorney as well as detailed organ-donation documents. Yet it remains steadfast in defense of the right to suicide as a part of the right to self-determination and is supportive of patients who make this choice.

To be sure, assisted suicide is not the only option open to terminally ill patients in Germany, nor is there clear evidence concerning its frequency. Reported suicide rates in Germany are not dramatically higher than in the Netherlands or the United States, though there is reason to think that many terminal-illness suicides in all countries are reported as deaths from the underlying disease. There is also increasing emphasis on help in dying that does not involve direct termination, and organizations like Omega, which offers hospice-style care and an extensive program of companionship, are attracting increasing attention. Nevertheless, the DGHS is a conspicuous, widely known organization, and many Germans appear to be aware that assisted suicide is available and not illegal even if they do not use its services.

OBJECTIONS TO THE THREE MODELS OF DYING

In response to the dilemmas raised by the new circumstances of death, in which the majority of the population in each of the advanced industrial nations dies of degenerative diseases after an extended period of terminal deterioration, different countries develop different practices. At this moment, the United States legally permits only withholding and withdrawal of treatment, though of course physician-assisted suicide and active euthanasia do occur. The Netherlands also openly permits voluntary active euthanasia, and although Germany rejects euthanasia, it permits non–physician-assisted suicide. To be sure, all of these practices are currently undergoing evolution, and in some ways they are becoming more alike: Germany is paying new attention to the rights of patients to execute advance directives and thus to have treatment withheld or withdrawn; the Royal Dutch Medical Association has urged physicians to encourage patients who request euthanasia to administer the lethal dose themselves, as a further protective of voluntary choice, and thus seems to favor physician-assisted suicide in preference to euthanasia; and, although the United States Supreme Court has ruled on the issue of physician-assisted suicide, it appears that this practice will become legal in at least some American states. Nevertheless, there remain substantial differences among these three countries in their approaches to dying, and while each recognizes advantages to its approach, there are also serious moral objections to be made to each of them, objections to be considered before resolving the issue of which practices our own culture ought to permit.

Objections to the German Practice

German law does not prohibit assisting suicide, but postwar German culture discourages physicians from taking any active role in death. This gives rise to distinctive moral problems. For one thing, it appears that there can be little professional help or review provided for patients' choices about suicide; because the patient makes this choice essentially outside the medical establishment, medical professionals are not in a position to detect or treat impaired judgment on the part of the patient, especially judgment impaired by depression. Similarly, if the patient must commit suicide assisted only by persons outside the medical profession, there are risks that the patient's diagnosis and prognosis will be inadequately confirmed, that the means chosen for suicide will be unreliable or inappropriately used, that the means used for suicide will fall into the hands of other persons, and that the patient will fail to recognize or be able to resist intrafamilial pressures and manipulation. After the 1992 scandal, even the DGHS itself was accused of promoting rather than simply supporting choices of suicide. Finally, as the DGHS now emphasizes, assistance in suicide can be a freely chosen option only in a legal context that also protects the many other choices a patient may make about how his or her life shall end, including those involving the withholding or withdrawal of treatment.

Objections to the Dutch Practice

The Dutch practice of physician-performed active voluntary euthanasia also raises a number of ethical issues, many of which have been discussed vigorously both in the Dutch press and in commentary on the Dutch practices from abroad. For one thing, it is sometimes said that the availability of physician-performed euthanasia creates a disincentive for providing good terminal care. There is no evidence that this is the case; on the contrary, Peter Admiraal, the anesthesiologist who has been perhaps the Netherlands' most vocal defender of voluntary active euthanasia, insists that pain should rarely or never be the occasion for euthanasia, as pain (in contrast to suffering) is comparatively easily treated.[13] In fact, pain is the primary reason for the request in only about 5 percent of cases. Instead, it is a refusal to endure the final stages of deterioration, both mental and physical, that primarily motivates the majority of requests.

It is also sometimes said that active euthanasia violates the Hippocratic oath. The original Greek version of the oath does prohibit the physician from giving a deadly drug, even when asked for it; but the original version also prohibits the physician from performing surgery and from taking fees for teaching medicine, neither of which prohibition has survived into contemporary medical practice. Dutch physicians often say that they see performing euthanasia—where it is genuinely requested by the patient and nothing else can be done to relieve the patient's condition—as part of their duty to the patient, not as a violation of it.

The Dutch are also often said to be at risk of starting down the slippery slope, that is, that the practice of voluntary active euthanasia for patients who meet the criteria will erode into practicing less-than-voluntary euthanasia on patients whose problems are not irremediable and perhaps by gradual degrees will develop into terminating the lives of people who are elderly, chronically ill, handicapped, mentally retarded, or otherwise regarded as undesirable. This risk is often expressed in vivid claims of widespread fear and wholesale slaughter—claims based on misinterpretation of the 1,000 cases of life-ending treatment mentioned earlier. However, the Dutch are now beginning to agonize over the problems of the incompetent patient, the mentally ill patient, the newborn with serious deficits, and other patients who cannot make voluntary choices, though these are largely understood as issues about withholding or withdrawing treatment, not about direct termination.[14]

What is not often understood is that this new and acutely painful area of reflection for the Dutch—withholding and withdrawing treatment from incompetent patients—has already led in the United States to the development of a vast, highly developed body of law: namely, that series of cases cited earlier in the chapter, beginning with Quinlan and culminating in Cruzan. Americans have been discussing these issues for a long time and have developed a broad set of practices that are regarded as routine in withholding and withdrawing treatment from persons who are no longer or were never competent. The Dutch see Americans as much further out on the slippery slope than they are, because Americans have already become accustomed to second-party choices that result in death for other people. Issues involving second-party choices are painful to the Dutch in a way they are not to us precisely because voluntariness is so central in the Dutch understanding of choices about dying. Concomitantly, the Dutch see the Americans' squeamishness about first-party choices—voluntary euthanasia, assisted suicide—as evidence that we are not genuinely committed to recognizing voluntary choice after all. For this reason, many Dutch commentators believe that the Americans are at a much greater risk of sliding down the slippery slope into involuntary killing than they are. I fear, I must add, that they are right about this.

Objections to the American Practice

The German, Dutch, and American practices all occur within similar conditions—in industrialized nations with highly developed medical systems where a majority of the population die of illnesses exhibiting characteristically extended downhill courses—but the issues raised by our own response to this situation, relying on withholding and withdrawal of treatment, may be even more disturbing than those of the Dutch or the Germans. We Americans often assume that our approach is "safer" because it involves only letting someone die, not killing him or her; but it, too, raises very troubling questions.

The first of these issues is a function of the fact that withdrawing and especially withholding treatment are typically less conspicuous, less pronounced, less evident kinds of actions than direct killing, even though they can equally well lead to death. Decisions about nontreatment have an invisibility that decisions about directly causing death do not have, even though they may have the same result, and hence there is a much wider range of occasions in which such decisions can be made. One can decline to treat a patient in many different ways, at many different times—by not providing oxygen, by not instituting dialysis, by not correcting electrolyte imbalances, and so on—all of which will cause the patient's death; open medical killing also brings about death but is much more overt and conspicuous. Consequently, letting die also invites many fewer protections. In contrast to the standard slippery-slope argument, which sees killing as riskier than letting die, the more realistic slippery-slope argument warns that because our culture relies primarily on decisions about nontreatment, grave decisions about living or dying are not as open to scrutiny as they are under more direct life-terminating practices and hence are more open to abuse.

Second, reliance on withholding and withdrawal of treatment invites rationing in an extremely strong way, in part because of the comparative invisibility of these decisions. When a health care provider does not offer a specific sort of care, it is not always possible to discern the motivation; the line between believing that it would not provide benefit to the patient and that it would not provide benefit worth the investment of resources in the patient can be very thin. This is a particular problem where health care financing is decentralized and profit-oriented, as in the United States, and where rationing decisions without benefit of principle are not always available for easy review.

Third, relying on withholding and withdrawal of treatment can often be cruel. It requires that the patient who is dying from one of the diseases that exhibits a characteristic extended, downhill course (as the majority of patients in the Netherlands, Germany, and the United States all do) must, in effect, wait to die until the absence of a certain treatment will cause death. For instance, the cancer patient who forgoes chemotherapy or surgery does not simply die from this choice; he or she continues to endure the downhill course of the cancer until the tumor finally destroys some crucial bodily function or organ. The patient with amyotrophic lateral sclerosis who decides in advance to decline respiratory support does not die at the time this choice is made but continues to endure increasing paralysis until breathing is impaired and suffocation occurs. We often try to ameliorate these situations by administering pain medication or symptom control at the same time we are withholding treatment, but these are all ways of disguising the fact that we are letting the disease kill the patient rather than directly bringing about death. But the ways diseases kill people are far more cruel than the ways physicians kill patients when performing euthanasia or assisting in suicide.

THE PROBLEM: A CHOICE OF CULTURES

Thus we see three similar cultures and countries and three similar sets of circumstances, but while much of medical practice in them is similar, they do offer three quite different basic options in approaching death. All three of these options generate moral problems; none of them, nor any others we might devise, is free of moral difficulty. But the question that faces us is this: Which of these options is best?

It is not possible to answer this question in a less-than-ideal world without some attention to the specific characteristics and deficiencies of the society in question. In asking which of these practices is best, we must ask which is best for us. That we currently employ one set of these options rather than others does not prove that it is best for us; the question is, would practices developed in other cultures or those not yet widespread in any culture be better for our own culture than that which has developed here? Thus, it is necessary to consider the differences between our own society and these European cultures that have real bearing on which model of approach to dying we ought to adopt.

First, notice that different cultures exhibit different degrees of closeness between physicians and patients—different patterns of contact and involvement. The German physician is sometimes said to be more distant and more authoritarian than the American physician; on the other hand, the Dutch physician is often said to be closer to his or her patients than either the American or the German is. In the Netherlands, basic primary care is provided by the general practitioner or family physician, who typically lives in the neighborhood, makes house calls frequently, and maintains an office in his or her own home. This physician usually also provides care for the other members of the patient's family and will remain the family's physician throughout his or her practice. Thus, the patient for whom euthanasia becomes an issue—say, the terminal cancer patient who has been hospitalized in the past but who has returned home to die—will be cared for by the trusted family physician on a regular basis. Indeed, for a patient in severe distress, the physician, supported by the visiting nurse, may make house calls as often as once a day, twice a day, or even more frequently (after all, the physician's office is right in the neighborhood) and is in continuous contact with the family. In contrast, the traditional American institution of the family doctor who makes house calls is rapidly becoming a thing of the past, and although some patients who die at home have access to hospice services and receive house calls from their long-term physician, many have no such long-term care and receive most of it from staff at a clinic or from house staff rotating through the services of a hospital. Some 78 percent of Americans die in institutions, 61 percent in hospitals and 17 percent in nursing homes; in the Netherlands, over 40 percent of deaths occur at home. The degree of continuing contact that the patient can have with a familiar, trusted physician and the degree of institutionalization clearly influence the nature of his or her dying and also play a role in whether physician-performed active euthanasia, assisted suicide, and/or withholding and withdrawing treatment is appropriate.

Second, the United States has a much more volatile legal climate than either the Netherlands or Germany; our medical system is increasingly litigious, much more so than that of any other country in the world. Fears of malpractice actions or criminal prosecution color much of what physicians do in managing the dying of their patients. We also tend to develop public policy through court decisions and to assume that the existence of a policy puts an end to any moral issue. A delicate legal and moral balance over the issue of euthanasia, as is the case in the Netherlands, would not be possible here.

Third, we in the United States have a very different financial climate in which to do our dying. Both the Netherlands and Germany, as well as every other industrialized nation except South Africa, have systems of national health insurance or national health care. Thus the patient is not directly responsible for the costs of treatment, and consequently the patient's choices about terminal care and/or euthanasia need not take personal financial considerations into account. Even for the patient who does have health insurance in the United States, many kinds of services are not covered, whereas the national health care or health insurance programs of many other countries have multiple relevant services, including at-home physician care, home-nursing care, home respite care, care in a nursing home or other long-term facility, dietitian care, rehabilitation care, physical therapy, psychological counseling, and so on. The patient in the United States needs to attend to the financial aspects of dying in a way that patients in many other countries do not, and in this country both the patient's choices and the recommendations of the physician are very often shaped by financial considerations.

There are many other differences between the United States, on the one hand, and the Netherlands and Germany, with their different options for dying, on the other.[15] There are differences in degrees of paternalism in the medical establishment and in racism, sexism, and ageism in the general culture, as well as awareness of a problematic historical past, especially Nazism. All of these and the previously mentioned factors influence the appropriateness or inappropriateness of practices such as active euthanasia and assisted suicide. For instance, the Netherlands' tradition of close physician-patient contact, its absence of malpractice-motivated medicine, and its provision of comprehensive health insurance, together with its comparative lack of racism and ageism and its experience in resistance to Nazism, suggest that this culture is able to permit the practice of voluntary active euthanasia, performed by physicians, without risking abuse. On the other hand, it is sometimes said that Germany still does not trust its physicians, remembering the example of Nazi experimentation, and given a comparatively authoritarian medical climate in which the contact between physician and patient is quite distanced, the population could not be comfortable with the practice of active euthanasia or physician-assisted suicide. There, only a wholly patient-controlled response to terminal situations, as in non–physician-assisted suicide, is a reasonable and prudent practice.

But what about the United States? This is a country where (1) sustained contact with a personal physician has been decreasing, (2) the risk of malpractice action is increasing, (3) much medical care is not insured, (4) many medical decisions are financial decisions as well, (5) racism has been on the rise, and (6) the public has not experienced direct contact with Nazism or similar totalitarian movements. Thus, the United States is in many respects an untrustworthy candidate for practicing active euthanasia. Given the pressures on individuals in an often atomized society, encouraging solo suicide, assisted if at all only by nonprofessionals, might well be open to considerable abuse too.

However, there are several additional differences between the United States and both the Netherlands and Germany that may seem relevant here. First, although the United States is indeed afflicted by a great deal of racism and sexism, it is also developing an increasingly strong tradition of independence in women. In many other countries, especially in the Far East and the Islamic countries, the role of women still involves much greater disempowerment and expectations of subservience; in contrast, the United States is particularly advanced—though, of course, it has a long way to go. The United States may even be ahead of the Netherlands and perhaps Germany in this respect. Whatever the case, this issue is of particular importance with respect to euthanasia, especially among elderly persons, because it is women whose life expectancies are longer than those of men and hence who are more likely to be confronted with late-life degenerative terminal conditions.

Second, American culture is more confrontational than many others, including Dutch culture. While the Netherlands prides itself rightly on a long tradition of rational discussion of public issues and on toleration of others' views and practices, the United States (and to some degree also Germany) tends to develop highly partisan, moralizing oppositional groups. In general, this is a disadvantage, but in the case of euthanasia it may serve to alert a public to issues and possibilities it might not otherwise consider, especially to the risks of abuse. Here the role of religious groups may be particularly strong, since in discouraging or prohibiting suicide and euthanasia (as many, though by no means all, religious groups do), they may invite their members to reinspect the reasons for such choices and encourage families, physicians, and health care institutions to provide adequate, humane alternatives.

Third, though this may at first seem to be a trivial difference, it is Americans who are particularly given to self-analysis. This tendency not only is evident in America's high rate of utilization of counseling services, including religious counseling, psychological counseling, and psychiatry, but also is more clearly evident in its popular culture: its diet of soap operas, situation comedies, and pop psychology books. It is here that the ordinary American absorbs models for analyzing his or her personal relationships and individual psychological characteristics. While, of course, things are changing and our cultural tastes are widely exported, the fact remains that the ordinary American's cultural diet contains more in the way of professional and do-it-yourself amateur psychology and self-analysis than anyone else's. This long tradition of self-analysis may put us in a better position for certain kinds of end-of-life practices than many other cultures: Despite whatever other deficiencies we have, we live in a culture that encourages us to inspect our own motives, anticipate the impact of our actions on others, and scrutinize our own relationships with others, including our physicians. This disposition is of importance in euthanasia contexts because euthanasia is the kind of fundamental choice about which one may have somewhat mixed motives, be subject to various interpersonal and situational pressures, and so on. If the voluntary character of these choices is to be protected, it may be a good thing to inhabit a culture in which self-inspection of one's own mental habits and motives is encouraged.

Finally, the United States population is characterized by a kind of do-it-yourself ethic, an ethic that devalues reliance on others and encourages individual initiative and responsibility. (To be sure, this ethic has been somewhat eclipsed in recent years and is little in evidence in the series of court cases cited earlier, but it is still part, I think, of the American character.) This ethic seems to be coupled with a sort of resistance to authority that perhaps also is basic to the American temperament. If this is really the case, Americans might be especially well-served by end-of-life practices that emphasize self-reliance and resistance to authority.

These, of course, are mere conjectures about features of American culture that would support appropriate use of euthanasia or assisted suicide. These are the features that one would want to reinforce should these practices become general, in part to minimize the effects of the negative features. But, of course, these positive features will differ from one country and culture to another, just as the negative features do. In each country, a different architecture of antecedent assumptions and cultural features develops around end-of-life issues, and in each country the practice of euthanasia, if it is to be free from abuse, must be adapted to the culture in which it takes place.

What, then, is appropriate for our own cultural situation? Physician-performed euthanasia, though not in itself morally wrong, is morally jeopardized where legal, time, and especially financial pressures on both patients and physicians are severe; thus, it is morally problematic in our culture in a way that it is not in the Netherlands. Solo suicide outside the institution of medicine (as in Germany) may be problematic in a country (like the United States) that has an increasingly alienated population, offers deteriorating and uneven social services, is increasingly racist and classist, and in other ways imposes unusual pressures on individuals, despite opportunities for self-analysis. Reliance only on withholding and withdrawing treatment (as in the United States) can be cruel, and its comparative invisibility invites erosion under cost-containment and other pressures. These are the three principal alternatives we have considered, but none of them seems wholly suited to our actual situation for dealing with the new fact that most of us die of extended-decline, deteriorative diseases. However, permitting physicians to supply patients with the means for ending their own lives (as permitted, or example, under Oregon's Measure 16) still grants physicians some control over the circumstances in which this can happen—only, for example, when the prognosis is genuinely grim and the alternatives for symptom control are poor—but leaves the fundamental decision about whether to use these means to the patient alone. It is up to the patient then—the independent, confrontational, self-analyzing, do-it-yourself, authority-resisting patient—and his or her advisors, including family members, clergy, the physician, and other health care providers, to be clear about whether he or she really wants to use these means or not. Thus, the physician is involved but not directly, and it is the patient's decision, although the patient is not making it alone. We live in an imperfect world, but of the alternatives for facing death—which we all eventually must—I think that the practice of permitting physician-assisted suicide is the one most nearly suited to the current state of our own flawed society. This is a model not yet central in any of the three countries examined here—the Netherlands, Germany, or the United States—but it is the one, I think, that suits us best.

NOTES

1. S. J. Olshansky and A. B. Ault, "The Fourth Stage of the Epidemiological Transition: The Age of Delayed Degenerative Diseases," *Milbank Memorial Fund Quarterly/Health and Society* 64 (1986): 355–91.
2. S. Miles and C. Gomez, *Protocols for Elective Use of Life-Sustaining Treatment* (New York: Springer-Verlag, 1988).
3. C. L. Sprung, "Changing Attitudes and Practices in Forgoing Life-Sustaining Treatments," *JAMA* 262 (1990): 2213.
4. N. G. Smedira et al., "Withholding and Withdrawal of Life Support from the Critically Ill," *New England Journal of Medicine* 322 (1990): 309–15.
5. *New York Times,* 23 July 1990, A13.
6. P. J. van der Maas et al., "Euthanasia and Other Medical Decisions Concerning the End of Life," *Lancet* 338 (1991): 669–74. Published in full in English as a special issue of *Health Policy,* 22, no. 1–2 (1992).
7. G. van der Wal et al., "Euthanasie en hulp bij zelfdoding door artsen in de thuissituatie, parts 1 and 2," *Nederlands Tijdschrift voor Geneesekunde* 135 (1991): 1593–98, 1600–03.
8. P. J. van der Maas et al., "Euthanasia, Physician-Assisted Suicide, and Other Medical Practices Involving the End of Life in the Netherlands, 1990–1995," *New England Journal of Medicine* 335 (1996): 1699–1705.
9. G. van der Wal et al., "Evaluation of the Notification Procedure for Physician-Assisted Death in the Netherlands," *New England Journal of Medicine* 335 (1996): 1706–11.
10. E. Borst-Eilers, "Euthanasia in the Netherlands: Brief Historical Review and Present Situation," in Robert I. Misbin, ed., *Euthanasia: The Good of the Patient, the Good of Society* (Frederick, MD: University Publishing Group, 1992): 59.
11. Van der Maas et al., "Euthanasia and Other Medical Decisions Concerning the End of Life," 673.
12. Van der Maas et al., "Euthanasia, Physician-Assisted Suicide, and Other Medical Practices," 1705.
13. P. Admiraal, "Euthanasia in a General Hospital" (paper read at the Eighth World Congress of the International Federation of Right-to-Die Societies, Maastricht, Holland, June 8, 1990).
14. H. ten Have, "Coma: Controversy and Consensus," *Newsletter of the European Society for Philosophy of Medicine and Health Care* (May 1990): 19–20.
15. See two of my chapters, "A Dozen Caveats Concerning the Discussion of Euthanasia in the Netherlands," and "Assisted Suicide: Can We Learn from Germany?" both in my *Least Worst Death* (New York and London: Oxford University Press, 1994): 130–44, 254–70.

Chapter 29

The Problem with Futility

Robert D. Truog, Joel E. Frader, and Allan S. Brett

"Futility" is one of the newest additions to the lexicon of bioethics. Physicians, ethicists, and members of the media are increasingly concerned about patients and families who insist on receiving life-sustaining treatment that others judge to be futile. A clear understanding of futility has proved to be elusive, however. Many clinicians view futility the way one judge viewed pornography: they may not be able to define it, but they know it when they see it.[1]

The notion of futile medical treatment may go back to the time of Hippocrates, who allegedly advised physicians "to refuse to treat those who are overmastered by their diseases, realizing that in such cases medicine is powerless."[2] More recently, the concept has appeared frequently in court decisions and policy statements.[3] The so-called Baby Doe law exempts physicians from providing treatment that would be "virtually futile."[4] The Council on Ethical and Judicial Affairs of the American Medical Association (AMA) recently concluded that physicians have no obligation to obtain consent for a do not resuscitate (DNR) order when cardiopulmonary resuscitation (CPR) is deemed futile.[5] The fact that this concept has appeared in law and policy may seem to indicate that it is clearly understood and widely accepted. In reality, however, the notion of futility hides many deep and serious ambiguities that threaten its legitimacy as a rationale for limiting treatment.

PARADIGMS OF FUTILITY

Contemporary discussions of futility have centered primarily on cases involving patients in a persistent vegetative state and those involving the use of CPR. A third type of case, involving organ-replacement technology, has received little attention but is helpful to our understanding of futility.

Futility and the Persistent Vegetative State

The first type of scenario involving the question of futility is represented by the recent Minnesota case of Helga Wanglie.[6] Mrs. Wanglie was an 86-year-old woman who had been dependent on mechanical ventilation and in a persistent vegetative state for more than a year. Her husband insisted that she believed in maintaining life at all cost, and that "when she was ready to go . . . the good Lord would call her."[7] Her physicians, on the other hand, believed that the continued use of mechanical ventilation and intensive care was futile. When attempts to transfer her elsewhere failed, they sought to

---

Source: Reprinted with permission from R. D. Truog, A. S. Brett, and J. Frader, The Problem with Futility, *The New England Journal of Medicine*, Vol. 326, No. 23, pp. 1560–1564, Copyright 1992, Massachusetts Medical Society. All rights reserved.

have a court appoint an independent conservator with responsibility for making medical decisions on her behalf. The judge denied this petition and reaffirmed the authority of her husband as legal surrogate. Three days later, Mrs. Wanglie died.

Cases like that of Mrs. Wanglie seldom reach the courts, but they are probably not rare. A similar case involving a child with severe brain damage was concluded with a settlement favorable to the family before a judicial decision.[8]

Futility in Cases Involving CPR

The second prototypical scenario involves the use of DNR orders. Although the techniques of CPR were originally intended only for use after acute, reversible cardiac arrests, the current practice is to use CPR in all situations unless there is a direct order to the contrary. Since cardiac arrest is the final event in all terminal illness, everyone is eventually a candidate for this medical procedure. DNR orders were developed to spare patients from aggressive attempts at revival when imminent death is anticipated and inevitable. Nevertheless, patients or families sometimes request CPR even when caregivers believe such attempts would be futile. Some have argued that in these circumstances a physician should be able to enact a DNR order without the consent of the patient or family.[9]

Futility and Organ-Replacement Technology

Although the bioethical debate over the question of futility has been most concerned with cases involving CPR and the treatment of patients in a persistent vegetative state, a third type of futility-related judgment has gone essentially unchallenged. It involves the increasingly large number of interventions that could possibly prolong the life of virtually any dying patient. For example, extracorporeal membrane oxygenation can replace heart and lung function for up to several weeks. Physicians now use this intervention when they expect organ systems eventually to recover or while they await organs for transplantation. However, it could prolong the life of almost anyone with cardiorespiratory failure, reversible or not. Patients thus kept alive may remain conscious and capable of communicating. Caregivers do not now offer this therapy to terminally ill patients, presumably because it would be futile. This judgment has gone largely unchallenged, yet it is not obvious why a clinician's unilateral decision not to use "futile" extracorporeal membrane oxygenation is inherently different from a decision not to use "futile" CPR or "futile" intensive care. If all three treatments can be characterized as objectively futile, then unilateral decisions not to offer them should be equally justified.

As it is used in these three cases, the concept of futility obscures many ambiguities and assumptions. These can be usefully grouped into two categories: problems of value and problems of probability.

FUTILITY AND VALUES

It is meaningless simply to say that an intervention is futile; one must always ask, "Futile in relation to what?" The medical literature provides many examples in which the importance of identifying the goals of treatment has not been fully appreciated. The effectiveness of CPR, for example, is often discussed in terms of whether patients who require the procedure can survive long enough to be discharged from the hospital.[10] This definition of success usually implies that short-term survival is a goal not worth pursuing. Patients or family members may value the additional hours of life differently, however. Indeed, physicians and other caregivers have repeatedly been shown to be poor judges of patients' preferences with regard to intensive care.[11]

Schneiderman and colleagues have argued that treatments that merely preserve permanent unconsciousness or that cannot end dependence on intensive medical care should be considered futile.[12] Although society may eventually endorse decisions to override the previously expressed wishes of patients or the desires of surrogates who demand such treatments, it does not follow that the treatments are futile. Mr. Wanglie would have rejected this conclusion, and there is no reason to dismiss his view out of hand. The decision that certain goals are not worth pursuing is best seen as involving a conflict of values rather than a question of futility.

Certainly in this context, the plurality of values in our society makes agreement on the concept of futility difficult if not impossible. Several groups have therefore attempted to arrive at a value-free understanding of the concept.[13] The most promising candidate thus far is the notion of "physiologic futility." As the guidelines on the termination of life-sustaining treatment prepared by the Hastings Center state, if a treatment is "clearly futile in achieving its physiological objective and so offer[s] no physiological benefit to the patient, the professional has no obligation to provide it."[14] For example, the physiologic objective of mechanical ventilation is to maintain adequate ventilation and oxygenation in the presence of respiratory failure, and the physiologic objective of CPR is to maintain adequate cardiac output and respiration in the presence of cardiorespiratory failure. The New York State Task Force on Life and the Law mistakenly concludes that CPR is physiologically futile when it will "be unsuccessful in restoring cardiac and respiratory function or [when] the patient will experience repeated arrest in a short time period before death occurs."[15] CPR is physiologically futile only when it is impossible to perform effective cardiac massage and ventilation (such as in the presence of cardiac rupture or severe outflow obstruction). Saying that CPR is physiologically futile when it will be unsuccessful in restoring cardiac function is like saying that mechanical ventilation is physiologically futile if it cannot restore respiratory function. The immediate physiologic effect of the intervention differs from the broader and more uncertain question of prognosis.

Physiologic futility, understood in narrow terms, comes close to providing a value-free understanding of futility. Unfortunately, it applies to a very small number of real cases involving CPR. Similarly, since in the case of Mrs. Wanglie mechanical ventilation could maintain adequate oxygenation and ventilation, her treatment could not be considered futile in the physiologic sense. Even the use of extracorporeal membrane oxygenation in terminally ill patients cannot be considered physiologically futile, since it can maintain circulation and ventilation. The concept of physiologic futility therefore falls short of providing guidance in most cases resembling those described above.

FUTILITY AND STATISTICAL UNCERTAINTY

In most medical situations, there is no such thing as never. Futility is almost always a matter of probability. But what statistical cutoff point should be chosen as the threshold for determining futility? The statement from the Council on Ethical and Judicial Affairs of the AMA concludes that physicians have no obligation to provide futile CPR, but it fails to specify any level of statistical certainty at which the judgment is warranted.[16] The AMA statement fails to acknowledge that this is even an issue. Should each physician decide independently what probability of success should be considered to indicate futility?

Even if we could agree on a statistical cutoff point for determining futility, physicians are often highly unreliable in estimating the likelihood of success of a therapeutic intervention. Psychological research[17] has shown that estimates of probability are susceptible to "severe and systematic errors."[18] Empirical studies have corroborated the limitations of clinical assessment in estimating both prognosis[19] and diagnosis.[20] Even in theory, statistical inferences about what might happen to groups of patients do not permit accurate predictions of what will happen to the next such patient. In addition, the tendency to remember cases that are unusual or bizarre predisposes physicians to make decisions on the basis of their experiences with "miraculous" cures or unexpected tragedies.

Schneiderman and colleagues recently argued that a treatment should be considered futile when 100 consecutive patients do not respond to it.[21] But how similar must the patients be? In assessing the efficacy of mechanical ventilation to treat pneumonia, for example, is it sufficient simply to recall the 100 most recent patients who received artificial ventilation for pneumonia? Or must this group be stratified according to age, etiologic organism, or coexisting illness? Clearly, many of these factors will make an important difference.

FUTILITY AND RESOURCE ALLOCATION

Although medical practice has increasingly emphasized patients' autonomy, there is growing pressure on physicians to slow the increase in health care costs by foreclosing some options. Thus, we have a tension between the value of autonomy, exercised in the form of consent to use or omit various interventions, and the desirability of a more Spartan approach to the consumption of medical resources. We promote patients' freedom to request whatever the medical menu has to offer, but we also require that interventions be guided by considerations of cost and the likelihood of benefit.[22] Unfortunately, there is no consensus about what constitutes a just method of balancing the preferences of individual patients against the diverse needs of society.

To some, the concept of futility provides at least a partial solution to this dilemma: It offers a reason to limit therapy without the need to define a fair procedure for allocating resources. This approach allows treatments to be denied on the grounds that they are simply not indicated, apart from the matter of cost. Despite its attractions, there are good reasons why we should not use this concept to solve problems of allocation.

First, arguments based on the futility concept conceal many statistical and value-laden assumptions, whereas strategies based on resource allocation force these assumptions to be stated explicitly. Societies may choose to limit the use of therapies that may be of value and have a reasonable likelihood of success in some cases. For example, the much discussed Oregon plan for allocating Medicaid funds[23] seeks to reflect community values in ranking various health care goals (placing preventive care ahead of cosmetic surgery, for example). Since rationing policies make explicit the values and probabilities that futility-based arguments leave implicit, it is clearly preferable to develop and adopt them rather than use futility arguments as a cover for limiting the availability of scarce and expensive resources.

Another problem with invoking the idea of futility in the debate over allocation is that we have no reason to believe that it is applicable in enough cases to make a difference in the scarcity of medical resources. Although it may be true that beds in the intensive-care unit (especially those used for extracorporeal membrane oxygenation) are relatively scarce, it seems unlikely that patients similar to Helga Wanglie occupy an important fraction of those beds, let alone account for a major proportion of the cost of medical care in the United States. From a macroeconomic perspective at least, we must remain skeptical that an appeal to the idea of futility will get us very far.

MOVING BEYOND FUTILITY

Our rejection of futility as a useful concept does not imply that we endorse patients' unrestricted demands for interventions such as those described in our prototypical scenarios. On the contrary, when providers oppose such demands they are usually acting from a profound sense that further treatment would be fundamentally wrong. Our task is to take account of that sense of wrongness without resorting to unilateral, provider-initiated declarations of futility.

In many of the situations in which questions of futility arise, providers believe that the treatment in question would not be in the patient's interests, even from the patient's perspective, and that any insistence by the patient (or surrogate) on further interventions is based on faulty reasoning, unrealistic expectations, or psychological factors, such as denial or guilt. In these circumstances, providers are obligated to make every effort to clarify precisely what the patient intends to achieve with continued treatment. If the patient's goals appear to reflect unrealistic expectations about the probable course of the underlying illness or the probable effect of medical interventions, providers should attempt to correct those impressions. Because inadequate or insensitive communication by providers probably accounts for a substantial proportion of unrealistic requests, such discussions will successfully resolve many conflicts.[24] Empirical studies of ethics consultations have demonstrated precisely this point.[25]

Although this appeal to the patient's interests may seem to contain some of the same ambiguities as arguments using the concept of futility, there is a subtle but important distinction between the two. Judgments about what is in the patient's interest are properly grounded in the patient's perspective, whereas judgments cast in the language of futility falsely assume that there is an objective and dispassionate standard for determining benefits and burdens. Nevertheless, even after providers make sustained attempts to clarify patients' preferences, some patients or surrogates will continue to demand life-sustaining interventions when the caregivers feel deeply troubled about providing them. In many such cases, unrestrained deference to the wishes of the patient or surrogate conflicts with two other values that do not require a unilateral judgment of the futility of treatment: professional ideals and social consensus.

The ideals of medical professionals include respect for patients' wishes, to be sure, but they also include other values, such as compassionate action and the minimization of suffering. Consider, for example, a bedridden victim of multiple strokes who has contractures and bedsores and who "communicates" only by moaning or grimacing when touched. Physicians asked to perform chest compressions, institute mechanical ventilation, or use other life-sustaining interventions in such a patient may regard these actions as cruel and inhumane.[26] Moreover, physicians and other caregivers have a legitimate interest in seeing that their knowledge and skills are used wisely and effectively. For example, if surgeons were repeatedly pressured to perform operations that they believed to be inappropriate, they would certainly suffer a loss of dignity and sense of purpose. Although appealing to professional ideals can serve as a convenient means of protecting the interests of physicians at the expense of patients' values, these ideals are legitimate factors to weigh against other values. To dismiss this perspective as irrelevant in decision making is to deny an essential part of what it means to practice medicine.

Although we believe that health care professionals should not be required to take part in care that violates their own morals, the law in this area remains uncertain. On the one hand, courts have upheld a state interest in protecting the ethical integrity of the medical profession. This may provide some basis for protecting doctors who wish to refrain from cruel or inhumane treatment, despite the wishes of the patient or surrogate.[27] On the other hand, in the two cases that have led to court decisions (those of Helga Wanglie and of Jane Doe in Atlanta)[28] the judges upheld the surrogates' decision-making authority. Clearly, this area of the law remains to be defined.

Finally, social consensus is yet another expression of the values at stake in some medical decisions. In a pluralistic society, differences in personal values and interests occasionally run so deep that they cannot be resolved by the introduction of additional facts or by further private debate. At certain critical junctures, the resolution of these conflicts may require an explicit public process of social decision making.[29] Social consensus has been sought, for example, to address the issue of fair allocation of resources.[30] The involvement of society is also essential when the most highly charged questions of morality are at stake, as in the increasingly heated debate over euthanasia.[31]

In the prototypical scenarios described at the outset of this chapter, an ongoing attempt to achieve social consensus is perhaps most conspicuous with regard to the prolongation of life for patients in a persistent vegetative state. From a legal perspective, the relevant decisions began with the case of Karen Quinlan[32] and have extended through that of Nancy Cruzan.[33] These cases have increased awareness of the ethical issues raised by the situation of patients in a persistent vegetative state and have helped to consolidate the view that it is acceptable to withdraw life-sustaining treatment from patients in such a state. Controversy does remain about who has the ultimate authority to make these decisions. Some hold that the choice must remain with the patient or surrogate, whereas others believe that under some circumstances this prerogative may be overridden. For example, the Hastings Center[34] and the Society of Critical Care Medicine[35] have concluded that providing intensive care to patients in a persistent vegetative state is generally a misuse of resources, and the President's Commission stated that such patients should be removed from life support if such action is necessary to benefit another patient who is not in a persistent vegetative state.[36] It is unclear how this debate will conclude, but the confluence of medical, legal, and ethical thinking about the persistent vegetative state is an example of how social consensus may evolve.

In summary, the Wanglie case demonstrates how the resolution of these conflicts must proceed on many levels. Most such cases will benefit from sustained attempts to clarify the patient's values and the likelihood of the various relevant outcomes and to improve communication with patients or their surrogates. When this approach fails, physicians and other caregivers should ask themselves whether the care requested is consistent with their professional ethics and ideals. When these ideals appear to be violated, either alternative venues for such care should be found or the conflict should be addressed in a public forum. This broader review could be provided through institutional mechanisms, such as the hospital's ethics committee, or by the courts. The public scrutiny that attends such cases will further the debate over the appropriate use of medical resources and foster the development of consensus through legislation and public policy.

CONCLUSION

In outlining the perspectives of the principal stakeholders—patients and their surrogates, physicians, and society—we have avoided the construction of a rigid formula for resolving conflicts over interventions frequently regarded as futile. Because of clinical heterogeneity, pluralistic values, and the evolutionary nature of social consensus, most clinical decision making on behalf of critically ill patients defies reduction to universally applicable principles.

The notion of futility generally fails to provide an ethically coherent ground for limiting life-sustaining treatment, except in circumstances in which narrowly defined physiologic futility can be plausibly invoked. Futility has been conceptualized as an objective entity independent of the patient's or surrogate's perspective, but differences in values and the variable probabilities of clinical outcomes undermine its basis. Furthermore, assertions of futility may camouflage judgments of comparative worth that are implicit in debates about the allocation of resources. In short, the problem with futility is that its promise of objectivity can rarely be fulfilled. The rapid advance of the language of futility into the jargon of bioethics should be followed by an equally rapid retreat.

NOTES

1. *Jacobellis v. State of Ohio,* 84 S. Ct. 1676 (1964).
2. Hippocrates, "The Art," in *Ethics in Medicine: Historical Perspectives and Contemporary Concerns* (Cambridge, Mass.: MIT Press, 1976), 6–7.
3. A. M. Capron, In re *Helga Wanglie, Hastings Center Report* 21, no. 5 (1991): 26–28; J. D. Lantos et al., "The Illusion of Futility in Clinical Practice," *American Journal of Medicine* 87 (1989): 81–84; "Standards for Cardiopulmonary Resuscitation (CPR) and Emergency Cardiac Care (EEC): V. Medicolegal Considerations and Recommendations," *JAMA* 227, suppl. (1974): 864–66; "Appendix A: The Proposed Legislation," in *Do Not Resuscitate Orders: The Proposed Legislation and Report of the New York State Task Force on Life and the Law*, 2d ed. (New York: New York State Task Force on Life and the Law, 1986), 83.
4. 1984 Amendments to the Child Abuse Prevention and Treatment Act, Public Law 98-457, 1984.
5. American Medical Association, "Council on Ethical and Judicial Affairs, Guidelines for the Appropriate Use of

Do-Not-Resuscitate Orders," *JAMA* 265 (1991): 1868–71.

6. S. H. Miles, "Informed Demand for 'Non-beneficial' Medical Treatment," *New England Journal of Medicine* 325 (1991): 512–15.
7. "Brain-damaged Woman at Center of Lawsuit over Life-Support Dies," *New York Times,* 5 July 1991, A8.
8. J. J. Paris et al., "Physicians' Refusal of Requested Treatment: The Case of Baby L," *New England Journal of Medicine* 322 (1990): 1012–15.
9. L. J. Blackhall, "Must We Always Use CPR?" *New England Journal of Medicine* 317 (1987): 1281–85; J. C. Hackler and F. C. Hiller, "Family Consent to Orders Not to Resuscitate: Reconsidering Hospital Policy," *JAMA* 264 (1990): 1281–83; D. J. Murphy, "Do-Not-Resuscitate Orders: Time for Reappraisal in Long-Term-Care Institutions," *JAMA* 260 (1988): 2098–2101.
10. S. E. Bedell et al., "Survival after Cardiopulmonary Resuscitation in the Hospital," *New England Journal of Medicine* 309 (1983): 569–76.
11. M. Denis et al., "A Comparison of Patient, Family, and Physician Assessments of the Value of Medical Intensive Care," *Critical Care Medicine* 16 (1988): 594–600; M. Denis et al., "A Comparison of Patient, Family, and Nurse Evaluations of the Usefulness of Intensive Care," *Critical Care Medicine* 15 (1987): 138–43; M. Denis et al., "Patients' and Families' Preferences for Medical Intensive Care," *JAMA* 260 (1988): 797–802.
12. L. J. Schneiderman et al., "Medical Futility: Its Meaning and Ethical Implications," *Annals of Internal Medicine* 112 (1990): 949–54.
13. Hastings Center, *Guidelines on the Termination of Life-sustaining Treatment and the Care of the Dying* (Briarcliff Manor, N.Y.: Hastings Center, 1987), 32; "Appendix C: New York Public Health Law Article 29-B—Orders Not to Resuscitate," in *The Proposed Legislation and Report of the New York State Task Force on Life and the Law*, 2d ed. (New York: New York State Task Force on Life and the Law, 1986), 96.
14. Hastings Center, *Guidelines on the Termination of Life-sustaining Treatment and the Care of the Dying.*
15. "Appendix C: New York Public Health Law Article 29-B."
16. American Medical Association, "Council on Ethical and Judicial Affairs, Guidelines for the Appropriate Use of Do-Not-Resuscitate Orders."
17. A. Tversky and D. Kahneman, "Judgment under Uncertainty: Heuristics and Biases," *Science* 185 (1974): 1124–31; A. S. Elstein, "Clinical Judgment: Psychological Research and Medical Practice," *Science* 194 (1976): 696–700.
18. Tversky and Kahneman, "Judgment under Uncertainty."
19. R. M. Poses et al., "The Answer to 'What Are My Chances, Doctor?' Depends of Whom the Question Is Asked: Prognostic Disagreement and Inaccuracy for Critically Ill Patients," *Critical Care Medicine* 17 (1989): 827–33.
20. R. M. Poses et al., "The Accuracy of Experienced Physicians' Probability Estimates for Patients with Sore Throats: Implications for Decision Making," *JAMA* 254 (1985): 925–29.
21. Schneiderman et al., "Medical Futility."
22. H. Aaron and W. B. Schwartz, "Rationing Health Care: The Choice before Us," *Science* 247 (1990): 418–22.
23. D. M. Eddy, "What Is Going on in Oregon?" *JAMA* 260 (1991): 417–20.
24. Murphy, "Do-Not-Resuscitate Orders"; S. J. Youngner, "Who Defines Utility?" *JAMA* 260 (1988): 2094–95.
25. T. A. Brennan, "Ethics Committees and Decisions to Limit Care: The Experience at the Massachusetts General Hospital," *JAMA* 260 (1988): 803–7; J. La Pluma, "Consultations in Clinical Ethics: Issues and Questions in 27 Cases," *Western Journal of Medicine* 146 (1987): 633–37.
26. S. Braithwaite and D. C. Thomasma, "New Guidelines on Forgoing Life-sustaining Treatment in Incompetent Patients: An Anticruelty Policy," *Annals of Internal Medicine* 104 (1986): 711–15.
27. A. Meisel, *The Right to Die* (New York: Wiley, 1989), 104.
28. In re: *Doe,* Civil Action No. D93064 (Fulton County, Ga., October 17, 1991).
29. D. Callahan, "Medical Futility, Medical Necessity: The-Problem-without-a-Name," *Hastings Center Report* 21, no. 4 (1991): 30–35.
30. Eddy, "What Is Going on in Oregon?"
31. R. I. Misbin, "Physicians' Aid in Dying," *New England Journal of Medicine* 325 (1991): 1307–11.
32. In the *Matter of Karen Ann Quinlan, an Alleged Incompetent,* 355 A.2d 647; or 70 NJ 10, March 31, 1976.
33. G. J. Annas, "Nancy Cruzan and the Right to Die," *New England Journal of Medicine* 323 (1990): 670–73.
34. Hastings Center, *Guidelines on the Termination of Life-sustaining Treatment and the Care of the Dying*, 112.
35. Society of Critical Care Medicine, Task Force on Ethics, "Consensus Report on the Ethics of Forgoing Life-sustaining Treatments in the Critically Ill," *Critical Care Medicine* 18 (1990): 1435–39.
36. President's Commission for the Study of Ethical Problems in Medicine and Biomedical and Behavioral Research, *Deciding to Forgo Life-sustaining Treatment: Ethical, Medical, and Legal Issues in Treatment Decisions* (Washington, D.C.: U.S. Government Printing Office, 1983), 188–89.

CHAPTER 30

Is It Time To Abandon Brain Death?

Robert D. Truog

Over the past several decades, the concept of brain death has become well entrenched within the practice of medicine. At a practical level, this concept has been successful in delineating widely accepted ethical and legal boundaries for the procurement of vital organs for transplantation. Despite this success, however, there have been persistent concerns over whether the concept is theoretically coherent and internally consistent.[1] Indeed, some have concluded that the concept is fundamentally flawed, and that it represents only a "superficial and fragile consensus."[2] In this analysis I will identify the sources of these inconsistencies, and suggest that the best resolution to these issues may be to abandon the concept of brain death altogether.

DEFINITIONS, CONCEPTS, AND TESTS

In its seminal work, *Defining Death,* the President's Commission for the Study of Ethical Problems in Medicine and Biomedical and Behavioral Research articulated a formulation of brain death that has come to be known as the "whole-brain standard."[3] In the Uniform Determination of Death Act, the President's Commission specified two criteria for determining death: (1) irreversible cessation of circulatory and respiratory functions, or (2) irreversible cessation of all functions of the entire brain, including the brainstem.

Neurologist James Bernat has been influential in defending and refining this standard. Along with others, he has recognized that analysis of the concept of brain death must begin by differentiating among three distinct levels. At the most general level, the concept must involve a *definition.* Next, *criteria* must be specified to determine when the definition has been fulfilled. Finally, *tests* must be available for evaluating whether the criteria have been satisfied.[4] As clarified by Bernat and colleagues, therefore, the concept of death under the whole brain formulation can be outlined as follows:[5]

> *Definition of Death:* The "permanent cessation of functioning of the organism as a whole."
>
> *Criterion for Death:* The "permanent cessation of functioning of the entire brain."
>
> *Tests for death:* Two distinct sets of tests are available and acceptable for determining that the criterion is fulfilled:
>
> (1) The cardiorespiratory standard is the traditional approach for determining death and relies upon documenting the prolonged absence of circulation or respiration. These tests fulfill the criterion, according to

Source: Reprinted with permission from R. D. Truog, Is It Time to Abandon Brain Death? *Hastings Center Report* Vol. 27, No. 1, pp. 29–37, © 1997, The Hastings Center.

Bernat, since the prolonged absence of these vital signs is diagnostic for the permanent loss of all brain function.

(2) The neurological standard consists of a battery of tests and procedures, including establishment of an etiology sufficient to account for the loss of all brain functions, diagnosing the presence of coma, documenting apnea and the absence of brainstem reflexes, excluding reversible conditions, and showing the persistence of these findings over a sufficient period of time.[6]

CRITIQUE OF THE CURRENT FORMULATION OF BRAIN DEATH

Is this a coherent account of the concept of brain death? To answer this question, one must determine whether each level of analysis is consistent with the others. In other words, individuals who fulfill the tests must also fulfill the criterion, and those who satisfy the criterion must also satisfy the definition.[7]

First, regarding the tests-criterion relationship, there is evidence that many individuals who fulfill all of the tests for brain death do not have the "permanent cessation of functioning of the entire brain." In particular, many of these individuals retain clear evidence of integrated brain function at the level of the brainstem and midbrain, and may have evidence of cortical function.

For example, many patients who fulfill the tests for the diagnosis of brain death continue to exhibit intact neurohumoral function. Between 22 percent and 100 percent of brain-dead patients in different series have been found to retain free-water homeostasis through the neurologically mediated secretion of arginine vasopressin, as evidenced by serum hormonal levels and the absence of diabetes insipidus.[8] Since the brain is the only source of the regulated secretion of arginine vasopressin, patients without diabetes insipidus do not have the loss of all brain function. Neurologically regulated secretion of other hormones is also quite common.[9]

In addition, the tests for the diagnosis of brain death require the patient not to be hypothermic.[10] This caveat is a particularly confusing Catch 22, since the absence of hypothermia generally indicates the continuation of neurologically mediated temperature homeostasis. The circularity of this reasoning can be clinically problematic, since hypothermic patients cannot be diagnosed as brain-dead but the absence of hypothermia is itself evidence of brain function.

Furthermore, studies have shown that many patients (20 percent in one series) who fulfill the tests for brain death continue to show electrical activity on their electroencephalograms.[11] While there is no way to determine how often this electrical activity represents true "function" (which would be incompatible with the criterion for brain death), in at least some cases the activity observed seems fully compatible with function.[12]

Finally, clinicians have observed that patients who fulfill the tests for brain death frequently respond to surgical incision at the time of organ procurement with a significant rise in both heart rate and blood pressure. This suggests that integrated neurological function at a supraspinal level may be present in at least some patients diagnosed as brain-dead.[13] This evidence points to the conclusion that there is a significant disparity between the standard tests used to make the diagnosis of brain death and the criterion these tests are purported to fulfill. Faced with these facts, even supporters of the current statutes acknowledge that the criterion of "whole-brain" death is only an "approximation."[14]

If the tests for determining brain death are incompatible with the current criterion, then one way of solving the problem would be to require tests that always correlate with the "permanent cessation of functioning of the entire brain." Two options have been considered in this regard. The first would require tests that correlate with the actual destruction of the brain, since complete destruction would, of course, be incompatible with any degree of brain function. Only by satisfying these tests, some have argued, could we be assured that all functions of the entire brain have totally and permanently ceased.[15] But is there a constellation of clinical and laboratory tests that correlate with this degree of destruction? Unfortunately, a study of over 500 patients with both coma and apnea (including 146 autopsies for neuropathologic correlation) showed that "it was not possible to verify that a diagnosis made prior to cardiac arrest by any set or subset of criteria would invariably correlate with a diffusely destroyed brain."[16] On the basis of these data, a definition that required total brain destruction could only be confirmed at autopsy. Clearly, a condition that could only be determined after death could never be a requirement for declaring death.

Another way of modifying the tests to conform with the criterion would be to rely solely upon the cardiorespiratory standard for determining death. This standard would certainly identify the permanent cessation of all brain function (thereby fulfilling the criterion), since it is well established by common knowledge that prolonged absence of circulation and respiration results in the death of the entire brain (and every other organ). In addition, fulfillment of these tests would also convincingly demonstrate the cessation of function of the organism as a whole (thereby fulfilling the definition). Unfortunately, this approach for resolving the problem would also make it virtually impossible to obtain vital organs in a viable condition for transplantation, since under current laws it is generally necessary for these organs to be removed from a heart-beating donor.

These inconsistencies between the tests and the criterion are therefore not easily resolvable. In addition to these problems, there are also inconsistencies between the criterion and the definition. As outlined above, the whole-brain concept assumes that the "permanent cessation of functioning of the entire brain" (the criterion) necessarily implies the "permanent cessation of functioning of the organism as a whole" (the definition). Conceptually, this relationship assumes the principle that the brain is responsible for maintaining the body's homeostasis, and that without brain function the organism rapidly disintegrates. In the past, this relationship was demonstrated by showing that individuals who fulfilled the tests for the diagnosis of brain death inevitably had a cardiac arrest within a short period of time, even if they were provided with mechanical ventilation and intensive care.[17] Indeed, this assumption had been considered one of the linchpins in the ethical justification for the concept of brain death.[18] For example, in the largest empirical study of brain death ever performed, a collaborative group working under the auspices of the National Institutes of Health sought to specify the necessary tests for diagnosing brain death by attempting to identify a constellation of neurological findings that would inevitably predict the development of a cardiac arrest within three months, regardless of the level or intensity of support provided.[19]

This approach to defining brain death in terms of neurological findings that predict the development of cardiac arrest is plagued by both logical and scientific problems, however. First, it confuses a prognosis with a diagnosis. Demonstrating that a certain class of patients will suffer a cardiac arrest within a defined period of time certainly proves that they are *dying,* but it says nothing about whether they are *dead.*[20] This conceptual mistake can be clearly appreciated if one considers individuals who are dying of conditions not associated with severe neurological impairment. If a constellation of tests could identify a subgroup of patients with metastatic cancer who invariably suffered a cardiac arrest within a short period of time, for example, we would certainly be comfortable in concluding that they were dying, but we clearly could not claim that they were already dead.

Second, this view relies upon the intuitive notion that the brain is the principal organ of the body, the "integrating" organ whose functions cannot be replaced by any other organ or by artificial means. Up through the early 1980s, this view was supported by numerous studies showing that almost all patients who fulfilled the usual battery of tests for brain death suffered a cardiac arrest within several weeks.[21]

The loss of homeostatic equilibrium that is empirically observed in brain-dead patients is almost certainly the result of their progressive loss of integrated neurohumoral and autonomic function. Over the past several decades, however, intensive-care units (ICUs) have become increasingly sophisticated "surrogate brainstems," replacing the respiratory functions as well as the hormonal and other regulator activities of the damaged neuraxis.[22] This technology is presently utilized in those tragic cases in which a pregnant woman is diagnosed as brain-dead and an attempt is made to maintain her somatic existence until the fetus reaches a viable gestation, as well as for prolonging the organ viability of brain-dead patients awaiting organ procurement.[23] Although the functions of the brainstem are considerably more complex than those of the heart or the lungs, in theory (and increasingly in practice) they are entirely replaceable by modern technology. In terms of maintaining homeostatic functions, therefore, the brain is no more irreplaceable than any of the other vital organs. A definition of death predicated upon the "inevitable" development of a cardiac arrest within a short period of time is therefore inadequate, since this empirical "fact" is no longer true. In other words, cardiac arrest is inevitable only if it is allowed to occur, just as respiratory arrest in brain-dead patients is inevitable only if they are not provided with mechanical ventilation. This gradual development in technical expertise has unwittingly undermined one of the central ethical justifications for the whole-brain criterion of death.

In summary, then, the whole-brain concept is plagued by internal inconsistencies in both the tests-criterion and the criterion-definition relationships, and these problems cannot be easily solved. In addition, there is evidence that this lack of conceptual clarity has contributed to misunderstandings about the concept among both clinicians and laypersons. For example, Stuart Youngner and colleagues found that only 35 percent of physicians and nurses who were likely to be involved in organ procurement for transplantation correctly identified the legal and medical criteria for determining death.[24] Indeed, most of the respondents used inconsistent concepts of death, and a substantial minority misunderstood the criterion to be the permanent loss of consciousness, which the President's Commission had specifically rejected, in part because it would have classified anencephalic newborns and patients in a vegetative state as dead. In other words, medical professionals who were otherwise knowledgeable and sophisticated were generally confused about the concept of brain death. In an editorial accompanying this study, Dan Wikler and Alan Weisbard claimed that this confusion was "appropriate," given the lack of philosophical coherence in the concept itself.[25] In another study, a survey of Swedes found that laypersons were more willing to consent to autopsies than to organ donation for themselves or a close relative. In seeking an explanation for these findings, the authors reported that "the fear of not being dead during the removal of organs, reported by 22 percent of those undecided toward organ donation, was related to the uncertainty surrounding brain death."[26]

On one hand, these difficulties with the concept might be deemed to be so esoteric and theoretical that they should play no role in driving the policy debate about how to define death and procure organs for transplantation. This has certainly been the predominant view up to now. In many other circumstances, theoretical issues have taken a back seat to practical matters when it comes to determining public policy. For example, the question of whether tomatoes should be considered a vegetable or a fruit for purposes of taxation was said to hinge little upon the biological facts of the matter, but to turn primarily upon the political and economic issues at stake.[27] If this view is applied to the concept of brain death, then the best public policy would be that which best served the public's interest, regardless of theoretical concerns.

On the other hand, medicine has a long and respected history of continually seeking to refine the theoretical and conceptual underpinnings of its practice. While the impact of scientific and philosophical views upon social policy and public perception must be taken seriously, they cannot be the sole forces driving the debate. Given the evidence demonstrating a lack of coherence in the whole-brain death formulation and the confusion that is apparent among medical professionals, there is ample reason to prompt a look at alternatives to our current approach.

ALTERNATIVE APPROACHES TO THE WHOLE-BRAIN FORMULATION

Alternatives to the whole-brain death formulation fall into two general categories. One approach is to emphasize the overriding importance of those functions of the brain that support the phenomenon of consciousness and to claim that individuals who have permanently suffered the loss of all consciousness are dead. This is known as the "higher-brain" criterion. The other approach is to return to the traditional tests for determining death, that is, the permanent loss of circulation and respiration. As noted above, this latter strategy could fit well with Bernat's formulation of the definition of death, since adoption of the cardiorespiratory standard as the test for determining death is consistent with both the criterion and the definition. The problem with this potential solution is that it would virtually eliminate the possibility of procuring vital organs from heart-beating donors under our present system of law and ethics, since current requirements insist that organs be removed only from individuals who have been declared dead (the "dead donor rule").[28] Consideration of this latter view would therefore be feasible only if it could be linked to fundamental changes in the permissible limits of organ procurement.

The Higher-Brain Formulation

The higher-brain criterion for death holds that maintaining the potential for consciousness is the critical function of the brain relevant to questions of life and death. Under this definition, all individuals who are permanently unconscious would be considered to be dead. Included in this category would be (1) patients who fulfill the cardiorespiratory standard, (2) those who fulfill the current tests for whole brain death, (3) those diagnosed as being in a permanent vegetative state, and (4) newborns with anencephaly. Various versions of this view have been defended by many philosophers, and arguments have been advanced from moral as well as ontological perspectives.[29] In addition, this view correlates very well with many common-sense opinions about personal identity. To take a stock philosophical illustration, for example, consider the typical reaction of a person who has undergone a hypothetical "brain switch" procedure, where one's brain is transplanted into another's body, and vice versa. Virtually anyone presented with this scenario will say that "what matters" for their existence now resides in the new body, even though an outside observer would insist that it is the person's old body that "appears" to be the original person. Thought experiments like this one illustrate that we typically identify ourselves with our experience of consciousness, and this observation forms the basis of the claim that the permanent absence of consciousness should be seen as representing the death of the person.

Implementation of this standard would present certain problems, however. First, is it possible to diagnose the state of permanent unconsciousness with the high level of certainty required for the determination of death? More specifically, is it currently possible to definitively diagnose the permanent vegetative state and anencephaly? A Multi-Society Task Force recently outlined guidelines for diagnosis of permanent vegetative state and claimed that sufficient data are now available to make the diagnosis of permanent vegetative state in appropriate patients with a high degree of certainty.[30] On the other hand, case reports of patients who met these criteria but who later recovered a higher degree of neurological functioning suggest that use of the term "permanent" may be overstating the degree of diagnostic certainty that is currently possible. This would be an especially important issue in the context of diagnosing death, where false positive diagnoses would be particularly problematic.[31] Similarly, while the Medical Task Force on Anencephaly has concluded that most cases of anencephaly can be diagnosed by a competent clinician without significant uncertainty, others have emphasized the ambiguities inherent in evaluating this condition.[32]

Another line of criticism is that the higher-brain approach assumes the definition of death should reflect the death of the *person,* rather than the death of the *organism.*[33] By focusing on the person, this theory does not account for what is common to the death of all organisms, such as humans, frogs, or trees. Since we do not know what it would mean to talk about the permanent loss of consciousness of frogs or trees, then this approach to death may appear to be idiosyncratic. In response, higher-brain theorists believe that it is critical to define death within the context of the specific subject under consideration. For example, we may speak of the death of an ancient civilization, the death of a species, or the death of a particular system of belief. In each case, the definition of death will be different and must be appropriate to the subject in order for the concept to make any sense. Following this line of reasoning, the higher-brain approach is correct precisely because it seeks to identify what is uniquely relevant to the death of a person.

Aside from these diagnostic and philosophical concerns, however, perhaps the greatest objections to the higher-brain formulation emerge from the implications of treating breathing patients as if they are dead. For example, if patients in a permanent vegetative state were considered to be dead, then they should logically be considered suitable for burial. Yet all of these patients breathe, and some of them "live" for many years.[34] The thought of burying or cremating a breathing individual, even if unconscious, would be unthinkable for many people, creating a significant barrier to acceptance of this view into public policy.[35]

One way of avoiding this implication would be to utilize a "lethal injection" before cremation or burial to terminate cardiac and respiratory function. This would not be euthanasia, since the individual would be declared dead before the injection. The purpose of the injection would be purely "aesthetic." This practice could even be viewed as simply an extension of our current protocols, where the vital functions of patients diagnosed as brain-dead are terminated prior to burial, either by discontinuing mechanical ventilation or by removing their heart and/or lungs during the process of organ procurement. While this line of argumentation has a certain logical persuasiveness, it nevertheless fails to address the central fact that most people find it counterintuitive to perceive a breathing patient as "dead." Wikler has suggested that this attitude is likely to change over time, and that eventually society will come to accept that the body of a patient in a permanent vegetative state is simply that person's "living remains."[36] This optimism about higher-brain death is reminiscent of the comments by the President's Commission regarding whole brain death: "Although undeniably disconcerting for many people, the confusion created in personal perception by a determination of 'brain death' does not . . . provide a basis for an ethical objection to discontinuing medical measures on these dead bodies any more than on other dead bodies."[37] Nevertheless, at the present time any inclination toward a higher-brain death standard remains primarily in the realm of philosophers and not policy makers.

Return to the Traditional Cardiorespiratory Standard

In contrast to the higher-brain concept of death, the other main alternative to our current approach would involve moving in the opposite direction and abandoning the diagnosis of brain death altogether. This would involve returning to the traditional approach to determining death, that is, the cardiorespiratory standard. In evaluating the wisdom of "turning back the clock," it is helpful to retrace the development of the concept of brain death back to 1968 and the conclusions of the Ad Hoc Committee that developed the Harvard Criteria for the diagnosis of brain death. They began by claiming:

> There are two reasons why there is need for a definition [of brain death]: (1) Improvements in resuscitative and

> supportive measures have led to increased efforts to save those who are desperately injured. Sometimes these efforts have only partial success so that the result is an individual whose heart continues to beat but whose brain is irreversibly damaged. The burden is great on patients who suffer permanent loss of intellect, on their families, and on those in need of hospital beds already occupied by these comatose patients. (2) Obsolete criteria for the definition of death can lead to controversy in obtaining organs for transplantation.[38]

These two issues can be subdivided into at least four distinct questions:

1. When is it permissible to withdraw life support from patients with irreversible neurological damage for the benefit of the patient?
2. When is it permissible to withdraw life support from patients with irreversible neurological damage for the benefit of society, where the benefit is either in the form of economic savings or to make an ICU bed available for someone with a better prognosis?
3. When is it permissible to remove organs from a patient for transplantation?
4. When is a patient ready to be cremated or buried?

The Harvard Committee chose to address all of these questions with a single answer, that is, the determination of brain death. Each of these questions involves unique theoretical issues, however, and each raises a different set of concerns. By analyzing the concept of brain death in terms of the separate questions that led to its development, alternatives to brain death may be considered.

Withdrawal of life support. The Harvard Committee clearly viewed the diagnosis of brain death as a necessary condition for the withdrawal of life support: "It should be emphasized that we recommend the patient be declared dead before any effort is made to take him off a respirator . . . [since] otherwise, the physicians would be turning off the respirator on a person who is, in the present strict, technical application of law, still alive" (p. 339).

The ethical and legal mandates that surround the withdrawal of life support have changed dramatically since the recommendations of the Harvard Committee. Numerous court decisions and consensus statements have emphasized the rights of patients or their surrogates to demand the withdrawal of life-sustaining treatments, including mechanical ventilation. In the practice of critical care medicine today, patients are rarely diagnosed as brain-dead solely for the purpose of discontinuing mechanical ventilation. When patients are not candidates for organ transplantation, either because of medical contraindications or lack of consent, families are informed of the dismal prognosis, and artificial ventilation is withdrawn. While the diagnosis of brain death was once critical in allowing physicians to discontinue life-sustaining treatments, decision making about these important questions is now appropriately centered around the patient's previously stated wishes and judgments about the patient's best interest. Questions about the definition of death have become virtually irrelevant to these deliberations.

Allocation of scarce resources. The Harvard Committee alluded to its concerns about having patients with a hopeless prognosis occupying ICU beds. In the years since that report, this issue has become even more pressing. The diagnosis of brain death, however, is of little significance in helping to resolve these issues. Even considering the unusual cases where families refuse to have the ventilator removed from a brain-dead patient, the overall impact of the diagnosis of brain death upon scarce ICU resources is minimal. Much more important to the current debate over the just allocation of ICU resources are patients with less severe degrees of neurological dysfunction, such as patients in a permanent vegetative state or individuals with advanced dementia. Again, the diagnosis of brain death is of little relevance to this central concern of the Harvard Committee.

Organ transplantation. Without question, the most important reason for the continued use of brain death criteria is the need for transplantable organs. Yet even here, the requirement for brain death may be doing more harm than good. The need for organs is expanding at an ever-increasing rate, while the number of available organs has essentially plateaued. In an effort to expand the limited pool of organs, several attempts have been made to circumvent the usual restrictions of brain death on organ procurement.

At the University of Pittsburgh, for example, a new protocol allows critically ill patients or their surrogates to offer their organs for donation after the withdrawal of life-support, even though the patients never meet brain death criteria.[39] Suitable patients are taken to the operating room, where intravascular monitors are placed and the patient is "prepped and draped" for surgical incision. Life-support is then withdrawn, and the patient is monitored for the development of cardiac arrest. Assuming this occurs within a short period of time, the attending physician waits until there have been two minutes of pulselessness, and then pronounces the patient dead. The transplant team then enters the operating room and immediately removes the organs for transplantation.

This novel approach has a number of problems when viewed from within the traditional framework. For example, after the patient is pronounced dead, why should the team rush to remove the organs? If the Pittsburgh team truly believes that the patient is dead, why not begin chest compressions and mechanical ventilation, insert cannulae to place the patient on full cardiopulmonary bypass, and remove the organs in a more controlled fashion? Presumably, this is not done because two minutes of pulselessness is almost certainly not long enough to ensure the development of brain death.[40] It is even conceivable that patients managed in this way could regain consciousness during the process of organ procurement while supported with cardiopulmonary bypass, despite having already been diagnosed as "dead." In other words, the reluctance of the Pittsburgh team to extend their protocol in ways that would be acceptable for dead patients could be an indication that the patients may really not be dead after all.

A similar attempt to circumvent the usual restrictions on organ procurement was recently attempted with anencephalic newborns at Loma Linda University. Again, the protocol involved manipulation of the dying process, with mechanical ventilation being instituted and maintained solely for the purpose of preserving the organs until criteria for brain death could be documented. The results were disappointing, and the investigators concluded that "it is usually not feasible, with the restrictions of current law, to procure solid organs for transplantation from anencephalic infants."[41]

Why do these protocols strike many commentators as contrived and even somewhat bizarre? The motives of the individuals involved are certainly commendable: They want to offer the benefits of transplantable organs to individuals who desperately need them. In addition, they are seeking to obtain organs only from individuals who cannot be harmed by the procurement and only in those situations where the patient or a surrogate requests the donation. The problem with these protocols lies not with the motive but with the method and justification. By manipulating both the process and the definition of death, these protocols give the appearance that the physicians involved are only too willing to draw the boundary between life and death wherever it happens to maximize the chances for organ procurement.

How can the legitimate desire to increase the supply of transplantable organs be reconciled with the need to maintain a clear and simple distinction between the living and the dead? One way would be to abandon the requirement for the death of the donor prior to organ procurement and, instead, focus upon alternative and perhaps more fundamental ethical criteria to constrain the procurement of organs, such as the principles of consent and nonmaleficence.[42]

For example, policies could be changed such that organ procurement would be permitted only with the consent of the donor or appropriate surrogate and only when doing so would not harm the donor. Individuals who could not be harmed by the procedure would include those who are permanently and irreversibly unconscious (patients in a persistent vegetative state or newborns with anencephaly) and those who are imminently and irreversibly dying.

The American Medical Association's Council on Ethical and Judicial Affairs recently proposed (but has subsequently retracted) a position consistent with this approach.[43] The council stated that, "It is ethically permissible to consider the anencephalic as a potential organ donor, although still alive under the current definition of death," if, among other requirements, the diagnosis is certain and the parents give their permission. The council concluded, "It is normally required that the donor be legally dead before removal of their life-necessary organs . . . The use of the anencephalic neonate as a live donor is a limited exception to the general standard because of the fact that the infant has never experienced, and will never experience, consciousness" (pp. 1617–18).

This alternative approach to organ procurement would require substantial changes in the law. The process of organ procurement would have to be legitimated as a form of justified killing, rather than just as the dissection of a corpse. There is certainly precedent in the law for recognizing instances of justified killing. The concept is also not an anathema to the public, as evidenced by the growing support for euthanasia, another practice that would have to be legally construed as a form of justified killing. Even now, surveys show that one-third of physicians and nurses do not believe brain-dead patients are actually dead but feel comfortable with the process of organ procurement because the patients are permanently unconscious and/or imminently dying.[44] In other words, many clinicians already seem to justify their actions on the basis of nonmaleficence and consent, rather than with the belief that the patients are actually dead.

This alternative approach would also eliminate the need for protocols like the one being used at the University of Pittsburgh, with its contrived and perhaps questionable approach to declaring death prior to organ procurement. Under the proposed system, qualified individuals who had given their consent could simply have their organs removed under general anesthesia, without first undergoing an orchestrated withdrawal of life support. Anencephalic newborns whose parents requested organ donation could likewise have the organs removed under general anesthesia, without the need to wait for the diagnosis of brain death.

The diagnosis of death. Seen in this light, the concept of brain death may have become obsolete. Certainly the diagnosis of brain death has been extremely useful during the last several decades, as society has struggled with a myriad of issues that were never encountered before the era of mechanical ventilation and organ transplantation. As society emerges from this transitional period, and as many of these issues are more clearly understood as questions that are inherently unrelated to the distinction between life and death, then the concept of brain death may no longer be useful or relevant. If this is the case, then it may be preferable to return to the traditional standard and limit tests for the determination of death to those based solely upon the permanent cessation of respiration and circulation. Even today we uniformly regard the cessation of respiration and circulation as the standard for determining when patients are ready to be cremated or buried.

Another advantage of a return to the traditional approach is that it would represent a "common denominator" in the definition of death that virtually all cultural groups and religious traditions would find acceptable.[45] Recently both New Jersey and New York have enacted statutes that recognize the objections of particular religious views to the concept of brain death. In New Jersey, physicians are prohibited from declaring brain death in persons who come from religious traditions that do not accept the concept.[46] Return to a cardiorespiratory standard would eliminate problems with these objections.

Linda Emanuel recently proposed a "bounded zone" definition of death that shares some features with the approach outlined here.[47] Her proposal would adopt the cardiorespiratory standard as a "lower bound" for determining death that would apply to all cases but would allow individuals to choose a definition of death that encompassed neurologic dysfunction up to the level of the permanent vegetative state (the "higher bound"). The practical implications of such a policy would be similar to some of those discussed here, in that it would (1) allow patients and surrogates to request organ donation when and if the patients were diagnosed with whole-brain death, permanent vegetative state, or anencephaly, and (2) it would permit rejection of the diagnosis of brain death by patients and surrogates opposed to the concept. Emanuel's proposal would not permit organ donation from terminal and imminently dying patients, however, prior to the diagnosis of death.

Despite these similarities, these two proposals differ markedly in the justifications used to support their conclusions. Emanuel follows the President's Commission in seeking to address several separate questions by reference to the diagnosis of death, whereas the approach suggested here would adopt a single and uniform definition of death, and then seek to resolve questions around organ donation on a different ethical and legal foundation.

Emanuel's proposal also provides another illustration of the problems encountered when a variety of diverse issues all hinge upon the definition of death. Under her scheme, some individuals would undoubtedly opt for a definition of death based on the "higher bound" of the permanent vegetative state in order to permit the donation of their vital organs if they should develop this condition. However, few of these individuals would probably agree to being cremated while still breathing, even if they were vegetative. Most likely, they would not want to be cremated until after they had sustained a cardiorespiratory arrest. Once again, this creates the awkward and confusing necessity of diagnosing death for one purpose (organ donation) but not for another (cremation). Only by abandoning the concept of brain death is it possible to adopt a definition of death that is valid for all purposes, while separating questions of organ donation from dependence upon the life/death dichotomy.

TURNING BACK

The tension between the need to maintain workable and practical standards for the procurement of transplantable organs and our desire to have a conceptually coherent account of death is an issue that must be given serious attention. Resolving these inconsistencies by moving toward a higher-brain definition of death would most likely create additional practical problems regarding accurate diagnosis as well as introduce concepts that are highly counterintuitive to the general public. Uncoupling the link between organ transplantation and brain death, on the other hand, offers a number of advantages. By shifting the ethical foundations for organ donation to the principles of nonmaleficence and consent, the pool of potential donors may be substantially increased. In addition, by reverting to a simpler and more traditional definition of death, the long-standing debate over fundamental inconsistencies in the concept of brain death may finally be resolved.

The most difficult challenge for this proposal would be to gain acceptance of the view that killing may sometimes be a justifiable necessity for procuring transplantable organs. Careful attention to the principles of consent and nonmaleficence should provide an adequate bulwark against slippery slope concerns that this practice would be extended in unforeseen and unacceptable ways. Just as the euthanasia debate often seems to turn less upon abstract theoretical concerns and more upon the empirical question of whether guidelines for assisted dying would be abused, so the success of this proposal could also rest upon factual questions of societal acceptance and whether this approach would erode respect for human life and the integrity of clinicians. While the answers to these questions are not known, the potential benefits of this proposal make it worthy of continued discussion and debate.

ACKNOWLEDGMENTS

The author thanks numerous friends and colleagues for critical readings of the manuscript, with special acknowledgments to Dan Wikler and Linda Emanuel.

NOTES

1. Some of the more notable critiques include R. M. Veatch, "The Whole-Brain-Oriented Concept of Death: An Outmoded Philosophical Formulation," *Journal of Thanatology* 3 (1975): 13–30; M. B. Green and D. Wikler, "Brain Death and Personal Identity," *Philosophy and Public Affairs* 9 (1980): 105–33; S. J. Youngner and E. T. Bartlett, "Human Death and High Technology: The Failure of the Whole-Brain Formulations," *Annals of Internal Medicine* 99 (1983): 252–58; A. Halevy and B. Brody, "Brain Death: Reconciling Definitions, Criteria, and Tests," *Annals of Internal Medicine* 119 (1993): 519–25.
2. S. J. Youngner, "Defining Death: A Superficial and Fragile Consensus," *Archives of Neurology* 49 (1992): 570–72.
3. President's Commission for the Study of Ethical Problems in Medicine and Biomedical and Behavioral Research, *Defining Death* (Washington, D.C.: U.S. Government Printing Office, 1981).
4. K. Gervais has been especially articulate in defining these levels. See K. G. Gervais, *Redefining Death* (New Haven: Yale University Press, 1986); "Advancing the Definition of Death: A Philosophical Essay," *Medical Humanities Review* 3, no. 2 (1989): 7–19.
5. J. L. Bernat, C. M. Culver, and B. Gert, "On the Definition and Criterion of Death," *Annals of Internal Medicine* 94 (1981): 389–94; J. L. Bernat, "How Much of the Brain Must Die in Brain Death?" *Journal of Clinical Ethics* 3 (1992): 21–26.
6. Report of the Medical Consultants on the Diagnosis of Death, "Guidelines for the Determination of Death," *JAMA* 246 (1981): 2184–86.
7. Aspects of this analysis have been explored previously in, R. D. Truog and J. C. Fackler, "Rethinking Brain Death," *Critical Care Medicine* 20 (1992): 1705–13; Halevy and Brody, "Brain Death."
8. H. Schrader et al., "Changes of Pituitary Hormones in Brain Death," *Acta Neurochirurgica* 52 (1980): 239–48; K. M. Outwater and M. A. Rockoff, "Diabetes Insipidus Accompanying Brain Death in Children," *Neurology* 34 (1984): 1243–46; J. C. Fackler, J. C. Troncoso, and F. R. Gioia, "Age-Specific Characteristics of Brain Death in Children," *American Journal of Diseases of Children* 142 (1988): 999–1003.
9. Schrader et al., "Changes of Pituitary Hormones in Brain Death"; H. J. Gramm et al., "Acute Endocrine Failure after Brain Death," *Transplantation* 54 (1992): 851–57.
10. Report of Medical Consultants on the Diagnosis of Death, "Guidelines for the Determination of Death," p. 339.
11. M. M. Grigg et al., "Electroencephalographic Activity after Brain Death," *Archives of Neurology* 44 (1987): 948–54; A. E. Walker, *Cerebral Death,* 2nd ed. (Baltimore: Urban & Schwarzenberg, 1981), pp. 89–90; and C. Pallis, "ABC of Brain Stem Death. The Arguments about the EEG," *British Medical Journal [Clinical Research]* 286 (1983): 284–87.
12. E. Rodin et al., "Brainstem Death," *Clinical Electroencephalography* 16 (1985): 63–71.
13. R. C. Wetzel et al., "Hemodynamic Responses in Brain Dead Organ Donor Patients," *Anesthesia and Analgesia* 64 (1985): 125–28; S. H. Pennefather, J. H. Dark, and R. E. Bullock, "Haemodynamic Responses to Surgery in Brain-Dead Organ Donors," *Anaesthesia* 48 (1993): 1034–38; and D. J. Hill, R. Munglani, and D. Sapsford, "Haemodynamic Responses to Surgery in Brain-Dead Organ Donors," *Anaesthesia* 49 (1994): 835–36.
14. Bernat, "How Much of the Brain Must Die in Brain Death?"
15. P. A. Byrne, S. O'Reilly, and P. M. Quay, "Brain Death—An Opposing Viewpoint," *JAMA* 242 (1979): 1985–90.
16. G. F. Molinari, "The NINCDS Collaborative Study of Brain Death: A Historical Perspective," in U.S. Department of Health and Human Services, *NINCDS monograph No. 24. NIH publication No. 81-2286* (1980): 1–32.
17. Pallis, "ABC of Brain Stem Death," pp. 123–24; B. Jennett and C. Hessett, "Brain Death in Britain as Reflected in Renal Donors," *British Medical Journal* 283 (1981): 359–62; P. M. Black, "Brain Death (first of two parts)," *NEJM* 299 (1978): 338–44.
18. President's Commission, *Defining Death.*
19. "An Appraisal of the Criteria of Cerebral Death, A Summary Statement: A Collaborative Study," *JAMA* 237 (1977): 982–86.
20. Green and Wikler, "Brain Death and Personal Identity."
21. President's Commission, *Defining Death.*
22. Green and Wikler, "Brain Death and Personal Identity"; Daniel Wikler, "Brain Death: A Durable Consensus?" *Bioethics* 7 (1993): 239–46.
23. D. R. Field et al., "Maternal Brain Death During Pregnancy: Medical and Ethical Issues," *JAMA* 260 (1988): 816–22; M. Washida et al., "Beneficial Effect of Combined 3,5,3'-Triiodothyronine and Vasopressin Administration on Hepatic Energy Status and Systemic Hemodynamics after Brain Death," *Transplantation* 54 (1992): 44–49.
24. S. J. Youngner et al., "'Brain Death' and Organ Retrieval: A Cross-Sectional Survey of Knowledge and

Concepts among Health Professionals," *JAMA* 261 (1989): 2205–10.

25. D. Wikler and A. J. Weisbard, "Appropriate Confusion over 'Brain Death,'" *JAMA* 261 (1989): 2246.
26. M. Sanner, "A Comparison of Public Attitudes toward Autopsy, Organ Donation, and Anatomic Dissection: A Swedish Survey," *JAMA* 271 (1994): 284–88, at 287.
27. Green and Wikler, "Brain Death and Personal Identity."
28. R. M. Arnold and S. J. Youngner, "The Dead Donor Rule: Should We Stretch It, Bend It, or Abandon It?" *Kennedy Institute of Ethics Journal* 3 (1993): 263–78.
29. Some of the many works defending this view include: Green and Wikler, "Brain Death and Personal Identity"; Gervais, *Redefining Death*; Truog and Fackler, "Rethinking Brain Death"; and R. M. Veatch, *Death, Dying, and the Biological Revolution* (New Haven: Yale University Press, 1989).
30. The Multi-Society Task Force on PVS, "Medical Aspects of the Persistent Vegetative State," *NEJM* 330 (1994): 1499–1508 and 1572–79; D. A. Shewmon, "Anencephaly: Selected Medical Aspects," *Hastings Center Report* 18, no. 5 (1988): 11–19.
31. N. L. Childs and W. N. Mercer, "Brief Report: Late Improvement in Consciousness after Post-Traumatic Vegetative State," *NEJM* 334 (1996): 24–25; J. L. Bernat, "The Boundaries of the Persistent Vegetative State," *Journal of Clinical Ethics* 3 (1992): 176–80.
32. Medical Task Force on Anencephaly, "The Infant with Anencephaly," *NEJM* 322 (1990): 669–74; Shewmon, "Anencephaly: Selected Medical Aspects."
33. J. R. Botkin and S. G. Post, "Confusion in the Determination of Death: Distinguishing Philosophy from Physiology," *Perspectives in Biology and Medicine* 36 (1993): 129–38.
34. The Multi-Society Task Force on PVS, "Medical Aspects of the Persistent Vegetative State."
35. M. Angell, "After Quinlan: The Dilemmas of the Persistent Vegetative State," *NEJM* 330 (1994): 1524–25.
36. Wikler, "Brain Death: A Durable Consensus?"
37. President's Commission, *Defining Death,* p. 84.
38. Report of the Ad Hoc Committee of the Harvard Medical School to Examine the Definition of Brain Death, "A Definition of Irreversible Coma," *JAMA* 205 (1968): 337–40.
39. "University of Pittsburgh Medical Center Policy and Procedure Manual: Management of Terminally Ill Patients Who May Become Organ Donors after Death," *Kennedy Institute of Ethics Journal* 3 (1993): A1–A15; S. Youngner and R. Arnold, "Ethical, Psychosocial, and Public Policy Implications of Procuring Organs from Non-Heart-Beating Cadaver Donors," *JAMA* 269 (1993): 2769–74. Of note, the June 1993 issue of the *Kennedy Institute of Ethics of Journal* is devoted to this topic in its entirety.
40. J. Lynn, "Are the Patients Who Become Organ Donors Under the Pittsburgh Protocol for 'Non-Heart-Beating Donors' Really Dead?" *Kennedy Institute of Ethics Journal* 3 (1993): 167–78.
41. J. L. Peabody, J. R. Emery, and Stephen Ashwal, "Experience with Anencephalic Infants as Prospective Organ Donors," *NEJM* 321 (1989): 344–50.
42. See for example, N. Fost, "The New Body Snatchers: On Scott's 'The Body as Property,'" *American Bar Foundation Research Journal* 3 (1983): 718–32; J. A. Robertson, "Relaxing the Death Standard for Organ Donation in Pediatric Situations," in *Organ Substitution Technology: Ethical, Legal, and Public Policy Issues,* ed. D. Mathieu (Boulder, Colo.: Westview Press, 1988), pp. 69–76; Arnold and Youngner, "The Dead Donor Rule."
43. AMA Council on Ethical and Judicial Affairs, "The Use of Anencephalic Neonates as Organ Donors," *JAMA* 273 (1995): 1614–18. After extensive debate among AMA members, the Council retracted this position statement. See C. W. Plows, "Reconsideration of AMA Opinion on Anencephalic Neonates as Organ Donors," *JAMA* 275 (1996): 443–44.
44. Youngner et al., "'Brain Death' and Organ Retrieval."
45. J. Nudeshima, "Obstacles to Brain Death and Organ Transplantation in Japan," *Lancet* 338 (1991): 1063–64.
46. R. S. Olick, "Brain Death, Religious Freedom, and Public Policy: New Jersey's Landmark Legislative Initiative," *Kennedy Institute of Ethics Journal* 1 (1991): 275–88.
47. L. L. Emanuel, "Reexamining Death: The Asymptotic Model and a Bounded Zone Definition," *Hastings Center Report* 25, no. 4 (1995): 27–35.

CHAPTER 31

Waste Not, Want Not: Communities and Presumed Consent

Erich H. Loewy

When a man dies he is disposed of by burial, by cremation, or by other means. His remains are kept but briefly, and only a memory of his days persists. As the reality of being yields its fruits to memory, symbolism, often expressed in private or public ritual, takes its place. It is a time to reflect, to take stock, to grieve for what might have been or to rejoice in what was; it is a time when men confront their own mortality and their own brief stay. Grief, if it is to be tempered by compassion instead of turned only inward toward the self ("my loss," "my grief," "my mortality"), involves awareness of the mortality, suffering, and tenuous existence of others.

Burial and cremation, then, dispose of what only briefly remains and inevitably decays. Society does not bury, cremate, or dispose of memory but seeks to enhance and fortify remembrance by symbolism expressed in concrete ritual. Whatever act is chosen may be meaningful and fitting to that end. Burying, cremating, or otherwise disposing of the remains is hallowed in tradition and confirmed in fact. The methods of disposition evolve over time and differ in diverse cultures, serving the ends of the living rather than that which is beyond benefit or harm. Life, indeed, is for the living, and so are the rites and rituals that mark its passage.

The dead serve the living by providing a period of reflection, of realization, and ultimately of self-renewal. Dissection and autopsy of the remains, until recent times, were the only ways that the dead could make a contribution to the living. And as important as dissection and autopsy continue to be, they rarely involve an immediate life-saving measure needed by someone living in order to function or stay alive. However, things have changed today. The dead, rather than contributing to the living in a rather indirect manner, are able to make critical contributions to living persons. These contributions do not diminish the dead. In fact, they can indeed enhance the symbolism and symbolic value of transition for the living.

The dead, today, are often vitally needed by the living in more than a symbolic sense. They are needed both to increase our knowledge of life processes and disease through doing careful autopsies, and to enhance the life of the living in a very concrete manner by tissue and organ donation. To destroy a resource critically needed by a living person and entirely useless to another seems morally odd.

This chapter will examine the following topics involved in the issue of tissue waste: (1) the problem of tissue waste as it has developed through history and the problem today; (2) community, justice, and mutual obligation; (3) scarce resources and organs donation; (4) objections to the customary salvage of organs; and (5) a possible resolution of this problem.

THE PROBLEM TODAY

The idea of using tissues and organs is not new; however, the reality is. The miraculous transplantation of organs was spoken of in medieval times, and a sixteenth-century picture by Fernando del Rincon hanging in the Prado shows a sacristan whose leg had become gangrenous receiving a new leg from a black man, presumably a slave. (The instrument of consent and the outcome of this venture are unfortunately not stated!) Despite the apocryphal stories (and the probably equally apocryphal story of Pope Innocent VIII's "transfusion" in 1492),[1] there is no evidence that tissue transfers took place prior to the seventeenth century, when Richard Lower, in England, first transfused blood from one animal to another.[2] In Paris shortly thereafter, Denys first transfused animal blood into humans. A failure of one such procedure and a suit brought by the patient's widow (who, it was later found, had murdered her husband and blamed the physician)[3] soured physicians, and no further attempts occurred until 1818, when Blundell at Guy's Hospital first transfused blood from human to human. From then on, transfusions (tissue transplants in their own right) were carried out, some meeting with success, others unaccountably resulting in disaster. It was not until Landsteiner in 1900 described blood groups and he and Wiener made further refinements in 1940 that these disasters were understood and safe blood transfusions became a reality.[4] Successful skin grafting and early transplantation occurred in the late nineteenth and early twentieth century. Ullman in Vienna[5] and Alexis Carrel in New York[6] first successfully transplanted the kidney of one animal into another in 1902. Transplants of other organs, blood vessels, and limbs soon followed.[7]

Successful transplants from nontwins, or at least from nonrelated donors, awaited a better understanding of the immune process and, where needed, its relatively safe suppression. Tissue transplants, other than corneas (not usually subject to rejection) and blood (transfusable since the development of blood grouping), have become a reality only in very recent times. Now, however, the transplantation of kidneys, hearts (or hearts and lungs), livers, and corneas, as well as bones and sometimes skin, is an everyday event. Each newly dead could potentially restore sight to two sightless persons, renal function to two dialysis-dependent persons, liver function to one person in liver failure, and heart or heart-lung function to another on the brink of death—aside from serving as a possible donor of other tissues. Scarcity of organs, partly due to an archaic and inefficient retrieval system, is the limiting factor. Throughout this country only about 10 or 15 percent of suitable donors ever become actual ones, and even these rarely end up donating fully.[8]

There are three possible ways of looking at organ retrieval. We can (1) consider the use of cadaver organs immoral and forbid it altogether, (2) allow the donation of organs, or (3) routinely salvage organs regardless of consent or dissent. The first possibility is neither a moral nor a legal option. It slams the door on life or function and permits needless death to occur. The second possibility, voluntarism, comes in two forms: Either we can make nongiving the norm and giving a supererogatory act or we can establish giving as the norm and allow dissent in unusual cases. The third possibility, taking useful cadaver organs under all circumstances, would require neither assent nor permit dissent.

In America today, voluntarism of the first kind described above is the established norm. A person declared brain dead (by a procedure that keeps the retrieval team distinct from the team caring for a donor) serves as a donor after valid instruments of donation have been executed and accepted. The process, criteria, and validity of declaring persons brain dead have been established in ethics and in law.[9] Premortem donation is legally accepted in all states.[10] In theory, such instruments when properly executed are the only vehicle of donation needed; in practice, partly because of the ever present fear of litigation, no team is willing to harvest organs in the face of objections by the next of kin.[11] When no instrument has been executed, donation can be made by the next of kin. However, the hospital staff is often loath to request donation. The newly dead who might be a suitable donor is generally a young person unexpectedly visited by disaster.

As a result, the family is stunned.[12] It is a time when emotions run high and when rational deliberation is unlikely to occur. Hopes, fears, grief, guilt, superstition, and just plain fatigue mitigate against a dispassionate decision.[13] The process of organ donation will prolong the ordeal and will extend the time when family and staff are obliged to remain in a state of confusion, anguish, and fatigue.

Voluntarism of the second part, called *presumed consent,* shifts the burden. It allows physicians and hospitals to remove and transplant needed organs unless the decedent prior to death has objected or, when there is no express wish, the next of kin after death specifically objects. In case of conflict, the decedent's wishes have primacy over those of the family.[14] This kind of consent is extensively used and readily understood throughout much of the world. It still leaves much to be desired, because teams in hospitals not actively engaged in transplants have shown a tendency to place salvage low in their scale of priorities.[15] Salvaging potentially useful organs from all brain-dead patients, regardless of assent or dissent, is enticing from a purely utilitarian perspective, but it smacks of autocracy. Its moral justifiability in a given community depends, as we shall see, largely on how that community conceives of itself.

COMMUNITY, JUSTICE, AND MUTUAL OBLIGATION

The way in which we view communities underlies our concept of justice, our sense of mutual obligation, and ultimately our laws and procedures.[16] The notion that members of communities are bound only by the duty to refrain from harming one another is critically different from the notion that they are united by far more than this. In communities where the sole duty is to refrain from harm, freedom is likely to be a condition of morality (a "side constraint," as Nozick would have it)[17] rather than a value. It, therefore, cannot be negotiated or limited in any way. Freedom for any individual should be restricted only to the extent that it directly interferes with another's freedom. The sole legitimate power of the community is to enforce and defend individual freedom. Beyond the duty to refrain from harming one another, persons have the freedom, although not the duty, to help each other. Except when such help is freely and explicitly agreed upon by mutual contract, they have no obligation to respond to their neighbors' problems.[18]

A collection of individuals living together cannot long endure if it is not united by certain ways of behaving toward each other.[19] The duty to refrain from harming one another is essential for coexistence. Individuals must avoid killing or injuring each other and must refrain from other clearly injurious acts. But refraining from harm, by itself, is insufficient for maintaining what we ordinarily think of as a community. A community, in ordinary thinking, demands common goals toward which all members work (besides working toward their individual goals). A community is cemented by the inclination of its members to aid each other. A "minimalist ethic" is insufficient.[20] If a community is to endure, perfect duties (duties where no discretion is allowed, such as the duty to refrain from harming others) must be leavened by imperfect duties (duties where discretion or inclination is allowed, such as the duty of benevolence, which one can fulfill by helping this, that, or the other person).[21]

The two views of community described above entail starkly differing consequences. If one views freedom as the absolute condition of morality and community members as bound only by duties of noninterference, one will refuse to tax the affluent for the benefit of the poor, be unwilling to ensure the safety (or free availability) of drugs, and be inclined to allow men to sell themselves freely into slavery. Freedom would no longer be a bargaining chip. Instead of being a fundamental communal value, one promulgated, secured, and safeguarded by the community, freedom becomes an untouchable absolute. As such, it too easily leads to the domination of the weak by the strong, the poor by the rich.[22] Communities in which freedom is an absolute have their moral views fixed; no room exists for development, where freedom is concerned.

If, on the other hand, one views freedom as a fundamental societal value (but a value nonetheless), other consequences follow. One can, for example, tax the rich, set standards of safety, and limit the term of subjugation of one person to another. In such communities, the principle that one can (or even should) ameliorate gross inequities will be generally held. Obligations to others are far more complex and more fruitful. Such a view permits and even facilitates experimentation, growth, and evolution.

Our notion of the nature of communities underlies our view of what is and what is not just. If by justice we mean giving each person his or her due, we are left with the question of what that due might be.[23]

The pure individualist, who holds freedom to be a side constraint and who therefore sees a community as united only by duties of noninterference, perceives justice to consist purely of allowing every member as much opportunity for achieving whatever is desired as is consonant with everyone else having the same opportunity. For example, a neighbor in need must be allowed the opportunity to seek freely food or other goods as long as in so doing that opportunity for others is not diminished.

Those who see in community an association of people united by more than this will affirm that a neighbor's want creates certain positive obligations. They will readily acknowledge that discharging such obligations inevitably must diminish untrammeled freedom and attenuate individual liberty. Yet the obligation to help one's less fortunate neighbor becomes obvious for those who conceive of communities in this way.

Justice, as John Dewey has pointed out, is not an end in itself.[24] It is a means for facilitating communal life as well as individual opportunity, and its content will, therefore, vary with history. Justice, like all other human concepts and activities, is biologically grounded and must adapt and support survival and growth. If we affirm communities to be united by more than mere duties of noninterference, we allow adaptation and growth to occur and we see justice and the attendant obligations as dynamic and evolving. Obligations are not strictly bound or circumscribed. They vary with time, with circumstance, and with technical advances, as well as with a community's vision of the good life—which itself changes and will ever change.

SCARCE RESOURCES AND ORGAN DONATIONS

Scarcity is a relative matter. Medical resources are often scarce today because of an increase in costs and because society seems less willing to allocate more funds to health care. Whether this need be so is another matter. The availability of medical resources as ordinarily conceived is generally a societal construct, for it is ultimately society that allocates, or fails to allocate, necessary funds. Resources, for the most part, are renewable, obtainable, and limited in their availability only by our reluctance to allocate sufficient funds for them. Even the most expensive goods can be made available by the expenditure of more funds.

Goods that are unrenewable, however, are a different matter. Once used up, they cannot then be created. There is an unbridgeable gap between what is extremely expensive and hard to produce and what is priceless and not possible to make. The problem is similar to that of dealing with the infinite or eternal on human terms. No number, no matter how large, no length of time, however great, serves as a stepping stone to the infinite or the eternal. The difference between the eternal and the transitory, the infinite and the finite, the unrenewable and the renewable is like an impenetrable barrier.[25]

Intuitively, most people would hold that destroying resources useless to the one destroying them but critically needed by another is morally wrong. Our view on this, of course, depends upon our view of communities. Disposing of food down my disposal while my neighbor starves may not be nice, but it is not morally blameworthy if a community is only united by the duty to refrain from harm. (Taking food away from my neighbor, of course, would be morally wrong.) If, however, a community entails obligations beyond refraining from harm, destroying a meal while my neighbor goes hungry becomes morally problematic. If, furthermore, my neighbor would be certain to die without this food, its destruction would surely be a blameworthy act.

Cadaver organs differ radically from most other resources in a number of pertinent ways. First, organs cannot be renewed (although they could certainly be made far more readily available and be less wasted than they are today). Second, they are of vital use to the living persons whose organs they are, but aside from being potentially transplantable they are of use to others only under exceptional circumstances. Third, when organs are of use to other living persons, they are critical to the continuance of these persons' lives or functioning. Fourth, organs are not, once a person is dead, the property of any specific other person, except perhaps for purposes of burial (and then such property rights are hedged) or organ donation.[26] Finally, cadaver organs were (up to the time of death) organic parts of living, breathing, and thinking persons, members of a community sharing in their values, hopes, and aspirations and united with it by a social contract. As such, such organs are of symbolic value to others and to the community.

OBJECTIONS TO CUSTOMARY SALVAGE

The idea of transplanting the organs of the newly dead into the living makes some persons uncomfortable. This uneasiness is related to a not unreasonable fear of technocracy and an aversion to the philosophy so prevalent today that holds that what can be done ought to be done.[27] The fear of "mutilation" and notions of wholeness, as well as the fear that making body parts interchangeable between individuals will serve to make individuals be looked upon as themselves (complex) organs to be disposed of by others at will, are central to the issue of transplantation.[28] It has also been feared that diluting the respect for natural symbols (such as newly dead bodies) will weaken the important communal respect for symbols.[29] A long religious tradition that endows the physical remains with mystic qualities beyond the symbolic often helps to sustain such fears.[30]

The argument from wholeness essentially takes the following form. The first premise is that capriciously removing a part of an organism (say, hacking off an ear merely for the sake of doing this) not only is irrational behavior but is unacceptable mutilation.[31] Persons are their body's stewards and are compelled not to treat their body in injurious ways. (A hidden premise often is that this is offensive to God.) Second, persons are justified in removing a part of their body threatening the integrity of the whole.[32] Assuming the notion of stewardship is correct, such self-mutilation is not only permissible but perhaps mandatory. Third, mutilation of the body by removing a part is impermissible for any reason (even to help one's neighbor) other than to preserve the integrity of the whole body of which it is a part. Fourth, totality to be preserved persists intact when a person dies. (This harkens back to issues dealing with resurrection.) The conclusion is that donation of organs is impermissible.

The fear that allowing the invasion of one body for the sake of another will create a society less mindful of individual rights is connected with the argument from wholeness.[33] It can take the following argumentative form. First, a person's wholeness may be disrupted only for the sake of preserving the person's own integrity. Second, communities and their members relate to each other in ways substantially different from the relationship of individuals to their parts. Third, although one might hope for more, individuals are bound together within communities by the duty to refrain from harming others and not by any other duties. Fourth, if one allows people to be invaded for the sake of other people or of the community as a whole, one is apt to produce a state of affairs in which a person is perceived as merely another organ of the community and is disposable for the needs of the state. Since this state of affairs is undesirable, organ transplantation should not be allowed to be customary.

It can be added to the above argument that making organ retrieval customary, even if not mandatory, reduces property rights, dispels an opportunity for generosity, dilutes a laudatory communal urge, and unduly burdens families in their hour of grief.[34] Customarily salvaging tissues and organs (even when dissent is permitted and accepted) will lessen communal respect for other symbols and hence for the reality that they represent.[35] A society geared only to reality and unmindful of its symbols may, it is feared, become callous and uncaring.

Those who see a community as a group of people united merely by duties of noninterference, and who hold absolute freedom to be the necessary condition of morality and justice, will look askance at a society in which tissues and organs are routinely taken, even if the possibility of dissent were to remain. They would argue that in a community where noninterference is the only moral principle, the only reasonable presumption is that members will refrain from harming each other, not that they will act to benefit each other. Since no act of beneficence should be presupposed or in any way mandated, to presume consent to organ donation would, they feel, violate the basic notion of respect for others.[36] Some, no doubt, would find it laudatory to donate organs. They would see such donation as a supererogatory instance of generosity rather than as a duty or as an instance of justice.

A POSSIBLE RESOLUTION

Failure to use the organs and tissues of the newly dead for persons whose future life or function is dependent upon them seems, at the very least, wasteful. And yet, the idea of affording persons no choice in the disposition of their own or their relatives' remains seems almost as repugnant. We balance feeling against fact, symbol against reality, and ultimately we stand in danger of committing one grievous wrong to prevent another.[37] Objections to making organ donation customary basically rely on fears of violating symbols. The fear of destroying wholeness, the fear of mutilation, the equating of cadaver organs with those of living persons and the consequent fear for the security of the living, and finally the fear that allowing the invasion of one body for the sake of another will weaken individual rights, all depend on a confusion of symbol with reality or on mistakenly holding that symbol and reality have equal value.

Symbols come into being as the epiphenomena of a reality that they come to represent. Symbols, wherever found, relate to reality. They may outlast it or become distorted and hard to recognize. Nevertheless, symbols must either represent reality or, as happens occasionally, be derived from yet another symbol that itself is ultimately grounded in reality. But symbols are not reality itself. Confounding a symbol with the reality it represents, or holding it to have the same value, ultimately distorts reality. When symbols rather than the thing they stand for assume primary value, the sentiment of benevolence is replaced by sentimentality.

Communities are cemented together by sentiments of mutual benevolence. Communities consist of individuals affected by each other's needs. Sentiments of benevolence are related to respect for such needs. Respect for the newly dead is symbolic of respect for the living. In respecting the grief of relatives, we respect the relatives as well as the object of their grief. But that respect may be increased, rather than lessened, by using newly dead as a bridge to continued life for the living. Symbols change and adapt with reality, not, it is hoped, the other way around. When we make refusal instead of assent the norm and forgo using the tissues of the newly dead to build these bridges because we fear violating a symbol, we create a new and distorted reality, a reality without substance. And, what is worse, we impair the reality of the sick out of respect for mere symbolism.

Symbols comfort the bereaved. They stand for the person that was as well as for ideals and aspirations. Symbols allow the abrupt transition from life to death to be softened, and in a sense they postpone the moment of loss. The newly dead, no longer really here, are honored in memory and through symbols. Many objects and acts can be symbols or be symbolic. What is symbolic at a given time or to a given individual may be meaningless at other times or to other persons. The type of symbols we use are an expression of the "education and discipline of the feelings."[38]

Communities consist of persons with individual troubles. If just communities are conceived of as caring communities, then we must presume that caring will be expressed in meaningful ways by their individual members. Building bridges by using the newly dead to give life and function to the living creates new symbols of love and caring. Routinely taking the organs and tissues of the newly dead to serve the critical need of others is to presume the newly dead to have been members of the same caring community as the currently living. Presuming the newly dead not to have cared about their neighbors' needs, not to have wanted to serve as the bridge to life and function for others, is hardly to show respect for them. Instead of violating a symbol, presuming consent may allow symbols to evolve. Seeing in the cadaver a holy object not to be "violated" for fear of violating a symbol neglects two important facts—that the cadaver has still viable organs and tissues and that the life of another member of the community depends on these very organs and tissues. Seeing in the cadaver a bridge to life for another changes the form of the symbolism but does not destroy it. Cadavers still can be seen as holy objects in their own right and with their own purpose. In so doing, respect for the newly dead is fully expressed.

Unless we are to resort to arguments involving mysticism or belief in an afterlife, arguments of which the premises can be neither refuted nor proven, no one can reasonably hold that the dead are diminished by anything done to them after death. Harm, if possible, is purely symbolic. Even when the reputation or "memory" of the dead is impaired, the dead are not injured in themselves. Gratuitous injuries done to reputation or memory or other forms of disrespect shown to the dead constitute harm done to the community (by dragging a role model into the dirt or by gratuitously violating a symbol and thereby blunting sensitivity) and to the nearest kin. But it is not harm done to the deceased in the sense that harm can be visited upon the living.[39] Symbols manifest the reality for which they stand. The bereaved tend to remember the deceased in positive ways: They remember intelligence, beauty, and generosity; they generally fail to dwell on stupidity, ugliness, and greed. They do this because the traits of intelligence, beauty, and generosity are valued in our peculiar community and the others are not. Respect for the dead, it seems, would be shown by presuming the dead to have shared fully in what the community considers to be positive traits.

When all is said and done, we are still confronted with the problem of wasting as little tissue from the newly dead as possible while meaningfully showing respect for the symbolism so dear to some members of our community. If one were to salvage all organs regardless of assent or dissent, a maximal supply could be obtained. This would be done at the price of seriously discomforting those members of community who belong to a moral enclave that considers the use of such organs to be reprehensible. (Their objections should probably preclude their receiving organs should the need arise, a rule which would be hard to implement!) But our larger community has no such strictures. Most members of a just community would, in the cold light of day, affirm their belief that it is just to give to living persons who critically need them the organs from cadavers, which have no use for them.[40] Presumed consent merely affirms this. To presume to be the case what is unlikely to be the case (i.e., refusal of consent) is not rational. And of course a policy of presumed consent would respect dissent if it were explicitly expressed.

Presumed consent as the instrument of donation has, furthermore, an educational effect. By affirming the values of the community, it tends to emphasize societal norms and to weave them more solidly into the fabric of community expectations while continuing to exhibit that respect for peculiar beliefs that a pluralistic community demands. Families, "heavily burdened in their hour of grief,"[41] will be less likely to be afflicted by the fear of violating imagined communal symbols while still able, by dissenting, to apply standards peculiar to their own moral enclave or to their own moral conscience. Making the donation of organs a supererogatory act subtly suggests that nongiving rather than giving is the norm; it suggests the value of symbol over reality and lends a hand to the ascendency of sentimentality (which values the symbol more than what the symbol represents). Making the donation of organs a societal norm (while allowing dissent) suggests that the just community is a caring community in which sentiment inclines its members to build bridges for the living. It helps to educate, discipline, and channel feelings and thus to create new symbols of caring and respect.

NOTES

1. J. L. Joughin, "Blood Transfusion in 1492," *Journal of the American Medical Association* 62 (1914): 553–54.
2. F. H. Garrison, *An Introduction to the History of Medicine* (Philadelphia, Pa.: W.B. Saunders, 1929).
3. C. Singer and E. A. Underwood, *A Short History of Medicine* (New York: Oxford University Press, 1962).
4. Ibid.
5. E. Ullman, "Experimentelle Nierentransplantation," *Wien Klin Wochenschr* 15 (1908): 281–82.
6. A. Carrell, "Results of the Transplantation of Blood Vessels, Organs and Limbs," *Journal of the American Medical Association* 51 (1908): 1662–67.
7. S. N. Chatterjee, ed., *Organ Transplantation* (London: John Wright PSG, 1982).
8. S. J. Youngner et al., "Psychosocial and Ethical Implications of Organ Retrieval," *New England Journal of Medicine* 313 (1985): 321–32; A. L. Caplan, "Organ Procurement: It's Not in the Cards," *Hastings Center Report* 14, no. 5 (1984): 9–12; Medical News, "The Organ Procurement Problem: Many Causes, No Easy Solutions," *Journal of the American Medical Association* 254 (1985): 3285–88.
9. Ad Hoc Committee of the Harvard Medical School to Examine the Definition of Brain Death, "A Definition of Irreversible Coma; Report of the Ad Hoc Committee of the Harvard Medical School to Examine the Definition of Brain Death." *Journal of the American Medical Association* 205 (1968): 337–40; B. Green and D. Winkler, "Brain Death and Personal Identity," *Philosophy and Public Affairs* 9, no. 2 (1980): 104–33; President's Commission for the Study of Ethical Problems in Medicine and Biomedical and Behavioral Research, *Defining Death: A Report on the Medical, Legal and Ethical Issues in the Determination of Death* (Washington, D.C.: U.S. Government Printing Office, 1981); F. Plum and J. Posner, *The Diagnosis of Stupor and Coma,* 3d ed. (Philadelphia, Pa.: Davis Publishing, 1980); E. L. Pallis, "ABC of Brain Stem Death," *British Medical Journal* 285 (1982): 1409–12; F. Plum, "Prognosis in Severe Brain Damage and Diagnosis of Brain Death," in *Cecil's Textbook of Medicine,* 17th ed., ed. J. B. Wyngarden and L. H. Smith (Philadelphia, Pa.: W.B. Saunders, 1985).
10. A. M. Sadler, B. L. Sadler, and E. B. Stason, "The Uniform Anatomical Gift Act," *Journal of the American Medical Association* 206 (1968): 2501–6.
11. T. D. Overcast et al., "Problems in the Identification of Potential Organ Donors," *Journal of the American Medical Association* 251 (1984): 1559–62.
12. P. Ramsey, *The Patient as Person* (New Haven, Conn.: Yale University Press, 1970).
13. E. H. Loewy, "Presumed Consent in Organ Donation: An Almost Binding Duty," in *Covenants of Life: Essays in Honor of Paul Ramsey,* ed. K. E. Vaux (Urbana, Ill.: University of Illinois Press, 1987).
14. C. Perry, "The Right of Public Access to Cadaver Organs," *Social Science and Medicine* 15 (1981): 163–66; J. Dukeminier and D. Sanders, "Organ Transplantation: A Proposal for Routine Salvage of Cadaver Organs," *New England Journal of Medicine* 269 (1968): 413–19; J. L. Muyskens, "An Alternative Policy for Obtaining Cadaver Organs for Transplantation," *Philosophy and Public Affairs* 8, no. 1 (1978): 88–99; E. H. Loewy, "Presumed Consent in Organ Donation: Values and Means in the Distribution of a Scarce Resource," in *Ethical Dilemmas in Modern Medicine: A Physician's Viewpoint* (Lewiston, N.Y.: Edwin Mellen Press, 1986).
15. F. P. Stuart, F. J. Veith, and R. E. Cranford, "Brain Death Laws and Patterns of Consent to Remove Organs from Cadavers in the United States and 28 Other Countries," *Transplantation* 31, no. 4 (1981): 238–44; Report of the Swedish Committee on Defining Death, *The Concept of Death* (Stockholm: Swedish Ministry of Health and Social Affairs, 1984).
16. E. H. Loewy, "Communities, Obligation and Health-Care," *Social Science and Medicine* 25, no. 7 (1987): 783–91.
17. R. Nozick, *Anarchy, State and Utopia* (New York: Basic Books, 1974).

18. H. T. Englehardt, *Foundations of Bioethics* (New York: Oxford University Press, 1986).

19. J. P. Reeder, "Beneficence, Supererogation and Role Duty," in *Beneficence and Health Care,* ed. E. E. Shelp (Dordrecht, Holland: D. Reidel, 1982).

20. D. Callahan, "Minimalist Ethics," *Hastings Center Report* 11, no. 5 (1981): 19–25.

21. I. Kant, *Foundations of the Metaphysics of Morals,* trans. L. W. Beck (Indianapolis, Ind.: Bobbs-Merrill, 1978).

22. R. Niebuhr, "Rationing and Democracy," in *Love and Justice,* ed. D. R. Robertson (Philadelphia, Pa.: Westminster Press, 1957).

23. Aristotle, *Nicomachean Ethics,* trans. M. Ostwald (Indianapolis, Ind.: Bobbs-Merrill, 1962); W. K. Franken, "The Concept of Social Justice," in *Social Justice,* ed. R. B. Brandt (Englewood Cliffs, N.J.: Prentice-Hall, 1962).

24. J. Dewey, *Theory of the Moral Life* (New York: Holt, Rinehart & Winston, 1960).

25. E. H. Loewy, "Drunks, Livers and Values: Should Social Value Judgments Enter into Transplant Decisions," *Journal of Clinical Gastroenterology* 9, no. 4 (1987): 436–41.

26. Perry, "Public Access to Cadaver Organs."

27. Loewy, "Presumed Consent in Organ Donation."

28. Ramsey, *Patient as Person.*

29. W. May, "Attitudes towards the Newly Dead," *Hastings Center Report* 1, no. 1 (1973); 3–13.

30. Ramsey, *Patient as Person*; Loewy, "Presumed Consent in Organ Donation"; May, "Attitudes towards the Newly Dead."

31. B. Gert, *The Moral Rules* (New York: Harper & Row, 1973).

32. G. Kelly, "The Morality of Mutilation: Towards a Revision of the Treatist," *Theological Studies* 17, no. 3 (1952): 332–48.

33. Ramsey, *Patient as Person.*

34. Ibid.

35. May, "Attitudes towards the Newly Dead."

36. Englehardt, *Foundations of Bioethics.*

37. J. Feinberg, "The Mistreatment of Dead Bodies," *Hastings Center Report* 15, no. 1 (1985): 31–37.

38. M. Tanner, "Sentimentality," *Proceedings of the Aristotelian Society* 77 (1977): 127–47.

39. E. Partridge, "Posthumous Interests and Posthumous Respect," *Ethics* 91 (1981): 243–64.

40. C. E. Koop, "Increasing the Supply of Solid Organs for Transplantation," *Public Health Report* 98, no. 6 (1983): 566–72.

41. Ramsey, *Patient as Person.*

Part IV

Justice and Economics in Health Care

Chapter 32

Intergenerational Justice: Is It Possible?

Myles N. Sheehan

In the United States, the fastest growing segment of the population is those individuals 85 years of age and older. Not only are the oldest old increasing, there is a marked shift in the demographics of the United States, with the proportion of people 65 and over expected to rise from the 1994 level of 12.6 percent[1] to over 21 percent by 2030.[2] The increasing number of elderly individuals will have a marked effect on the nature of health care and health care expenditures. It is not clear how the United States, or other Western nations with similar demographic changes, will be able to pay for the needs of an increasingly aged population. Nor is it clear how a society can balance a variety of communal needs among the generations, given finite resources and a decreased percentage of the population in the active work force. The aging of society raises not only issues of economics but underlying questions about what is fair and what generations owe each other in both monetary resources and personal care. These are issues of justice between generations.

Is intergenerational justice possible? Can the children, the young adults, the middle-aged, the young old, and the frail elderly all exist in one society so that all groups have legitimate needs met in an equitable manner? There is no easy answer. Any attempt to consider the question requires a careful look at the multiple facets of the question. This chapter will examine the issue of intergenerational justice. First, the meaning of justice will be explored to reveal some of its complexity and consider why it can be difficult to define, much less attain. Second, a particular perspective on justice will be used to reflect on what generations owe to each other. The perspective that will be offered comes from the Roman Catholic tradition. Although this may seem a narrow approach to a broad and contentious issue in a secular and pluralistic society, I will argue that listening to a distinctive voice on justice that has rich intellectual and theological resources can provide guidance even to those who disagree with particular points. Third, and very briefly, some concrete suggestions will be offered as to how our society may come closer to grappling with intergenerational justice.

THE COMPLEXITY OF JUSTICE

Justice is one of the most elusive terms in ethics. A seemingly straightforward definition of justice is that individuals receive what is their due. Most people have an intuitive sense of what constitutes clearly just or unjust behavior and what it means to refer to a person as being just or unjust. Yet, attempting to pin down those intuitions raises difficulties. Three points stand out.

First, justice requires procedures and rules to guarantee fair relationships within a society. But it also requires individuals who act justly. In ethics, justice is both a principle and a central virtue. As a principle, justice consists of policies, decisions, procedures, and rules that regulate interaction and provide for a society where people are treated fairly. Fair treatment requires, at a minimum, actions that are in accord with rules and procedures that are applied in an even-handed manner. As a virtue, however, justice describes a habitual manner of acting justly. Just as a runner grows in speed and endurance by the habitual act of a daily run, a just person grows in the virtue of justice by acting justly. In considering the virtues, Aristotle notes that justice, alone among the virtues, does not have a mean. Courage and temperance are both virtues and they both have a mean. One can be foolhardy and bold and go beyond the mean of courage. One can be excessively temperate, stingy and cowardly, and thus go beyond the mean of temperance. A just individual, however, cannot be too just. Likewise, individuals and societies should not stop at a minimal standard of procedural justice (although even that in a world marked by flagrant injustice is praiseworthy), but should exercise care and concern in habitual actions to ensure that individuals receive what is due to them. Justice as a principle and justice as a virtue are not in conflict. Rather, our human sense of justice expects more than fair rules; it expects institutions and individuals that perseveringly act with fairness to create a society where fairness is the standard of personal interaction. Justice is demanding.

Second, in striving to fulfill the demands of justice, it can be difficult to balance the needs of society versus the needs of an individual. How does one balance the common good against the desires of the individual? How does one create conditions of fairness that allow for a just distribution of society's goods, provide equal access to opportunity, and rectify past injustice? In tackling the problem of intergenerational justice, the principal issue is distributive justice, deciding fairly who gets what from a societal pot of resources that are finite. Health care is a leading issue in distributive justice. It is one of the many items that needs to be balanced in finding the meaning of justice between generations. How does one balance the costs and benefits of neonatal intensive-care units for very premature infants versus rehabilitative and preventive care for older persons? Conversely, how does one justify aggressive surgical and intensive care for the very old when, in the United States, for example, many children are not adequately immunized? Intergenerational justice, however, is more than the allocation of health care resources. There are other competing goods. How does health care for the elderly balance with the need for schools and programs for children? How do we care for the poor and sick while maintaining and developing a social infrastructure that allows for highways, police, clean water, and a variety of other services that make life possible and provide the necessary conditions for human flourishing? Compounding these knotty problems of allocation on a grand scale is the consideration of how decisions will affect individuals. Where is justice when one faces the realization that allocation decisions mean that an individual may be told no to a therapy that could possibly benefit her or him for an otherwise fatal illness?

Third, our quandaries over justice, competing goods, and the macro and micro issues of allocation decisions point to a lack of consensus over the obligations owed by one member of a society to another. Questions about neonatal intensive-care units versus preventive services for senior citizens are very hard to answer when there is little framework in American society to express mutual obligations. In the United States, there is a framework of law that aims to protect individuals from unwanted interference, coercion, violence, and disruption of life, but there is little that defines positive obligations. Justice is more than being free to live one's life free of interference and facing just punishment for violating the freedom of others. Justice, especially when considered as a virtue, requires concern for others. When we examine intergenerational justice, justice must meet the needs of those who are suffering and need help, make sure future generations are educated to deal with the complexity of life, and attempt to secure a decent minimum so that young and old have a fair shot at those things that allow human flourishing.

If nothing else, the three points suggest a conclusion about justice and point to a fundamental confusion: Justice means different things to different people. It is problematic, at best, to decide what is just when a community has a variety of competing versions of justice. Justice often seems a matter of opinion rather than a reflection of communally accepted truths. As Alasdair MacIntyre comments: "When Aristotle praised justice as the first virtue of political life, he did so in such a way as to suggest that a community which lacks practical agreement on a conception of justice must also lack the necessary basis for political community. But the lack of such a basis must therefore threaten our own society."[3] Although one may not agree with the somewhat apocalyptic vision of MacIntyre, it is reasonable to suggest that the lack of a shared framework for understanding justice makes it unlikely that justice will be seen as a reality by all the members of a society. It is unlikely that justice can ever be perfect for all individuals in a society. Yet the greater the shared understanding of foundational truths about justice, the higher the chances that individuals will agree on a procedural framework for justice as well as judgments about when justice is achieved and when it falls short.

Looking to a shared communal vision of justice is not without risk. A communal acceptance of what is "right" and what is "true" may ignore dissenting voices. The legitimate concerns of individuals and small groups may be crushed by the majority. Common moral agreement can slide into totalitarianism. Despite that fear, it is worth listening to distinctive voices regarding a vision of justice. Paying attention to communities that make up the patchwork quilt of the United States can, by appreciating some of the major themes in that variegated fabric, provide a service to a nation that values pluralism.

In facing the problems that the aging of our culture poses for industrialized nations, a research program at the Hastings Center neatly raised the issues of community, the individual, the need for consensus, and the dangers of enforcing consensus.

> A paradox in the life of individuals is that they must find their own personal meanings for life and death—for youth, adulthood, and old age—and yet they cannot well do this without the help of the larger community of which they are a part. Even in countries without strong individualistic traditions, or where the value of solidarity is still prized, few societies any longer presume to instruct their citizens on how they should understand their own lives, a function once performed by religious traditions or homogeneous value systems. Historically, there is some evidence to suggest that those traditions and systems did help the elderly to make sense of their lives, usually by placing them in some larger context of religious, cultural, and generational transcendence.
>
> Is it desirable to seek, once again, some degree of consensus on the meaning of old age for individual lives? Is it possible? The case against such an effort can seem compelling: in pluralistic societies, where the value of religious and philosophical freedom is prized, it is inappropriate, even hazardous to seek for some common meaning. All too quickly a consensus on meaning can become an instrument of repression. Yet it is no less true that the secular citizens of modern societies find it extraordinarily hard to create personal meaning in a culture that does not allow, or encourage, its citizens to talk openly and comfortably with each other about the crucial phases of human life. Nor is it clear how government and other social institutions will come to prize and support the elderly if there seems to be a studied cultural indifference to the deeper issues that aging poses for the self-understanding of the old. . . . It is most appropriate for private institutions to help the elderly develop their

> own sense of personal meaning in their lives.[4]

In what follows, I will attempt to develop a response to issues of intergenerational justice from my own apprehension of an institutional perspective, that of the Roman Catholic Church. I am a priest, a Jesuit, and a physician who specializes in internal medicine and geriatrics. There is no formal Roman Catholic position on justice between generations. In a presentation of a Roman Catholic approach to this issue, I will refer to Scripture, the teachings of popes and bishops, and the perspective of theologians. Inevitably, my citations and emphases will reflect areas of greater familiarity to me and my own particular biases. This exercise, however, is more than idiosyncratic.

As the lengthy citation above notes—albeit ironically from my perspective by the use of the past tense—religious tradition is an important shaper of the meaning of justice, aging, and obligations between generations. Authentic religion continues to perform the function of instructing individuals in understanding the meaning of their lives. The Roman Catholic tradition is, arguably, one of the dominant voices of the world's religious traditions. Although I cannot fully capture the richness of that voice, I hope to give a sense of the kind of tune it sings.

A ROMAN CATHOLIC PERSPECTIVE

A Catholic perspective on justice between generations relies on three sources: Scripture, the living tradition of the Church as expressed by the teaching of the Magisterium, and the input of social and natural science. Sacred Scripture provides a privileged place from which to begin an examination of this perspective. Three texts from the Hebrew Scriptures provide rich resources for considering aging and intergenerational justice: the fourth commandment of the Decalogue, a selection from Isaiah 65, and Psalm 71.

The fourth of the Ten Commandments, "Honor your father and your mother," is one of the central texts that serve as a foundation for the understanding that the young have obligations to the old: "Honor your father and your mother, as the Lord your God has commanded you, that you may have a long life and prosperity in the land which the Lord, your God, is giving you" (Dt 5:16).[5] One must be cautious in interpreting the nature of obligations imposed by this commandment. The command is to honor father and mother. There is no explicit command to care for the elderly in general, only parents. Neither is there a definition of the meaning of honoring one's parents. The commandment was originally received by a nomadic people who were heading to Canaan as part of their historical journey to establish a promised land, Israel. In the context of ancient Israel and the Hebrew people, the point of the commandment is that one's parents are to be cared for in old age, not thrown out of the family dwelling when old age or illness makes them unable to make a significant contribution to the household by hunting, farming, or the performance of household duties. What does this text say to contemporary Americans or citizens of other industrialized, technologically advanced nations? Although one can reasonably judge that the commandment urges respect, care, and concern for parents, it is difficult to translate this into specific duties or obligations. It is especially difficult when parents may live to a very old age, chronic illness and disability can persist for years, and families are small, often with all the adult children of older parents working outside the home. The lack of a blueprint in how to apply the commandment, however, does not annul its relevance. At the least, it suggests children are responsible, in some measure, for elderly parents, and provides a mandate for care between generations.

The prophetic texts of the Hebrew Scriptures often indict current misdeeds while holding out a vision of a society where God's justice is established. In the book of the prophet Isaiah, the author depicts a new heavens and a new earth, where the generations live in harmony with each other and with God's creation:

> Lo, I am about to create new heavens and a new earth; the things of the past

> shall not be remembered or come to mind. Instead there shall always be rejoicing and happenings in what I create; for I create Jerusalem to be a joy and its people to be a delight; I will rejoice in Jerusalem and exult in my people. No longer shall the sound of weeping be heard there, or the sound of crying; No longer shall there be in it an infant who lives but a few days, or an old man who does not round out his full lifetime; He dies a mere youth who reaches but a hundred years, and he who fails of a hundred shall be thought accursed. . . . As the years of a tree, so the years of my people; and my chosen ones shall enjoy the produce of their hands. They shall not toil in vain, nor beget children for sudden destruction. . . . The wolf and the lamb shall graze alike, and the lion shall eat hay like the ox. . . . None shall hurt or destroy on my holy mountain, says the LORD. (Is 65:17–20, 22–23a, 25)

The passage from Isaiah depicts a world where the beauty of God's original creation has been restored: Lion and lamb are friends, not predator and prey, and the old and young live together in peace, enjoying the good things of life. The key is a world where harmony is restored: between generations, between peoples, and in nature. This type of vision is idyllic and utopian. Humans have not experienced this type of intergenerational harmony, long life, or total peace. Indeed, the passage is clear that this type of world will come about only from the direct creative intervention of God. Even if not fully achievable by human effort, however, the vision of longevity, an end to infant mortality and premature death, and a life rich with peace does provide contemporary Americans with a clear message that sudden death, dying infants, and lives spent in desperation are not what God desires. Like the text of the fourth commandment, this passage does not give a blueprint that details social obligations but is a proclamation of the way things should be. Harmony between generations is part of the Biblical perspective.

A third text from the Hebrew Scriptures, Psalm 71, provides a highly personal account of an old man's perspective on justice during a time of troubles. Psalm 71 is the prayer of an old man who is threatened by enemies. Clearly, his world is not "the new heavens and new earth" of the text from Isaiah. It may be that Psalm 71 is meant to evoke the prayers of King David in his final years as he faced palace intrigue and struggles over succession. The identity of the psalmist, however, is less important than the perspective it brings on aging, justice, the relations between generations, and the relationship with God.

> 1. In you, LORD, I take refuge, let me never be put to shame.
>
> 2. In your justice rescue and deliver me; listen to me and save me!
>
> 3. Be my rock and refuge, my secure stronghold; for you are my rock and fortress.
>
> 4. My God, rescue me from the power of the wicked, from the clutches of the violent.
>
> 5. You are my hope, Lord; my trust, GOD, from my youth.
>
> 6. On you I depend since birth; from my mother's womb you are my strength; my hope in you never wavers.
>
> 7. I have become a portent to many, but you are my strong refuge!
>
> 8. My mouth shall be filled with your praise, shall sing your glory every day.
>
> 9. Do not cast me aside in my old age; as my strength fails, do not forsake me.
>
> 10. For my enemies speak against me; they watch and plot against me.
>
> 11. They say, "God has abandoned that one. Pursue, seize the wretch! No one will come to the rescue!"
>
> 12. God, do not stand far from me; my God, hasten to help me.
>
> 13. Bring a shameful end to those who attack me; Cover with contempt and scorn those who seek my ruin.
>
> 14. I will always hope in you and add to all your praise.

> 15. My mouth shall proclaim your just deeds, day after day your acts of deliverance, though I cannot number them all.
>
> 16. I will speak of the mighty works of the LORD; O GOD, I will tell of your singular justice.
>
> 17. God, you have taught me from my youth; to this day I proclaim your wondrous deeds.
>
> 18. Now that I am old and gray, do not forsake me, God, That I may proclaim your might to all generations yet to come,
>
> 19. Your power and justice, God, to the highest heaven. You have done great things O GOD, who is your equal?
>
> 20. You have sent me many bitter afflictions, but once more revive me. From the watery depths of the earth once more raise me up.
>
> 21. Restore my honor; turn and comfort me.
>
> 22. That I may praise you with the lyre for your faithfulness, my God, And sing to you with the harp, O Holy One of Israel!
>
> 23. My lips will shout for joy as I sing your praise; my soul, too, which you have redeemed.
>
> 24. Yes, my tongue shall recount your justice day by day. For those who sought my ruin will have been shamed and disgraced.

The psalmist begs not to be cast aside in old age nor forsaken because of physical weakness. There is a clear link between the justice of God and the way an old man is treated in times of trouble. A just God will rescue and deliver him (v. 2). God's care and positive response to the prayer of this old man will be seen as another of God's mighty works of justice (vv. 15–16). The unstated assumption is that the rescue of the elderly psalmist will be part of the legacy of justice and liberation that God has brought about in the paradigmatic mighty deed for Israel: the rescue from slavery in Egypt and the passage of the Exodus to the Promised Land. Along with the confident assurance of God's justice and care for an old man, the psalmist asserts that his life, now approaching its end, is linked with the generations: God has been his help since even before birth, God will help him now that he is old. It is the duty of the old man to proclaim God's might "to generations yet to come" (vv. 18–19). Although the psalmist is very concerned with his personal plight, he is not self-obsessed. He is aware of his place in the generations and sees his life in continuity with the past and knows that he has a contribution to make to the future. The psalm emphasizes that justice requires attention to the elderly and their troubles. Those who pursue the old and hound them are not just wicked, they are an affront to the Divine order and are to be seen as rebels against God (vv. 10–13). God's justice demands that the elderly be treated with care and respect. At the very least, this psalm strongly asserts that a just society is one where the old are treated fairly. It also presents a vision of aging that views the last portion of life not as a time of withdrawal and isolation from society but as a period of completion. The aged psalmist lives his life in the context of the generations and sees a vocation to transmit the knowledge of God and his people's religious traditions to the young and the generations of the future.

This selection of texts, admittedly brief and not representing the full voice of the Hebrew Scriptures, provides the outlines of a perspective on aging and the demands of justice. Three points stand out. First, and most obvious, God is concerned about what happens to older persons. The commandments require care of older parents, the prophets speak of a new creation where the old round out their lives in peace, and the psalmist links divine justice with the fate of an old man. Second, there are obligations between generations. Children are commanded to care for parents. The old have the responsibility to transmit the traditions and faith of the people to a new generation. Third, harmony between young and old is part of God's plan. God's redeemed world is where lion and lamb are together and a person of 100 years enjoys the presence of a newborn infant. None of these three points tells us how to deal with our own contemporary concerns, for example, balancing health care costs for the elderly versus educational needs. But they do provide the insight that the task of caring among generations is one in which God has a stake, there are obligations, and harmony is the goal.

The teaching and ministry of Jesus as proclaimed in the Gospels are not explicit in what the young and old owe one another. But there are numerous examples of Jesus' teaching regarding relations between individuals in society as well as his own personal example of reaching out to persons who are isolated, sick, and somehow estranged from the larger community. One can extrapolate four points about intergenerational obligations and what it means for old and young to give each other their due.

First, young and old are called to recognize each other as neighbor. The parable of the Good Samaritan comes as Jesus' response to a lawyer who asks "Who is my neighbor?" (Lk 10:29). In the parable, a Samaritan, a member of an ethnic minority that had mutually poor relations with their Jewish neighbors, helps a Jewish traveler left wounded and robbed by the side of the road after two of his Jewish countrymen pass by without rendering assistance. The implication of the story is that "neighbors" are those in need and those who recognize that need. Being a neighbor to the individual who needs help is part of the duty to love God: "You shall love the Lord, your God, with all your heart, with all your being, with all your strength, and with all your mind, and you shall love your neighbor as yourself" (Lk 10:27). The love of God demands that young help old and old help young: generations are not isolated but are neighbors one to another.

Second, the poor are special objects of God's concern, and thus justice demands that the poor have a privileged place in distributing society's resources: "Blessed are you who are poor, for the kingdom of God is yours. Blessed are you who are now hungry, for you will be satisfied" (Lk 6:20–21). Jesus shows special attention to widows, usually older women who would be particularly vulnerable without income, husband, or family to protect them in society. He tells a parable about a persistent widow faced with a legal problem and a dishonest judge. The conclusion of the parable points out God's concern with justice for the "chosen ones," those who struggle in a community that may not respect them because of age, sex, or social standing: "Will not God then secure the rights of his chosen ones who call out to him day and night? Will he be slow to answer them? I tell you, he will see to it that justice is done for them speedily" (Lk 18:7–8a). Intergenerational justice in the light of these teachings requires attention to those who are on the margins. It is not simply young and old that are the concern, but looking at the needs of the poor and weak.

Third, Jesus' own ministry of healing provides a remarkable witness of the necessity to provide physical and spiritual support for those who are sick. Jesus cures the blind, lepers, the epileptic, the deaf, and dumb. Illness is removed, as is the separation from the larger community that illness imposes on those who are sick. In Jesus' time, many of the people he touched and healed were considered ritually impure. The physical burden was compounded by religious and social isolation. Restoration to bodily health brought restoration to the community. In our day, many may feel uncomfortable with the miraculous nature of Jesus' ministry, uncertain of its meaning and suspicious of a seemingly non-scientific credulity about disease and physical healing. In thinking about what the miracles might suggest for intergenerational justice, however, there is a clear thread that the legacy of Jesus is to bring those who are isolated by illness into human contact. The issue is not one of age but of the burden of illness: physical, spiritual, and social. Those who are sick, regardless of age, require reweaving into the social fabric that has been torn by the experience of illness.

Fourth, mercy is an absolute requirement in structuring relationships between individuals and, by extension, within a society. It is not simply a suggestion that one care for one's neighbor, assist the poor, or reach out to the sick. It is the criterion for salvation or damnation. In Matthew's gospel, Jesus teaches that the final judgment by which individuals will be destined for eternal reward or eternal punishment will rest on how women and men have chosen to act with the hungry, the poor, the sick, the homeless, and the prisoner.

> When the Son of Man comes in his glory, and all the angels with him, he will sit upon his glorious throne, and all the nations will be assembled before him. And he will separate them one from another, as a shepherd separates the sheep from the goats. He will place the sheep on his right and the goats on his left. Then the king will say to those on his right, "Come, you who are blessed by my Father. Inherit the kingdom prepared for you from the foundation of the world. For I was hungry and you gave me food, I was thirsty and you gave me drink, a stranger and you welcomed me, naked and you clothed me, ill and you cared for me, in prison and you visited me." Then the righteous will answer him and say, "Lord, when did we see you hungry and feed you, or thirsty and give you drink? When did we see you a stranger and welcome you, or naked and clothe you? When did we see you ill or in prison, and visit you?" And the king will say to them in reply, "Amen, I say to you, whatever you did for one of these least brothers of mine, you did for me." (Mt 25: 31–41)

These four points suggest an important conclusion about intergenerational justice: the Gospels do not assert a particular need for the young to care for the old or the old to care for the young. The Gospels are not focused on age and generational obligation. The call is more for human solidarity across generations rather than a priority of claims of one generation on another. There is no age-based standard. Rather, the call to mercy and justice that can be heard in the message of Jesus' life and teaching is one of recognizing neediness and suffering regardless of particular details. Jesus asserts that God demands care for young and old, man and woman, when the individual is suffering. The response that Jesus embodies is one of personal contact, meeting immediate needs (food for the hungry, clothes for the naked), and bringing isolated people back into a network of human relationships. Intergenerational justice demands care across, within, and beyond generations.

A strong assertion of obligations between generations; requirements for young and old to care each for the other; the necessity of a social framework where individuals work harmoniously to meet the needs of the members of society; and morally binding demands to reach out to the suffering, the sick, and the poor are scriptural underpinnings of any Catholic approach to intergenerational justice. The strongly normative tone of these statements and the implication that justice is an absolute requirement of individuals and society may be somewhat off-putting for contemporary Americans. Individual freedom without constraint and the ability to determine right and wrong based on each one's own tastes and experience are sometimes absolutized. As the U.S. Supreme Court wrote in its 1992 decision reaffirming a woman's right to abortion: "At the heart of liberty is the right to define one's own concept of existence, of meaning, of the universe and of the mystery of human life."[6]

The Church, however, finds liberty not in an individualistic creation of meaning and the universe but in its faith that humanity has been created by God and that God loves and cares about humanity with a love and care so profound that in order to redeem humanity from its failings God took human form and suffered and died: "For God so loved the world that he gave his only Son, so that everyone who believes in him might not perish but have eternal life" (Jn 3:16). In taking this faith as the basis for human existence, there is an absolute grounding of meaning and the mystery of human life. Although the exact dictates of justice are not explicitly spelled out in this revelation, the existence of right and wrong is not found simply in personal choice but in relation to the meaning of humans as made, loved, and redeemed by a God who commands love and service to both God and neighbor. Justice and obligation within a society is not simply what an individual feels like. From a Catholic perspective, the attitude conveyed by the Supreme Court in *Planned Parenthood v. Casey* denies the possibility of truth because it is relativized to individual choice. It rends a community that would work together and replaces it with a version of freedom that is so solipsistic that obligations within a society are negated to a minimum. A passage from the Catechism of the Catholic Church, quoting Pope John Paul II, describes a very different basis of society and social obligations than that inherent in the Supreme Court decision:

> Every institution is inspired, at least implicitly, by a vision of man and his destiny, from which it derives the point of reference for its judgment, its hierarchy of values, its line of conduct. Most societies have formed their institutions in the recognition of a certain preeminence of man over things. Only the divinely revealed religion has clearly recognized man's origin and destiny in God, the Creator and Redeemer. The Church invites political authorities to measure their judgments and decisions against this inspired truth about God and man: 'Societies not recognizing this vision or rejecting it in the name of their independence from God are brought to seek their criteria and goal in themselves or borrow from them some ideology. Since they do not admit that one can defend an objective criterion of good and evil, they arrogate to themselves an explicit totalitarian power over man and his destiny, as history shows.[7]

It is very clear that many Americans would not find this viewpoint congenial. Many could also point to times in the history of the Church that, despite its protests about an absolute criterion of good and evil, the Church itself has been seen as possessing totalitarian power and contributing to human suffering. Recognizing these serious objections and the failures of the Church to fulfill its perceived mission, there remains the task of moving from the biblical foundations to the outlines of principles with which a vision of intergenerational justice can be sketched, albeit roughly and incompletely.

In keeping with the assertion of an absolute truth that is part of Catholic teaching, freedom and justice are found not in individual self-assertion but in a recognition of personal responsibility and desire to respond to God. Individuals are free to deny this responsibility or to reject the notion of God. The Church, however, would assert that the fullness of human dignity comes when people realize who they are in the light of revelation. Instead of individuals who are bent on pursuing their own personal agenda for happiness and pleasure, there are goals of love of God, love of neighbor, and a recognition of duties to care for those who are in need of assistance. In considering intergenerational justice, three themes should be emphasized: a connectedness between generations, a recognition of the value of human life, the priority of mercy.

Why should a young person care about the old? Why should a young man take time away from study or recreation to assist an elderly neighbor in his apartment building? Why should an older woman who has spent her life raising children and caring for others volunteer to help in a day-care center or tutor underprivileged children? In Catholic social teaching the answer is clear: We are our brother's and sister's keepers. Although an assertion of human solidarity and being "our brother's keeper" does not specify the details of how we exercise that mutual care, freedom and human dignity are found in our choices to care for each other rather than in an assertion of personal independence that denies a network of social and community relationships:

> Yes, every man is his "brother's keeper," because God entrusts us to

> one another. And it is also in view of this entrusting that God gives everyone freedom, a freedom which possesses an inherently relational dimension. This is a great gift of the Creator, placed as it is at the service of the person and of his fulfillment through the gift of self and openness to others.[8]

If justice is to exist between generations, then the central question for differing age groups is not, "How can I get from others what is my due?" but, "How can I work to make sure that others receive what they need?" The old and the young are to look to serve each other, not just to satisfy their own desires. Generational selfishness is excluded in a Catholic vision of human solidarity.

Human solidarity, however, has its limits and there are many whose legitimate needs in justice are often ignored. It is not selfish to recognize that one is being treated in an unjust manner and to work to right that wrong. If intergenerational justice is to become a reality, there must be a willingness to listen to those who feel that they are not receiving their due. In the words of the National Conference of Catholic Bishops in their 1985 pastoral letter on economic justice, "The justice of a community is measured by its treatment of the powerless in society."[9] Considering Jesus' emphasis on the poor, the sick, and those not in the mainstream of society as people who need special concern and attention, finding justice between generations will require the voices of those who may often be silenced when the rich, the strong, and the healthy are in control. Hearing the voice of the voiceless is crucial if justice and the common good are to flourish: "We seek to include and as we work for the common good, our world cannot become more just if left to the vision of a few. Inclusion without voice is a puppet's role; it leaves both the marginalized as powerless as children and those who think they speak for all as deaf as before."[10] Intergenerational justice will require a method wherein different groups can hear the voices of others. It must operate from an attitude of prudent cooperation rather than hostility.

Catholic teaching emphasizes the value of human life in any consideration of justice. In a social context where individuality is prized over community and the weak and poor have few ways to be heard, then human life is at risk. There can be no justice if society encourages the destruction of the unborn, the disabled, the chronically ill, or the aged. Working to build justice between generations will require methods to care for the weak and disabled. It will be necessary to provide for competent nursing care, housing, and the basic materials needed to maintain human dignity, warmth, and cleanliness. This will have an economic and social cost. Many forces in our current society are resistant to the notion that they should contribute to the care of others unable to fend for themselves. As John Paul II writes:

> We are confronted today by an even larger reality, which can be described as a veritable structure of sin. This reality is characterized by the emergence of a culture which denies solidarity and in many cases takes the form of a veritable "culture of death." This culture is actively fostered by powerful cultural, economic and political currents which encourage an idea of society excessively concerned with efficiency. Looking at the situation from this point of view, it is possible to speak in a certain sense of a war of the powerful against the weak: a life which would require greater acceptance, love and care is considered useless, or held to be an intolerable burden, and is therefore rejected in one way or another. A person who, because of illness, handicap or, more simply, just by existing, compromises the well being or life-style of those who are more favored tends to be looked upon as an enemy to be

> resisted or eliminated. In this way a kind of "conspiracy against life" is unleashed.[11]

Catholic teaching on the value of human life is not a mandate that all types of aggressive medical interventions are required. Such a viewpoint could destroy the legitimate needs of younger people faced with crippling medical costs for high-technology medical care for an exploding older population. While vigorously defending the sacredness of human life and maintaining a strict prohibition of the deliberate destruction of human life, the Church does not hold human life to have ultimate value. With the understanding that earthly existence is a prelude to eternal life after death, justice between generations does not require that individuals work to keep those who are seriously ill alive at all costs. It is wrong to kill people. It is, however, not required to bankrupt a nation and shortchange younger individuals in misguided and burdensome medical interventions of questionable benefit:

> Certainly, there is a moral obligation to care for oneself and to allow oneself to be cared for, but this duty must take account of concrete circumstances. It needs to be determined whether the means of treatment available are objectively proportionate to the prospects for improvement. To forgo extraordinary or disproportionate means is not the equivalent of suicide or euthanasia; it rather expresses acceptance of the human condition in the face of death.[12]

In formulating the elements of intergenerational justice, human life needs to be protected and preserved. But that does not imply a wholesale acceptance of financing extraordinarily expensive interventions for individual life extension when confronted with serious illness. Health care is at the service of the human community.

Intergenerational justice will require not only respect for life and care between generations but also the need for mercy. Mercy tempers procedures and rules. It bends the hearts of people and society to recognize ways to care in circumstances that challenge our assumptions, stretch our perceptions, and touch our hearts. The National Conference of Catholic Bishops wrote in a 1981 pastoral on health care:

> An essential element of our religious tradition regarding human rights is the understanding that the works of mercy and the works of justice are inseparable. . . . The works of mercy call Christians to engage themselves in direct efforts to alleviate the misery of the afflicted. The works of justice require that Christians involve themselves in sustained struggle to correct any unjust social, political and economic structures which are the causes of suffering. . . . Because we believe in the dignity of the person, we must embrace every chance to help and to liberate, to heal the wounded world as Jesus taught us. Our hands must be the strong and gentle hands of Christ, reaching out in mercy and justice, touching individual persons, but also touching the social conditions that hinder the wholeness which is God's desire for humanity.[13]

It may be that attempts to find a strict and equitable distribution of resources and services between generations will require limits on the types and amount of health care that are provided. But there always must be the provision of care that will aim at limiting physical suffering and not allowing the person to be abandoned in the experience of illness. Much is made in the contemporary press when individuals are denied access to an experimental medical procedure or very expensive therapy. Our hearts go out to the individual, often a mother or young child. We need to affirm the instinct to care for the person we see who is suffering while recognizing that costs and results may require us to forgo some expenses for individuals to provide more resources for the health of a community. Mercy allows for compassion and care while not requiring that mercy be expressed with intensive-care units or the use of aggressive therapies. Mercy recognizes that individuals can suffer from a lack of care and preventive services that we never see if we focus only on the spectacular tragedy. Intergenerational justice in a society of finite resources will require limits, but it does not require a limit on compassion. Compassion can be expressed by human care and concern, even if it does not cheat death or create a medical miracle. Intergenerational justice will require less emphasis on technology as a mode of interaction and a return to communication and personal attention.

SOME PRACTICAL SUGGESTIONS ON POLICY

In attempting to formulate a Catholic perspective on intergenerational justice, a number of noble themes have been sounded. Basic questions remain about how these themes could be translated into policy or become part of the ethos of a society. Certainly, it is unlikely that the United States will adopt Roman Catholic social teaching as the basis of public policy. But a perspective that urges solidarity, compassion, mercy, attention to the poor, the recognition of intergenerational obligations and the need to consider the common good can be an eloquent voice in a nation that honors pluralism. What are some of the practical suggestions that would help to enflesh the viewpoint on intergenerational justice that flows from the Church's tradition? The six points that follow sketch, with very broad strokes, a preliminary view.

First, universal access to health care with a guaranteed minimum of benefits must be ensured. As the National Conference of Catholic Bishops wrote:

> Every person has a basic right to health care. This right flows from the sanctity of human life and the dignity that belongs to all human persons, who are made in the image of God. It implies that access to health care which is necessary and suitable for the proper development and maintenance of life must be provided for all people, regardless of economic, social or legal status.[14]

Second, the package of benefits needs to take into account the voices not just of the healthy and the rich but to consider the views of the chronically ill and the poor. Third, age should not be the determining factor in access to health care, but there must also be a recognition that age is a marker for the end of life, that death is part of that life and is not to be ceaselessly resisted. Fourth, human life is to be protected and valued. The deliberate killing of the sick or unborn is forbidden. The recognition of death as a natural process, however, means that the benefits and burdens of treatments need to be considered and not every treatment must be provided. Fifth, health care needs to take its place in the context of other needs. In listening to a variety of voices about what is a basic minimum in health care, there must be a discussion of a basic minimum of food, housing, clothing, and education. Sixth, the need for public discussion and dialogue about what constitutes the common good in society and the role of the individual will be crucial. The great difficulty about working for justice and distributing societal goods is that some individuals will feel that they are not receiving what is their due. Careful attention must be given to build a society that realizes that constraints may be necessary for the common good but also develops effective ways to show care and compassion for those who may face limitations of treatment.

These six points are sweeping and may raise more questions than answers about the practical issues involved in formulating policy and encouraging reflection that fosters the realization of intergenerational justice. The points do outline some of the broad and vexing problems that will need to be tackled if achieving justice is a goal of the American nation. Voices from the Roman Catholic tradition can bring a particular perspective on justice between generations. Dialogue with other communities, cultures, and traditions that make up the United States is an important part of considering intergenerational justice. It is past time for the dialogue to begin.

NOTES

1. P. S. German, "Demography of Aging," in *Geriatrics Review Syllabus: A Core Curriculum in Geriatric Medicine,* 3d ed., ed. D. B. Reuben et al. (Dubuque, Iowa: Kendall Hunt Publishing, 1996), 1.
2. S. A. Gaylord, "Demography of Aging," in *Geriatrics Review Syllabus: A Core Curriculum in Geriatric Medicine,* ed. J. C. Beck (New York: American Geriatrics Society, 1991), 1.
3. A. MacIntyre, *After Virtue,* 2d ed. (Notre Dame: University of Notre Dame Press, 1984), 244.
4. R. ter Muellen and C. D. Topinkova, "What Do We Owe the Elderly?" *Hastings Center Report* 24 (1994): S11.
5. All citations from Scripture are from *The New American Bible,* including the revised New Testament and the revised Psalms.
6. U.S. Supreme Court, *Planned Parenthood v. Casey,* 1992.
7. Catechism of the Catholic Church, no 2244, quoting John Paul II, *Encyclical Letter, Centesimus Annus* (1 May 1991): 45, 46.
8. John Paul II, *Encyclical Letter, Evangelium Vitae* (25 March 1995), 19.
9. National Conference of Catholic Bishops, *Pastoral Letter on Catholic Social Teaching and the U.S. Economy,* second draft, no. 44 (Washington, D.C.: Office of Publishing and Promotion Services, United States Catholic Conference, 1985).
10. J. F. Keenan, *Virtues for Ordinary Christians* (Kansas City: Sheed and Ward, 1997), 69.
11. John Paul II, *Encyclical Letter, Evangelium Vitae,* 12.
12. Ibid., 65.
13. United States Catholic Conference, *Health and Health Care: A Pastoral Letter of the American Catholic Bishops* (Washington, D.C.: Office of Publishing and Promotion Services, United States Catholic Conference, 1981), 6.
14. Ibid., 17–18.

Chapter 33

Gender and Health Insurance

Steven Miles and Kara Parker

INTRODUCTION

Although there is increased awareness of gender-related issues in health care, for example, participation in research or in the provision of clinical care,[1] there is less awareness of how private insurance,[2] Medicare,[3] and Medicaid[4] differently serve women and men. Explicit sex discrimination in health insurance is unjustifiable. Even so, men and women have different life spans and patterns of illnesses; thus identical coverage of health services may not equitably serve both sexes. Furthermore, gender differences in vocational, familial, or political roles, or in economic status affect opportunities to obtain insurance or influence insurance design. It is important to consider these biological and social differences between men and women as changes in private and public insurance are occurring or are being considered.

Aggregate statistics camouflage differences in how men and women are insured. At any time, a smaller percentage of women than men are uninsured (13.7 percent versus 16.6 percent) because the relatively greater number of women than men who are over 65 receive Medicare and because women are poorer than men and thus more likely to have means-tested public insurance (16 percent of all women versus 11.9 percent) of men.[5] Women are as likely as men to have private insurance (59.7 percent versus 62.5 percent), including pension and Medicare supplements, though women are more likely to be covered by a spouse's policies or to purchase partial or more costly individual policies.

NONELDERLY ADULTS AND PRIVATE INSURANCE

Women work for less pay, in smaller firms, at lower rank, with fewer benefits, less union participation, and more part-time work than men: All of these factors reduce the numbers of women with job-based insurance.[6] Men working full-time are more likely to have employer-paid insurance than are women (68.3 percent versus 60.5 percent), as are those working part-time or discontinuously (25.6 percent versus 16.6 percent; 18.8 percent versus 9.8 percent). Men's advantage exists even after adjusting for skills, education, pay, or union participation.[7] Insurance for higher-wage (more often male) workers involves greater coverage and a larger employer contribution, both of which constitute larger tax-free supplements to men's incomes.[8]

Women are more likely than men to change jobs for childbearing or family reasons. This makes them vulnerable to becoming ineligible for private insurance or to facing higher premiums for conditions acquired during interrupted

---

Source: Reprinted with permission from Miles and Parker, Men, Women, and Health Insurance, *The New England Journal of Medicine,* Vol. 336, No. 3, pp. 218–221,

private policies[9] and adversely affects eligibility for pension-based insurance.[10] Though women and men between 25 and 54 years old are as likely to lose employer-based insurance in shifting to new jobs (49 percent insured before, 30 percent after), women's new jobs pay less than men's (median: $306 versus $459 per week). A fourth of men's and half of women's new jobs pay less than poverty-level wages. Though women are less able to pay for insurance without an employer contribution or group discount, they are more likely to be eligible for Medicaid, especially if they have children.[11] Thus, of all workers with interrupted employment, more men than women (51 versus 35 percent) are uninsured for at least a month after changing jobs.[12] A woman's insurance is improved by marriage to a "breadwinner"[13] at the cost of her vulnerability to becoming uninsured or uninsurable after divorce or an adverse change in her husband's job.[14]

Though women are only slightly more likely than men to be underinsured for catastrophic illness or for unaffordable health expenses, private policies for less-well-off working women have important limits. Child coverage, critical for women single parents, is rare.[15] A 1993 study found that 7 percent of companies with fewer than 100 employees did not cover obstetric services that were covered by nearly all of the larger health plans. Mammograms were covered by three-fourths of typical job policies but were covered by all health maintenance organization (HMO) policies that served only 20 percent of employees. A fourth of typical job insurance plans did not cover Papanicolaou tests; 10 percent did not cover abortion.[16] A quarter to half of insurers ask women if they have been victims of domestic violence. An insurer justified excluding or charging higher premiums to such women by equating them with "diabetic[s] not taking their medication."[17]

Persons between 55 and 64 years old constitute 14 percent of nonelderly people, but they have a high incidence of acute and chronic disease and use a third of all surgeries and hospital days used by persons under 65 years old. Uninsured people of this age tend to be unmarried, unemployed, and poor, and to have chronic, often nondisabling conditions for which they underuse health care.[18] A review of 1986 data found that women face twice as many uninsurance spells, mostly because of an abrupt income fall and privately purchased insurance lapse. Insurance is repurchased when income later rises.[19] Less than 30 percent of 55- to 65-year-olds without private insurance are eligible for Medicaid.[20]

ELDERLY ADULTS AND INSURANCE

There is a regressive relationship among older women's longevity, resources, and chronic health care needs.[21] Though women are 59 percent of persons over 65, they are 72 percent of poor elderly people[22] and have a third more postretirement years. They are half as likely to have pensions (24 percent versus 46 percent), and their pensions are half as much.[23] Women's longevity, given that they are four times as likely to depend on husbands' pensions or insurance, means that they risk becoming uninsured.[24] Dying men are three times as likely to leave an impoverished spouse. Single women tend to purchase home care that men get from spouses.

Medicare serves men better than women. It covers hospital costs well but has poorer coverage for nursing-home care, community services, outpatient medications, preventive-health exams, and adaptive aids. Women have more chronic illness and more disabled days, and use 14 percent more physician visits, 18 percent more prescriptions, and 60 percent more formal community or home care services. Older men use 5 percent more hospital care; women use two to six times more nursing-home days.[25] Even though women on Medicare are older than men, Medicare pays 12 percent more per year for male beneficiaries.[26]

Pension or Medigap insurance does not offset men's Medicare advantage.[27] Men are more likely to have pension-based policies than women are, and women use their more meager personal resources to buy Medigap policies.[28]

Pension policies have lower hospital copayments; easier eligibility for home and nursing-home care; and better coverage for physician services, medications, and mental health and routine vision, hearing, and dental care than Medigap policies.[29] After a finding that Medicare reimbursements were much higher for comparably difficult procedures (e.g., genital biopsies, pelvic surgery) on men than women, the federal government has promised to adjust reimbursement formulas in 1997.[30] A study of the 10 most common illnesses for which there is a treatment consensus in persons with Medicare and Medigap coverage found that three of the four illnesses with the highest out-of-pocket costs (e.g., arthritis) were more common in women. Four of five treatments with the lowest out-of-pocket costs (e.g., lung cancer) were more common in men.[31] Reimbursements for mental health and rehabilitation should be similarly examined. A fourth of Medicare enrollees lack supplemental policies, and this number, especially among women, is growing.[32]

MEDICAID: OLD AND YOUNG WOMEN COMPETE

Medicaid is often the last resort for people who cannot afford health insurance.[33] Pregnant women and children account for half of the recent growth in beneficiaries but for only 9 percent of its large cost growth, which is due to a smaller number of disabled or chronically ill people, especially those in nursing homes.[34] In 1994, women made up 59 percent of Medicaid recipients.

Many forces are pushing women to Medicaid.[35] Employers' retreats from providing health insurance are most often in job types or salary levels that are more often occupied by women.[36] Young women who are priced out of insurance, who are underinsured, or who are deprived of insurance by work roles, divorce, or responsibilities for children enroll in Medicaid for themselves or their children. Women who are chronically ill or who are single parents of chronically ill children are less likely than other women to enter the work force if it means that they must give up Medicaid.[37] Older women with fewer pension or personal resources turn to Medicaid for payment of services not covered by Medicare and are four times as likely as men to use Medicaid for nursing-home care.[38] Thus, increasingly more older, frail women[39] compete with increasing numbers of uninsured working-age women and children.

States that are facing federal cuts in Medicare or Medicaid will try to avoid absorbing the transferred health care costs as employers within those states also try to avoid higher charges from providers who are trying to compensate for having less public revenue. These strategies to manage federal cuts may disproportionately and adversely affect women as nursing-home residents, as chronically ill elderly, as poor people, as single parents for children, or as less adequately workplace-insured employees.

DISCUSSION

Unequal health insurance is inevitable as long as our nation relies on insurance subsystems that are not collectively accountable to a universal, equitable access to health care. Women's increasingly disadvantaged access to private insurance reflects their lower pay and lower work status; employers are less often providing insurance to employees at the bottom of the pay scale. But, this is not the whole story. It may be that men's relatively greater seniority as insurers, employers, union officials, or public office holders (and perhaps a policy-making insensitivity to how gender and sex affect health care need and financing) may partly explain why Medicare and private insurance better fit men's needs and financing. Furthermore, though women who are married to working husbands have better insurance before and after retirement, women's deteriorating access to private insurance may also reveal the inadequacy of insurance systems that are designed for a more economically homogeneous society with more restricted roles for men and women in households, as parents or as partners.

Unequal health insurance for men and women reveals the fundamental problem of a regressively financed health care system with unequal opportunities for participating in insurance policy making. Looking at health care through gender and the life cycle should not invite a distracting debate about whether health dollars should be equally divided between men and women but rather how to equitably meet individual needs. Similar issues face men and women who are poor, chronically ill, or disadvantaged by discrimination. Women are such a large and diverse "class" that solutions to their problems would necessarily remedy similar problems for other disadvantaged persons as well.

Proposals for reforming the design or financing of health insurance might be discussed in terms of a "gender impact" to consider how they (1) equitably serve the health needs of men and women given their differing financial resources, (2) reduce unequal access to adequate coverage by private insurance, and (3) reduce vulnerable dependence on public entitlement programs. For example, medical savings accounts might be considered as to whether they (1) offer women equitable opportunities to have basic primary, preventive, and obstetric health care; (2) offset disadvantages women face in employer-based health insurance; and (3) offer equal opportunities to save and shelter income from taxes. The present system for financing health care shows that this will not happen naturally.

NOTES

1. C. M. Clancy and C. T. Massion, "American Women's Health Care: A Patchwork with Gaps," *JAMA* 268 (1992): 1918–20.
2. J. K. Iglehart, "The American Health Care System: Private Insurance," *New England Journal of Medicine* 326 (1992): 1715–20.
3. J. K. Iglehart, "The American Health Care System: Medicare," *New England Journal of Medicine* 327 (1992): 1467–72.
4. J. K. Iglehart, "The American Health Care System: Medicaid," *New England Journal of Medicine* 328 (1995): 896–900.
5. R. L. Bennefield, *Current Population Reports: Who Loses Coverage and for How Long?* (Washington, D.C.: United States Bureau of the Census, 1995); *id., Current Population Reports: Health Insurance Coverage—1994* (Washington, D.C.: United States Bureau of the Census, 1996).
6. J. R. Tallon and R. Block, "Changing Patterns of Health Insurance Coverage: Special Concerns for Women," *Women and Health* 12, no. 3–4 (1988): 119–36; N. S. Jecker, "Can an Employer-Based Health Insurance System Be Just?" *Journal of Health, Politics, Policy, and Law* 18 (1993): 657–73; K. Seccombe, "Employer Sponsored Medical Benefits: The Influence of Occupational Characteristics and Gender," *Sociological Quarterly* 34 (1993): 557–80.
7. Tallon and Block, "Changing Patterns of Health Insurance Coverage"; Jecker, "Can an Employer-Based Insurance System Be Just?"; Seccombe, "Employer Sponsored Medical Benefits"; K. Seccombe and L. Beeghley, "Gender and Medical Insurance: A Test of Human Capital Theory," *Gender and Society* 6 (1992): 283–300.
8. Agency for Health Care Policy and Research, National Medical Expenditure Survey, "Employment Related Health Insurance in 1987," no. 43 (April 1995).
9. A. L. Schorr, "Job Turnover: A Problem with Employer Based Health Care," *New England Journal of Medicine* 323 (1990): 543–45.
10. Agency for Health Care Policy and Research, National Medical Expenditure Survey, "Retirees: Employment-Related Health Insurance," no. 4 (February 1992).
11. U.S. Department of Commerce, "Dynamics of Economic Well-being: Labor Force 1991 to 1993" (August 1995).
12. Bennefield, *Current Population Reports: Who Loses Coverage and for How Long?*
13. Seccombe, "Employer Sponsored Medical Benefits."
14. Seccombe and Beeghley, "Gender and Medical Insurance."
15. P. F. Hort and J. S. Banthin, "New Estimates of the Underinsured Younger Than Sixty-five Years," *JAMA* 274 (1995): 1302–6.
16. Alan Guttmacher Institute, *Uneven and Unequal: Insurance Coverage and Reproductive Health Services* (New York: Alan Guttmacher Institute, 1993).
17. J. Brienza, "Lawmakers Seek to Help Battered Women Get Insurance," *Trial* 32, no. 4 (1996): 14.
18. G. A. Jenson, "The Dynamics of Health Insurance among the Near Elderly," *Medical Care* 30 (1992): 598–614.
19. Ibid.
20. Agency for Health Care Policy and Research, National Medical Expenditure Survey, "Retirees: Medicaid and

Other Public Health Insurance Coverage," no. 6 (March 1992).

21. R. N. Butler, "On Behalf of Older Women," *New England Journal of Medicine* 334 (1996): 794–96.
22. R. Stone, "The Feminization of Poverty among the Elderly," *Women's Studies Quarterly* 17, no. 1–2 (1989): 20–34; S. Sofaer and E. Abel, "Older Women's Health and Financial Vulnerability: Implications of the Medicare Benefit Structure," *Women and Health* 16, no. 3 (1990): 47–67.
23. J. Dimeo, "Women Receive the Short End When It Comes to Their Retirement Pension Incomes," *Pension World* (October 1992): 28.
24. Agency for Health Care Policy and Research, National Medical Expenditure Survey, "Retirees: Employment-Related Health Insurance"; Department of Health and Human Services, "Prescribed Medicines: A Summary of Use and Expenditures by Medicare Beneficiaries," DHHS no. (PHS) 89-3448, National Medical Expenditure Survey Research Findings 3, Agency for Health Care Policy and Research (Rockville, MD: Public Health Service).
25. Butler, "On Behalf of Older Women"; Dimeo, "Women Receive the Short End When It Comes to Their Retirement Pension Incomes"; Department of Health and Human Services, "Prescribed Medicines"; Department of Health and Human Services, "Use of Home and Community Services by Persons Age Sixty-five and Older with Functional Difficulties," DHHS no. (PHS) 90-3466, National Medical Expenditure Survey Research Findings 5, Agency for Health Care Policy and Research (Rockville, MD: Public Health Service); M. A. Cohen et al., "Long Term Care Insurance and Medicaid," *Health Affairs* (Fall 1994): 127–39.
26. *Medicare and Medicaid: Statistical Supplement,* 1995 W731, H434.
27. Sofaer and Abel, "Older Women's Health and Financial Vulnerability."
28. M. A. Morrisey, "Retiree Health Benefits," *Annu. Rev. Public Health* 14 (1993): 271–92.
29. G. A. Jensen and M. A. Morrisey, "Employer-Sponsored Postretirement Health Benefits: Not Your Mother's Medigap Plan," *Gerontologist* 32 (1992): 693–703.
30. P. Chernouy and C. Nadolski, "Underreimbursement of Obstetric and Gynecologic Invasive Services by the Resource-Based Relative Value Scale," *Obstet. Gynecol.* 87 (1996): 328–31; W. B. Harer, "Gender Bias in Health Care Services Valuations," *Obstet. Gynecol.* 87 (1996): 453–54.
31. Harer, "Gender Bias in Health Care Services Valuations."
32. A. C. Monheit and C. L. Schur, "Health Insurance Coverage of Retired Persons," DHHS no. (PHS) 89-3444, National Medical Expenditure Survey Findings 2, Agency for Health Care Policy and Research (Rockville, MD: Public Health Service).
33. Iglehart, "The American Health Care System: Medicaid."
34. J. Holahan et al., *The Changing Composition of Health Insurance Coverage in the United States* (Washington, D.C.: Urban Institute, 1995).
35. Butler, "On Behalf of Older Women."
36. Holahan et al., *The Changing Composition of Health Insurance Coverage in the United States.*
37. B. L. Wolfe and S. C. Hill, "The Effect of Health on the Work Effort of Single Mothers," *Journal of Human Resources* 30 (1995): 42–62.
38. Department of Health and Human Services, National Medical Expenditure Survey, "Prescribed Medicines."
39. T. A. Coughlin et al., "State Responses to the Medicaid Spending Crisis: 1988–1992," *Journal of Health, Policy, Politics, and Law* 19 (1994): 837–64.

Chapter 34

Is Rationing of Health Care Ethically Defensible?

Chris Hackler

INTRODUCTION

Expenditures for health care constitute a significant portion of the budgets of all industrialized nations. Without conscious measures to control medical spending, it tends to grow more rapidly than the general rate of economic growth. Increasing demand and the high cost of new medical technologies are only two factors driving health care inflation. In some countries, such as the United States and South Africa, substantial portions of the population face difficulty in obtaining medical care. Correcting this situation will mean even greater demand for health care services. It would seem that the only way to expand coverage while holding costs near current levels would be to reduce per-capita spending. The problem in the United States becomes even more acute when we plan for the future. Early in the twenty-first century, when the average age of the population will increase dramatically, pressures on both health care and retirement programs will be formidable. Unless we find some way to reduce the level of health care spending, at least government health care spending, there may be little left to fund other essential social services. Health care spending is a serious and growing problem for which we must find a solution that is both economically sound and ethically just.

The most difficult, painful, and divisive debates about this problem today, at least in the United States, revolve around the issue of rationing. Some say we must never ration health care and that physicians certainly must not do such a thing. Others maintain that soaring health expenditures require us to place significant limits on medical spending, denying some medical services that are both beneficial and desired. Still others claim that we are already rationing health care, either by market forces or by denying inclusion or coverage in public programs for the poor. This debate certainly involves serious substantive issues, but some of it also results from unclarity about the term *rationing.*

WHAT IS RATIONING?

In the strict sense of the term, we are not rationing health care and never have. To ration generally means to give equal portions of a scarce good to everybody. A clear example of rationing is the allotment of goods such as rubber, sugar, gasoline, or gunpowder that are needed in wartime. The amount needed by the military is set aside, and the remainder is allocated to citizens in equal shares. The term is also used for the fixed (and equal) amounts of food that soldiers are given in battle. Rationing in this sense, which is the common or dictionary definition, does not apply to health care. We have

---

Source: Adapted with permission from C. Hackler, Is Rationing of Health Care Ethically Defensible? Gesundsheitsoeconomica 1995, Austrian Society for Health Economics.

never considered giving our citizens fixed allotments of health care—so many days of hospitalization, so many visits to the doctor, a fixed amount of money to spend on health care, or any such thing. An essential point is that rationing in the ordinary sense is not practiced as a way to save money or decrease expenditures. Rather, it is a response to a real physical scarcity of goods for consumption. The shortage may be the result of diversion to war efforts or to export for foreign capital, or it may result from natural events such as crop failures or earthquakes. We have no comparable shortage of medical goods or services in the United States or Western Europe, so it is not obvious why *rationing* would be the term chosen to refer to some of our attempts to limit health care spending.

Rationing is essentially a method of distributing resources outside the market system. We in the United States are ambivalent about the status of health care. We think of it both as a commodity to be marketed and as a social good that we ought to supply to those unable to procure it for themselves. The result is a complex patchwork of a "system" that leaves many without adequate access to care. That millions of our citizens are not getting the health care they need because they cannot afford it is a deplorable fact and a serious ethical and political problem, but it may be confusing to describe the situation, as many do, as "rationing by price."[1]

One of the first uses of the term in the context of health care was by Aaron and Schwartz.[2] According to them, rationing occurs when "not all care expected to be beneficial is provided to all patients." This is surely too broad a definition of rationing. If this is the meaning of the term, then almost everything is rationed. Most of us would be benefited by a new automobile, a new suit of clothes, and perhaps even by extensive cosmetic surgery! Treatment for infertility by in vitro fertilization is rarely provided to patients who cannot pay for it, but it seems odd to say it is being rationed. Aaron and Schwartz claim that denying any potentially beneficial care means that "the value of care is being weighed against its costs, explicitly or implicitly."[3] This seems to equate rationing with cost-benefit analysis, that is, basing the decision whether to provide a certain treatment not just on whether it would be of any benefit, but whether the benefits would be proportional to the cost of the treatment.[4] Cost-benefit analysis is certainly a potential strategy to reduce health care spending, but it is not rationing in the customary sense.

A number of practices resemble rationing and are frequently so labeled. Three of these are distribution of scarce goods, prioritization of services, and allocation of financial resources. Distribution of organs for transplantation is a clear example of the first. Transplantable organs are an absolutely scarce resource (that is, there is no way to produce enough to satisfy all needs). Choices must be made concerning who will get a given organ and who will not. We all agree that it is ethically acceptable that someone be denied the organ, because only one can have it, and it is better that someone gets it than that no one gets it. It is not possible for all to share equally in the limited resources, which is the ordinary sense of rationing, but it is possible and ethically necessary to distribute organs fairly. Since someone is denied access to the organ, some will call it rationing, but the expression "just distribution of scarce goods" is quite adequate and less misleading.

The practice of triage in the emergency room is an example of prioritizing access to care. A scarce resource, in this case physician and staff time, is distributed according to urgency of need. This is sometimes referred to as rationing, though it bears almost no resemblance to ordinary rationing. Everybody is served; it is only the order that is at issue. *Prioritizing* is a perfectly serviceable term and more accurate in describing the practice than is *rationing.* Again, nobody questions the ethical propriety of this practice, since the alternative policy of "first come, first served" would lead to much poorer aggregate outcomes.

Allocation of scarce resources is also often referred to as rationing. Allocating resources means dividing or apportioning them among competing interests. When there is a scarcity of a given resource, then a scheme must be devised to allocate among potential recipients in a way that is efficient, fair, and socially desirable. Rationing in the usual sense, that is, handing out equal shares, is one possible scheme but not necessarily the best, certainly not in health care.

Money is a scarce resource, though not in the same way that transplantable organs are. As a society, we can always find more money to meet the needs of a given group, but we do so at the expense of competing interests. There is a growing consensus that we are spending too much on health care and neglecting other important social needs, and that we must find ways to limit health care spending that are ethically acceptable. We may try to reduce waste and inefficiency, reduce the level of compensation for services, and so on. But the most direct way to limit spending is to limit consumption or utilization. There are roughly two strategies for limiting utilization: to eliminate some of the kinds of services offered, or to limit access to the services (or both). If access is to be limited, the next step is to find an acceptable way to determine who will gain access to the available services. One way to do this is by chance, either first come, first served, or some kind of lottery. Another way is to identify criteria on the basis of which access will be granted. It may be urgency of medical need, potential for medical benefit, potential for quantity or quality of life, or any combination of factors. It is here that we are most inclined to speak of rationing, but notice that the situation is quite similar to the distribution of transplantable organs; we have too little to go around and must distribute what we have on the basis of criteria that are fair to all. The big difference, and one that calls for ethical justification, is that the scarcity is a matter of policy, a deliberate choice we have made in the allocation of social resources. If the services no longer available are ineffective or of little benefit, the policy will be relatively easy to justify. If the services, however, are of significant benefit, the task of justification will be more difficult.

Though it should be understood as a special use of the term, let us use *rationing of health care* for the present purpose to refer to policies and procedures that result in individuals' being denied services that would be of significant medical benefit to them for reasons other than absolute scarcity or inability to pay (again, lack of access because of inability to pay is also a serious ethical issue but a different one both conceptually and ethically). There are two aspects to rationing so understood: policies that restrict the availability of services, and the implementation of those policies by individual gatekeepers who deny patients access to particular services. We turn now to the ethical justification of rationing so understood.

IS RATIONING ETHICALLY JUSTIFIABLE?

The case for the general possibility of rationing health care is quite simple. Life and health are basic goods, and we have a very strong social claim on the means necessary to sustain them. But however strong the claim, they must compete with other social goods that in the long run may be more important to the flourishing of the community. Under certain circumstances to be discussed below, we may limit the funds devoted to health care in order to invest in such things as education and cultural enrichment, without which life and health would be hollow possessions, as well as such things as prisons and police activities, which are necessary to the very preservation of the community. To deny that rationing could ever be justified, it would seem necessary to hold that health (or life) is an absolute good or that our moral claim on the means to health is always stronger that any competing claim or need. To compromise that claim for essentially economic reasons could be seen as putting a price on human life, thus contradicting the Kantian maxim that life has not a price but a dignity, that is, an inner value that takes it out of the realm of things to which we can assign a comparative value or price. We will return to this issue later.

The case for rationing of health care in principle is simple, but that does not mean it will be easy to justify particular rationing schemes. What would be the important considerations in deciding whether a given proposal to ration health care were justifiable? Let us attempt to answer that question by trying to construct an ideal set of conditions sufficient to justify rationing. After surveying that list, we shall consider how these ideal conditions might be realized in the real world:

1. There are other equally important needs competing for scarce resources.
2. There are no alternative ways to produce equivalent savings.
3. Savings from denied services will benefit other patients or be invested in equally important social needs.
4. Policies and procedures for limiting access to treatment are applied equitably to all.
5. Limits are self-imposed through democratic processes.

If all these conditions were met, then rationing of health care would clearly be justifiable. The trouble is that they are only imperfectly met in the real world, and the degree of approximation varies from place to place. We will have to decide in each case how close to the ideal we must be before a given rationing scheme would be justifiable. There are real budget pressures and competing needs that we must somehow resolve. It is not helpful to insist on the perfect realization of ideal conditions before adopting a policy to deal with a pressing problem. With this in mind, let us examine the above criteria in greater detail and discuss briefly the problems in satisfying them under various social arrangements.

JUSTIFYING RATIONING IN THE REAL WORLD

First there must be equally important needs competing for scarce resources. The appropriate level of funding for such things as education, housing, and national defense will need to be addressed in concrete terms in a given social context. Is the military budget too big? Are we wasting money on inefficient administrative programs? These are important questions to raise, but, in the end, I believe we will still find far more needs than we can fulfill at current budget levels. In addition, the constant development of new and expensive medical technologies and the aging of the population will continue to increase both the demand for health care and the cost of providing it.

Rationing of care is by no means the only way to control health care costs. Before rationing is implemented, every reasonable effort should be made to reduce waste and inefficiency within the system. Unnecessary services should be eliminated and duplication of resources minimized. This is surely easier in more centrally organized systems such as those of Great Britain and Canada than in the fragmented system of the United States. In the United States, there is far more expensive equipment than necessary because of competition among hospitals. Each institution has its own magnetic resonance imaging machine, though it sits unused much of the time. Since the hospital must pay for the machine, the charge for the procedure is artificially high. There are 10,000 mammogram machines in the United States, but 2,000 would satisfy current demand and 5,000 would satisfy all potential demand if everyone for whom it is recommended had the procedure.[5] Inefficient deployment of resources is a serious structural problem that is difficult to attack in a decentralized and fragmented system.

Another structural problem for the justification of rationing within the United States system concerns the proper transfer of savings. The justice of the practice of distributing organs for transplantation is apparent because we can see that someone benefits from the organ that is denied to someone else. It is likewise important in the justification of health care rationing that savings stay within the system and benefit other patients, though the trade-offs may be less visible. The trade-offs are much easier to accomplish and to demonstrate in a unified system than in a fragmented one. It is quite possible for savings to be directed to the salaries of health care or insurance company executives or to corporate profits. As private hospitals and health maintenance organizations increase their share of the United States health care system, the potential for misdirection of savings grows. Where we have insufficient guarantees against such results, we have a strong argument against rationing measures.

The fourth item on the list of ideal conditions for rationing is equitable application of rationing policies. If one person sacrifices a beneficial and desired treatment, then others in the same situation should make the same sacrifice. Once again, this criterion is much more easily satisfied within a unified system than a fragmented one. If the system is unified, then the same policies should apply to everyone. If there are many separate and independent units, there is no assurance that their policies will be similar. Similarity of policies, however, is not the only issue. Policies need to be applied similarly by individual physicians within the same system. Because the traditional role of the physician is patient advocate, an understandable temptation will be to "game the system" for one's own patients, that is, bend, manipulate, or bypass rules that deny a needed resource. Since clinical judgment is necessary in any rationing scheme, we probably will have to live with this problem and just try to minimize it.

The fifth ideal condition for rationing is that limits to health care are freely adopted rather than imposed. Clearly it is better to be denied a service because of a policy one has adopted rather than because of a policy that has been imposed by others. There are two ways in which limits can be self-imposed: by participating in the formation of policies and by accepting the results of the process. Direct citizen participation in policy making can be cumbersome, but it was an important element in the development of Oregon's prioritized list of health care procedures.[6] Rationing policies developed openly by politically accountable representatives would also carry a presumptive legitimacy that secretly developed plans would lack.

In addition to the process of development, the fairness of the result is of great importance. If limits are to be freely adopted in the sense of accepted, they must be perceived as fair by those who are affected. It will be no small task to create policies universally perceived as just, especially in nations with diverse populations and historic inequities. It would be difficult enough if there were general agreement on the criteria for making rationing decisions, but the American philosopher Norman Daniels has argued persuasively that there is no consensus on this matter and that none is likely. In distributing organs for transplantation, for example, should we favor those who will live longest and thus benefit most, or should we give each individual a fair chance by means of a lottery? We have neither consensus nor a demonstrable theory that would yield a convincing answer to the question. Nor is there consensus on the matter of aggregating benefits. Prolonging a life for a year has a higher priority than providing routine dental care for one person, but if the funds saved by allowing the person to die can provide dental care for 600 people during that year, is that an appropriate trade-off? We do not now have answers to these questions, and there is no good reason to think a philosophical theory is about to be produced that will enable us to resolve such issues with confidence.[7]

It is unfortunate that such fundamental issues are unresolved, but it need not paralyze public policy. We do not have a theory that guides our trade-offs in other areas of social policy either, but we manage to make difficult decisions nonetheless. We should not expect a system that everyone agrees is perfectly just. What we should expect is a system that is openly created, tries to be fair and succeeds in large measure, and is open to continual improvement. Designing a workable system that is "just enough"[8] is a matter not only of ethics, but also of economics, history, psychology, and politics.

WHO MAKES RATIONING DECISIONS?

The realization that we do not have an adequate and agreed-upon theoretical basis for rationing decisions makes more poignant the issue of who is making the decisions and how they are made. It was suggested above that open procedures that are broadly inclusive are best. There is an opposite view that deserves consideration. In their book *Tragic Choices,* Guido Calabresi and Philip Bobbit argue that public involvement in rationing decisions would be unwise. Every open society adheres to a set of fundamental values that is not internally consistent; that is, the values may come into conflict with one another. Tragic choices are those that bare the inconsistencies and force us to choose between cherished values, thus eroding our commitment to the dishonored value. Rationing decisions are among the most dangerous of tragic choices because they expose our willingness to make trade-offs with human life and in some sense to set a price on it, thus compromising our commitment to the Kantian principle that human life does not have a price but rather, a dignity that gives it inestimable value and incomparable worth.[9]

Of course we regularly make public-policy decisions that in effect price human life, but only if they are the lives of unknown future individuals. We may refuse to invest in mine safety, knowing that lives will be lost as a result, but we will pay whatever it takes to rescue a trapped miner. To do otherwise would be to acknowledge our willingness to price life. But that is the essence of rationing decisions, so the argument goes. They will expose the conditional nature of our commitment to the sanctity and equality of human life. In addition to being psychologically painful to individuals, there may be two truly serious consequences: We may become too willing to price and trade in human life, and social cohesion may suffer. Our shared values provide the moral foundation of social collaboration. As tragic choices expose the contradictions among our values and erode our commitments to them, the foundation will begin to crumble. To preserve social cohesion, according to Calabresi and Bobbit, societies must mask their tragic choices. A policy-making elite should make rationing decisions. They will be sophisticated enough to realize that necessary compromises do not truly diminish the value of life, whereas the larger group "may not be able to make such nice distinctions."[10]

While we should be sobered by the possibility that public participation in rationing decisions might produce moral and political decay, it is by no means clear that this would result. It is an empirical claim for which evidence is scant. In fact we have no more evidence for this pessimistic and antiutopian vision than we do for the idealistic strain in Rousseau's view of democracy (Rousseau was, characteristically, capable of deep pessimism at the same time). The primary value of democracy for Rousseau was not what it does *for* us (by producing good laws), but what it does *to* us. By participating as a member of the Sovereign an individual's "faculties so unfold themselves by being exercised, his ideas are so extended, his sentiments so exalted, and his whole mind so enlarged and refined," that he is transformed "from a circumscribed and stupid animal into an intelligent being and a man."[11]

Surely the truth lies somewhere between the deep skepticism of Calabresi and Bobbit and the soaring faith of Rousseau in human reason. It would be wrong to rely solely on any one source for rationing policies. Open and democratic procedures should be employed, though their exact nature and role in the overall process is not clear. Citizen opinions and preferences should be taken into account, though the actual formulation of policies must be done by policy experts (a point acknowledged by Rousseau as well, in the figure of the Legislator). The potential role of citizen groups is very much an open question that deserves further study.

An important lesson to learn from Calabresi and Bobbit, however, is that we should frame the debate in such a way that allegiance to the basic conflicting values is preserved as much as possible, consistent with effective and responsible decision making.[12] Although choices may need to be formulated in terms of monetary value, this does not mean that the ultimate trade is lives for money. Money is only the medium of exchange that allows us to purchase one good at the expense of another. The real trade is, for example, the last two remaining months of a person's life that would cost $200,000 to prolong for the many infant lives to be saved by a citywide inoculation program that would cost $200,000. Thus understood, it is not life for money but life for life, which is still in a sense a tragic choice, but one that is perhaps not so ethically suspect or socially corrosive.

SUMMARY

Rapidly increasing spending on health care may threaten a society's economic and cultural vitality by decreasing savings and investment and draining funds from other social services. Governments are seeking to limit the growth of health spending by promoting greater efficiency and limiting reimbursement for physician and hospital services. A further step is to limit utilization of services, first by discouraging marginally beneficial treatments, and then, if necessary, by denying some costly treatments that would be of substantial benefit. Adopting policies that limit access to treatments of significant medical benefit is commonly called *rationing* of health care, though this use is somewhat at odds with the ordinary meaning of the word. Rationing will be defensible to the extent that funding is truly needed for other essential social goods and services, that alternative ways of limiting medical spending have been attempted, that money saved will be directed to more compelling needs, and that limits are applied equitably to everyone. It is also important that limits be self-imposed in the sense that they are openly developed and generally accepted as fair. Accepting rationing will be painful because it calls into question our conviction that human life is priceless. We must guard against the potentially corrosive effects of overtly making comparative judgments about human lives.

NOTES

1. For example, L. Churchill uses this terminology in his excellent book *Rationing Health Care in America* (Notre Dame, Ind.: University of Notre Dame Press, 1987), 14.
2. H. J. Aaron and W. B. Schwartz, *The Painful Prescription: Rationing Hospital Care* (Washington, D.C.: The Brookings Institution, 1984).
3. Ibid.
4. M. D. Reagan, "Health Care Rationing: What Does It Mean?" *New England Journal of Medicine* 319, no. 17 (27 October 1988): 1150.
5. M. L. Brown et al., "Is the Supply of Mammography Machines Outstripping Need and Demand? An Economic Analysis," *Annals of Internal Medicine* 113 (1990): 547–52.
6. M. Brannigan, "Oregon's Experiment," *Health Care Analysis* 1, no. 1 (1993): 15–28.
7. N. Daniels, "Rationing Fairly: Programmatic Considerations," *Bioethics* 7, no. 2–3 (1993): 224–32.
8. I borrow this term from L. M. Fleck, who has used it in a number of works. See, e.g., "Just Caring: Lessons from Oregon and Canada" in *Health Care for an Aging Population,* ed. C. Hackler (Albany, N.Y.: State University of New York Press, 1994), 193.
9. J.-J. Rousseau, *The Social Contract* (New York: E.P. Dutton, 1913).
10. G. Calabresi and P. Bobbit, *Tragic Choices* (New York: W. W. Norton & Company, 1978), 69.
11. Rousseau, *The Social Contract.*
12. J. L. Nelson, "Publicity and Pricelessness," *The Journal of Medicine and Philosophy* 19, no. 4 (August 1994): 340.

CHAPTER 35

The Social Obligations of Health Care Practitioners

David T. Ozar

Almost everyone would agree that when one makes a voluntary commitment to act in a certain way for a specific individual or group, one thereby comes to have an *obligation* to so act. Thus, health care practitioners certainly do have some social obligations, namely the obligations to specific individuals and groups that each has voluntarily undertaken. We can also speak meaningfully of a general, underlying social obligation that all humans, including health care practitioners, have to keep the commitments they make.

But are there other kinds of obligations that health care practitioners have toward others? Do they have any obligations toward others that are not dependent on their voluntary commitments to specific individuals and groups but are incumbent on them for other reasons? It is obligations of this sort (if there are any) that will be referred to as *social obligations* throughout the remainder of this chapter. The aim of the chapter is to inquire whether health care practitioners have any such obligations.

The first step will be to examine several answers to the following question: Do human beings in general have any obligations toward other humans that are not dependent on their voluntary commitments to specific individuals and groups but are incumbent on them for other reasons? If the answer to this question is yes, then health care practitioners will have some social obligations (in our sense of the term) simply because they are members of the human community. If the answer is no, then the only social obligations that health care practitioners could have would be obligations specifically due to their roles as health care practitioners. The first part of this chapter examines several important accounts of the foundations of social obligation.

In either case, whether the first question is answered yes or no, the second step will be to ask whether health care practitioners have any social obligations specifically due to their roles as health care practitioners. If the answer to either the first or the second question is yes, then a third question must be asked: When health care practitioners' social obligations come into conflict with one another or with the obligations toward specific individuals and groups that health care practitioners have voluntarily undertaken (especially their obligations towards specific patients), how should such conflicts be resolved?

GENERAL SOCIAL OBLIGATIONS

Libertarianism

Do human beings in general have any obligations toward other humans that are not dependent on their voluntary commitments to specific individuals and groups but are incumbent on them for other reasons? One important answer to this question holds that we have obligations only to specific individuals with whom we deal and no obligations beyond those. The most frequent defense of this answer rests on the claim that there is, at bottom, only one fundamental rule of morality for all relations between persons. This rule is: Respect people's liberty. That is, do not interfere with people's efforts to choose, act, and live in accord with their own values, goals, ideals, or principles provided only that their actions in turn respect the comparable liberty of others. (In practice, this view of our obligations toward others primarily concerns the interactions of competent adults. Other principles are taken to govern the dealings of competent adults with other humans who are not at the time competent. Other principles also govern the special circumstance in which someone is deliberately violating his or her own or another person's liberty.)

This approach to morality has several names, the most distinctive being *libertarianism.* Libertarianism does not recognize any obligations between persons beyond the original obligation to respect others' liberty and those obligations that have been voluntarily undertaken by the persons involved. Consequently, there is no general category of social obligations that are incumbent upon all human beings (or all competent human beings), but only such obligations as human beings actually undertake in their voluntary dealings with other human beings (plus the fundamental obligation to respect others' liberty).

But could it not be the case that people undertake obligations to "society"? From one perspective it is hard to see how this could be the case, because it is hard to see what "undertaking an obligation to society" could mean. When I agree to act in a certain way for someone's benefit, undertaking an obligation toward him or her, there is a "someone" who benefits and who, in most instances, undertakes to act in a certain way toward me in return. But both elements of this common relationship seem to be lacking in regard to "obligations toward society." *Who* is the beneficiary of the action that I commit myself to perform? *Who* is it who might act for my benefit in some way in return? *Society,* one version of libertarianism would argue, is simply a word we use to refer generically to all the people in a given place who interact with each other, undertaking thousands of obligations to act for one another in thousands of different ways, but none of them undertaking to act in some way for the benefit of *all* the rest. From this point of view, there is nothing concrete enough in the idea of society to enable us to make good sense of "undertaking an obligation toward society."

So in this version of libertarianism, there are no general social obligations that all humans have beyond the fundamental rule to respect others' liberty. Nor is there something called "society" to which they might undertake obligations by their voluntary acts. Instead there are only the dealings of individual humans with other specific individuals and groups, dealings that tend to generate freely chosen commitments and their concomitant obligations. There are no social obligations (in our sense of the term).

But there is another way to look at the notion of society within the libertarian tradition. John Locke, a famous seventeenth-century British political philosopher, claimed that when a group of people voluntarily place the use of force—for the punishment of wrongdoers among them (e.g., those who violate others' liberty) and for protection from external enemies—into the hands of a select few, then the whole group form themselves by doing so into a new kind of actor within the human community, a collective actor that Locke calls "civil society." They do this by each voluntarily contracting with all the others to be governed by the decisions of the majority; that is, they agree, in the "social contract" that establishes civil society, to be obligated to carry out these majority decisions.

There is much more to be said about all this, of course. For a civil society cannot function effectively without establishing a government that makes and enforces laws in the name of the whole group and that is supported from the property of the whole group. There are also some important limitations, Locke argues, on the range of decisions by the majority (or its government) that are obligatory for the citizens. In particular, citizens have no obligation under the original social contract to give up their property to the society or its government for the improvement, for example, of anyone's life or living conditions. In the original social contract they have committed their property only to the extent needed to prevent crime, to try, convict, and punish wrongdoers, and to protect the society from external enemies. Since taking a person's property is violating his or her liberty and other takings were not originally agreed to, all other takings of property must be specifically and voluntarily agreed to either directly or through the people's representatives in the government.

What is important for our purpose is that there is here a notion of society as a thing toward which an individual person can have obligations by reason of participation in the original social contract. Each member of the community participates in this contract either directly by choosing to participate in a society's political life or, Locke also holds, simply by living there and enjoying the benefits of the society's increased social and economic potential. Thus everyone who lives within a political community has obligations, which are clearly social obligations in our sense, to obey the laws of the land and to contribute from his or her property for the maintenance of the society's appropriate legislative, executive, judicial, and military activities. But beyond providing what the decisions of the majority properly require, no one in a Lockean civil society has any other obligations except the fundamental obligation to respect others' liberty and such obligations to specific individuals and groups as each one might voluntarily undertake.

There are many other traditions of moral reflection that, like the Lockean version of libertarianism, begin with an understanding of human obligations generally and draw out from it an understanding of significant obligations to society. Three of these are, like the two versions of libertarianism already discussed, important modes of moral and social reflection in contemporary American society. Unlike the Libertarian model, each of them holds that humans *do* have social obligations simply by reason of their membership in the human community. Each also claims that our social obligations are more fundamental and more inclusive than the social obligations acknowledged in Lockean libertarianism. The three traditions we shall examine are the golden rule tradition, the utilitarian or value-maximizing tradition, and the human rights tradition.

These three traditions differ from one another in many ways. But about one thing they agree, namely, that the picture of human beings that is found in both versions of libertarianism is seriously flawed because it omits something essential. All three of these views hold that libertarianism, in both its versions, is mistaken in presupposing that social relationships are something "added on" to already complete human beings. For all three of these traditions, a human being's relationships with other humans are part of the essential and intrinsic makeup of that human being. Although there are humans who do not actualize this aspect of their humanity to any great extent, that is to be viewed as a deficit in their lives. Their relative isolation should not be taken as the norm of full humanness.

Furthermore, when we are talking about obligations—about how people ought to act—the social aspect of human beings must be included in the account. It is not surprising, then, that each of these traditions has an important place for social obligations within its account of morality.

The Golden Rule

The core of the golden rule tradition is the principle that what is right (or wrong) for one person in a given situation is similarly right (or wrong) for any other person in an identical situation. Many philosophers call this the *principle of universality*. With regard to an action that has an impact on another person, for that action to be morally defensible, it must be the case that the actor would choose, and could reasonably choose, to be the "recipient" of an identical action by someone else under identical circumstances. In short, "Do unto others as you would have them do unto you."

The golden rule, developed into a more abstract and generalized rule of morality by the eighteenth-century German philosopher Immanuel Kant, was held by him to be an unavoidable requirement of rationality itself. The alternative, he argued, was to live by contradictions. A contemporary version of this approach, developed by the Harvard philosopher John Rawls, urges that any social, legal, or economic regime that we choose to live under must be such that it would be chosen over alternative regimes by everyone who might live under it, even by those who might benefit the least. It must be reasonable for the latter to say, "This is the best social system of those that could really come into being under the present circumstances." Many contemporary social systems appear to fail this test miserably.

One implication of the golden rule tradition is that every human has an obligation to support only such social, political, legal, and economic structures as could reasonably be chosen (as the best structures actually available at the time) by everyone who has to live under them, even those in the least desirable social positions. This conclusion applies not only to the choice of a whole social system but also to each rule and structure of social, political, legal, and economic life. One important social obligation implied by the golden rule tradition is that each of us must attend to the impact of such structures on *everyone in the community* whenever we select and support these structures, both directly through voting or other political action and indirectly through our acceptance and toleration of what happens to be produced by the political process and other processes of social change.

Moreover, as Rawls argues in detail, a social system constructed on this sort of golden rule principle will place a high premium on *equality,* both equality of civil and political liberty as well as equality of property and of access to the resources on which ordinary life depends. This is because many social structures that lead to unequal distributions of resources make the condition of the people on the bottom of the social ladder worse off. According to the golden rule principle, however, such inequalities will be moral only when they yield—by motivating some people to produce more and by implementing structures to distribute the results appropriately—a better situation for the people on the bottom as well as for everyone else. Consequently the Lockean prohibition against property being taken from some citizens by the government in order to secure or improve the well-being of others (except to fund the proper activities of government) is at odds with the golden rule tradition. Our obligation to take account of the impact of our institutions on everyone in the society will certainly require that, if there are enough resources to do so, we must direct our society's resources toward filling the basic needs of every citizen.

The implications of the Golden Rule tradition for social obligations on the part of health care practitioners are threefold. First, as in the Lockean version of libertarianism, all members of the community are obligated to obey and contribute their property to support properly conducted activities of government.

Second, in contrast to Lockean libertarianism, all members of the community are obligated to work for the restructuring of all or part of the social system insofar as it falls short of taking adequate account of the least well-off within it. They have this obligation not by reason of having made commitments to these persons, or to the whole community in some sort of "social contract," but by reason of the character of sound moral reasoning, indeed of rationality itself.

Third, since every member of the community is obligated to work for a proper social system insofar as he or she has opportunity and since health care practitioners have greater influence than many other groups over the community's use of resources to meet people's health care needs, they are obligated to use their greater influence to ensure that the least well off receive health care to the extent and in a manner consistent with golden rule principles. Health care practitioners are not obligated in this respect for any reason that does not apply to everyone else; all are obligated to work for a proper social system insofar as they have the opportunity. But because of health care practitioners' generally greater influence in medical matters, they are, if not "more obligated," ordinarily obligated to do more.

Utilitarianism

Another tradition, the utilitarian or value-maximizing tradition, also is concerned with taking account of everyone in the society. Although the term *utilitarian* is used in many ways, some even derogatory, it refers historically to the tradition that holds that an action is morally obligatory if it is the one (of all available alternatives) that maximizes the realization of value in the lives of those affected. Thus, when my actions are expected to affect others, it is incumbent on me to weigh the positive values and also the pain, loss, and disvalue that my actions may bring about for each of the persons affected—myself and everyone else. What I ought to do is the available action that will bring about the greatest net value. Like the golden rule tradition, the utilitarian tradition claims there is a "socialness" of obligation in every action that might affect someone else.

The best known defenders of the utilitarian or value-maximizing tradition have argued strongly for representative government as the most effective means of securing the social, political, legal, and economic structures that would maximize values for a given society. Our fundamental obligation to attend to the effects of our actions on everyone entails that we are obligated to obey and support proper activities of government and to work for the restructuring of the whole social system or any of its parts that fail to bring about the greatest net value, among alternatives available at the time, for everyone who is affected. In this respect, the implications of the utilitarian tradition are much like those of the golden rule tradition. Especially in the contemporary versions of this tradition, great emphasis is placed on equality of civil and political liberties because of their crucial role in securing for everyone the best possible social system.

The utilitarian tradition explicitly acknowledges that the pains of some may have to be tragically accepted in particular situations in which the best realization of value for everyone affected makes them unavoidable. But it is also concerned in a special way with the condition of persons whose needs are greatest or are least met in any given social situation. Most theorists in this tradition believe that the use of a given amount of resources to relieve pain and meet people's basic needs constitutes a greater realization of value than the use of the same measure of resources to produce positive benefits and pleasures for persons not in pain or persons whose basic needs are already met. So the Lockean prohibition against property being taken from some citizens by the government in order to secure or improve the well-being of others (except to fund the proper activities of government) is also rejected by the utilitarian tradition, unless in particular cases the "transfer costs," which must include the lost sense of security of those whose property is taken, come to outweigh the benefit of the transfer.

The Human Rights Tradition

Another tradition approaches moral obligations in terms of human rights. Every member of the human community is possessed of a fundamental worth or dignity that implies obligations on the part of everyone else to respect it. There are many different accounts of the rights that derive from this fundamental dignity or worth and many different accounts of the obligations that these rights entail. Some thinkers see these rights and obligations solely in terms of noninterference by others in the free choices and the freely chosen actions of a person, in a manner that closely parallels the libertarian tradition. But many others claim that respect for human worth or dignity requires the acknowledgment not only of the civil and political rights that secure a person's ability to participate, at least to some extent, in a structure of representative government but also of rights to the resources necessary to fill each person's basic needs. This second, more expansive human rights approach would hold for rights to basic nutrition, housing, and clothing, as well as basic health care, in any social situation with sufficient resources to provide for them. Like the golden rule and the utilitarian traditions, this version of the human rights tradition opposes libertarian constraints on government's taking of property to secure or improve the well-being of other members of a society.

According to the human rights tradition, many of our most basic obligations to others derive not from any voluntary agreements we have made with them, but simply from their worth and dignity as fellow human beings. We may be able to fulfill some of these obligations to our fellow humans on a one-by-one basis. But many of them cannot be fulfilled without actions directed at changing the structures of human societies. Consequently, particularly in the more expansive version of the human rights tradition (as in the golden rule and the utilitarian traditions), everyone in the community has obligations, each according to his or her opportunity, to work for an appropriate social system, restructuring it in whole or in part insofar as it falls short.

The human rights, golden rule, and utilitarian traditions also have much more to say about the social obligations of humans generally (there are important variants of each of these approaches to morality that have not been considered here). But, as this brief summary has made clear, all three traditions can be seen to argue that we do have obligations to others over and above the obligations to specific individuals and groups that we voluntarily undertake and over and above the obligations stressed in Lockean libertarianism to obey and support appropriate actions of any government acting in the name of the majority. We have obligations in regard to the development, and if necessary, the restructuring, of an appropriate system of social structures, and we have particular obligations in regard to meeting people's basic needs and rectifying the condition of those who are least benefited by the social system. (Each of these obligations is also frequently discussed as an obligation of *social justice.* But since the concept of justice is itself used in a variety of distinct ways, each of which requires thoughtful exposition and reflection, it has seemed simpler to focus here on the substance of these obligations and on the reasons proposed for them in the several traditions of moral reflection that have been discussed.)

If one of these three accounts of morality and social obligation is correct, then obviously health care practitioners have these social obligations, as do the rest of their fellow humans.

THE SOCIAL OBLIGATIONS OF HEALTH CARE PRACTITIONERS

We now need to ask if health care practitioners have any social obligations specifically due to their roles as health care practitioners. As was said at the outset, health care practitioners obviously have whatever obligations to specific individuals and groups that each has voluntarily undertaken. But again our question here is about social obligations, that is, obligations to others that are incumbent upon health care practitioners for other reasons.

The key notion here is the notion of *profession.* Is it the case that in choosing to be health care professionals, people undertake obligations to others over and above their voluntary obligations to the specific individuals and groups, especially patients and colleagues, with whom they deal?

One view of the professional in health care takes health care practice to be no different in principle from the activity of any producer selling his or her wares in the marketplace. The health care practitioner has a product to sell and makes mutually agreed upon arrangements with any interested purchasers. Beyond the fundamental obligation not to coerce, cheat, or defraud purchasers (i.e., the producer must respect the liberty of others in the marketplace), the health care practitioner has no obligations to patients or anyone else other than the obligations he or she voluntarily undertakes with specific individuals or groups. Let us call this the "commercial picture" of health care practice.

In contrast with this picture is the "normative picture" of the health care professions. In the normative picture, the health care practitioner has joined a group of persons who have made, both individually and collectively, a set of commitments to the community at large. They have undertaken certain obligations, not by means of commitments to specific individuals or groups, but by means of a commitment to the whole larger community whom they, as a group of experts, serve. We shall survey these obligations in a moment, but first we need to describe in more detail the general circumstances surrounding the relationships between the health care professions and the larger community and between health care professionals and their patients.

The most characteristic feature of a profession is its expertise in a matter of great importance to the community at large. Moreover, the kind of expertise that we associate with a profession is also unavoidably exclusive. It involves knowledge and experience sufficiently esoteric that neither one can be gained effectively except under the direction of someone who is already an expert in the field. Consequently only the experts are in a position to recognize if another practitioner is expert or not and only they can give a timely judgment (i.e., before irreparable damage has been done) of the quality of a particular instance of professional practice.

Since the larger community is dependent upon such experts for effective health care, which it values greatly, it is in the community's interest, both individually and collectively, to place health care decisions to a significant extent into the hands of these experts. But to do so is to grant a great deal of power to the experts. Nevertheless the community does this, not only granting to health care professionals a great deal of decision-making power over people's well-being, but entrusting to these professionals the task of supervising how this power is used.

Compare the power granted to health care professionals with, for example, the power granted to politicians in government. The community grants to politicians power over people's well-being without fully trusting the politicians to use it well or to supervise the exercise of such power. Instead the community supports a complex and inefficient system of checks and balances within government, periodic elections, a nosy free press, and other structures to maintain close supervision of the politicians' performance. But for health care professionals, no such close scrutiny or persistent distrust is maintained.

How then does the community at large assure itself that so much power will not be abused by health care professionals? The answer is by instituting health care *professions* (as professions are understood in the normative picture). Each profession and each individual professional is committed to using this power according to norms mutually acceptable to the community and the expert group, norms that assure the community that the experts will use the power in such a way as to secure the well-being of the people whom they serve.

According to this normative picture of the health care professions, then, each health care practitioner clearly has important social obligations. We can describe these obligations briefly under seven headings: (1) expertise, (2) individual and collective control of practice, (3) relationship to clients, (4) central values, (5) impact on cultural values, (6) distribution of care, and (7) sacrifice and the limits of professional obligation.

Expertise. The original reason for granting special decision-making power to health care professionals is their expertise. Obviously one important social obligation of a health care practitioner, then, is to maintain and improve his or her expertise and to work effectively to maintain and improve the expertise of other members of the profession and of the profession as a whole.

Individual and Collective Control. Because of the importance of health care to the community, and because of the necessarily exclusive character of the expertise needed to provide such care effectively, the community grants to the profession as a group—and individual patients grant to individual members of the profession—an amazing degree of unsupervised control over details of their work. For their part, the members of the health care professions are obligated by their commitments as professionals to use this power, not primarily for their own aggrandizement, but for the well-being of their patients. In the same way, the power given the profession as a whole—in its task of training and certifying new practitioners, in its relations with other groups, and in its management of its own internal affairs—must be used not just to benefit the members, but primarily to benefit their patients.

Relationship to Clients. There are many models of the relationship of a professional to patients and other clients. Of these, some place clients in the position of passive receivers of assistance, without any significant voice in matters that profoundly affect their lives and well-being. Others place the practitioner simply at the service of the patient's or client's ends. Others strongly affirm the moral status of patient and practitioner alike. Health care professionals are obligated to choose thoughtfully from among these models and to work to establish a proper relationship between themselves and their patients in daily practice. There can be little doubt that it is the last, collaborative view that constitutes the norm for practitioner–patient relationships in contemporary American society.

Central Values. Every professional group ascribes to certain ranked values and uses them to resolve complex issues of priorities within the setting of actual practice. Each of the health care professions is obligated to identify thoughtfully the central values of its specific form of practice, and health care professionals are obligated to guide their professional practice in accord with these values.

Among the values proposed as central for the health care professions are life, i.e., continued biological life; health, both as the experience of well-being and as conformity to physiological and statistical norms; relief of pain and discomfort; maximal functioning, relative both to the capacities of the species and to the capacities of the individual; autonomous decision making by the patient whenever possible; advocacy of the patients' values to the greatest extent possible, including whenever the patient is not competent; maintenance of the profession's preferred patterns of practice; aesthetic considerations; and understanding, self-care, and health maintenance by the patient.

Impact on Cultural Values. Many professionals, by reason of the authority of their expertise in the eyes of the larger community and by reason of the importance of the benefits their practice secures for the larger community, have an impact on the larger community beyond securing these benefits. The impact particularly affects the community's collective priorities regarding certain means helpful in achieving the benefits that the professions' practice secures. Thus, for example, the emphasis within contemporary medicine on crisis intervention and cure and the relative lack of emphasis, until very recently, on health education, health maintenance, and prevention have over the years produced a comparable set of priorities regarding health care in the minds of large segments of the public. The members of the health care professions have an obligation to be sensitive to this broader, "cultural" impact on the larger community and to direct it thoughtfully insofar as it is in their power, both individually and collectively.

Distribution of Care. The broad social, economic, and legal structures that largely determine how resources (both health care and other kinds of resources) are distributed within the society and within the health care system itself ought ideally to be guided by general principles of social obligation like those discussed in the first part of this chapter. Health care practitioners' particular obligations in the application of such general principles, based on their generally greater influence on questions of health care distribution, have already been mentioned. In addition, all health care practitioners make decisions within care settings that also impact on the distribution of health care resources. Do the health care professions' or the health care professionals' commitments to the larger community include a commitment to support a particular principle or pattern of distribution?

Many members of the health professions would argue that health professionals' commitments have nothing to say about the ethics of distributing resources. Mark Siegler has argued, however, that every physician is committed, by reason of his or her profession, to respond to patients' health care needs in proportion to need and therefore to also work for systems of distribution that make sufficient resources available to physicians so that they can fulfill this commitment. The question is a difficult one. But at least we can say that each health care practitioner is obligated to examine his or her professional conscience carefully in order to determine if the commitment that is the basis of his or her professional obligations has any implications specifically in regard to the distribution of health care resources.

Sacrifice and the Limits of Professional Obligation. Besides these important categories of social obligation—which derive from the health care practitioner's commitment as a professional if the normative picture of professions is accepted—it is important to note that any coherent account of professions will entail that there are limits to professional obligation. There are areas of a health care professional's life that are not subject to the norms of professional life. There are conflicts between professional obligations that cannot be resolved from within the norms of the profession. There are flaws in each profession and consequent obligations to work to rectify them rather than to blindly follow them. There may be complicated reservations in a health care practitioner's affiliation with a profession known to be flawed in significant ways. There may well be times when a practitioner's obligation as a professional is clear-cut, but he or she recognizes a more fundamental obligation, grounded in a more fundamental rule of morality, that overrides it—the professional equivalent of conscientious refusal or civil disobedience.

Every category mentioned in this part of the chapter presents a set of possible social obligations that the health care practitioner ought to examine carefully. Professionals' views about the nature of professions and about the specific obligations that flow from professions will differ. But the possibility that the health care practitioner's professional commitment gives rise to a significant class of social obligations cannot be lightly set aside.

MANAGED CARE

During most of the twentieth century, the distribution of health care resources has been the result of agreements between individual or institutional health care providers and the patients whom they serve. From midcentury on, these agreements have been mediated through health insurance plans of various sorts; but up until the early 1980s, those who managed these plans made little effort to shape the decisions that patients and providers made and therefore had little direct impact on the use or distribution of health care resources. By the late 1980s, however, concern that the use of health care resources needed to be constrained was widespread, and the American health care system began undergoing a major change. In the new system, the economic power of insurers and of a new class of brokers of health care was increasingly brought to bear to limit rising health care costs. The traditional dialogue between provider and patient about what could and should be done for the patient increasingly took place within parameters on available treatments established by insurers' and brokers' contracts with patients, providers, and each other. Moreover, in the interest of constraining health care costs, the insurers and brokers began to link limitations of treatment for patients with the economic self-interest of providers. The various elements of this new economic environment are collectively referred to as "managed care."

If health care professionals have no obligations besides those created by explicit contractual agreements, then these changes in the economic climate of health care have no special moral significance. But if the categories sketched in the previous section represent additional obligations undertaken by persons who choose to become health care professionals, then managed care raises new and often very challenging ethical questions for these persons.

Professionals always have opportunities to use their professional expertise to further their own well-being at the expense of those whom they serve. This is one of the chief reasons that a society opts for the normative picture of professions and trains its professionals according to it, so the society can depend on professionals to be committed to using their expertise first in the interests of others rather than themselves. But the new entrepreneurial environment of health care in the late twentieth century has created new pressures and challenges for the health professional committed to putting his or her patient's well-being first. At least three of these challenges relate directly to the professional-patient relationship; others concern health professionals' obligations in relation to the larger social system.

First, health care providers are almost always better informed than their patients about the contractual parameters established by the patients' insurers and relevant brokers for particular types of care. Consequently, the long-standing obligation of health care professionals to provide capable patients with full information on which to base well-considered judgments about their treatment must now also extend to information about the parameters of the care available to the patient. In addition to the benefits and risks of a treatment that are in the nature of things, health care professionals now must often explain financial limits on treatment as well. In this role, moreover, the health professional will often seem to the patient more like a representative of the absent third-party payer than a concerned collaborator with the patient in health care decisions. This can make the achievement of an appropriate practitioner-patient relationship all the more difficult.

A second obligation of health professionals that is significantly affected by managed care is their obligation to act as advocates for their patients to the various bureaucracies within which health care is delivered. No longer focusing principally on the potential for depersonalization of patients within large institutions, health care professionals will now often have to advocate for patients with insurers and brokers interested in limiting care to reduce costs. They will have to spend time and effort to argue that a patient does indeed meet the insurer's or broker's criteria for a particular treatment or that this patient's situation falls within a relevant class of special cases or deserves special treatment for some other reason. Moreover, health care professionals will now find themselves much more frequently in circumstances in which a treatment that they and their patient both believe likely to be beneficial is nevertheless not available to the patient. Aggressive advocacy toward insurers and brokers and compassionate support for denied patients adds to the ethical challenges of the health professions.

Third, insurers and brokers of health care under managed care have been quick to design payment structures specifically aimed at manipulating health care professionals' self-interest in the direction of their offering patients more limited and cheaper forms of health care. But this fact does not relieve them of the basic obligation to put their patients' health care interests above their own economic interests. Properly weighing such pushes and pulls on their loyalty will make the ethical challenges of professional life even more difficult.

Some health professionals have held that it is simply not part of their role to be determining who gets what health care resources except insofar as they do so by proper judgments of patients' health care needs. But in fact every health professional's obligation to use his or her expertise to serve the needs of each patient has always been limited by the professional's obligation to respond to every patient in this way, with unavoidable limits therefore on what is possible for any one patient. In other words, health care professionals inevitably distribute their limited time, energy, and attention among a number of patients. So what is new about the managed care situation is not the fact that some health care resources are being treated as finite but the fact that the circumstances surrounding resources previously controlled by the provider and the patient are now being controlled and constrained by other parties as well. Nevertheless, as various groups within the society are excluded from access to the health care system by the workings of managed care, health care professionals may have a greater and greater obligation to work to change the system so no one's health care needs are overlooked.

The third parties in these encounters are, moreover, mostly private interests; they are, for example, insurance companies and health care brokers working for profit for their stockholders in the marketplace. They may take the view, therefore, that they have no special obligations to those with health care needs beyond what is explicitly contracted for. Several of the positions examined in earlier sections of this chapter hold, however, that such parties may still have special obligations to the whole society and to the members of the society in need of health care precisely because basic human needs are at stake in these matters. For this reason, health care professionals may in turn have special obligations to raise questions about basic human needs and to press third parties until they are answered properly.

But there is also another possibility that deserves notice. It is possible that the changes involved in managed care are not just the work of powerful private interests in the health care marketplace. That is, the elements of this economic restructuring of health care may be a signal of a far more fundamental change. It is possible that, as a society, we have reached the upper limit of the proportion of social resources we are willing to commit to health care, even if that requires that some categories of health care may have to be less available or forgone altogether. If so, then the American health care system may be in the process of shifting from an ideal of the "best health care possible" to one in which, at least in some categories of health care, the ideal will be "adequate or good enough health care."

So complex a change in social priorities is difficult to discern in a short time. But if such a shift does come to pass, then two of the special obligations of health professionals mentioned in the preceding section will take on additional importance; namely, the obligation to properly influence and educate the larger community in relevant cultural values, and the obligation to influence social decisions about the distribution of health care resources.

If there is a shift from the ideal of the best possible health care in every area of health care practice to an acceptance of the more modest ideal of adequate health care in some areas, health care professionals will need to play a very important role in the wise and humane development of the operational criteria for adequate health care in whatever areas of care are governed by that standard. It will also be incumbent on health care professionals to influence the larger society to make sure that all persons' health care needs are attended to in any restructured health care economy. But several generations of health care professionals have been trained and deeply formed in an ethic of the best possible care. If there is a profound shift in social priorities so that an ethics of adequate health care is the society's chosen path for certain categories of care, this will surely be profoundly troubling to many health professionals trained in another view. Responding wisely and ethically to such a change, should it come to pass, would be one of the health professions' most difficult ethical challenges.

CONFLICT OF OBLIGATIONS

It seems that when obligations conflict, those grounded in more fundamental and more broadly based moral principles ought to take precedence over those grounded solely in our chosen commitments, unless special considerations grounded themselves in more fundamental, broadly based principles should indicate otherwise. Consequently, if conflicts between social obligations arise, those grounded in the fundamental principles sketched in the section "General Social Obligations" would take precedence over principles grounded in a person's commitment to a profession, with the exception just noted. Similarly, obligations of both these kinds would take precedence over obligations based on a person's particular voluntary commitments to specific individuals or groups, with the same exception. Consider the following case.

Case Example

You are a cardiologist practicing at University Hospital and also sit on its transplantation committee. You have a patient, Michael Plumner, a 45-year-old male who is afflicted with amyloidosis. The disease has focused its effects, for reasons unknown, on Plumner's heart. Several weeks ago you had to hospitalize him because of his deteriorating heart function, which now resembles that of a victim of advanced cardiomyopathy. His only hope of survival is a heart transplant, a procedure that is available at University Hospital. Plumner is now in the category of "most urgent" organ recipients for a heart, along with two patients suffering from cardiomyopathy.

You and Plumner have had many conversations about his disease. He has indicated how he wishes his care to be handled in many respects. Among other things, he has asked you to promise him that, in the event of his death, you will remind his family firmly of his wish to give his body to medical researchers studying amyloidosis; and you have so promised. He has also offered you a large financial bonus if you would use your position on the hospital's transplantation committee, which selects recipients of transplant organs, to make sure that the first available heart with a favorable tissue match will be given to him. How does the ranking of social obligations just proposed apply to your obligations in this situation?

First, consider your promise to Plumner. Obligations based on fundamental principles of morality and obligations based on professional commitment are to take precedence over obligations based on a person's particular voluntary commitments to specific individuals. But neither of the former sets of obligations would seem to conflict with your speaking firmly to Plumner's family about the disposition of his body. In addition, neither set of obligations would seem to *require* such action on your part (as it might if Plumner's disease was highly contagious and research on it was much more urgently needed). Therefore, if Plumner's family resisted offering his body for research, you might—if you had not made a promise to him about it—justifiably refrain from pressuring them. But given your voluntary commitment to Plumner to do so, you would be obligated in this case to speak forcefully to them about it.

What about Plumner's proposal that you use your position and influence to secure him the next available organ in return for a sizeable financial reward? If you had voluntarily agreed to such an arrangement, would you be obligated to carry it out? By the same token, is this a kind of arrangement to which you could morally commit yourself? The answer to these questions seems quite clearly to be no. The reasons are twofold. First, it seems clear that the obligations that a physician undertakes as a member of the medical profession preclude acting as an advocate for a patient specifically for financial gain rather than on the basis of the relationship between patient and professional.

Second, the moral criteria that should be used in determining the distribution of scarce lifesaving resources, including organs for transplant, should be determined on the basis of fundamental moral principles, not by whatever particular personal or business arrangements happen to be made between individuals. For both reasons, it would be morally unjustifiable for a physician to make a commitment like that proposed by Plumner, and it would also be immoral for a physician who improperly made such an agreement to carry it out. The priority here is again that obligations founded on the commitment to a profession or on fundamental principles of morality should take precedence over obligations based solely on voluntary agreements with specific individuals.

Finally, having assumed that you would not agree to Plumner's proposal, let us consider how you should act when Plumner's case comes before the transplantation committee. Let us suppose that among the many professional obligations that you would have toward a patient is a genuine obligation to act as the patient's advocate within the complex bureaucracy of the health care system. Since you sit on the transplantation committee, you are involved in the decision as to whether Plumner or one of the other two equally urgent patients should receive the next donor heart (assuming equally successful tissue matches). May you prefer Plumner to the others on the basis of your professional obligation to act as your patient's advocate within the system?

If it is true that the criteria that should be used in allocating scarce lifesaving resources should be determined on the basis of fundamental moral principles, then unless these principles proved to be neutral between Plumner and the other patients under consideration, you would be obligated to set aside your advocacy of Plumner, as his physician, while you played your role in the deliberations of the transplantation committee. The reason for this, it is proposed here, is that obligations grounded in fundamental moral principles are to take precedence over obligations grounded in professional commitment.

This case is only one example of how the various obligations examined above should be ranked. It would take many cases to examine carefully the comparative moral importance of all the elements of social obligation that have been discussed. In addition, the proposed manner of ranking social obligations will remain largely abstract until each health care practitioner has reflected carefully on the foundations of social obligation sketched in the first section above and determined in thoughtful reflection that one of them, some consistent combination of them, or some other foundation is the correct basis of social morality. The practitioner will also need to identify the commercial picture, the normative picture, or some other portrayal of professions and professional obligation as the most accurate representation of professional commitment.

At that point, the thoughtful reader will be able to begin to identify his or her most important social obligations as a health care practitioner and to carry on the enterprise, undoubtedly already begun, of living up to them. The aim of this chapter has not been to offer final answers to these questions but to explain a variety of positions and categories to facilitate the reader's own careful reflection.

BIBLIOGRAPHY

Libertarianism

Englehardt, H. Tristram. *The Foundation of Bioethics.* Oxford: Oxford University Press, 1986.

Locke, John. *Two Treatises of Government.* 1690.

Machan, Tibor, ed. *The Libertarian Reader.* Totowa, N.J.: Rowman & Allenheld, 1982.

The Golden Rule Tradition

Daniels, Norman. *Just Health Care.* New York: Cambridge University Press, 1985.

Kant, Immanuel. *Foundations of the Metaphysics of Morals,* trans. Lewis Beck White (New York: Bobbs-Merrill, 1959).

Murphy, Jeffrey. *Kant: The Philosopher of Right.* New York: Macmillan, 1970.

Rawls, John. *A Theory of Justice.* Cambridge, Mass.: Belknap Press of Harvard University Press, 1971.

The Utilitarian or Value-Maximizing Tradition

Bentham, Jeremy. *Introduction to the Principles of Morals and Legislation.* 1789.

Mill, John Stuart. *Utilitarianism.* 1863.

President's Commission for the Study of Ethical Problems in Medicine and Biomedical and Behavioral Research. *Securing Access to Health Care.* Washington, D.C.: U.S. Government Printing Office, 1983.

The Human Rights Tradition

Ramsey, Paul. *The Patient as Person.* New Haven, Conn.: Yale University Press, 1970.

Shue, Henry. *Basic Rights.* Princeton, N.J.: Princeton University Press, 1980.

Veatch, Robert. *A Theory of Medical Ethics.* New York: Basic Books, 1981.

Werhane, P., A. Gini, and D. Ozar, eds. *Philosophical Issues in Human Rights.* New York: Random House, 1985.

Professions and Professional Obligations

Bayles, Michael. *Professional Ethics.* Belmont, Calif.: Wadsworth, 1981.

Camenisch, Paul. *Grounding Professional Ethics in a Pluralistic Society.* New York: Haven, 1983.

Freidson, Eliot. *Profession of Medicine.* New York: Harper & Row, 1970.

Jonsen, Albert, Mark Siegler, and William Winslade. *Clinical Ethics.* New York: Macmillan, 1982.

Ozar, David. "Patients' Autonomy: Three Models of the Professional-Lay Relationship in Medicine." *Theoretical Medicine* 5 (1984): 61–68.

———. "Social Ethics, The Philosophy of Medicine, and Professional Responsibility," *Theoretical Medicine* 6 (1985): 281–94.

———. "The Demands of Profession and Their Limits." In *Professional Commitment: Issues and Ethics in Nursing,* edited by M. Smith and C. Quinn. Philadelphia: Saunders, 1987.

Pellegrino, Edmund and David Thomasma. *A Philosophical Basis of Medical Practice.* Oxford: Oxford University Press, 1981.

Siegler, Mark. "A Physician's Perspective on a Right to Health Care," *Journal of the American Medical Association* 244 (1980): 1591–96.

Starr, Paul. *The Social Transformation of American Medicine.* New York: Basic Books, 1982.

CHAPTER 36

Social Systems and Professional Responsibility

Arlene Gruber

Suggestions have been made that new models of autonomy and bioethics are needed because the acute care model is too limited in scope to address the issues in home care and chronic illness.[1] Since acute care bioethics addresses issues within a narrow physician–individual patient framework, it is believed that issues involving broader systems—the family, the community, and the general society—are poorly served. Talk of "models" implies the existence of discrete systems of patient care. Such systems do not exist. Although acute care illness and chronic illness differ in some of their characteristics, the individuals experiencing these illnesses share the need for a response to their specific personal and social challenges, whether they are short or long term.

One of the professions involved in home care—and indeed one that since its inception has been involved in working with clients in community settings—is social work. Among its core values are client self-determination, maximum realization of each individual's potential within the context of social responsibility, and a strong social welfare system (defined as the organized norms and institutions by which we care for one another). Since these values are also the issues any "new ethics model" should deal with, this chapter draws upon the social work framework used in addressing professional responsibility. This is not an ethical decision-making framework but a mindset of the profession in its relationships with individual clients and with society. Another way of stating this is that the mindset is the profession's lived understanding of its societal job assignment and core values. Since a profession's framework or mindset determines the material chosen to be used in the ethical decision-making process (e.g., the facts of the case, the values of all parties involved, etc.), the understanding professionals have of their profession's framework is crucial to their ability to make sense of the dilemmas they face. Instead of a call for new models of autonomy and bioethics, the call should be for health care professionals to gain a clearer understanding of the complexity of their relationships with and responsibilities to patients, families, and society.

A NEW MODEL OF AUTONOMY?

For a number of years in the recent past, medical literature, which has included serious discussions of health care ethics, focused on the patient's right to be included in the medical decision-making process. This attention to autonomy was, to a great degree, a reaction to medicine's commitment to physician beneficence, which unfortunately evolved from acting in the patient's best interest to paternalistically intervening without knowledge and consideration of the patient's values, goals, and wishes.

Originally, autonomy was defined as the freedom to choose among available options and act upon the choices made.[2] *Autonomy* was treated as synonymous with *self-determination* by some authors[3] and by the social work profession. In the acute care model, the physician-patient relationship is understood to be a time-limited contractual relationship entered into by rational, self-interested individuals; the contract outlines the rights and responsibilities of each party. Autonomy, as a condition in the contract, ensures that the patient is made an active participant in the medical decision-making process, is given the necessary information to make crucial medical decisions, and is not coerced into making decisions based more on the physician's values than on his or her own. There is concern that this contractual model of the professional-patient relationship could limit the responsibilities of the professional if he or she accepts as morally obligatory only those responsibilities mutually agreed upon. "It elevates isolation and separation as the necessary starting point of human commitment"[4] with the extreme possibility that professional responsibility would end when patient autonomy was proclaimed.

The contractual model, it is argued, may be functional in the acute care setting, where patients need to protect themselves from professionals who have superior knowledge, power, and authority and whose values and goals may differ from those of the patients. However, since professionals caring for the elderly and chronically ill must address social and not just medical issues, and since they are likely to be confronted with numerous autonomous individuals and community agencies, the call is for an "accommodating" or "negotiating" autonomy that can mediate competing interests and varied responsibilities.[5] The concern seems to be that an empowering and rights-enhancing patient-centered ethic of autonomy blocks the possibility of allowing patients to think and act as communal, interdependent people.

Because of these concerns about the emphasis on individualism and its seeming inapplicability to the needs of systems, autonomy has been redefined as a "cluster of notions including self determination, freedom, independence, liberty of choice and action";[6] an "internally problematic concept having several polarities";[7] "a goal toward which people strive, which never really exists";[8] an ideal that must be "reconceptualized in terms that are relevant to the world of long-term care";[9] and the "responsible use of freedom [which is] diminished whenever one ignores, evades, or slights one's responsibilities."[10]

Additionally, there is particular concern that even families have begun framing their moral dilemmas as conflicts between the competing values of caring and autonomy rather than interpreting them as difficulties that arise in family relationships.[11] Since the demand for equal consideration by family members is perceived to be a legitimate one, it has been suggested that it may be morally correct "for a physician to sacrifice the interests of her patient to those of nonpatients"; the patient must realize that, as a member of a family, he or she is "morally required to make decisions on the basis of thinking about what is best for all concerned," not only what is good for him or her. It is no longer considered acceptable to advocate that "the interests of family members should be irrelevant or should take a backseat to the interests of the patient."[12]

THE SOCIAL WORK PERSPECTIVE

The difficulty experienced by professionals in weighing autonomy and beneficence; the difficulty of determining whether or not it is appropriate to persuade, cajole, or act paternalistically when a patient's decision is considered to be unwise or appears to go against previously stated values; the guilt or sadness felt when a patient's choice has been overridden—all of these factors led people to question the validity of autonomy or the possibility that it can be honored. Hence also the modified definitions, the "linguistic contortions,"[13] believed necessary to maintain the viability of the concept.

Self-determination—determination of oneself by oneself—is rejected by some as a legitimate goal, because they cannot make sense of the notion that they should be asked to accept socially unacceptable decisions or behaviors. But this is precisely why autonomy is so perplexing, why it is given so much attention. There is no problem accepting the *acceptable,* but reminders are necessary regarding the protection, if not the acceptance, of that which deviates from social norms.

It is feared that to accept self-determination in its literal meaning would jeopardize its status as a professional value. If a client chooses to behave illegally or immorally, the professional must either allow the unacceptable act or prevent it. It is possible for the professional to mistakenly believe that adherence to self-determination as an important value requires him or her to act complicitly—to support or at least refrain from preventing the illegal or immoral behavior.

Another example of linguistic contortion is Bart Collopy's six polarities of autonomy: decisional versus executional autonomy, direct versus delegated autonomy, competent versus incapacitated autonomy, authentic versus inauthentic autonomy, immediate versus long-range autonomy, and negative versus positive autonomy.[14] These are not, however, all sets of contrary qualities: A person can exercise decisional and executional autonomy, address immediate and long-range issues, and have his or her negative right and positive right to freedom recognized. The cases Collopy uses to illustrate the polarities merely show that at times decisional autonomy can be present when executional autonomy is not, that care should be taken not to give automatic priority to either immediate or long-range considerations, and that honoring negative freedom without attempting to enhance that freedom through positive intervention can result in neglect.

The points Collopy makes are important, but the language used in making them is unfortunate: Autonomy is not authentic; authenticity is a characteristic of an autonomous choice or of an autonomous person. Autonomy is not competent; a certain type of competence is required for autonomous decision making. Autonomy is not immediate or long range; consequences are immediate or long range. Collopy mistakes criteria for determining whether or not a person can or should be allowed to exercise his or her right as modifiers of the right. Aspects *external* to the right or value or principle of autonomy are presented as if they were *internal* to it.

It is important, therefore, that self-determination or autonomy be understood and accepted as a qualified particular right that certain persons possess under certain conditions. It is a particular, not a universal, right because it is possessed by a limited class of persons (e.g., decisionally incapacitated persons are excluded). It is a qualified, not an absolute, right because it may justifiably be suspended in certain situations (e.g., when the interests of others are adversely affected to an unacceptable degree). Qualified particular rights are the most troublesome for professionals because the decision regarding who will qualify for the right and the decision as to whether or not the right will be suspended are more often than not judgment calls.[15] But once health care professionals accept the fact that they are dealing with a qualified particular right, the problems that are inevitably experienced with autonomy can be put in the proper perspective. They are *accompanying*, not inherent, problems. They are problems that exist because of the complexity of human relationships, not because of the complexity of the concept.

If professional ethics is viewed in the context of the individual professional and his or her clients (as has been suggested of medicine in the ethics literature), the social context of autonomous choice can easily be overlooked. The social worker, however, treats the client-in-situation. This means that the client is never viewed as an isolated individual; whatever problem the client brings to the professional for resolution exists in his or her relationships with family members, the health care team, the immediate community, and society as a whole. The treatment (be it psychotherapy, a discharge plan from the hospital, or long-term home care) involves working with the client as a member of various social systems all of whom have rights.

> A live and struggling client is vividly before us, and we feel keenly our responsibility to his concerns and to his self-determination. But the fact that he is our client does not place him in a preferred ethical realm, with a higher

> order of claim . . . the thoughtful worker is alert to the others who will be affected by whatever the immediate business may be. . . . It is a test of professional maturity for a social worker to show his genuine concern for a client while making clear that he does not identify with the client's partisanship.[16]

In this context, the responsibility of the professional does not end when the patient declares his or her autonomy in the acute or long-term setting, for autonomy or self-determination is not a condition of contract. It is, rather, part of the human condition. It is too important to be misunderstood. Having open discussions about the difficulties professionals have with autonomy is not a mistake; leaving people with the impression that social factors somehow dilute autonomy is. Care must be taken to ensure that self-determination is not "defined out of existence."[17]

A NEW BIOETHICS

The call for a new bioethics is in part a call for a better understanding of the human and social significance of chronic illness. In the acute care model, the physician attempts to protect the patient's interests by keeping the patient free from sickness and disease; the physician's intervention is predominantly focused on the patient's illness. In chronic care, the physician helps the patient to integrate the illness and its effects into his or her life. One of the physician's roles is to protect the integrity of self while changes take place.

> The primary obligation of chronic care medicine, then, is not to protect the person's interests in the sense of keeping them from being affected by illness . . . but rather, to assist the person in keeping the transformative power of illness under control, to integrate new subjective interests (wants) and new objective interests (needs) into a coherent and satisfying life.[18]

Achieving a satisfying life is dependent to a great degree upon maintaining good relationships with family members, professional caregivers, and society. The family provides, at the very least, love and emotional support; the professional caregivers provide available community resources; and society provides recognition and acceptance of the needs of the chronically ill and the elderly through social policy and funding.

In reality, the ability of a disabled or elderly individual to continue to live according to his or her needs and values is often challenged by the needs and values of others. In the first section of this chapter, the weighing of competing choices was addressed. In this section, the issue is the provision of additional options the lack of which diminishes the quality of the individual's life. Jennings states that it is "not whether public and community services should be provided to supplement family care, but what goals these family assistance programs should serve and what moral aspects of family relationships we want to preserve and strengthen as we publicly assist families with their caregiving responsibilities."[19]

Some believe that "for children living in a modern system of social welfare, the consequences of failing in one's filial duties are usually less dramatic, and the strength of the duties is correspondingly weaker."[20] This is not the case. Since in home care a higher priority is still placed on the "medical" issues than on the social issues, the gap between need and available community-funded resources (home health aides, homemaking services) is great.

Therefore, two concerns for professionals are (1) the making of decisions regarding the fair distribution of health care resources while at the same time acting as a patient advocate, and (2) the necessity of intervening in family systems. How these concerns are addressed will depend upon whether the physician views the patient as an isolated individual to whom allegiance is owed or as a member of numerous social systems, each of which has legitimate demands.

A more appropriate way of phrasing this is that how these issues are addressed will depend upon the physician's view of him- or herself in relationship to his or her patients. As in the discussion of autonomy, the suggestion is that, rather than a new bioethics, what is needed is an accurate understanding of professional responsibility.

THE MORAL UNIVERSE OF PROFESSIONS

Professions are occupations that have been granted a special status in and by society. They address societal needs whose importance is recognized not only by those individuals who are experiencing those needs but by society as a whole. The suggestion has been made that no matter what the societal job assignment (the specific need addressed), each profession focuses only on a limited aspect of the total well-being of its clients.[21] The job assignment or aspect of well-being determines one of the profession's central values. (For example, medicine's job assignment is health; a central or core value, the job assignment value it shares with society, is also health.) And because they are a part of the social arrangement that provides individuals with goods, services, and opportunities necessary to lead full and productive lives, professions and their members are moral instrumentalities of society.[22]

Professional morality is a type of role morality that narrows the "moral universe"[23] of each profession, allowing its members to give greater or lesser weight to some values than is usually given in private morality. "The complexity of the moral world is thereby reduced and made manageable . . . by parcelling out responses to given situations in such a way that no profession is sensitive to *all* situations or has available to it a full range of responses."[24]

For example, when treating a patient, the physician in the acute care model (if this model is understood correctly) focuses primarily, if not exclusively, on illness. The physician might recognize that a patient has an illness-related social issue and that another profession (social work) with another societal job assignment should be consulted to address that issue, but the physician's involvement is still with "health" or "illness." The physician's moral universe includes only those factors necessary for the physician and the patient to make medical decisions.

THE SOCIAL WORK PERSPECTIVE

The societal job assignment of social work is the mediation of the person's need to be a full and productive member of the relevant social systems and the ability of those systems to provide the means for integrating its members and enriching their social contribution. This is done in settings (hospitals, schools, mental health agencies, the community) that are designed to harmonize individual needs and social resources. One of social work's responsibilities is to develop and strengthen the social welfare system (which includes health care).

Therefore the social worker who receives a referral from a physician will address not only the specific problem for which the consult was called but will recommend that all needs discussed during the psychosocial assessment process be addressed either by that social worker or by professionals in other agencies. The social worker's mediating function results in a focus on the client's *general* well-being (e.g., the client's physical and mental health, the client's finances, possible legal issues and family problems, etc.).

As a consequence, the social worker's moral universe is not a narrow one. Rather, the social worker's professional relationship draws him or her into the life of the client as a person with conflicting roles, complex obligations, and value dilemmas.[25]

The social worker must assist clients in acknowledging their responsibilities to individuals and social systems that exist outside of the professional-client relationship. The client's responsibilities to others are grounded in his or her membership as a moral agent in various social systems; the professional's responsibilities are grounded in his or her profession's relationship to society and its individual members through its function or job assignment and its core values.

Professional commitments must not be perceived as being

> made only to a select few clients, to the professionals' contract partners. They can be met only by professions and professionals who understand that their commitment as professionals is also a commitment to the total society and who will therefore involve themselves actively . . . even aggressively in such matters as . . . the just distribution of medical . . . services, and access to health . . . care on the basis of need.[26]

If, as Jennings suggests, the physician is to become involved in helping patients integrate new wants and needs into a coherent and satisfying life, the physician's moral universe must expand to include not just issues relating to discrete decisions regarding illness but those that relate to the patient as whole person. Inherent in the suggestion that decisions must be made regarding the extent of family assistance programs and the moral aspects of family relationships is the suggestion that individuals will make those decisions. The physician, in choosing to be among those individuals, must recognize and accept the necessity of intervening in family and societal systems.

The question is not *whether* professionals, including physicians, have the moral authority to intervene in the family system and the family's style of caregiving but *how* they should exercise that moral authority. The question is not whether professionals, including physicians, should detach the ethical concerns about the distribution of resources from the ethics of individual patient care but how they should weigh two competing but legitimate responsibilities. Here again it is possible to mistakenly assume that because carrying out the responsibilities is difficult, the responsibilities do not really exist.

CONCLUSION

An examination of the reasons given for believing that new models of autonomy and bioethics need to be developed suggests that instead health care professionals need a better understanding of their responsibilities to clients in the context of social roles and social systems. Certain dilemmas that appear to be new are in fact just easier to avoid in acute care than in home care. It is, for example, much easier to focus on the decisions and social needs of a single individual than it is to weigh the needs of the family, the community, and the general society.

It is also much easier to demand that decisions be made by someone other than the practitioner (e.g., let society decide whether or not homemaking services should be provided for individuals over the age of 80, or let another profession be solely responsible for family issues). This allows the professional to, with clear conscience, act according to specific policies without having to give any thought to the rules of common morality upon which the policies are grounded. In some cases, it also allows the professional *not* to act because of supposed boundaries between professions erected on the misperceived notion that there exist discrete sets of professional responsibilities. A narrow moral universe can be very attractive because it limits the range of necessary interventions; it does not, however, serve the best interests of the patients or society.

NOTES

1. B. Collopy et al., "The Ethics of Home Care: Autonomy and Accommodation," *Hastings Center Report* 20, no. 2, suppl. (1990); B. Jennings et al., "Ethical Challenges of Chronic Illness," *Hastings Center Report* 18, no. 1, suppl. (1991).
2. S. Gadow, "Medicine, Ethics, and the Elderly," *Gerontologist* 20 (1980): 683.
3. T. L. Beauchamp and L. B. McCullough, *Medical Ethics: The Moral Responsibilities of Physicians* (Englewood Cliffs, N.J.: Prentice-Hall, 1984), 42.
4. D. Callahan, "Autonomy: A Moral Good, Not a Moral Obsession," *Hastings Center Report* 14, no. 5 (1984): 41.
5. Collopy et al., "The Ethics of Home Care"; H.R. Moody, "From Informed Consent to Negotiated

Consent," *Gerontologist* 28, suppl. (1988): 65–70.

6. B. J. Collopy, "Autonomy in Long Term Care: Some Crucial Distinctions," *Gerontologist* 28, suppl. (1988): 10.
7. Ibid., 11.
8. E. Cassell, "Life as a Work of Art," *Hastings Center Report* 14, no. 5 (1984): 36.
9. Moody, "From Informed Consent to Negotiated Consent," 64.
10. J. Hardwig, "What about the Family?" *Hastings Center Report* 20, no. 2 (1990): 8.
11. P. G. Clark, "Ethical Dimensions of Quality of Life in Aging: Autonomy vs. Collectivism in the United States and Canada," *Gerontologist* 31 (1991): 633.
12. Hardwig, "What about the Family?" 5, 6.
13. F. E. McDermott, "Against the Persuasive Definition of Client Self Determination," in *Self Determination in Social Work*, ed. F. E. McDermott (London: Routledge and Kegan Paul, 1975), 131.
14. Collopy, "Autonomy in Long Term Care."
15. C. L. Clark and S. Asquith, *Social Work and Social Philosophy: A Guide for Practice* (London: Routledge and Kegan Paul, 1985).
16. S. Bernstein, "Conflict, Self-Determination, and Social Work," in *Values in Social Work: A Re-examination,* Monograph 9 (New York: National Association of Social Workers, 1967), 73.
17. McDermott, "Against the Persuasive Definition of Client Self Determination," 136.
18. Jennings et al., "Ethical Challenges of Chronic Illness," 11.
19. Ibid., 14.
20. S. Selig, et al., "Ethical Dimensions of Intergenerational Reciprocity: Implications for Practice," *Gerontologist* 31 (1991): 626.
21. D. Ozar, "Professions and Their Ethics: The Foundations of Professional Obligation" (Unpublished manuscript).
22. P. F. Camenisch, *Grounding Professional Ethics in a Pluralistic Society* (New York: Haven Publications, 1983), 54.
23. G. J. Postema, "Moral Responsibility in Professional Ethics," in *Profits and Professions: Essays in Business and Professional Ethics,* ed. W. L. Robison et al. (Clifton, N.J.: Humana Press, 1983), 39.
24. D. Luban, *Lawyers and Justice: An Ethical Study* (Princeton, N.J.: Princeton University Press, 1988), 127.
25. R. T. Constable, "Relations and Membership: Foundations for Ethical Thinking in Social Work," *Social Thought* 15, no. 3–4 (1989): 63.
26. P. F. Camenisch, "On Being a Professional, Morally Speaking," in *Professional Ideals,* ed. A. Flores. (Belmont, Calif.: Wadsworth, 1984), 25.

CHAPTER 37

Equality and Inequality in American Health Care

Charles J. Dougherty

INEQUALITIES, BORN AND MADE

Among the most profound inequalities of life is the fact of illness. Some of us are born healthy. Others are sickly from the start. Some inherit sound bodies. Others are heir to genetic mishaps and tragedies. Some enter early environments that preserve health and foster growth. Others have surroundings that undermine health and stunt growth. Some enter relationships that educate, nurture, and balance the mind. Others' early relationships deprive, abuse, and distort mental development. For some, physical and mental health at the outset make success and happiness in life distinct possibilities, even likelihoods. For others, childhood illness makes lifetime success and happiness remote possibilities, even impossibilities.

It is part of the human condition that these inequalities of health and illness continue throughout adult life. Genetics and early development account for some of the differences, perhaps a great many. Some adult variation is shaped by individual choice, the most familiar and least understood human experience. Often the distribution of health and illness cannot be accounted for at all, or accounted for only by those placeholders for explanation—accident, luck, and fate.

But in the particular human condition of contemporary America, there are social realities that help to account for a great deal of the disparities of health and illness. Chief among these conditions are socioeconomic status and race. Americans living in or near poverty and members of minority groups, and especially those who are in both categories, have uniformly worse health status than other Americans. They are far more likely not to survive infancy, to be debilitated by disease and injury, and to die prematurely.[1]

Some features of the general human condition may play a role in these marked differences. It is not impossible that genetics plays some role in the very marked racial differences in American infant mortality rates, for example, even though there are plausible social explanations.[2] Poor and minority Americans are individuals, too. They make their own choices, even if the range of options they face are shaped by their cultures and circumstances. Their lives are also entangled with the unfathomables of accident, luck, and fate, though poverty and minority membership plainly affect the rate of accidents, life's mixture of good and bad luck, and the fates of individuals.

A central role in determining states of health and illness is played by two fundamental American realities, one inherently malign, the other a positive and important value in its proper place but disabling in its presently hypertrophic expression. The first reality is racism. In spite of considerable strides in the legal arena, de facto

---

Source: Reprinted courtesy of the Kettering Foundation from *Freedom and Equality: Humanities Perspectives on Health Care, Crime, and the U.S. Economy,* ©1992.

racism remains a characteristic feature of the American scene. It skews the distribution of illness through the inequality of living and working conditions that it breeds; through the violence that has become part of the fabric of many minority neighborhoods; through the poor education, unemployment, and absence of the two-parent family that marks much of the minority experience; and, most important, through the barriers to health care created by lack of health insurance and primary care in the inner cities.

The value that helps to explain the health experience of many poor minority Americans is the disproportionate emphasis placed on individual freedom in American society. Individual freedom is a genuinely important value; its rebirth in formerly Communist nations is one of the triumphs of the age. But excessive individual freedom in the health care domain has left the United States alone among major industrial nations in failing to create a national health care system that ensures basic care for all citizens. Instead of the community service it is elsewhere, health care in America is largely a commodity produced and marketed for profit.[3] Instead of making access to the basics a matter of right as it is elsewhere, health care in America is generally available to those who can pay and to the insured.

These facts are linked to the value of freedom in three ways. First, American providers and payers have succeeded in their insistence on professional and marketplace freedoms—the claim of a right to treat health care as a matter of commerce. Doctors, hospitals, insurers, drug companies, and producers of medical goods all demand and have secured wide entrepreneurial freedom. Second, consumers have refused to relinquish the freedom to choose their own package of insurance coverage, individually and through employment groups. Specters of waiting lists, lowered quality, and bureaucratic incompetence are invoked at the mere mention of a national health care plan, in spite of the generally favorable experience with such arrangements in the industrial democracies of Europe, Canada, East Asia, and Australia. Finally, citizens have refused to pay the taxes that a system of universal coverage would entail because higher taxes mean less discretionary wealth and that, in turn, means less individual freedom.

Unfortunately, racism and an exaggerated emphasis on freedom work together in the United States to reinforce the inequalities of health and illness. An inevitable implication of freedom is inequality of outcomes. When the value of freedom dominates, some choose well and win; some choose poorly and lose. Some businesses prosper; some go bankrupt. When the value of freedom dominates health care, some individuals have a regular source of health care; some don't. And this inevitable implication of freedom is socially acceptable to majority Americans so long as the some who don't have access to care are largely members of racial minorities, whose lot in life apparently matters less.[4]

BUILDING EQUALITY

Both racism and an exaggerated concept of freedom can be confronted by efforts to increase equality in American life generally. For a number of reasons, greater equality is especially important in health care.

Matters of Fact

In fact, humans are fundamentally equal in several ways essential to health care. The human body, though differing in its many expressions, operates on the same general principles, knowledge of which makes health care itself possible. Every body has the same biological structure, the same range of functions, and the same general needs. Each is subject to the same set of diseases and disabilities. Bodies differ, of course, in gender and age, relative strength, and resistance to disease. But these differences are minor compared to the similarities, the equalities, of human bodies from a health care perspective.

A similar point can be made about the human mind. In daily encounters attention is drawn to the diversities of culture and personality and how they create differences in worldview and behavior. Yet from a health care perspective, these differences must be set against the context of the larger similarities of the human mind. Though circumstances and experiences shape people in distinctive ways, humans share, by and large, a common mental experience. The same set of desires—for affection, honor, and productive activity, for example—and the same list of fears—of failure, abandonment, injury, and death, for example—are part of the human scene across time and place. This is what makes great literature possible: It transcends the limits of time and place to speak with authority about the constants of human experience. Even extreme cases of mental illness—autism, depression, multiple personality disorder—are thought by mental health professionals to be exaggerated expressions of mental experiences common to all or to be dysfunctions in the brain, part of our common bodily inheritance. Thus, in spite of the diversity that appears, at a more reflective level the equality of mind is a fact.

The final and most critical equality central to health care is the fact of death and anticipation of it. Alone among species, humans are capable of understanding their personal mortality and of conceiving life as a temporal trajectory with a beginning and an end. Health care deals intimately with death, fear of death, and the myriad conditions that cause death and provoke fear of it. Though the nature and circumstances of individuals' deaths vary greatly, one universal fact, one ultimately equalizing fact, remains: We each know that we must die.

In addition to these facts about human equality, there are two other considerations that argue for greater equality in health care. Both are grounded in the negative consequences of inequality—one at the personal level of health care, the other at the social level.

Equalizing Advocacy

At the personal core of health care is the doctor-patient relationship. In the Hippocratic oath, the doctor-patient relationship became the occasion for the first explicit discussion in the West of the ethical dimensions of a professional role.[5] The reason for this ethical focus is clear. The relationship between a doctor and a patient is one of marked inequality. The typical patient enters a therapeutic encounter with anxiety and often with pain and dysfunction. He or she relies on the doctor to address these forms of suffering with competence and compassion. Except for subjective experience and personal history, the doctor knows more about the patient's body and mind than the patient does—more about the present state of his or her illness and health, more about various strategies for confronting illness and preserving health, and more about likely outcomes. Because of this inequality in knowledge, doctors have tremendous authority. Even in this age of mandatory second opinions, the medical advice of a doctor with whom there is a personal relationship is irresistible to most Americans. Moreover, doctors have legal authority to control access to contemporary medical resources to a large degree. About 70 percent of all tests and treatments in American health care require a doctor's order.[6]

There are equalizing strategies to redress this imbalance in the doctor-patient relationship. On the side of the doctor, a moral duty is recognized to put the interests of patients first and to protect them from harm. This fiduciary obligation is meant to protect patients from the exploitation possible by virtue of the disparity of knowledge and power in therapeutic relationships. On the side of the patient, the requirement that providers obtain informed consent before all major tests and treatments represents a major equalizing innovation in the second half of the twentieth century. This right protects patient autonomy and checks doctors' tendency toward paternalism.[7]

But there are reasons why both doctors' fiduciary responsibility and patients' right to informed consent may fail to reestablish the human equality routinely lost in the doctor-patient relationship. Multiple new conflicts of interest have developed in the entrepreneurial climate that has pervaded American medicine for the last two decades.[8] An aggressive "let the buyer beware" attitude now competes with the traditional professional mandate to "first, do no harm" to patients. At the same time, in many care settings informed consent is an empty formality of signing legal documents. It does not reach its moral goal of ensuring that patients are genuine partners in therapy.

A third equalizing strategy can both strengthen doctors' commitment to their fiduciary responsibility and secure the moral meaning of patients' right to informed consent. That strategy is to ensure that every American has access to a primary health care provider—a family practice doctor or nurse practitioner, for example—who can serve as a personal point of entry into the health care system and as a professional advocate for the patient throughout his or her care. It is precisely here, in the widely absent primary care network, that the American health care delivery system shows one of its most conspicuous failures.[9] Millions of Americans—largely the poor and members of minority groups—have no primary health care provider. They avoid and delay needed care and rely when they must on the nearest hospital emergency room. Every inner-city emergency room is filled with patients who could have been seen for their conditions in the office of a primary care provider. Not only is office care by a primary provider likely to be more comprehensive, continuous, and personal than that available in the emergency room, but it is also significantly cheaper. The tertiary care provided to those without primary care is often superb from a technological perspective. There is access through the emergency rooms of major urban teaching hospitals to some of the best medical technology in the world. But without the equalizing influence of a primary care advocate, this social arrangement yields comparatively poor outcomes overall and offers therapeutic encounters that many of the least well off Americans find deeply alienating.[10]

National Self-Interest

The social consideration that underscores the need for greater equality in the health care system is national self-interest. Great Britain's history of health care reform is illustrative by way of counterexample. Britain began a national health insurance program in 1911 in order to maintain a healthier and more productive work force and army. Lloyd George crystallized the issue: "You can not maintain an A-1 empire with a C-3 population."[11] During World War II, when Britain faced the bleakest of prospects, a national health service was promised as a way of defining a community of aspiration in the midst of a national calamity.[12] In both cases, equalizing health care reforms were rooted in national self-interest.

For its own national interest, the United States needs a work force that can produce the wealth needed to support an affluent culture. The United States also needs a health care financing system that allows the nation to compete effectively with other economies around the world. But there are many indications that the present health care system's inequalities are working against achievement of these two requisites of a robust society.

By all estimations the future work force of the United States will be composed increasingly of minority Americans. Yet these are just the individuals that have the hardest time accessing the health care system appropriately. They are disproportionately represented among the uninsured and underinsured.[13] Moreover, they have worse health status not only in terms of infant mortality and average lifespan but also in terms of morbidity. They experience, for example, more bed disability days, more chronic illnesses, and a self-reported health status lower than the nonpoor majority population.[14] As U.S. industry comes to be more and more dependent on minority Americans, the work force will also be less and less healthy. This trend will make the United States less competitive with other advanced democracies whose working people are all covered by some form of national health care plan.

In addition to this general cost of inequality in the health care arena, there are other specific burdens produced by the way Americans finance and deliver care. First, it is becoming clear that one of the factors accounting for the emergence of costly and demoralizing patterns of welfare dependency over the last 20 years is lack of universal health coverage.[15] A single mother contemplating leaving welfare to return to work, for example, must weigh not only the prospect of netting less money from the private sector than from welfare; she must also weigh the prospect of losing health insurance for herself and her children since welfare and Medicaid eligibility are linked in most states and many low-wage jobs, especially in the small business sector, offer no health insurance fringe benefits. Illness or likelihood of illness on the part of parent or children becomes an almost unassailable argument for staying on welfare.

Second, one of the hallmarks of a successful modern service economy is the ability to accommodate rapid change, to bring new kinds of services and products into the market quickly. This in turn requires a mobile work force, one filled with individuals willing to change jobs with some frequency over a working lifetime. But the American choice to link health insurance status to employment—rather than to citizenship or residency, for example—is beginning to work against American business by creating structural barriers to job mobility.[16] Competition in the private health insurance industry has generated a socially perverse incentive: the need to avoid covering those who are ill or who are at high risk of becoming ill. Therefore many insurers have adopted preexisting illness exclusions for new employees. These exclusions from coverage in turn provide a strong disincentive against changing jobs for working people who have had serious illnesses themselves or in their families. A new job may mean the loss of insurance coverage for just the condition that will most likely require treatment. This self-destructive consequence of the health insurance system is taking its toll not only on the poor and minorities. Many working Americans of all descriptions simply cannot afford to change jobs.

Finally, the inequalities in the U.S. health care system have made the problem of escalating health care costs virtually intractable. In spite of the fact that millions are uninsured and underinsured and in spite of mediocre achievement on key vital statistics, the United States spends more on health care than any other nation in the world—more in absolute dollars, more per capita, and more as a percentage of gross national product (GNP). The U.S. Department of Commerce projects that the nation will devote 14 percent of GNP to health care in 1992.[17] There is a deep irony here. Americans' stress on freedom and suspicion of government has prevented development of a national health care program. But comparative international experience suggests that the way to contain overall health care costs is by global governmental budgeting through a national health care program. Refusal to establish such a program has meant that American health care has become more and more a corporate enterprise, a matter of business. But this has fed the cost spiral and hurt business generally. Costly measures to protect and increase market shares of insured patients have been implemented by hospitals, nursing homes, and doctors' groups. Health care advertising has exploded in the last decade, for example, creating an entirely new set of costs wholly unrelated to the care of patients. While inner-city and rural hospitals and clinics have closed, overcapacity has been constructed in America's suburbs, duplicating expensive technology and feeding patterns of overutilization. In the absence of the discipline of an overall budget, expensive and intrusive administrative measures have been relied on to "micromanage" the behavior of providers. As a result many U.S. businesses are fighting unmanageable cost increases in their employee benefits packages. At the same time, these businesses are competing against foreign companies whose governments have national health care programs that allow them to contain health care costs better and to spread them more equally than in the United States.[18]

Greater equality is therefore an appropriate prescription for some of what ails American health care. It fits with the broader equalities of human experience, equalities touched intimately by health care. It can also help to address the negative consequences of inequality in therapeutic relationships and some of the system's failures that most jeopardize the nation's self-interest.

JUSTICE, PRUDENCE, AND EQUALITY

How much equality is appropriate for the American health care system? It is impossible to achieve equality in health status or in the outcome of health care interventions since the causes of health and illness are so varied and individual circumstances so complex. But greater equality in access to health care is a reasonable goal.

Strict Equality of Treatment

The simplest, most egalitarian formulation for health care access is to mandate the same treatment for all conditions that are substantially similar. The obvious way to embody this formula in a system of care is through construction of a national health service that provides equal treatment to all, treating everyone the same who has the same medical condition, without regard to other considerations such as wealth or race.

But there is a serious value problem with the strict equality of such a national health service. While the exaggerated expression of freedom deserves rejection, there is a legitimate and important range to this value. Recognition of the importance of freedom entails the acceptance of some measure of inequality. If freedom is allowed in the health care system, then some similar conditions will be treated differently. This can occur because some have greater wealth to purchase more or better care and insurance for it, or because those with even moderate wealth prioritize the purchase of health care and insurance higher than their neighbors do. It would certainly be curious, if not wrong, were Americans permitted the inequalities of freedom everywhere in the economy except in health care. Moreover, the practical measures that would be necessary to prevent Americans from buying services outside an egalitarian national health service would be Draconian.

Thus achievement of more equality in health care is an important goal, but strict equality of status and outcome is unattainable and strict equality of treatment undesirable. How much equality then is an appropriate goal for American health care? A response to this question can be focused around two considerations: the amount of equality that is required by justice and the amount of equality that is politically prudent.

Justice and the Social Contract

A theory of social or distributive justice provides an account of the minimal arrangements required by morality. Alternately put, a theory of justice provides a framework for articulating the social rights of individuals, in this case, the health care that individuals deserve as a matter of right.

There are many competing accounts of social or distributive justice, but one of the most persuasive is the social contract theory. In its various forms, this theory can be found in the writings of Plato and on the pages of contemporary writing in philosophy and jurisprudence.[19] The core insight of the tradition is that justice is grounded in an implicit contract or promise individuals make to one another by virtue of living together in society. Since no such promise has ever been made explicitly by all members of any society, the central conceptual challenge of social contract theory has been to give an intelligible interpretation to the notion of a morally binding promise never actually made.

One contemporary version of social contract theory, that of John Rawls, holds that the character of the social contract can be defined by imagining what would be promised by individuals about to enter a new society together if those original people were conceived to be reasonable and free of biases.[20] These hypothetical people can be conceived to be reasonable by assuming that they are able to understand what is in their own interest generally and able to select appropriate means to attain it. They can be conceived to be free of biases by assuming they are denied knowledge of their own particular interests, the knowledge that draws real people toward selfishness.

A Supernatural Lottery

The mechanics of this Rawlsian scheme are complex, but the main insight can be clarified through the use of a simple if fanciful scenario. Imagine that God, an all-powerful being, calls together a group of angels, that is, a group of intelligent spiritual beings without bodies. Because the angels have no bodies, they are not differentiated by gender, race, or ethnicity. There are no stronger or weaker angels, no healthier or sicker, no older or younger. Without bodies the angels also have no differing social and economic circumstances; angels are not richer or poorer. God informs the assembled angels that they will all become humans and be placed on earth to live together. Each will be given a specific human body in a random process God calls the "natural lottery." Thus they will be assigned genders and separated into different racial and ethnic groups by lot. The bodies they receive in the natural lottery will make some of them strong, others weak; some healthy, some sick and dying; some young, some old. Because their bodies will be situated in differing social and economic circumstances, some angels will be wealthy and well-placed, others poor and marginalized.

But God is also all-merciful. Before the natural lottery begins, the angels are allowed to agree among themselves on the social arrangements that will structure their human lives together. God assures them that whatever social arrangements they agree to will be made binding elements of justice on earth. In essence, God creates the conditions for a social contract: reasonable and nonbiased agents agreeing on the kind of society they will accept.

How would angels deliberate about society in anticipation of the natural lottery? Not knowing their gender, race, or ethnic group, they will reject sexism, racism, and discrimination. Each angel knows that he or she has a chance of suffering considerably under such arrangements. Similarly, they will reject differential treatment of the young and old, strong and weak, rich and poor whenever those differences are likely to make their lot in life worse than it otherwise would be. They will, however, allow differences that work to everyone's advantage regardless of what lot he or she draws. The negotiating strategy each angel will adopt is straightforward: Agree only to social arrangements that will make my future human life the best life it can be, even if my draw in the natural lottery gives me one of the worst lives.

When the angels reach the health care question, their strategy will remain the same. Knowing the health-related inequalities of human life, they realize that they may be among those who have severe medical needs. Moreover, they know that virtually all people need health care sometime. Consequently, they will insist on universal access to health care. Unless all are covered, each risks being among those who are left out. Presuming that they also know that a society's medical demands can become financially endless, they will agree to put some limits on the care to which all have a right. No society can afford to provide all health care services to everyone, as this would be incompatible with the enjoyment of other economic goods. Thus, they will agree that everyone should be guaranteed a right to a basic package of health care. They will not agree to providing everything that health care might offer, but they will agree to establishing a decent minimal level of care for all.

What is the ethical implication of this fanciful tale? It shows that when we imagine ourselves to be reasonable and free of biases we see that the social contract must include a health care system that covers everyone for a basic package of care. But justice is a normative concept. It requires that we be as reasonable and as free of biases as possible. Therefore justice requires a health care system equal enough to provide everyone with the basics.

This scenario also illustrates an important point about moral psychology. Real lives are lived after the natural lottery, so to speak. We each know our own situation. By definition, most of us are members of the majority. Most Americans are white and nonpoor. Most of us are insured for a basic package of health care. Knowledge of their own situations thus blinds the majority of Americans to the injustice worked by the inequalities of the present health system. But when a hypothetical situation creates the possibility that anyone may be among the millions of uninsured and underserved Americans, the injustice of the situation becomes transparent. Thus, the thought experiment of a supernatural lottery accomplishes a movement fundamental to moral psychology. It requires that present social arrangements be assessed from others' points of view. It accomplishes the reciprocity of perspective central to the golden rule. It thereby describes the moral minimum that justice demands.

Playing, Paying, and National Health Insurance

This requirement of justice could be satisfied by any number of different health care arrangements. Since this is a minimal ethical requirement, the easiest way for Americans to satisfy it would be to make the fewest necessary changes in the present United States health care system. Most nonelderly Americans now receive their health care coverage as a fringe benefit through their employment. A program already exists—Medicaid—that is designed to provide financial assistance to (some of) those who are not otherwise insured and cannot pay for their own health care. Thus, the easiest practical way to satisfy the moral demands of justice is by spreading employment-based coverage as far as possible and then covering those who remain uncovered by an expanded Medicaid program. Generally speaking, this is the "play-or-pay" approach to health care reform: Mandate that all employers cover all their employees with health insurance or pay a tax (generally about 7 percent of payroll) into a pool to fund government coverage in an expanded Medicaid program.[21]

If successful, play-or-pay would erase the extreme inequality created by a system that allows millions to go completely uncovered and to face financial barriers to care. It would, however, leave in place the inequalities of a clearly two-tiered health care system of relatively comprehensive coverage for those insured at work (though wide variations may be expected) and a minimal package of basic coverage for those in the government program.

Play-or-pay would achieve moral decency. But just as it is often prudent for individuals to go beyond what is required by respect for another's rights, it can also be prudent for a society to do more than what justice demands. Considerations of justice define the ethical floor below which society should not fall, but a successful social structure needs more than a floor. Another reform alternative goes further than play-or-pay in the direction of equality and can contribute to building a more successful American society: a national health insurance program with a single payer, funded by progressive taxation and designed to cover the vast majority of Americans.[22] Although this direction for reform creates more equality than justice alone demands, there are several prudential considerations that make this alternative preferable to play-or-pay.

First, there are technical problems with play-or-pay that are avoided by national health insurance. Imposition on small businesses of an insurance mandate (play) or a new tax (pay) will create a severe economic burden that will drive many businesses out of business. This will create more unemployment, swelling the numbers of those dependent on Medicaid and triggering an increase in the tax rate imposed under the pay option. At the same time, many large businesses that have been playing (insuring their employees) may opt to pay the tax instead, either because it is cheaper or because it frees them from the labor friction produced by the management of health care benefits. This will also put more Americans into the Medicaid program and lead to additional pressure on the pay option tax rate.

This double movement of small and large businesses to the pay side of play-or-pay may indirectly create a form of national health insurance for many, perhaps most, Americans. But there will be an important difference. If the United States "backs into" national health insurance this way, the insurance pool that results from the expanding pay option of play-or-pay will not be supported financially by companies that continue to play. These will include companies with insurance costs lower than the tax mandated under the pay option—generally companies with younger, healthier, low-risk work forces. But this will entail a system with private insurance for the cheap to insure, public insurance for the expensive to insure. This is a policy formula bound to create financial disaster for the public program.

Play-or-pay also holds little promise for serious cost control. Most specific play-or-pay proposals try to restrain spending with measures intended to micromanage providers' behavior, a strategy that has failed over the last decade. The one approach with an international track record of restraining costs is global budgeting, just what a national health insurance program would have to do.

A play-or-pay arrangement would not of itself be capable of addressing the main evidence of de facto racism in the American system: the evacuation of health care providers and resources from the minority-dominated inner cities. By contrast, a national health insurance program would have available many strategies to attract health care providers and resources to these underserved populations and help ensure that they have the primary care advocates they need. For example, a national health insurance program could enhance fee-for-service payments to providers in designated low-income areas or pay risk-adjusted capitated rates to organized provider networks to draw services to populations with greater needs.

Serious political problems will result from the two-tiered structure of the play-or-pay approach. Admittedly, even a national health insurance program would leave room for a second tier. Americans could buy health care services outside the national package because such freedom is an important value and the practical implications of forbidding it are too ominous. But the two tiers of a national health insurance program would be fundamentally different from those generated by play-or-pay. Under a national health insurance program, disincentives could be put in place (no tax benefits, for example) to keep individual purchases of noncovered services to a minimum. When new services are demanded by a large segment of the public, these services could be folded into the national program. Thus, recourse to care outside the national plan could be made a marginal activity, perhaps accounting for less than 10 percent of total health care spending. By contrast, play-or-pay will create a substantial two-tiered system. Depending on how many employers elect the pay option, the percentage covered under the Medicaid tier might range from 20 percent to more than half the population. Moreover, while the small second tier outside a national health insurance program would likely be composed of very wealthy Americans, the substantial second tier of play-or-pay would be composed disproportionately of poor and minority Americans.

The significance of this speculation about the size and character of a second tier of health care is political: Programs for the poor tend to become poor programs, underfunded and low in quality. On the other hand, if the middle class is served by a national health insurance program, it will be adequately funded and will sustain high quality. This point is clear in the history and present condition of Medicare, the program for all elderly Americans, and Medicaid, the program for the poor. Medicare, in spite of its many problems, works effectively and is defended vigorously by politicians. Medicaid is a public policy disaster and a political orphan.

Equality and Community

This observation about politics leads to the last prudential consideration that supports establishment of greater equality in health care than justice alone requires. Politics is not only about the power to create programs and to ensure that they are adequately funded and well-run. It is also about symbols. Politics is one of the arenas in which Americans symbolize the balance the nation strikes between self-interested and other-regarding motives, between the forces of individualism and those of the common good. It is where the solidarity of citizens is fragmented or reinforced. In politics, the national identity is reshaped through the public assignment of priorities to the competing values of freedom and equality.

Different arguments can be made about how much emphasis these opposing forces should be given in various endeavors of public and private life. But whatever balance is struck elsewhere, in health care there should be more emphasis on other-regarding motives, more stress on the common good, greater social solidarity, and a higher priority on equality. In health care, life and death and the quality of the experience in between are literally at stake. It is an arena in which altruistic care for those in need is not exceptional behavior but the rule. In health care, the well-being of the public is an explicit responsibility. Through health care, serious efforts are made to correct some of the worst inequalities of the natural lottery and to adjust more favorably the unfathomables of accident, luck, and fate. Because of these features, the health care policies of a nation can define a sense of community capable of transcending divisions of race and socioeconomic status. Through the health care system, it is possible to assert in the most concrete of terms that every American life is worthy, that every American is equally valuable.

Because of America's racism and exaggerated emphasis on the value of freedom, the nation stands in need of a renewed sense of community. Health care is a symbolically important place to strive for it. Commitment to greater equality than justice itself requires through construction of a national health insurance program is one way to attain it. At this time in the nation's life, it may be one of the few practical opportunities available for the reconstruction of a sense of American community.

NOTES

1. C. J. Dougherty, *American Health Care: Realities, Rights, and Reforms* (New York: Oxford University Press, 1988), 3–19.
2. P. Wise and D. Pursley, "Infant Mortality as a Social Mirror," *New England Journal of Medicine* 326 (1992): 1558–59.
3. C. J. Dougherty, "The Cost of Commercial Medicine," *Theoretical Medicine* 11 (1990): 275–86.
4. On the racial dimensions of national health policy, see J. Califano, "The Challenge to the Health Care System," in *Health Care for the Poor and Elderly: Meeting the Challenge*, ed. D. Yaggy (Durham, N.C.: Duke University Press, 1984), 45–57. On racism and medical education, see J. Holloman, Jr., "Access to Health Care," in *Securing Access to Health Care,* vol. 2, President's Commission for the Study of Ethical Problems in Medicine and Biomedical and Behavioral Research (Washington, D.C.: U.S. Government Printing Office, 1983), 79–106.
5. Hippocrates, *Hippocratic Writings,* ed. G. E. R. Lloyd (New York: Penguin, 1986).
6. A. Relman, "The New Medical-Industrial Complex," *New England Journal of Medicine* 303 (1980): 963–65.
7. T. Beauchamp and J. Childress, *Principles of Biomedical Ethics,* 3d ed. (New York: Oxford University Press, 1991), 307–65.
8. R. M. Green, "Medical Joint-Venturing: An Ethical Perspective," *Hastings Center Report* (1990): 22–26.
9. G. Moore, "Let's Provide Primary Care to All Americans—Now!" *JAMA* 265 (1991): 2108–9.
10. D. Brooks et al., "Medical Apartheid," *JAMA* 266 (1991): 2447–49.
11. P. Starr, *The Social Transformation of American Medicine* (New York: Basic Books, 1982), 239.
12. H. Aaron and W. Schwartz, *The Painful Prescription* (Washington, D.C.: Brookings Institution, 1984), 13.
13. Dougherty, *American Health Care*, 11–12; T. Bodenheimer, "Underinsurance in America," *New England Journal of Medicine* 327 (1992): 274–77.
14. American Medical Association, Council on Ethical and Judicial Affairs, "Black-White Disparities in Health Care," *JAMA* 263 (1990): 2344–46; Dougherty, *American Health Care,* 4–8.
15. E. Eckholm, "Solutions on Welfare: They All Cost Money," *New York Times*, 26 July 1992, 1.
16. Bodenheimer, "Underinsurance in America," 275.
17. U.S. Department of Commerce, *U.S. Industrial Outlook, 1992,* GPO #S/N 003-009-005-97-3 (Washington, D.C.: U.S. Department of Commerce, 1992).
18. U.S. General Accounting Office, *Health Care Spending*

Control: France, Germany, and Japan, GAO/HRD-92-9 (Washington, D.C.: U.S. General Accounting Office, 1991); A. McGuire et al., *Providing Health Care: The Economics of Alternative Systems of Finance and Delivery* (New York: Oxford University Press, 1991).

19. Plato, *Crito*, in *Plato: The Collected Works,* ed. E. Hamilton and H. Cairns (Princeton, N.J.: Princeton University Press, 1969), 35–39; see also, for example, P. McCormick, *Social Contract and Political Obligation* (New York: Garland, 1987).

20. J. Rawls, *A Theory of Justice* (Cambridge, Mass.: Harvard University Press, 1971).

21. Play-or-pay proposals include John D. Rockefeller IV, "The Pepper Commission Report on Comprehensive Health Care," *New England Journal of Medicine* 323 (1990): 1005–7; "Excellent Health Care for All Americans and At Reasonable Cost," in *Report of the National Leadership Coalition on Health Care Reform* (Washington, D.C.: National Leadership Coalition on Health Care Reform, 1991).

22. On national health insurance, see D. Himmelstein and S. Woolhandler, "A National Health Program for the United States: A Physicians' Proposal," *New England Journal of Medicine* 320 (1989): 102–8; Catholic Health Association, *Setting Relationships Right: A Working Proposal for Systemic Healthcare Reform* (St. Louis: Catholic Health Association, 1992); E. R. Brown, "Health USA: A National Health Care Program for the United States," *JAMA* 267 (1992): 552–58; C. J. Dougherty, "An Axiology for National Health Insurance," *Law, Medicine and Health Care* (Spring–Summer, 1992): 82–91.

PART V

Institutional Issues

Chapter 38

Rationing Health Care: The Ethics of Medical Gatekeeping

Edmund D. Pellegrino

An ethically perilous line of reasoning is gaining wide currency in our country today. It starts with a legitimate concern for rising health care costs, finds them uncontrollable by any means except some form of rationing, and concludes that the physician must become the "gatekeeper," the designated guardian of society's resources. By negative and positive financial incentives, it is reasoned, the physician can be forced to conserve tests, treatments, operations, hospitalization, and referrals for consultation. In this way, costs will presumably be cut by the elimination of "unnecessary" medical care.

There are three ways in which the physician can function as gatekeeper: One is morally mandatory, one is morally questionable, and one is morally indefensible.

The first form of gatekeeping is the traditional function imposed by the responsibility to practice rational medicine, i.e., to use only those diagnostic and therapeutic modalities beneficial and effective for the patient. The proper exercise of traditional gatekeeping is not only morally imperative but economically sound.

The second form of gatekeeping, negative gatekeeping, usually occurs within some form of prepayment system in which the physician is expected to limit access to health care services. For a physician to take on this role is morally dubious, because it generates a conflict between the traditional responsibilities of the physician as a primary advocate of the patient and his or her new responsibilities as guardian of society's resources. Under certain carefully defined conditions of economic necessity and moral monitoring, a negative gatekeeping role might be morally justifiable.

The third form of gatekeeping is positive gatekeeping. In positive gatekeeping, the physician encourages the use of health care facilities and services for personal or corporate profit. This is an indefensible form of gatekeeping for which no moral justification can be mustered.

This chapter delineates the nature of the ethical dilemmas of gatekeeping from the viewpoint of the patient's interests. It concludes that it is in the interest of society to preserve the integrity of the physician's primary responsibility to his or her patient, that rationing may not be as inevitable as generally supposed, and that rationing is morally valid only if other means of cost containment have been exhausted.

THE DE FACTO CONFLICT OF INTEREST

When the first physician requested a fee for his services, economics and conflict of interest entered medicine.[1] Ever since, physicians' fees and the degree to which physicians could equate necessity for their services with maintaining

Source: Reprinted with permission from E. D. Pellegrino, Rationing Health Care: The Ethics of Medical Gatekeeping, *Journal of Contemporary Health Law and Policy,* Vol. 2, pp. 23–38, © 1986, The Catholic University School of Law.

their own income have been sources of suspicion and contention between physicians and patients.

This de facto conflict of interest is difficult or impossible to eliminate given the fact that physicians must earn a living to support their families and are entitled to the same access to material goods as others. What mitigates the conflict is the ethical commitment of the physician to the patient's good, which can be conceived of as a commitment to the principle of beneficence.[2] This principle has been the central one of medical ethics. It is implicit in the Hippocratic Oath, the ancient codes of India and China, and the ethics of Thomas Percival (which inspired the American Medical Association's first code and all subsequent ones). Beneficence means acting on behalf of, in the interest of, or as an advocate of the patient. It has always implied some degree of effacement of the physician's self-interest in favor of the interests of the patient. Indeed, this effacement is what distinguishes a true profession from a business or craft.[3] And it is the expectation that physicians will by and large practice some degree of self-effacement that warrants the trust that society and individual patients place in them. It is also the physician's public commitment to service beyond self-interest that constitutes the real entry of the medical graduate into the profession. The awarding of a medical degree only signifies successful completion of a course of study. But the oath the physician takes is a public act of commitment to the special way of life and the special obligations demanded by the nature of medicine.[4]

Ethical commitments can, and do, mitigate the conflicts of interest inherent in medical practice, but they do not eliminate them—except perhaps in the heroic examples of self-sacrifice we expect only of saints and martyrs. Even if the physician's financial incentives are reduced, other motives can conflict with the care owed the patient, i.e., prestige, power, professional advancement, self-indulgence, unionization, and family obligations. These can be just as detrimental to the patient's well-being as the physician's monetary interests.

While there has always been some irreducible quantum of self-interest in medicine, rarely, if ever, has self-interest been socially sanctioned, morally legitimated, or encouraged in the way it is in the rationing approach to cost containment. Today, the physician's self-interest is deliberately used by policy makers to restrict the availability, accessibility, and quality of services to the patient. It is against this background—that is, how they accentuate the de facto conflict of interest in medicine—that the several forms of gatekeeping, licit and illicit, must be examined.

THREE FORMS OF GATEKEEPING

Morally Obligatory Gatekeeping: The Traditional Role

There is in the nature of the medical transaction an unavoidable gatekeeping function that the physician has always exercised and, indeed, is under compulsion to exercise in a morally defensible way. The unavoidable fact is that the physician recommends what tests, treatments, medications, operations, consultations, periods of hospitalization, nursing home, etc., the patient needs. Today physicians are responsible for 75 percent of all our health and medical care expenditures.

This fact imposes a serious positive moral duty on the physician to use both the individual patient's and society's resources optimally. In the case of the individual patient, the physician has the obligation, inherent in his or her promise to act for the patient's welfare, to use only those measures appropriate to the cure of the patient or alleviation of the patient's suffering. What the physician recommends must be *effective* (i.e., it must materially modify the natural history of the disease) and it must also be beneficial (i.e., it must be to the patient's benefit). Some measures are highly effective—like treatments for pneumonia—but may not be always beneficial if they prolong unnecessarily the act of dying and thus impose the burden of futility and expense without benefit for the patient. There are also treatments that benefit the patient but are not effective in altering the ultimate course of the disease, e.g., pain relief, nursing or home care, artificial feedings, etc. The same applies to diagnostic procedures.

Physicians, therefore, have a legitimate and morally binding responsibility to function as gatekeepers. They must use their knowledge to practice competent, scientifically rational medicine. Their guidelines should be *diagnostic elegance* (i.e., using the right degree of economy of means in diagnosis) and *therapeutic parsimony* (i.e., providing just those treatments that are demonstrably beneficial and effective). In this way, the physician automatically fulfills economic and moral obligations. He or she simultaneously avoids unnecessary risk to the patient from dubious treatment and conserves the patient's financial resources, and society's as well.

This form of gatekeeping entails no conflict with the patient's good. Economics and ethics, individual and social good, and doctors' and patients' interests are congruent. In this morally obligatory and traditional gatekeeper role, physicians use their de facto position to advance the good of their patients. In contrast, two new forms of gatekeeping have been introduced, each open to serious ethical objection because their primary intent is economic benefit, not the well-being of patients.

The Negative Gatekeeper Role

In the "negative" version of the gatekeeper role, the physician is placed under constraints of self-interest to restrict the use of medical services of all kinds, but particularly those that are most expensive. A variety of measures is used, each of which interjects economic considerations into the physician's clinical decisions and limits his or her discretionary latitude in making decisions.

One way this occurs is through the diagnosis-related group (DRG) program, which assigns to well over 400 disease categories a fixed sum or fixed number of days of hospitalization. If the actual number of days of hospitalization (or tests, etc.) exceeds the allotted sum or number, the institution or the physician "loses" the difference; if the number of days of hospitalization (or tests, etc.) is less than the allotted sum or number, the institution or physician makes a "profit." In other plans, the physician or institution contracts to provide care for some prescribed number of patients for a fixed annual sum. Again, if the total costs of care exceed the contracted amount, the provider bears the loss; if the costs are less, the provider makes a profit. Variations on these themes are several. They need not be detailed here. The essence of each plan is to motivate the provider to limit access to care by appealing to the provider's self-interest.[5]

With all these plans, the physician becomes the focus of incentives and disincentives in several ways—as a private practitioner when the physician hospitalizes a patient under the DRG system and as the employee or partner in a prepayment insurance plan, like a health maintenance organization (HMO), independent practice association (IPA), or primary care network (PCN). Increasingly in each case the physician's economic efficiency is monitored and deviations from the norm are rewarded or punished. The rewards may be in the form of profit sharing, bonuses, promotion in the organization, or other perquisites and preferments. The disincentives are loss of profit, limits on admitting privileges, or nonrenewal of coemployment contract. In some instances, productivity and efficiency schedules, "pass through" criteria, and other quantitative measures (not only of cost containment but of profit making) are used to evaluate the physician's performance.

The major pressure in these plans at present is upon the primary care physician, the first contact member of the health care system who makes the majority of decisions about entry into the system. The primary care physician may be a family practitioner, general internist, or pediatrician. The primary care physician has the greatest influence over access to expensive resources of hospitalization, testing, and consulting. For this reason, many prepayment plans insist that the patient must stay with one primary care physician within the system lest he or she shop around for one who might be more compliant. Gradually, as pressures for cost containment increase, the consultant and tertiary care specialists will very likely also be included as gatekeepers, with constraints and criteria suited to the nature of their specialties.

The Positive Gatekeeper Role

The "positive" form of gatekeeping is less well-defined and not usually explicitly formalized. In this version, the physician is constrained to increase rather than decrease access to services. However, the purpose here is not containing costs but enhancing profits. For those who can pay, the latest and most expensive diagnostic or therapeutic services are made available; services are provided based on market "demand" rather than medical need. The aim is to "penetrate" or "dominate" the market and to eliminate services that are not profitable. Increasing the demand for services is an implicit goal, and the physician becomes virtually a salesman. We see this most blatantly expressed in the TV and newspaper advertisements soliciting clients for elective surgery and all sorts of other services, some beneficial and some quite useless.

As positive gatekeepers, physicians use their position of control over access to medical care for their own financial advantage or for that of their employers. They share in the profit directly if they are owners of or investors in the service provided or they are rewarded by pay increases, advancement, etc., if they are employees.

THE ETHICAL ISSUES IN MEDICAL GATEKEEPING

Ethical Issues in Negative Gatekeeping

Both the positive and negative forms of gatekeeping exploit the de facto position of the physician as the conduit through which patients gain access to services. The purposes to be served by such gatekeeping are not entirely consistent with the patient's interests. Ethical issues arise inasmuch as these purposes reduce the trust the patient places in the physician as the patient's primary agent, minister, and advocate.

Efforts at cost containment are not in themselves unethical, and, as noted above, they are morally mandatory when they are in the best interests of the patient. They violate those interests if, for whatever reason, they deny needed services or induce the patient to demand, or the physician to provide, unneeded services. The ethical dilemmas of gatekeeping therefore arise out of the way economic incentives and disincentives modify the physician's freedom to act in the patient's behalf. While in the past the physician was largely responsible for defining "necessary" and "unnecessary" care, those determinations are now formularized by policy. In applying the formulas, the physician becomes the agent of the hospital or the system rather than the patient. Furthermore, the medical criteria used to determine necessary treatment are subject to modification or veto by economic considerations.

Many of the ethical dilemmas are illustrated in the Medicare prospective payment system now in force in the majority of states. In this system, the cost-base per diem reimbursement system of the past is replaced by a prospective payment system (PPS) based in fixed prices for 471 DRGs. The initial motivation behind this transition was to improve quality of care by linking quality of care directly to reimbursement. It was reasoned that the DRG system would also cut costs by causing a closer scrutiny of care aimed especially at limiting "unnecessary" tests, drugs, procedures, and hospitalization. Besides being economically wasteful, unneeded care is also dangerous to patients.

These cost containment measures are not intrinsically unethical. Certainly we cannot consider them unethical simply because they limit the physician's latitude in decision making. Rather, it is the effect of this limitation on the patient that is ethically crucial, and it is the moral responsibility of the physician operating within such a system to be concerned about this effect when it appears to be harmful to the patient.

The difficulty in the application of present DRG policies arises in the determination of what is necessary for quality care for a particular patient. In a system based on "average" lengths of stay for each disease, individual patients may suffer, since no disease manifests itself in the same way in every patient. As a result, disease entities are treated rather than individual patients, and the original goal (i.e., quality care) is compromised, sometimes dangerously.

Two tendencies deleterious to patients are already apparent in the way the DRG system is being administered in many hospitals. One is that patients are being discharged "quicker and sicker." The second is that extra funds are not being provided to those who need lengthier stays, etc., than the DRG allows. In both instances it is often the frail elderly patient who suffers—sent "home" with no adequate provision for posthospital care such as nursing home care, home care, etc. In fact, the trend of public policy at the moment is to curtail payment for nonhospital and long-term care, further aggravating the harm done by premature discharge.

In prospective payment systems, the physician is automatically a negative gatekeeper. To the extent that there is greater scrutiny of the quality of care rendered and that unnecessary care is avoided, the good of the patient is served. But when the system harms the patient, the question of the physician's primary duty arises. If the physician is primarily the patient's advocate, agent, and minister, then the physician must protect the patient's interests against the system, even with some risk or damage to the physician's own interests.

There is also pressure in prospective payment plans to disfavor or disenfranchise the sicker patients, those with chronic illness and those who need the more expensive kinds of care. Less admirable still is the way cost containment can be used consciously or unconsciously to justify the denial of services to those troublesome or obnoxious patients whom physicians prefer not to see—the neurotics, the "complainers," or the "hypochondriacs."

Another deleterious effect of negative gatekeeping is to foster the wrong kind of competition among providers. Instead of competition to provide the highest quality care (as judged by the standards of rational medicine), there is competition to compile the best records in terms of savings, productivity, efficiency, short hospital stays, or least number of procedures done.

To be effective, many prospective payment plans insist that patients must be locked into care by one primary care physician. The choice of physicians and the freedom to change physicians is severely limited. The most sensitive aspect of the healing relationship, the confidence one must have in one's personal physician, is thus ignored or compromised. Especially in regard to chronic or recurrent illness, this confidence is essential to effective care.

All of these factors converge to drive the physician's interests into conflict with the patient's. Such conflicts are heightened by the rather drastic changes occurring in the economics of the medical profession, which are making the physician more vulnerable to economic pressure. There is today an oversupply of physicians in urban areas and in many specialties.[6] Many physicians now graduate with debts due to the cost of their education in the neighborhood of $100,000. On top of this, expensive malpractice premiums must be paid before any physician dares risk even a day of medical practice. Consequently, competition from corporately owned and operated clinics can force even conscientious physicians into "survival" tactics of questionable morality.

The result is that many young and even older physicians are being driven into salaried group practices and automatically become negative gatekeepers. The physician's independence, as Paul Starr has shown, is rapidly eroding, and with it the physician's ability to withstand the institutional and corporate strictures inconsistent with his or her judgment about what is good for the patient.[7] It is becoming ever more costly personally and financially for even the most morally sensitive physician to practice the effacement of self-interest that medical ethics requires.

Ethical Issues in Positive Gatekeeping

The ethical conflicts in the positive form of gatekeeping are less subtle and more explicit. Here the profit motive is primary: The transaction between physician and patient becomes a commodity transaction. The physician is an independent entrepreneur or the hired agent of entrepreneurs and investors who themselves have no connection with the traditions of medical ethics. The physician thus begins to practice the ethics of the marketplace, to think of his or her relationship with the patient not as a covenant or trust but as a business and contractual relationship. Ethics becomes not a matter of obligations or virtue but a matter of legality. The metaphors of business and law replace those of ethics. Medical knowledge becomes proprietary, the doctor's private property to be sold to whom the doctor chooses at whatever price and under whatever conditions the doctor chooses.

The dependence, anxiety, lack of knowledge, and vulnerability of the sick person are exploited for personal profit. It is easy to exploit this vulnerability to encourage unnecessary cosmetic surgeries, hysterectomies, CAT scans, sonograms, fiber optic endoscopies, etc. The patient is led to believe he or she is getting "the latest and the best." All of this is inconsistent with even the most primordial concept of stewardship of patient interests. The moral questionableness is more obvious than in the negative form of gatekeeping. The patient becomes primarily a source of income. The crasser financial motives that have motivated the most selfish physicians are legitimated and even given social sanction.

For the positive form of gatekeeping there is not, as there may be for the negative form, any plausible moral justification. Some argue the profit motive is necessary for medical progress, for maintaining quality of service, or even for funding charitable care. It would be unrealistic to deny that for some physicians these are the only effective motives and that some good can come of them. But ultimately the profit motive erodes the ethical sensitivities and standards of the profession. When a conflict occurs between profit and patient welfare, patient welfare is sure to suffer in the end. Unrestrained monetary instinct corrupts medicine as surely as does an unrestrained instinct for power or prestige.

SOME SOCIAL-ETHICAL CONCOMITANTS OF RATIONING

The negative and the positive gatekeeper roles both involve ethical consequences for society. Both tolerate and indeed foster two or more levels of quality and availability of health care. Affluent persons can buy whatever they need or want. Affluent "outliers" can afford to supplement what a DRG plan allows. Prepayment plans and organizations seek eagerly to enroll such persons. The less affluent and the poor do not have such easy access to care. They may or may not be assured a so-called adequate level of care. "Adequacy" is always vaguely defined. On any definition, the gap between the health care provided to the rich and poor will widen. The poor and the lower economic strata of the middle class will be relegated to public hospitals. We have spent two decades trying to eliminate these institutions and the disparate levels of care they imply. Now it seems they must be reestablished and financed.

The differences in the care provided in public and private hospitals extend beyond mere conveniences, plushness of accommodations, or frills. Anyone whose experience, like the author's, goes back to the large municipal hospitals of several decades ago will know that the differences are nontrivial. The efforts of the last two decades to undo the injustices of a multilevel system of health care are being reversed by the move toward rationing, cost containment, and gatekeeping.

A different kind of social-ethical issue arises if we ask whether it is defensible for society to transpose its responsibility for rationing onto the physician. Are not the criteria for when and how to ration the responsibility of all of us? In situations of extreme economic exigency, rationing could be justified. But the criteria for rationing and the principle of justice to be followed should rest with society, not with physicians. There is no assurance that a physician is any fairer or juster than others in deciding who shall receive so crucially important a resource as health care. Do we as a society really want to give this kind of power to physicians?

A very careful balance between the relative place of societally determined criteria for rationing and the latitude allowed physicians in making rationing decisions must be struck. Society may wish to use the DRG mechanism as a way of expressing its value choices. But can physicians accept the resulting criteria if they violate the physicians' prime duty to act as patient advocates?

Because of the conflicts of interests they generate and the social injustice they foster, both positive gatekeeping and negative gatekeeping erode the commitment to the patient welfare that is mandatory in medical care. This commitment flows from the nature of illness and the promise of service made by individual physicians and by the profession as a whole. It has its basis in the empirical nature of the healing relationship, in particular, the fact that a sick person—dependent, vulnerable, exploitable—must seek out the help of another who has the knowledge, skill, and facilities needed to effect a cure. It is inevitably an unequal relationship in terms of freedom and power and one in which the stronger is obliged to protect the interests of the weaker.[8]

IS RATIONING INEVITABLE?

The only plausible justification for rationing is economic necessity. Some people have a fear that rising health care costs will seriously compromise the availability and accessibility of other goods our society needs to thrive—nutrition, housing, jobs, national security, etc. This fear is cited as justification for efforts to put some arbitrary ceiling on the percentage of gross national product dedicated to health care. But is the assumption of an impending national bankruptcy due to health care costs empirically sound? If it is, rationing might be justified. Then the ethical question becomes, under what conditions? If it is not, then rationing has no ethical sanction.

The main question concerns the truth or falsity of the initial premise in the argument for rationing as inevitable. This is a difficult question to answer, because comparable figures on national expenditures for other things our society wants are hard to come by. Moreover, whether there is a crisis or not depends very much on the value we place on other expenditures. Some of the data on health care costs that policy makers find distressing are the following.

The nation's total health care bill now exceeds $1 billion per day in the United States. The percentage of our gross national product going into health care is higher than for almost any other nation and it is increasing each year. Two and one-half billion dollars is spent on keeping 70,000 patients with chronic renal disease alive and $4.4 billion is spent on heart and liver transplants. Ten percent of all operating costs of a university hospital go into the last three to six months of life. Eighty percent of those who die do so in a hospital, as compared with 50 percent in 1949 and much lower percentages at the turn of the century. Each year 230,000 babies are born weighing less than 2,500 grams. Only half of them survive, and 15 percent of these end up with some residual defect. Two billion dollars per year are spent on neonatal intensive care units.

These and other figures have been cited by various advocates of rationing medical care for certain groups. Rationing for these groups is proposed on utilitarian, economic, and humanitarian grounds, i.e., to reduce the number of dependent, nonproductive members of society; to save money for other socially useful purposes or needs; or to prevent dooming the retarded and the disabled to lives of poor "quality." Some suggest that persons over a certain age should not be offered dialysis, that high-technology procedures like liver and heart transplants or even coronary bypasses should not be performed, that research in high-technology treatments like artificial hearts be halted, that babies under a certain cutoff weight should not be treated, that there should be a monetary limit on the expenditures for persons with terminal illnesses in the last few months of life, that those above a certain age should not be treated vigorously, etc.

These proposals deserve more critical examination than is possible here. They illustrate a range of policy options, all of which center on rationing expensive forms of care. Let it merely be noted that these expenditures should be compared with certain other expenditures that as a nation we make willingly, indeed sometimes avidly: $40 billion for alcohol, $30 billion for tobacco, $65 billion for cosmetics, $65 billion for advertising, $3.7 billion for potato chips, and unspecified billions for recreational handguns, illicit drugs, gambling, and various types of luxuries.[9]

What decisions would we make if we consciously compared these expenditures with those for health care? Is $2.5 billion too much to spend on keeping 70,000 people with renal disease alive (many of them leading active lives) or $4 billion to return people to active life by means of cardiac, liver, or renal transplants, which are becoming more effective each year? What about the 50 percent of underweight babies who *do* survive and the 85 percent of those who are not disabled or retarded? Can we decide what is "quality" life for another person, especially for an infant, whose values cannot possibly be known? How do we distinguish between futile and burdensome treatments and effective, though expensive, life-saving treatments? How do we protect the vulnerable—the old, the very young, the poor, and the socially outcast—from being discriminated against in rationing decisions? How do we know when research into high technology may turn out to be beneficial for all rather than for just a few?

How would we answer these questions if we considered health a higher value than some of the other things for which we make great expenditures without questioning them at all? Would we have to ask these questions at all if we could cut out truly unnecessary care, reduce inefficiencies in the care we now give, and establish some priority among the categories of care based on need, benefit, and effectiveness as seen from the patient's point of view?

If we address these questions in an orderly way, identifying the underlying values and making conscious choices, we might decide that rationing and lifeboat ethics are not warranted in this country today. It would take more space than this chapter permits to establish a position on these issues. The questions have yet to be examined with sufficient attention to their underlying value desiderata. This is a sensitive operation and one whose conclusions might prove embarrassing. How we make the choices required by rationing could well reveal more about the kind of people we are, and want to be, than we might wish.

NOTES

1. Fees for service—in goods, preferments, or money—are as old as medicine. Fees, their level, problems in collection, and the like are found in many of the books of the Hippocratic Corpus.
2. E. D. Pellegrino and D. Thomasma, *For the Patient's Good: The Restoration of Beneficence in Health Care* (New York: Oxford University Press, 1988). In this book Thomasma and I unpack the notion of patient good; we examine its components and the order of their moral importance.
3. H. Cushing, *Consecratio Medici and Other Papers* (1929). See also, Pellegrino, "What Is a Profession?" *Journal of Allied Health* 12 (1983): 168–76.
4. The Hippocratic Oath is still the most common public declaration of voluntary assumption of ethical obligations inherent in medicine. Other oaths like the so-called Oath of Maimonides, the Oath of Geneva, World Health Organization, etc., all carry the same message of commitment to the good of others.
5. Studies of the experiences with physician gatekeeping are beginning to appear. Samples of such studies are these: J. M. Eisenberg, "The Internist as Gatekeeper," *Annals of Internal Medicine,* 102, no. 1 (April 1985): 537–43; A. R. Somers, "And Who Shall be the Gatekeeper? The Role of the Physician in the Health Care Delivery System," *Inquiry* 20 (1983): 301–13; J. K. Inglehart, "Medicaid Turns to Prepaid Managed Care," *New England Journal of Medicine,* 308 (1983): 976–80; S. H. Moore, "Cost Containment Through Risk Sharing by Primary Care Physicians," *New England Journal of Medicine* 300 (1979): 1359–62. Some of the ethical ramifications of prepayment plans are outlined in *AMA News,* 2 January 1987.
6. *Summary Report of the Graduate Medical Education National Advisory Committee to the Secretary,* Department of Health and Human Services (Washington: U.S. Government Printing Office, 1980).
7. Paul Starr, *The Social Transformation of American Medicine* (New York: Basic Books, 1982), 514.
8. E. D. Pellegrino, "Toward a Reconstruction of Medical Morality: The Primacy of the Act of Profession and the Fact of Illness," *Journal of Medicine and Philosophy* 4, no. 1 (March 1979): 32–56.
9. Figures for national expenditures for goods, commodities and services are difficult to evaluate. For our purposes the important point is the relative order of magnitude of specific health and medical care expenditures as compared with other expenditures. For current statistics see: United States Department of Commerce, Bureau of Economic Analysis: Survey of Current Business (July issue annually).

Chapter 39

Multiculturalism, Bioethics, and End-of-Life Care: Case Narratives of Latino Cancer Patients

Patricia A. Marshall, Barbara A. Koenig, Donelle M. Barnes, and Anne J. Davis

In the last two decades, medical practices and procedures governing care at the end of life have changed considerably. Health providers, patients, and their families are now encouraged to anticipate and plan for end-of-life care and to participate actively in decision making. Traditionally, bioethics theory and practice have relied heavily on the Western philosophical principle of respect for persons to justify a model of end-of-life decision making that is focused on the rights and wishes of the individual patient. An important goal of bioethics innovations—such as advance care directives and open disclosure of prognosis—is to promote control of medical decision making at the end of life by an autonomous, fully informed patient.

Concurrent with the development of the field of bioethics and its growing influence on clinical practice, the United States was experiencing a profound increase in cultural diversity with important social and political consequences for health care delivery.[1] As a result of these demographic changes, encounters between patients and health professionals from diverse cultural backgrounds have become routine occurrences in the United States. This phenomenon is not limited to urban or metropolitan areas; crosscultural medical interactions also occur in rural districts of many states because of the influx of new immigrants and refugees.[2] Cultural and ethnic diversity is found even in regions that until recently were relatively homogeneous. Thus, in recent years, health providers have been more likely to practice medicine in social environments where value conflicts are commonplace. In these interactions, health care providers or their patients may represent ethnic minority, immigrant, or refugee populations.[3]

Despite the demographic reality of cultural diversity in the United States, until recently, ethical issues associated with cultural diversity in medical practice were, for the most part, ignored. Culture has been largely transparent within bioethics. The universal applicability of bioethics principles has been assumed. Yet, in the context of health care, an individual's cultural background provides an interpretive lens through which to examine perceptions of illness and health and response to medical treatment. Studies in the field of medical anthropology have shown that individuals of different ethnic backgrounds vary considerably in their perceptions and interpretations of symptoms, beliefs about appropriate treatments, reaction to pain and suffering, and understanding of the nature of the relationship between healer and patient.[4]

A number of authors have suggested that the notion of an informed, active decision maker may not be a universally held ideal of the good patient but rather, a very specific set of values based on a particular Western philosophical tradition.[5] In the United States, the "ideal" patient is a self-governing individual who is future oriented and willing to engage in frank discussions about difficult medical topics, including planning for his or her own death. The implications of cultural difference for bioethics practices at the end of life are significant. It is absolutely essential for health providers to recognize the importance of the particular cultural world in which a patient lives.

In this chapter, our goal is to explore why attention to cultural difference presents a fundamental challenge to the current paradigm of end-of-life decision-making practices in bioethics. First, we briefly review the literature on cultural diversity and end-of-life decision making with a particular focus on advance care planning and disclosure of medical information. These areas are important because they have been at the center of bioethics innovations over the past three decades. Second, we illustrate the importance of culture for end-of-life decision making using two cases involving Latino patients who are critically ill with cancer. These cases were collected during an ethnographic study of decision making at the end of life among ethnically diverse cancer patients and their families. The case narratives call attention to the need for a culturally sensitive approach to ethical decisions associated with end-of-life care. Finally, we discuss the implications for approaching cultural dimensions of decision making at the end of life. We are critical of policies and procedures that "essentialize" culture, leading to the perpetuation of ethnic stereotypes and diminished opportunities for cultural understanding in clinical settings.

CULTURAL DIVERSITY AND DECISIONS AT THE END OF LIFE: A REVIEW OF EMPIRICAL STUDIES

Medical practices surrounding death and dying in the United States have changed considerably during the last three decades. Traditionally, physicians were reluctant to inform patients about a diagnosis of terminal illness and discussions of advance care planning were uncommon. In the 1960s and 1970s, the movement toward respect for patient autonomy and patient rights had a significant impact on practices governing disclosure of terminal illness and on the development of advance directives such as the living will and durable power of attorney for health care. As Pellegrino observed, "In this context, truth telling is a necessary corollary, since human capability for autonomous choices cannot function if truth is withheld, falsified, or otherwise manipulated."[6] In the United States, competent patients now have a legally recognized right to be involved in decision-making processes, including the right to forgo treatment, even if refusal would lead to death. Health care providers are obligated to respect patients' wishes to withhold or withdraw all medical treatments—including cardiopulmonary resuscitation (CPR), mechanical ventilation, fluids and hydration, and antibiotics. Currently, the majority of physicians in the United States adhere to the accepted practice of disclosing a diagnosis of terminal illness to patients.[7] There is, however, greater variability regarding approaches to discussions of advance care planning.[8]

DISCLOSURE OF A DIAGNOSIS OF TERMINAL ILLNESS

Investigators have begun to assess the influence of ethnicity and cultural traditions on end-of-life care,[9] including the disclosure of a diagnosis of terminal illness.[10] In their comprehensive research on ethnicity and beliefs about patient autonomy, Blackhall and associates[11] found significant differences among ethnic groups in the Los Angeles area. Their sample included 800 individuals over 65 years of age (200 from each of the four cultural groups studied). African-Americans (88 percent) and European Americans (87 percent) were more likely than Mexican-Americans (65 percent) and Korean-Americans (47 percent) to believe that a patient should be told the diagnosis of metastatic cancer. European-Americans (69 percent) and African-Americans (63 percent) were also more likely than Mexican-Americans (48 percent) and Korean-Americans (35 percent) to believe that a patient should be told of a terminal prognosis. Additionally, Mexican-Americans and Korean-Americans were significantly more likely than European-Americans to support the view that doctors should not discuss death and dying with patients because it could be harmful. Rather than the patient autonomy model favored by African-Americans and European-Americans, Korean-Americans and Mexican-Americans were more likely to hold a family-centered model of medical decision making.

Orona, Koenig, and Davis also found a family-centered model of decision making in their ethnographic exploration of cultural aspects of nondisclosure among Chinese-American and Mexican-American cancer patients and their families: "Duty was defined by both Latino and Chinese relatives as protecting the patient . . . by making the remaining time comfortable and free of distress. Central to the protection was a need to keep information about the disease and prognosis from the patient."[12]

Other research supports the dominant bioethical paradigm that end-of-life care is firmly grounded in medical training. It is now widely accepted that physicians should disclose information about medical diagnosis and prognosis in a manner that is both truthful and compassionate. Good and associates interviewed 51 oncologists practicing in teaching hospitals in the United States. The oncologists expressed a strong desire for a partnership with the patient, emphasizing their belief that good communication strengthens the patient's experience of hope. Addressing the issue of disclosure, one oncologist stated,

> We want patients to have a good understanding, especially if we are going to be treating them. We need them to be, kind of, partners in what we are doing. So although we don't bludgeon people with the truth, I mean, ultimately you would like each patient to have the fullest understanding of the disease [that] they can tolerate.[13]

ADVANCE DIRECTIVES FOR END-OF-LIFE CARE

In addition to studies of ethnicity and disclosure of medical information, investigators have examined cultural differences associated with the reluctance to use advance care planning. Carrese and Rhodes,[14] for example, studied bioethics practices with 34 Navaho patients, health providers, and traditional healers. They found that 86 percent of the individuals interviewed considered discussion of advance care planning for near-death medical decisions a dangerous violation of Navaho values. Traditionally, Navaho culture emphasizes the importance of thinking and speaking in a positive way and the avoidance of thinking or speaking in a negative way. Discussion of end-of-life decision making or disclosure of a diagnosis of terminal illness would violate this proscriptive norm.

Findings from other studies suggest that European-Americans are more likely than other ethnic populations to complete a living will or durable power of attorney.[15] In a limited study of cultural value and end-of-life decisions, Klessig[16] found that African-Americans were more likely than Anglos to agree to initiate life support, but they were also more likely to disagree with stopping life support. In their study of end-of-life care in North Carolina, Garrett and colleagues[17] have demonstrated that European-Americans and African-Americans differ in their desires for life-sustaining treatment and in their willingness to complete advance directives. In a survey on the use of life-prolonging treatment in Miami, Caralis and associates found that significantly more African-American and Hispanic patients, "wanted their doctors to keep them alive regardless of how ill they were, while more . . . whites agreed to stop life-prolonging treatment under some circumstances."[18] Similarly, in a controlled study to promote the use of advance directives, Rubin and associates[19] reported that African-Americans and Hispanics were significantly less likely to complete a durable power of attorney for health care form than were non-Hispanic whites and Asians. In their study of the use of living wills in an elderly population, Stetler and associates[20] found that only 25 percent of the African-American population, compared to 86 percent of the Euro-American population, reported a desire to complete an advance directive.

In their comprehensive investigation, Blackhall and associates[21] found that Korean-Americans (28 percent) and Mexican-Americans (41 percent) were less likely than African-Americans (60 percent) or European-Americans (65 percent) to believe that the patient—as opposed to the family or physicians—should make decisions about the use of life-sustaining technologies. In a second report from the same study population, researchers[22] explored in depth the relationship between ethnicity and knowledge and the use of advance care planning. The rate of execution of advance care directives differed among Korean-American, Mexican-American, African-American, and European-American respondents who were able to correctly define a living will or durable power of attorney. Forty percent of the European-Americans possessed an advance directive, compared to 22 percent of the Mexican-Americans and 17 percent of the African-Americans; none of the Korean-Americans possessed an advance directive. Mexican-Americans were significantly more likely than European-Americans to support the view that doctors should not discuss death and dying with patients because it could be harmful; Mexican-Americans who were more acculturated, as measured by the Marin Short Acculturation Scale, were more likely to have an advance directive. In contrast to Mexican-American and Korean-American respondents, African-Americans reported more positive attitudes regarding advance care planning, yet were unlikely to possess an advance care planning document.

In their discussion of the striking differences between African-Americans' and European-Americans' knowledge of advance care planning documents such as durable power of attorney for health care, Blackhall and associates[23] note that all of the respondents were native English speakers born in the United States. However, 69 percent of the European-Americans compared with only 12 percent of the African-Americans were familiar with advance care documents. The researchers describe a pattern of information seeking that may help explain the difference in knowledge between the two groups. At one of their sites, seminars on advance care directives were theoretically available to the roughly equal numbers of African-Americans and European-Americans at the facility; however, at this site, 55 percent of the European-Americans, compared with 15 percent of the African-Americans, had knowledge of living wills. The researchers suggest that different ethnic groups may be differentially motivated to seek out information on advance directives. The concept of advance planning for medical treatment may be most compatible with European-Americans' underlying cultural beliefs and social expectations about health care treatment. The investigators report, for example, that when income and education were held constant, ethnicity still emerged as an independent factor in predicting possession of an advance care document. An alternative explanation is that African-Americans have been historically burdened with limited access to health care and may distrust the motivations of health care workers who propose advance care planning to limit overtreatment at life's end.[24]

The studies cited above show a consistent picture. Although there are regional variations within the United States, there appears to be a trend: Individuals from minority backgrounds are less likely to adopt the autonomy-based bioethics practices that have become standard practice in many United States hospitals and clinics. These individuals do not share the necessary assumptions—such as open disclosure of information about a poor prognosis—that are necessary background to making use of advance care planning documents. Either because of lack of interest, lack of cultural fit, or perhaps because of a fundamental mistrust of the health care system, members of United States minority groups make use of advance directives in significantly fewer numbers than do European-Americans.

Where, however, do these statistical findings lead us? Do we simply assume that there are cultural barriers to the use of advance directives and work toward educating clinicians and patients alike to their removal? How *should* clinicians and bioethicists take account of culture in their analyses? When working with a patient from a Korean or Mexican background, should the clinician infer that patients will not desire information about their prognosis or to execute a durable power of attorney for health care? Clearly, the use of empirical studies (such as those cited above) in a purely predictive fashion has many associated dangers. Not all individuals will follow a particular norm; intracultural variation is inevitable. But more dangerous still is the tendency to treat cultural background as a simple predictive variable. Cultural background will never correlate exactly with any specific behavior. Instead, we propose that a patient's cultural background must always be interpreted in a particular historical and political context.

CASE NARRATIVES

To illustrate the relevance of culture for decisions at the end of life, two case narratives involving Latino patients are presented. The individuals in these narratives—a man from El Salvador and a woman from Nicaragua—are participants in an ongoing ethnographic study of end-of-life decision making among a population of culturally diverse patients with end-stage cancer (see Acknowledgments at the end of the chapter). At the time of the interviews with these patients, both had been diagnosed with incurable cancer and a probable prognosis of approximately six months to live.

Patients in the Cultural Pluralism and Ethical Decision-Making Project were recruited from an outpatient clinic affiliated with a large, urban public hospital in California. Patients were asked to participate in the research after their primary health care provider, most often an oncologist or oncologist in training, verified that the patient's cancer was not considered curable by currently available treatment modalities and that the patient's prognosis for survival was likely to be less than six months. Individuals were assigned to cultural categories based on their self-identification as European-American, Hispanic or Latino, Chinese-American, and African-American. Study design and methods were approved by the institutional review board of the principal investigator's home institution. Study descriptions and consent documents were available in English, Spanish, and Chinese. Initial consent was obtained from the patient. The patient then gave consent for team members to contact family members and health care providers and to conduct chart reviews. Family members could then either consent or refuse for themselves.

Each case study includes a set of in-depth, semistructured interviews with the patient, two family members, and two members of the health care team (one physician and one nonphysician, e.g., social worker, nurse). The interviews varied in length between one half-hour to two hours, and averaged about 45 minutes. All interviews were audio-recorded and fully transcribed. Interviews conducted in Cantonese or Spanish were translated into English for analysis. Interviews with patients, family members, and health care providers were designed to elicit an illness narrative, which was then followed up with specific questions and probes dealing with end-of-life decision making.

The two case narratives presented involve self-identified Latinos, one male and one female. The cultural categories chosen for comparison conform generally to the population diversity of the clinic studied. From the beginning of the study, however, the researchers were forced to confront the serious limitations of conducting meaningful crosscultural comparisons using National Institutes of Health–mandated ethnic and racial categories.[25] The use of cultural categories presented difficulty in a number of ways. First, patients whose heritage was from Mexico or Central America self-identified according to their country of origin rather than in terms of a broad "Hispanic" or "Latino" category. Another difficulty was assigning patients from complex backgrounds to the study categories, for example, individuals of mixed background or Chinese immigrants who had lived extensively in Latin America. Since the majority of clinic patients from China were originally from Southern China, the Chinese-American sample was limited to speakers of Cantonese.

Case One: Mr. Samuel Hurtado

The first case highlights Mr. Samuel Hurtado, a 54-year-old Salvadorian who had been living in the United States for six years at the time of his interview. (All proper names are pseudonyms.) He has a high school education and has worked in a variety of jobs including tailoring and dishwashing. Mr. Hurtado says he speaks a little English but does not understand it very well. He uses an interpreter during his clinic visits, frequently either his daughter-in-law or a clinic-provided interpreter. He was diagnosed with multiple myeloma after suffering from back pain for several months, which then spread to several ribs. Before and after receiving his cancer diagnosis, Mr. Hurtado used a variety of therapies to treat both the pain and the cancer, including visits to a chiropractor and an acupuncturist, oral garlic and lemon juices, and intramuscular injections of pain medicine that he continues to buy in El Salvador. He has received repeated rounds of radiation and chemotherapy in California and El Salvador.

Mr. Hurtado reports that it was extremely difficult for him to accept the fact that his illness made it impossible for him to remain employed and, in his words, "productive." He expressed anger at the rehabilitation hospital staff who were unable to help him to return to "real work." Especially for male patients, the inability to continue to work appears to be a devastating loss, presumably because their sense of self-worth and financial independence is often tied to their occupation. Because of his illness, Mr. Hurtado was unable to provide financially for his wife and children; this had serious consequences for his familial relationships and obligations.

Mr. Hurtado displays a number of strategies for maintaining hope or expressing denial when he discusses his prognosis. For example, he says that the doctors told him that there was no cure and he believes that he has accepted the cancer. Yet, at another point in the conversation he says. "The disease is not going to kill me. I am going to defeat the disease. I have faith." The paradoxical expression of accepting the cancer and medical treatments while simultaneously believing in the possibility of a total cure is common among many of the patients involved in the study.

Mr. Hurtado states that no one has discussed resuscitation with him but goes on to suggest that if he had a heart attack, then he would want his doctor to let him die because he does not want to create problems for the family. Concern for his family's well-being was an important factor in his decisions, an orientation that was problematic for some providers who wanted the patients' needs and wishes to be the only consideration.

Mr. Hurtado denies that anyone has discussed advance directives with him and suggests that the issue has not come up because, "Perhaps they haven't seen the need to do so." The perception of readiness to discuss end-of-life issues with patients like Mr. Hurtado appeared to be quite different from both the average health care provider's time frame and the legally mandated time frame of offering this information at admission. Many patients assumed that treatment would continue as long as they were alive, thus making resuscitation or advance directive decisions unnecessary from their perspective. On the other hand, oncology health care providers routinely put off talking about advance directive issues until the patient is hospitalized or on the verge of a code situation, at which time the patient may be too sick to discuss his or her wishes. Many factors (not necessarily related to diversity) could contribute to the delay in speaking with patients about end-of life decisions, including time pressures or the discomfort experienced by some physicians when faced with the possibility of discussing death and dying.

Mr. Hurtado's daughter-in-law, who frequently translates for him during clinic visits, concurs with Mr. Hurtado's statements that his family refers to his illness as "cancer" and that everyone in the family knows about it. She goes on to relate what happened at the clinic visit when the oncologist first told her, as translator, to tell her father-in-law that he had approximately eight months to live. Because she was only a relative by marriage, she did not feel it was her place to give him that negative information, so she did not translate it but went home and told her husband what the doctor had said. Her husband told his mother, the patient's wife, who told the patient. Thus, Mr. Hurtado was eventually told what the physician had said but only through appropriate and acceptable family channels. The daughter-in-law also states that although the family members know that the father's prognosis is short and they discuss it among themselves, they do not discuss the prognosis with Mr. Hurtado. They do not want to "harm" him with the knowledge of his short life expectancy, believing that it is more merciful to withhold such painful information.

The daughter-in-law says that no health care provider has discussed advance directives with the patient while she was present but that resuscitation questions did come up during one visit. According to her, Mr. Hurtado was first questioned about his resuscitation wishes without a translator's being present, and he was upset because he thought they were telling him that he was going to die. At a subsequent visit, the daughter-in-law inquired about what had been said, and a nurse described her understanding of Mr. Hurtado's choice should he need to be resuscitated. The conflicting reports of whether or not a discussion about advance directives occurred with Mr. Hurtado, and the conflicting views about what exactly was said, illustrate how complicated it is to "speak the truth" about, in this case, advance care planning. There will always be multiple perspectives on events or discussions that take place in the course of planning for end-of-life care.

Mr. Hurtado's oncologist, Dr. Green, was interviewed about his perspective of the patient's decisions. When asked if Mr. Hurtado knew his prognosis, Dr. Green replied with information about the prognosis based on the diagnosis but never directly answered the question of whether or not Mr. Hurtado understood the prognosis.

Dr. Green acknowledges that he has not discussed advance directives or resuscitation issues with Mr. Hurtado. In direct conflict with the bioethics "ideal," he states repeatedly that resuscitation conversations do not come up at the clinic but usually are reserved for the hospital when the patient becomes critical. Dr. Green says, "We convince people to say they do not want to be resuscitated." The rationale is that it is hard on the family to see a patient "hooked up to machines," that most health providers do not believe it is necessary to maintain patients on life support machines indefinitely, and that long-term support on a ventilator or other machine is expensive. On the other hand, Dr. Green recognizes that patients do not want to feel abandoned and that they need hospice care, support groups, and health providers.

Mr. Hurtado's case narrative, which includes multiple voices, reveals the complexity of cultural background and the complicated way it is expressed in the course of routine cancer treatment. Discussions about end-of-life care and treatment decisions are shown to be embedded in the constraints of his everyday life, including his relationship with his family.

Case Two: Ms. Irene Guerrera

A second Latino case is Irene Guerrera, a 64-year-old woman who had lived in the United States over 20 years at the time of her interview. Ms. Guerrera, a Nicaraguan, had no formal education because she was raised "during the time of the Sandinistas" and there was no formal schooling available. She worked in domestic service in a private home until diagnosed with breast cancer with bone metastasis. Ms. Guerrera's closest support person is her employer, whom she describes as "family." Her only other family members live elsewhere in the United States or remain in Nicaragua.

Ms. Guerrera seems to be more assimilated into the dominant United States culture, perhaps because of the length of time she has spent in the United States. As a single woman, she describes herself as an "independent" decision maker and discusses her diagnosis openly with clinic oncologists, nurses, and social workers. On the other hand, when her sister was coming to visit, Ms. Guerrera revealed that she had not told her family in Nicaragua that she was sick and that she did not want them to know that she had cancer. The stigma of cancer drives some patients to protect their family members from knowledge of the diagnosis. Similarly, family members may attempt to protect the patient from learning the truth about a diagnosis of cancer. Neither approach conforms to the provider's ideal that everyone should know the diagnosis and be able to discuss it frankly. Ironically, this situation—one in which a patient appoints a nonfamily member as a proxy decision maker—should, theoretically, represent an ideal use of a durable power of attorney for health care.

Ms. Guerrera believes she will die from the disease; she is active in a cancer support group. Ms. Guerrera identifies herself as a Catholic, saying she is "very Catholic." She says that she will "die according to God's will." When accepting initial radiation and chemotherapy, she said, "Oh, well, let them do whatever God wants to do with me. Let's start the treatment." Some health care providers view religious beliefs, such as those expressed by Ms. Guerrera, as a potential road block to realistically "facing the facts."

In accordance with her refusal to be resuscitated, Ms. Guerrera does not want to be kept alive on machines. Her former employer is named as the person to make decisions for her if she is unable to do so. Her last wish is that she be able to return to Nicaragua to die, a frequent request among patients who were born outside the United States. Ms. Guerrera trusts her oncologist to tell her when it is time to return to Nicaragua.

Ms. Rolinsky, Ms. Guerrera's former employer, agrees that Ms. Guerrera is an independent decision maker, that she is aware of her grim prognosis, and that religion is helping the patient to cope. Ms. Rolinsky says that the patient's family views her as the alternate decision maker for Ms. Guerrera. However, to her knowledge, a legal document has not been signed naming her as Ms. Guerrera's durable power of attorney for health care. Ms. Rolinsky does not know if resuscitation has been discussed with the patient.

Ms. Guerrera's oncologist, Dr. Carlson, also agrees that Ms. Guerrera is an independent decision maker. He understands that Ms. Guerrera does not want to be resuscitated and that her primary wish is to return to Nicaragua to die. They have discussed these decisions openly and agreed that he will tell her, "when the game is up . . . when it's not worth doing [treatment] anymore."

In the meantime, Dr. Carlson's goal is to keep the patient alive as long as possible so that she can someday return to Nicaragua. He describes his approach to her therapy in this way: "We were going to take this huge risk with the treatment. This was a gamble. What were we going to do if she got some dreadful complication? . . . The risk I took was that if I killed her outright she would never get to go home and see everybody, and I would feel really bad."

Dr. Carlson's dilemma centers on the questions of how to give aggressive chemotherapy to keep Ms. Guerrera alive long term without "killing" her, thereby breaking his promise to tell Ms. Guerrera when it is time to go to Nicaragua.

Dr. Carlson indicates that durable power-of-attorney issues have only been briefly discussed and concedes that this issue is generally handled by the social worker. He says that Ms. Guerrera is unsure whom she would appoint as a proxy decision maker. In contrast, Ms. Guerrera, during interviews with the project team, had clearly identified her former employer as the surrogate decision maker.

As in Mr. Hurtado's case, Ms. Guerrera's narrative illustrates how her cultural background influences end-of-life decision making. However, a very different portrait emerges. Ms. Guerrera characterizes herself as self-reliant and independent, with a strong desire to be involved in the process of decision making about her medical treatment. In contrast, Mr. Hurtado's narrative reveals more "traditional" values concerning the need to protect the patient from information or decisions that might cause anxiety or discomfort. These two very distinct representations of the relationship between cultural background and end-of-life care call attention to the importance of recognizing intracultural variation and the limitations of broad ethnic categories such as "Latino" for predicting response to medical decision making.

DISCUSSION

Current practices governing end-of-life decision making rely on Western concepts that privilege respect for personal choice, occasionally in ways that harm individuals and families with different cultural backgrounds. In the multicultural environment of the United States, it is inevitable that there will be disagreements about the "correct" approach to death and dying. When misunderstandings occur, an individual's cultural background may be viewed as a barrier to scientific practice and patients may be blamed for their lack of cooperation with the medical team.[26] In addition to viewing cultural beliefs and values as obstacles to end-of-life decision making, too often ethnicity and cultural background are used as predictors of a patient's response to participation in medical decision making. This serves only to perpetuate superficial stereotypes that may seriously undermine patient care.[27] As the case narratives of Mr. Hurtado and Ms. Guerrera illustrate, there is considerable diversity in beliefs about end-of-life care among patients who appear to share a similar cultural heritage.

Greater sensitivity to the specific context of sociocultural background and its influence on end-of-life care is needed in both medical practice and clinical education. Patients should be evaluated as unique individuals, with particular biographical experiences, and with sharp attention to the context of family or other support systems.[28] Efforts to introduce and sustain educational programs on cultural difference and its relevance to patient care are vitally important.[29]

Elsewhere we have outlined in greater detail guidelines for a culturally sensitive approach to patients and families facing medical decisions at the end of life.[30] A number of factors are central to a successful model for respecting cultural difference in end-of-life care. These include but are not limited to the following: determination of the language used by patients and families to discuss their disease; elicitation of the patient's and family's understanding of the cause of and best treatment of the illness; consideration of the influence of gender and age; determination of who is considered to be the appropriate decision maker (including the option of joint, consensual decision making); consideration of religious beliefs; and recognition of the broader political and historical context that might impact patient care, such as unequal access to services or discrimination.

A research agenda is needed to explore the influences of particular sociocultural contexts on the response to medical decision making at the end of life. Quantitative surveys offer a useful starting point but ultimately limit insights into the complexity of the relationship between cultural background and end-of-life care. Ethnographic investigations, combined with quantitative methodologies, may be the most effective in providing a robust account of the end-of-life experiences of patients, families, and the health care providers who serve them.

ACKNOWLEDGMENTS

This program of research has been supported by a grant from the National Institutes of Health (R01 NR 02906) to Drs. Davis and Koenig. Koenig and Marshall's work on multiculturalism and bioethics has been supported by The Greenwall Foundation; we thank William Stubing for his support, both financial and personal. The Robert Wood Johnson Foundation provided financial support for an invitational meeting at the Hastings Center (September 16–17, 1996) called, "Culture, Bioethics, and End-of-Life Care: What Differences Make a Difference?" And finally, we wish to thank the patients, families, and health professionals whose participation made possible the research on which this paper is based. The contribution of patients and families—often during a time of great personal grief and stress—cannot be measured.

NOTES

1. B. A. Koenig and J. Gates-Williams, "Understanding Cultural Difference in Caring for Dying Patients," *Western Journal of Medicine* 163 (1995): 244–49.
2. P. A. Marshall, "Advanced Directives: Issues of Ethnic, Racial, and Cultural Diversity," in *Advance Directives: The Role of Health Care Professionals, Report of the Sixteenth Ross Roundtable on Medical Issues* (Columbus, Ohio: Ross Products Division, Abbott Laboratories, 1996), 25–30.
3. N. S. Jecker et al., "Caring for Patients in Cross-Cultural

Settings," *Hastings Center Report* 25 (1995): 6–14.

4. I. K. Zola, "Culture and Symptoms: An Analysis of Patients' Presenting Complaints," *American Sociology Review* 31 (1966): 615–30; B. Good and M. D. V. Good, "The Meaning of Symptoms: A Cultural Hermeneutic Model for Clinical Practice," in *The Relevance of Social Science for Medicine,* ed. L. Eisenberg and A. Kleinman (Dordrecht, The Netherlands: D. Reidel Publishing Co., 1981), 165–96; C. Hellman, *Culture, Health and Illness,* 3d ed. (Newton, Mass.: Butterfield and Heinmann, 1995).
5. B. Koenig, "Cultural Diversity in Decision-Making about Care at the End-of-Life," in *Dying, Decision-Making, and Appropriate Care* (Washington, D.C.: Institute of Medicine/National Academy of Sciences, 1993); B. Koenig and J. Gates-Williams, "Understanding Cultural Difference in Caring for Dying Patient"; Marshall, "Issues of Ethnic, Racial, and Cultural Diversity."
6. E. D. Pellegrino, "Is Truth Telling to the Patient a Cultural Artifact?" *JAMA* 268 (1992): 1734–35 (quote, 1734).
7. D. J. Klenow and G. A. Young, "Changes in Doctor/Patient Communication of a Terminal Prognosis: A Selective Review and Critique," *Death Studies* 11 (1987): 263–77; G. E. Dickenson and R. E. Tournier, "A Decade Beyond Medical School: A Longitudinal Study of Physicians' Attitudes toward Death and Terminally-Ill Patients," *Social Science and Medicine* 38 (1994): 1397–1400; D. H. Novack et al., "Changes in Physicians' Attitudes toward Telling the Cancer Patient," *JAMA* 241 (1979): 897–900.
8. M. Solomon et al., "Decisions Near the End of Life: Professional Views on Life Sustaining Treatment," *American Journal of Public Health* 83 (1993): 14–23; A. F. Connors et al., "A Controlled Trial to Improve Care for Seriously Ill Hospitalized Patients: The Study to Understand Prognoses and Preferences for Outcomes and Risks of Treatments (SUPPORT)," *JAMA* 274 (1995): 1591–98.
9. L. J. Blackhall et al., "Ethnicity and Attitudes toward Patient Autonomy," *JAMA* 274 (1995): 820–25; S. T. Murphy et al., "Ethnicity and Advance Care Directives," *Journal of Law, Medicine and Ethics* 24 (1996): 1008–17; P. V. Caralis et al., "The Influence of Ethnicity and Race on Attitudes toward Advance Directives, Life-Prolonging Treatments, and Euthanasia," *Journal of Clinical Ethics* 4 (1993): 155–65; S. Rubin et al., "Increasing the Completion of the Durable Power of Attorney for Health Care," *JAMA* 271 (1994): 209–12; G. P. Eleazer et al., "The Relationship between Ethnicity and Advance Directives in a Frail Older Population," *JAGS* 44 (1996): 938–48; Marshall, "Advance Directives: Issues of Ethnic, Racial, and Cultural Diversity"; J. Garrett et al., "Life-Sustaining Treatment during Terminal Illness: Who Wants What?" *Journal of General Internal Medicine* 8 (1993): 361–68.
10. L. M. Patcher, "Culture and Clinical Care: Folk Illness Beliefs and Behaviors and Their Implications for Health Care Delivery," *JAMA* 271 (1994): 690–94; N. S. Jecker et al., "Caring for Patients in Cross-Cultural Settings," *Hastings Center Report* 25 (1995): 6–14; R. D. Orr et al., "Cross-Cultural Considerations in Clinical Ethics Consultations," *Archives of Family Medicine* 4 (1995): 159–64; J. Carrese and L. Rhodes, "Western Bioethics on the Navaho Reservation," *Cambridge Quarterly of Healthcare Ethics* 3 (1994): 338–46.
11. Blackhall et al., "Ethnicity and Attitudes toward Patient Autonomy."
12. C. J. Orona et al., "Cultural Aspects of Nondisclosure," *Cambridge Quarterly of Healthcare Ethics* 3 (1994): 338–46.
13. M. D. Good et al., "American Oncology and the Discourse on Hope," *Culture Medicine Psychiatry* 14 (1990): 59–79.
14. Carrese and Rhodes, "Western Bioethics on the Navaho Reservation."
15. J. Klessig, "The Effect of Values and Culture on Life-Support Decision," *Western Journal of Medicine* 157 (1992): 316–22; Blackhall et al., "Ethnicity and Attitudes toward Patient Autonomy"; Caralis et al., "The Influence of Ethnicity and Race on Attitudes toward Advance Directives, Life-Prolonging Treatments, and Euthanasia"; Rubin et al., "Increasing the Completion of the Durable Power of Attorney for Health Care"; Garrett et al., "Life-Sustaining Treatment during Terminal Illness: Who Wants What?"
16. Klessig, "The Effect of Values and Culture on Life-Support Decision."
17. Garrett et al., "Life-Sustaining Treatment during Terminal Illness: Who Wants What?"
18. Caralis et al., "The Influence of Ethnicity and Race on Attitudes toward Advance Directives, Life-Prolonging Treatments, and Euthanasia."
19. Rubin et al., "Increasing the Completion of the Durable Power of Attorney for Health Care."
20. K. L. Stetler et al., "Living Will Completion in Older Adults," *Archives of Internal Medicine* 152 (1992): 954–59.
21. Blackhall et al., "Ethnicity and Attitudes toward Patient Autonomy."
22. Murphy et al., "Ethnicity and Advance Care Directives."
23. Blackhall et al., "Ethnicity and Attitudes toward Patient Autonomy."
24. A. Dula, "African American Suspicion of the System Is Justified," *Cambridge Quarterly of Healthcare Ethics* 3 (1994): 347–58; Marshall, "Advanced Directives: Issues of Ethnic, Racial, and Cultural Diversity."
25. See Koenig and Gates-William, "Understanding Cultural Difference in Caring for Dying Patient," for a fuller

discussion of the theoretical issues involved in crosscultural comparison; R. A. Habor et al., "Inconsistencies in Coding of Race and Ethnicity between Birth and Death in U.S. Infants," *JAMA* 267 (1992): 259–63; M. Lock, "The Concept of Race as an Ideological Construct," *Transcultural Psychiatric Research Review* 30 (1993): 203–27.

26. M. Lock, "Education and Self Reflection: Teaching about Culture, Health and Illness," in *Health and Cultures: Exploring the Relationships,* ed. R. Masi et al. (Oakville, Ontario: Mosau Press, 1993); P. A. Marshall and B. A. Koenig, "Anthropology and Bioethics: Perspectives on Culture, Medicine, and Morality," in *Medical Anthropology: Contemporary Theory and Methods,* 2d ed., ed. C. Sargent and T. Johnson (Praeger Publishing Co., 1996), 349–73.
27. Lock, "Education and Self Reflection: Teaching about Culture, Health and Illness."
28. Koenig and Gates-Williams, "Understanding Cultural Difference in Caring for Dying Patient."
29. R. Like et al., "Recommended Care Curriculum Guidelines on Culturally Sensitive and Competent Health Care," *Family Medicine* 28 (1996): 291–97.
30. Koenig and Gates-Williams, "Understanding Cultural Difference in Caring for Dying Patient"; Orr et al., "Cross-Cultural Considerations in Clinical Ethics Consultations"; Marshall, "Advanced Directives: Issues of Ethnic, Racial, and Cultural Diversity."

Chapter 40

Technology, Older Persons, and the Doctor-Patient Relationship

Myles N. Sheehan

An 84-year-old man with an independent life style begins to have bouts of chest pain and shortness of breath that restrict his activity. Gradually the pains increase in frequency and severity, and the man consults his physician, who makes the diagnosis of unstable angina and admits him to the hospital. Aggressive efforts to relieve the recurring episodes of chest pain are not effective. Where does the doctor go from here? One response, depending on the patient's wishes, is to proceed with coronary catheterization and angiography and, depending on the results of the angiogram, follow with angioplasty or coronary bypass surgery.

Many individuals might be deeply disturbed at the notion of an elderly man undergoing catheterization, bypass surgery, the concomitant intensive care, and the associated rehabilitation process. Why all this high technology to solve a problem? Where is the caring in this approach? How can our nation afford to use its resources on an old man when infant mortality rates are too high, our public educational system is the subject of much concern, and the infrastructure of the country needs extensive repair? After all, we want to live good lives of high quality, not be kept alive forever.

The patient's physician, likewise, may have qualms about which course to recommend. There are a number of possible adverse outcomes no matter what is done or not done. Could this case turn into one of those horrible disasters where someone is kept on machines when there is no hope for functional recovery? Maybe it is this man's time to die. What if the family becomes impossible and unrealistic, threatening and hostile if the results are less than perfect? Would a transfer to the university hospital be the best course, because it has more specialists and more sophisticated technology than the local hospital? Health care costs are out of control; should a physician recommend such an expensive approach for this old man? Does a doctor have to offer every possible therapy to every person, regardless of the likely benefits and risks?

Appropriate provision of medical care and use of technology is becoming a burdensome issue in American medicine. With the fastest growing segment of the population consisting of those 85 years and older, and demographic projections anticipating 21 percent of the population will be over 65 years of age in 2030 (rather than the 1980 figure of 11 percent), the need for some clarity in making decisions about technology in medicine is urgent.[1] As the case example illustrates, a variety of questions may be raised in attempts to come to such decisions. Disparate pressures are building that make it very hard to define the issues, much less answer the questions. In a country where some individuals insist on maximal medical care and the utmost in aggressive technological intervention, others are demanding the right to receive physician assistance in the committing of suicide. The moral arguments appear too confused, too varied, and too emotional for any individual health care professional to practice in a rational and coherent manner.

Alasdair MacIntyre, in his book *After Virtue,* notes the difficulty of reaching agreement on moral arguments in our society.[2] MacIntyre has a number of reasons that he offers as to why this is the case. Among them is what he terms the "conceptual incommensurability" of alternate positions in moral debate. Competing premises can be followed through to conclusions that are valid, yet we are unable to discern the truth of the arguments or logically choose one argument as better than another. The purpose of this chapter is to clarify issues in the debate concerning health care technology, especially in the medical care of the elderly, with the goal of assisting health care professionals in evaluating the use of technology in their own practice. Beginning with MacIntyre is appropriate for several reasons. The arguments surrounding technology use display the kind of conceptual incommensurability that he describes as characteristic of contemporary moral argument. Appeals to emotion often lurk beneath the surface of what appears to be highly logical argumentation. MacIntyre suggests that the rational basis for moral decision making (and coherent moral society) lies in determining the consistency of various positions within a shared vision of our common purpose or ends. Although complete agreement on shared purpose is unlikely, I will argue that physicians and the elderly for whom they care can frequently recognize common ends and make reasonable decisions about the use of technology.

TECHNOLOGY AND HUMAN RELATIONSHIPS

There is a clear sense of dissatisfaction with American medicine—a feeling that doctors use too much technology and are not responsive to the needs and desires of those whom they should help. There is much that is accurate in this sense of dissatisfaction. It is, however, too facile in its criticism of technology. Physicians are not the sole culprit in the way technology is used in medical care, and a critique of technology that considers only what is new, expensive, and mechanical is naive. Such criticism neglects the pervasive use of all sorts of technology throughout our lives and the ways technology influences human relationships, including those between doctors and patients. Greater clarity about individual decisions regarding technological application requires considerations of our societal responsibilities and relationships.[3] A personal narrative may help to make this point.

In late August 1991, Hurricane Bob brushed the eastern coast of the United States before crashing into Rhode Island, southeastern Massachusetts, and Cape Cod. My parents' year-round home is on Cape Cod. I was on vacation that week and had planned to take my mother and father away for a few days up to northern New Hampshire. We left early on the morning that Hurricane Bob hit New England. The traffic leaving the Cape was bad, and long delays led us to be caught in the approaching storm. The ride was terrible—blinding rains, strong winds, flooding on the roadways. Doggedly, I kept on driving and we arrived after a seven-hour drive, two and a half hours more than normal. The day after the storm, my parents, watching the morning television news programs and seeing the pictures of damage, were horrified and decided that we must return to the Cape to see if their home had survived. Thankfully, the damage to the house itself was minor, but the devastation to the area was tremendous. Several trees littered our lawn. A portion of the garage had been removed by a falling tree. Power and telephone lines were knocked down. We were without electricity for four days.

Life changed. We went to bed by nine or ten, the flickering light of the candles not enough to allow reading. We awoke early with the return of the sun. The electric stove would not work. Food had to be eaten fresh and prepared over a fire. There was no phone to call friends and relatives. There was no television to distract us. The feeling of isolation was profound. My parents and I had to interact in a different way than was our custom. The daylight became our good time together, working outside repairing damage and removing debris. The evenings were difficult, with a hurried meal in a darkening house. As night wore on, we were without the distractions of television and forced to sit quietly together in the candlelight, with long pauses in our conversation. Without a phone to speak to family and friends, nor television to tell us what was happening, we felt cut off from the world. We were pushed in on ourselves, separated from others, and made to feel our dependence on nature.

The experience of my family and the effects of Hurricane Bob may seem unrelated to the topic of technology and its application to life-threatening crises. There are, however, two points that are germane. First, the effects of the storm emphasized the pervasive nature of technology in the lives of modern Americans. Life was radically changed without power or communications. Second, the storm revealed how technology mediates relationships between people in our society. The lack of television or other distractions forced my parents and me to converse and interact in a way that is not our habit. The evenings became a time to tell stories, sit quietly, and maybe try to read by candlelight. We interacted directly with each other, without the mediating influence of the television or some other device.

An appreciation of how our lives are intertwined with technology and how technology mediates personal relationships leads to a crucial insight. A critique of technology in medicine is deficient if it treats medicine in isolation from the technological style of the larger culture in which the practice of medicine is embedded. The way medicine is practiced in our culture is part of the way our society lives. The hurricane highlighted the fact that technology need not be complex, new, or expensive. A telephone, a stove, and a refrigerator are all common appliances that are examples of technology. Likewise, technology in medicine is not simply gleaming magnetic resonance imaging scanners and the sophisticated hardware of an intensive-care unit. Technology has many forms, and the variety of forms technology takes in medicine must be acknowledged before an analysis of its use in the treatment of the seriously ill can be considered.

In medicine, as in every aspect of our lives, technology mediates relationships between individuals. A patient's visit to a physician involves a direct, personal encounter. The doctor speaks with the patient, learning the reason for the visit and asking questions to clarify the patient's complaint. There is a physical examination, with the doctor touching and probing the patient. The visit concludes with more conversation and with the doctor suggesting a course of action to be followed. But the encounter with the physician is rarely one of simply conversation and the touch of a physical examination. Instead, blood pressure is taken with a sphygmomanometer, eyes are inspected with an ophthalmoscope, ears examined with an otoscope, and heart and lungs auscultated with a stethoscope. An electrocardiogram may be done, and chances are the physician will have a sample of blood drawn for analysis. There may be X-rays taken or some other diagnostic imaging study performed. Frequently, the patient will receive a prescription to alleviate symptoms or cure the problem. The relationship between two people, doctor and patient, occurs not just through conversation and touch but through the mediation of diagnostic and therapeutic equipment of various kinds and the provision of a pharmaceutical preparation.

It may seem strange to refer to a simple office visit as a technological encounter. Recognition of the technological nature of even this basic interaction, however, may make it easier to be more discerning when considering the uses of the more complex and expensive machinery commonly mentioned in discussions of medical technology.[4] Technology changes the medical encounter. Listening to a patient's heart with a stethoscope is far different from pressing an ear against a patient's chest. A simple visit to the doctor for a routine complaint is filled with technology, even if it is familiar and not very flashy. Similarly, the use of so-called high-tech devices and procedures like ventilators or cardiac catheterizations still occurs within the context of a relationship between a doctor and a patient. To blame technology for the difficult problems we face in its application to the seriously ill misses the point. Technological interaction is the stuff of our society. What happened in the hurricane is only a rudimentary example of how our lives in this country are mediated by technology. The recognition of how pervasive technology is throughout medicine suggests that some of the dissatisfaction felt with medical care is not so much the fault of technology as of the quality of the relationship between doctor and patient.

Unfortunately, the use of technology can so dominate the encounter that it becomes the technical rather than the human that seems essential in the interaction. Again, this is not the exclusive problem of medicine. The hurricane forced me to relate to my parents on a different level because of the absence of distractions. There was no television to be our companion, and so we were forced to focus on each other. From the example of the hurricane, one can consider two types of relational styles. One could be called the personal, where people interact with each other. In the other type, the focus is on technology and the personal relationship serves only as an entree to the technological. It is not only in medicine that relationships meant to be personal and intimate are somehow changed for the worse by technology. In the evenings, families may sit together in front of the television. For some families, the TV serves as the focus to draw them together and provide common entertainment. In others, the TV itself is the focus of interaction, and individual family members exist together watching the screen but not conversing or speaking in any meaningful way with each other.

Likewise, in medicine, the use of technology can eliminate the personal. Going back to the example of the 84-year-old man with chest pains, his condition might evoke two different responses from his physician. The physician might begin by taking a careful history and performing a physical examination, judiciously supplemented by diagnostic and therapeutic interventions. The other response would be to truncate the history and physical examination and launch a diagnostic cascade: an electrocardiogram, a cardiac catheterization, and, depending on the result of these tests, an angioplasty or coronary bypass surgery. In any adequate evaluation of chest pain, much of the interaction involves technology. The use of these tests and therapeutic measures saves lives and lowers morbidity in certain instances. A diagnostic and treatment plan that uses technology as part of an ongoing interaction and conversation between physician and patient, however, is different from diagnosis and treatment based on tests and technical interventions. In the former, the individual is treated, whereas in the latter, one is treating the results of tests. In any given case, the end result may be the same but the doctor-patient relationship is fundamentally different: It changes from an encounter mediated by technology to an encounter that is primarily technological. The patient and physician do not interact so much as the patient becomes a kind of raw material for the technology to process.

The human outcome of these two types of encounters differs and reveals two possibilities for the place of technology in doctor-patient relationships: Technology can be used at the service of a doctor-patient relationship or technology can direct the encounter between doctor and patient. When a doctor interacts with a patient with care and attention for the individual, the two people are involved in a relationship that has as its goal the patient's well-being and health. (*Well-being* and *health* are admittedly vague terms, but I will not further define them.) The interaction between doctor and patient where the approach is not personal but a routine application of tests and treatments does not preclude taking the patient's well-being and health as a goal. It is, however, a relationship primarily directed toward producing a result—health—through the application of technological means. The patient may be made better by the application of technology, but the consequences are not always so benign. The physician has related not to the patient but rather to a symptom complex that, despite possibly superb and timely interventions, may remain problematic. The result is unsatisfactory. In a patient-oriented interaction, the nature of the relationship, which is geared toward well-being and improving function, provides the opportunity for a variety of personal responses by the two individuals despite an outcome that is not the one desired. In the interaction that relies on technology rather than personal relationship, a failure to cure means a failure in the relationship.

The replacement of personal encounter with technology is not solely the fault of physicians. Many patients labor under an illusion that the application of sophisticated diagnostic tests means they are being well cared for by their physician. Others feel that all medical problems require an aggressive technological approach and demand such care. Frequent and often vehement requests by a patient with chronic headaches for a computerized tomography (CT) scan to rule out a brain tumor, in the absence of clinical signs or historical details associated with brain neoplasms, is an example familiar to most practicing physicians. A suggestion that the headache may be related to difficulties at home or work may cause such a patient to "fire" the doctor if he or she will not perform the diagnostic study demanded. Patients, perhaps as much as physicians, are reluctant to enter into a personal relationship. Given that technology serves to distance people even within families, this reluctance to establish a personal relationship with a stranger is not surprising. Many assume that technology will clarify diagnosis and therapy, whereas careful history taking and suggestions about changes in one's lifestyle are perceived as a waste of time and an affront to privacy. There may be little appreciation that diagnostic testing, although providing more information, need not clarify treatment or prognosis. Diagnostic testing can, ironically, actually add to ambiguity by providing results that not only do little to change therapeutic options but actually confuse the clinical picture.

The strength of a personal type of doctor-patient relationship lies in its potential to deal with ambiguity and failure. The skillful application of technology does not guarantee a happy outcome. When one confronts care at the end of life, ambiguity frequently becomes an important element of the doctor-patient relationship no matter how skilled the physician. It may not be clear when someone will die, why they are doing poorly, what the results of sophisticated diagnostic tests mean prognostically, nor what treatment option, if any, is the best. The lack of a clear indication as to what is "the right thing to do" is a not uncommon event.

Physicians now practice medicine in a climate where decisions to institute, withhold, or withdraw life-sustaining technology are not limited to the patient-doctor relationship but are part of larger disputes within society. Many see medical technology as the culprit in current problems with the health care system. Our confusion about what to do with the use of technology in medicine, our difficulty in establishing priorities in health care, and our increasing demands for assisted suicide and euthanasia reflect underlying societal issues. In the past, physicians' decisions occurred within a framework of a relatively narrow group of treatment options that gave some promise of benefit. For many conditions, however, there was nothing that could be done and death could not be forestalled. We are now in the position of being able, in many cases, to hold death in abeyance even though our abilities to alter the underlying disease process or restore function to the sick person are limited.

The heart of the critique of the technological nature of American medicine lies in our fears as to what will happen to us when we become sick. More frightening than death is the contemplation of serious illness. Americans are afraid that technology will be used indiscriminately in their care rather than as a tool in the doctor-patient relationship. All of us are uneasy with the possibility of suffering alone without hope for the future. Most of us worry about being artificially maintained without any prospect of recovery. We fear that our physical pain will not be adequately treated. We are anxious over the possibility of decline and isolation. There is a mistrust of American medicine—of its commitment to limit suffering and not abandon the chronically sick to illness and death. Limiting the suffering of an individual and not abandoning him or her to illness cannot be accomplished merely by technological means. It requires the personal commitment of one person to another. Technology will inevitably be brought to bear in the encounter between doctor and patient, but suffering and isolation can only be relieved by compassion and personal contact.

Despite the best of medical care, we will all die. Our deaths may occur suddenly or after a brief period of illness, but for some there will be a long period of sickness, a chronic decline, and a gradual loss of function. Suffering can be of many kinds. The most obvious is related to physical pain. Less obvious but not less pernicious is the kind of suffering caused by the loss of independence, or the diminished ability to see and hear, or a combination of illness and frailty that results in isolation and loneliness. The varieties of suffering are multiple. Technology has a role in the treatment of suffering but only an instrumental role. Recall the example of the hurricane. Those in its wake were forced to confront each other. There was no longer a reassuring television to relate to. Instead, there were other people and dark nights and no telephones. One was thrown back on one's creatureliness: Notions of independence and the sense of removal from the natural world were radically challenged. Likewise, the experience of suffering strips an individual and forces reliance on others. A medical relationship based on technological interaction provides little succor in situations where cure is not possible, chronic illness results, and the experience of suffering becomes the major issue in the patient's life. A personal relationship with a physician provides the opportunity for relief of suffering through human interaction as well as the use of technology.

Relationship or not, when facing serious illness and the end of life, we are facing a situation laden with ambiguity. We all face decline and death but we do not know how or when or under what circumstances. The medical treatment we receive may cause us to live longer and in relative comfort or it may leave us simply lingering. We hope for care that is truly caring, attentive to our needs, our pain, and our loneliness. But we fear being left alone, either abandoned to illness without adequate medical attention or the recipient of medical care that is highly technical, depersonalized, and dehumanizing. We recognize that even with the best doctors and nurses there is no guarantee of good outcome. There remains the numbing and often suppressed knowledge that death cannot be denied. This seems to be our peculiar condition at the end of the twentieth century: We fear death and we fear what may be done to keep us living. Medical technology can extend our lives but sometimes it prolongs our lives beyond bearing. Death, to paraphrase Samuel Johnson, remarkably focuses our attention. Who will care for us and how will they show that care as we age and face the limits of our own mortality?

TECHNOLOGY, RELATIONSHIPS, AND CARING FOR THE ELDERLY

A crucial question is the meaning of caring in the use of technology. *Caring* is a word that can be much abused. It can be used to refer to sentimentality and to warm feelings that have little substance. Caring that is substantial and nontrivial is more hard-nosed: It is an attitude that lets caregivers face the patients who come their way, both successful agers and end-stage Alzheimer's patients, with a combination of technical excellence and compassion. Daniel Callahan's *Setting Limits* and *What Kind of Life?* have received much attention and acclaim for their proposals regarding health care, technology, medical expenditures, and care of the elderly.[5] According to Callahan, health expenditures should be directed toward the prevention of premature death and palliative care for those with chronic illness. After a reasonable life span, resources should not be directed to life extension or the curing of illness but to caring and limiting pain. Callahan, however, is mistaken in his views that caring is an inherently more limited venture than efforts aimed directly at cure.

The medical care of older persons is both challenging and poignant because of the unavoidable backdrop of mortality. There are instances where death is seen as a blessing, but it is also an occasion of apprehension and sorrow. Caring for those who, because of advancing years or progressive illness, are approaching the end of their lives requires a sensitivity to the fear that dying may provoke.[6] There is frequent unease caused by the recognition that one's time on this earth is coming to an end. Some elderly people fear that they will be abandoned to their fate and left to die alone. Physicians can be compassionate companions of the patients who struggle with these fears but they cannot cure them. The existential terror that such a recognition may trigger is not one that can be resolved by drugs, or technology, or resources other than those within the individual and those people and things that give meaning to the individual's life.

The clinician's obligation to limit suffering and not abandon patients may be best seen against the backdrop of these fears. Doctors can limit the suffering caused by confrontation with our existential finitude but cannot end it, unless they so drug their patients that self-consciousness is abolished. However, doctors can not only show compassion in the face of existential suffering but also use their skills and resources to control physical pain and not leave a patient abandoned. Abandonment can take a variety of forms. The most obvious would be neglecting an individual and leaving him or her alone to suffer. Abandonment can also be more subtle. A physician may well be physically present but not responsive to a patient's suffering. In the case of an older patient, this may take the form of easy assumptions about conditions not being treatable in the elderly, and consequent neglect of therapies that might have a chance of maintaining or restoring function. Conversely, a type of abandonment may occur when some physicians resort to a relentless high-technology diagnostic and therapeutic onslaught rather than carefully assessing the patient's wishes and best interests given the probable outcomes. The physician's commitment to limit suffering and not abandon is twofold. First, prior to the use of specifically medical knowledge, there must be sympathy for the patient as a person who is likely frightened and in pain. Second, medical skill and use of various therapeutic options ought to be directed toward the provision of care that relieves symptoms, restores function to the extent possible, and is consistent with the desires of the patient.

Callahan does an excellent job in establishing the attitude of caring that is prior to the distribution of resources. There is no doubt of his abundant compassion and good will in wishing that pain and suffering be limited: "At the center of caring should be a commitment never to avert its eyes from, or wash its hands of, someone who is in pain or is suffering, who is disabled or incompetent, who is retarded or demented; that is the most fundamental demand made upon us."[7] Callahan's thesis is that medical care has gone awry in a hunt for progress that emphasizes technological achievement rather than attending to personal caring. Our society is threatened by the growing burdens of health care cost, a burden fueled by unwholesome and unrealistic expectations that medicine can keep us young, restore health, and make us whole and vital regardless of age or illness.

Callahan's vision of health care for the elderly rests on his belief that aging individuals have life goals and sources of meaning that are specific to them as the elders of society. The elderly have a role in society that gives them meaning and respect:

> It should be the special role of the elderly to be the moral conservators of that which has been and the most active proponents of that which will be after they are no longer here. Their indispensable role as conservators is what generates what I believe ought to be the *primary* aspiration of the old, which is to serve the young and the future. Just as they were once the heirs of a society built by others, who passed on to them what they needed to keep it going, so are they likewise

> obliged to do the same for those who will follow them.[8]

The elderly deserve care. But older persons need to depart the stage of this life gracefully and not be caught up in an unseemly struggle to maintain their lives without regard for the society around them. Medicine must scale back its technological repertoire, not seek new cures and technologies and limit access to some therapies based on age.

Unfortunately, Callahan's discussion of caring is laced with unfair indictments of medicine and physicians: "Caring is just not the trait that is emphasized for physicians the way medical knowledge is. The technical skills they deploy are impersonal, directed to organ and system failures, not to the particularities of individual suffering."[9] Callahan overlooks the integral nature of the technical skills and resources used in caring for the particularities of individual suffering. Being a caring, competent doctor frequently requires the use of technology in ways that will limit a patient's suffering and not leave him or her abandoned to the experience of illness and ultimately death. Caring involves a willingness to listen to the patient's fears and suffering and to develop a response that will help that patient as a person who is requesting care. Sometimes that response will be emotional support; at other times it will involve medications and treatments for the underlying illnesses that create suffering and limit function. Sometimes it will involve aggressive therapy using invasive high technology because the alternative is a lingering and unhappy death. The technical side of caring requires considerable ingenuity; it is a response to the seemingly infinite variety of suffering that afflicts individuals. Callahan misses the point. For him "the individual need for cure is infinite in its possibilities, the need for caring is much more finite—there is always something we can do for each other. The possibilities of caring are, in that respect, far more self-contained than the possibilities of curing."[10] This statement is incoherent. If "there is always something we can do for each other," does that not imply an infinity of possibilities?

Callahan falsely believes that caring (without a curative intent) is a relatively circumscribed clinical exercise whereas treatment with curative intent means an infinite variety of expensive, aggressive, and often futile measures. Callahan reduces all doctor-patient relationships to a technological mode of encounter and ignores that the personal relationship can still employ high technology in delivering care. Part of acting rightly as a physician is listening to what patients say about what hurts them and makes their lives hard.

When the 84-year-old man in the example at the beginning of the chapter first went to see his physician, the physician was undoubtedly able to hear the suffering and fear that his relentless chest pain caused. Suffering in this instance has a face on it, the face of this old man. He knows the risk of myocardial infarction, and he may well state that he does not want to be in pain nor short of breath but that he is not afraid of dying. The physician knows that the myocardial infarction may not kill this man but may leave him debilitated and limit his ability to be independent. This is not the "greedy geezer" of ageist mythology who is somehow sapping the lifeblood of the young and living the high life on his Social Security check. How might the physician try to limit his suffering and not abandon him to myocardial ischemia and the specter of ongoing pain, infarction, and congestive heart failure? The physician could use his or her personal skill and knowledge and available social resources and recommend that the man proceed with cardiac catheterization and angioplasty or bypass grafting, depending on the results of the catheterization. Is this curing or caring? The man will die in a matter of years even if the operation is successful, so there should be no illusion that the physician is robbing the grim reaper. The physician should also realize, however, that unstable angina, recurrent myocardial infarction, and congestive heart failure are probably grimmer than death. Precipitous decline and loss of function with an unpleasant lingering period at death's door are hard to deal with, both emotionally and financially. Caring means the physician can sympathize with this man in his humanity, recognize the suffering caused by his illness, and be aware that unless aggressive treatment is offered the patient will be abandoned to a fate he finds intolerable and very few would want.

All the elderly who are sent to surgery for coronary bypass grafting, vascular reconstruction, prosthetic heart valves, and artificial joints will die one day. Myocardial ischemia, peripheral vascular disease, congestive heart failure, hip fractures, and degenerative joint disease are common sources of suffering in older patients. This inevitable fact of mortality does not imply that the appropriate response is to hold patients' hands and give analgesics while they experience myocardial infarction, suffer the pain of ischemic ulcers and gangrene, struggle with pulmonary edema, or become bedbound and crippled. Effective caring attempts to aid individuals by letting them know that resources and support are available for care, rehabilitation, and aggressive therapy if such provide some promise of relieving physical distress. There is no sharp dichotomy between caring and curing, nor is caring an inevitably more limited venture. Callahan's comment that the technical skills of physicians are often impersonally directed to organ systems rather than "the particularities of individual suffering" neglects the truth that the relief of suffering by physicians requires technical skills and resources to be directed toward the treatment of malfunctioning organs in an effort to render the whole person well.

CONCLUSION

The responsible use of technology in the care of the elderly is linked to our ability to emphasize the personal in doctor-patient relationships. Neither a reflexive use of high-technology equipment nor an automatic rejection of it on the basis of age is an appropriate response. This conclusion seemingly begs the question of the limits of technology use. Does a personal relationship between doctor and patient justify anything and everything in health care? No, but it sets the framework for what will be used by allowing decision making to be a shared process. Physicians need to cultivate the ability to speak with their patients about their wishes regarding life-sustaining technology. They should not reduce decision making to a process of mechanically fulfilling patient wishes but must supply the information that can make those wishes truly informed. Technology is not a list of items on a medical menu that are chosen at will. Rather, technology serves as a means to assist the doctor and patient in recognizing the patient's values and goals in health care. Within the context of the care of the elderly, physicians must determine two things: what nonabandonment and limiting suffering mean for each patient and the appropriate ways, personal and technological, to provide personal, attentive care.

This does not mean that there will be an end to societal conflict or that individual decision making will become easy. Some physicians will not be able to communicate with their patients and ascertain their goals and values. Other doctors will lack the prudence to choose wisely from the available technologies, the ones that provide real promise for assisting the elderly. Some older people will adopt an attitude that demands the aggressive use of all sorts of high-technology equipment regardless of the cost to themselves in terms of pain or suffering or the cost to other members of society because of the associated high price tag. One can describe a number of possible shortcomings. The underlying theme, however, of this chapter is that personal relationships and meaningful communication between individuals remain a possibility. In the context of those relationships and attempts to communicate, patients can talk to their doctors about what it is like to grow old, what they want from life, what they fear, and how they want to be cared for when their life is threatened by illness. Although there will remain questions, obscurity, and ambiguity, clarifying these basic questions will go a long way toward putting technology in its appropriate place in the relationship between the doctor and the older patient: as a tool for limiting suffering and providing the type of care the patient desires.

NOTES

1. B. J. Soldo and K. G. Manton, "Demography: Characteristics and Implications of an Aging Population," *Geriatric Medicine,* 2d ed., ed. J. W. Rowe and R. W. Besdine (Boston: Little, Brown, 1988).
2. A. MacIntyre, *After Virtue,* 2d ed. (Notre Dame, Ind.: University of Notre Dame Press, 1984).
3. P. R. Wolpe, "Medicine, Technology, and Lived Relations," *Perspectives in Biology and Medicine* 28 (1985): 314–22. Although I take a very different approach in this chapter and develop themes independently, I am indebted to Wolpe for his observations regarding the links between society, technology, medicine, and the physician-patient relationship.
4. M. MacGregor, "Technology and the Allocation of Resources," *New England Journal of Medicine* 320 (1989): 118–20.
5. D. Callahan, *Setting Limits* (New York: Simon and Schuster, 1987); D. Callahan, *What Kind of Life?* (New York: Simon and Schuster, 1990).
6. E. P. Seravalli, "The Dying Patient, The Physician, and the Fear of Death," *New England Journal of Medicine* 319 (1988): 1728–30.
7. Callahan, *What Kind of Life?* 145.
8. Callahan, *Setting Limits*, 43.
9. Callahan, *What Kind of Life?* 148.
10. Ibid., 145.

Chapter 41

Ethically Important Distinctions among Managed Care Organizations*

Kate T. Christensen

Due to society's need to control health care costs and the failure of legislated health care reform, managed care is expanding at a rapid rate and will soon be the predominate form of health care delivery.[1] When we take into account the growing momentum to bring Medicare and Medicaid under managed care,[2] it is apparent that managed care is a reality that most health care providers and patients will face, in one form or another.

The term *managed care* describes a diverse set of organizational forms. Wide variations in approach, financing, physician involvement, and philosophy exist among the different types of managed care organizations (MCOs). While many articles on the ethics of managed care acknowledge this variety, most analyses focus on the for-profit entities, paying less attention to the ethical distinctions among the different forms of managed care.[3] This paper discusses the key distinctions among MCO types, in particular the difference between for-profit and nonprofit plans, the relationship of the physician to the MCO, the incentives used to control costs, the incentives that improve patient care, and the organizational features that nurture the principled practice of medicine.

KEY DISTINCTIONS AMONG MCOs

For-Profit versus Nonprofit Managed Care

Although MCOs come in a bewildering array of structures, three crucial distinctions can be made among them: profit status, the relationship of physicians to the organization, and the nature of the capitation arrangement. The most important difference is between for-profit and nonprofit health plans. For-profit plans make up the fastest growing segment of the managed care market, are growing at a much faster rate than the nonprofits, and receive most of the business news attention.[4] Although all MCOs must generate surplus revenue to continue to operate, for-profit plans differ from nonprofit in that they trade their shares publicly and are not governed by the rules of charitable organizations.[5] As a result, their administrative costs as a percentage of total income tend to be much higher.

For-profit administrative costs often include extraordinarily large chief executive officer (CEO) salaries and bonuses, dividends to shareholders, and cash reserves for acquisition of competitors.[6] A 1994 survey in California, where 85 percent of the insured population belongs to a managed care plan, revealed a wide range between the total administrative expenses of MCOs. These expenses ran as high as 30.9 percent of total revenue in the for-profit MCOs,

---

*Based on an article in the *Journal of Law, Medicine & Ethics*, December 1995.

Source: Reprinted with permission from K. Christensen, Ethically Important Distinctions Among Managed Care Organizations, *Journal of Law, Medicine & Ethics,* Vol. 23, pp. 223–229, © 1995, American Society of Law, Medicine & Ethics.

but only 3.1 percent in the nonprofit organizations, like Kaiser Foundation Health Plan.[7] Other not-for-profit health plans also tend to have a larger share of income devoted to health services and a smaller profit/income ratio.[8] A more recent study by the California Medical Association of that state's health maintenance organizations (HMOs) demonstrated a similar trend: The largest portion of revenue spent on medical care was found in the nonprofit plans.[9]

This difference becomes ethically relevant when we consider the pressure on physicians to limit health care costs. Subscriber premiums or dues are set by the marketplace, and, because of direct competition between plans, the costs of the different plans tend to lie within a narrow range. Therefore, in order to create more profit for shareholders, the surplus is generated elsewhere. Part of it comes from reducing the amount spent on doctors, tests, treatments, and hospitalization.[10] Corner cutting, or erring on the side of doing less instead of more, is the feature of managed care that engenders the most concern. All MCOs keep costs down by decreasing the amount of money spent on unnecessary treatment or visits, making health care delivery more efficient. But between the area of clearly unnecessary treatment and the clearly necessary there is a margin of uncertainty. It stands to reason that physicians in an MCO that has both less to spend on patient care and stockholders to please will be under more pressure to keep this margin as narrow as possible.[11]

In one major review published in *Consumer Reports* in August 1996, the public came down solidly in favor of the nonprofit MCOs.[12] *Consumer Reports* polled more than 30,000 readers who were members of HMOs and preferred provider organizations (PPOs) for their opinions of their health plans, examined the data available comparing quality of care, and compared how tightly the various MCOs restricted physician discretion in patient care decisions. The top 11 plans were all not-for-profit, and the bottom of the list was made up of for-profit MCOs. Only future research will tell us whether such practices are also having a negative impact on clinical outcomes in patient care, such as rehospitalization rates and asthma mortality.[13]

Physicians and the MCO

Incentives

The second relevant distinction between MCO types is the relationship of the physician to the organization,[14] which manifests itself in the various incentives used to control patient care costs.[15] For physicians, incentives can influence their professional autonomy as well as their practice stability and quality of professional work life, which in turn impacts the quality of patient care in a variety of ways.[16]

All health care delivery systems have financial incentives that can influence physician behavior. Under the traditional fee-for-service (FFS) model, physicians are rewarded financially for overtreating patients.[17] And, because many patients believe that more health care is better health care, physicians have a further incentive to keep patients happy by doing more. This system (along with technological advances and increased public expectations) has led to spiraling health care costs and, at times, iatrogenic harm to patients. Few tests or procedures are entirely risk free, and incidental findings can cause unnecessary anxiety as well as further tests or procedures. Although FFS allows physicians more practice and administrative autonomy than any other system, this system is rapidly withering in the face of the massive growth and consolidation of MCOs, as well as the cost-containment measures to limit Medicare and Medicaid reimbursements. Many FFS physicians are now contracting with a variety of MCOs.[18]

For many years, Kaiser Permanente was the only large-scale private alternative to FFS in the United States. Now MCOs include a growing array of reimbursement and health care delivery systems. Many MCOs offer a number of different products to enrollees and employers, giving each a choice from a menu of managed care and traditional indemnity plans. The basic forms currently are the independent practice associations (IPAs), preferred provider organizations (PPOs), the

Table 41–1 The Financial Relationship of the Physician to the MCO

Practice Type	*Relationship of Physician to MCO*	*Physician Payment*	*Physician Involvement in Quality Assurance/ Utilization Review*
PPO	Physicians contract with MCO	Discounted FFS	High
IPA/network	Physicians contract with MCOs through IPA	Usually capitation	High
Group model	Group contracts with MCO	Capitation to group; salary with various incentives	High
Staff model	Physician is employee of MCO	Salary with various incentives	Low

group model HMOs (like Kaiser Permanente), and the staff model HMOs.

PPO physicians contract with the MCO and are usually paid on a FFS basis (see Table 41–1).[19] Fees are usually discounted deeply by the health plan, and, as a result, many FFS physicians have experienced declining incomes in the last five years.[20] Physicians in PPOs typically have contracts with a number of different MCOs and some indemnity plans. Because these physicians are still paid per service rendered, an inherent incentive arises to generate more health care costs by seeing patients more often and/or by ordering more tests and interventions (see Table 41–2).[21] These physicians also are exposed to sudden changes in their relationships with the health plan, such as contract termination and the subsequent loss of covered patients. Therefore, income security is lowest for this group of physicians, in particular for the subspecialists. Physicians in IPAs also contract with one or more MCOs, but are given organizational coherence and negotiating power by the IPA. They are usually reimbursed on a capitated basis.[22]

In the group model HMO, the physician is part of a group that contracts with the health plan.[23] Instead of receiving a fee for each service rendered, the group is paid a capitated amount by the health plan in advance of providing patient care services. The physicians are typically paid a basic salary plus a variety of financial incentives, such as bonuses. In contrast, physicians in staff model HMOs are employees of the MCO. They are salaried and are also paid a

Table 41–2 Spectrum of Physician Incentives*

	Traditional FFS	*Managed Care*
Compensation	Fee per service rendered	Fee per person enrolled (capitation)
General incentive	Do more, get more	Do less, get more
Examples of specific financial incentives	Direct reimbursement for patient care; income from laboratory or radiology services, partnership in hospital	Withhold part of income; capitation, direct or diffused; bonuses; threat of deselection

*This table is abstract, in that it does not take into account the many variations on these basic themes among MCOs.

variety of incentives—similar to group model physicians—designed to promote cost-effective medical care. Job security is often low in this group because of the employee status of the physicians. Some predict that the majority of physicians will be working for staff model HMOs in the future.[24]

Financial incentives common to many MCOs are the payment of bonuses from any unspent funds and withholding of portions of income, which may be paid out at the end of the year if certain cost-containment targets are met. Such targets may include keeping hospital utilization below a certain rate or limiting referrals to specialists. The larger the amount of the withheld income, the stronger the incentive to toe the line.[25] Laboratory and radiology costs are frequently deducted from the pooled funds as well.[26] In all but the group model HMOs, the threat of job loss or loss of one's patients also serves as a potent incentive to adhere to the MCO's rules.

Control over Clinical Practice: Utilization Review and Practice Guidelines

Another significant aspect of the relationship of physicians to MCOs is the degree of control physicians have over the administrative and clinical aspects of their practices. In IPAs and PPOs, income security may be low but physician autonomy over medical practice is high because physicians retain much of the traditional FFS prerogatives and practice format. Although practice autonomy is more restricted in group model HMOs than in IPAs or PPOs, physicians in IPAs, PPOs, and group model HMOs typically manage their own utilization review, quality assurance, and cost controls. Practice autonomy is usually lowest in the staff model HMOs, where utilization review and cost controls are usually managed and implemented by health plan administrators. Experience to date indicates that when control over the clinical aspects of practice rests with nonphysician administrators, the quality of patient care is threatened and physician morale plummets.[27]

Many physicians are happy to relinquish administrative responsibility for their medical practices, but are uncomfortable with losing control over the clinical aspects, such as utilization and quality management. Physicians in MCOs know that utilization review can be benign or malignant, depending on who is doing it and to what end. This is the nightmare of utilization review: A stranger in another city, who has no clinical experience, calls the doctor and tells her to discharge a patient, or denies approval for a test the physician deems necessary. When used in this way, utilization review can function as a barrier to patient care.[28] Physicians' job stress can be significantly increased by having to negotiate these hurdles on behalf of their patients.[29] That situation also raises a direct conflict of interest between physicians' duty to provide good patient care and their own financial well-being.[30]

However, when managed and implemented by physicians, utilization review can both promote better patient care (by minimizing unnecessary treatments or hospital stays) and save money. Utilization review should not put up barriers to good patient care, and, in the hands of physicians, it is less likely to do so.[31]

Similarly, practice guidelines can be imposed on physicians, as in many staff model MCOs, or developed and implemented by physicians, as in the group model MCOs.[32] When used inappropriately, such guidelines are applied as standards to measure, reward, and punish physician behavior.[33] But with physician involvement, this process serves as a useful extension of peer review and helps to maintain a high quality of care. When physicians are involved in the development and implementation of the guidelines, it is less likely that they will mistake guidelines for standards (which require more stringent outcomes studies and stricter enforcement)[34] and inappropriately use the guidelines to reward and punish.

Capitation

Another useful distinction among MCOs is the way members' premiums are distributed to the physicians.[35] Capitation forms the core financial process in all of the systems discussed above. In a capitated system, the pool of funds for the provision of services is collected by the health plan and then distributed in various ways, often called *risk sharing*. Some plans give a physician group the money (less administrative costs and, if applicable, profit), and the money is kept in a central pool to pay for health care services. Other plans give the funds to the physicians, or to small physician groups, and the physicians then keep whatever is left at the end of the period (monthly, quarterly, or yearly). The more individualized the capitation arrangement is in relation to the physician, the greater the ethical strain on his or her relationship with the patient.[36] For example, if a physician in a large group with a centralized fund orders an MRI to evaluate a young woman for multiple sclerosis, cost will not be a primary concern, because it is spread out over the group. If that same physician orders the MRI and the money comes out of his or her own capitated fund, it directly impacts that physician's income. The temptation to assign a heart murmur a benign status or to forgo a cardiology consult is greater if every penny spent comes out of the physician's own pocket. Most conscientious physicians will resist this temptation, but it injects an unnecessary "ethical stress" into the clinical encounter and may, in some cases, influence treatment decisions to the detriment of good patient care. Many HMOs now shy away from such direct capitation and instead capitate physicians as a group.

CONSEQUENCES OF MANAGED CARE FINANCIAL INCENTIVES

What are the possible consequences of capitation and other financial inducements to physicians to control costs? The most widely discussed is the temptation to withhold needed services.[37] Whether this really happens is hard to prove and has not been supported in the few studies that have examined it.[38] However, anecdotes about harm to patients from undertreatment abound, and this issue remains a primary concern of those who study managed care.[39] It may also be that a disincentive arises to retain ill patients in one's health plan or patient panel, as they will tend to cost more than they (or their employers) pay into the plan. This could endanger the care of patients with complex chronic illnesses, such as acquired immune deficiency syndrome (AIDS).[40]

The beneficial impact of managed care incentives includes the reduction of wasteful treatments, less iatrogenic harm to patients because of the avoidance of unnecessary tests and procedures, more emphasis on preventive care, the potential for better case management of very ill patients in an integrated setting,[41] and cost savings.[42] All of these benefits result in improvements in the quality of the care provided under managed care.[43] Although the degree of cost savings under managed care also has been contested,[44] this is the aspect of managed care that has propelled it to the forefront of health care delivery systems.

So far, I have focused primarily on the financial relationships that are intended to influence physician behavior and to decrease health care costs. But physicians are influenced by nonfinancial considerations as well.[45] What kinds of incentives exist that may balance or buffer the temptation to limit treatment for the physician's own pecuniary benefit?

The strongest forces that balance the temptation to undertreat are the principles most physicians acquired in medical school.[46] The most important and pervasive principle is the professional duty to benefit, and not to harm, their patients. Applying this principle in traditional FFS would counteract the temptation to overtreat. Under managed care, physicians will be less likely to withhold necessary treatments if their primary allegiance is to the patient's well-being.[47] Next in importance is the maintenance of the physician's professional and personal integrity, which again requires that they prevent harm to their patients. The approval of one's colleagues also exerts a strong effect on the behavior of many physicians and is why peer review is such a powerful tool to change physician behavior. If the philosophy and practice of the physician group reflect the primacy of good patient care over all other considerations, it is less likely that patients will suffer under managed care.[48] Reinforcing these principles in medical school and residency will be an important factor in maintaining good patient care as practiced in the managed care setting.

Health systems have mechanisms for reinforcing the principle of beneficence and for maintaining high-quality patient care, such as peer review and practice guidelines. These mechanisms, for example, give the physician feedback if he or she is not providing the quality of care that colleagues expect, or let a physician know, for example, if he or she is not ordering enough mammograms or vaccinations. The threat of malpractice is a reality in all treatment settings, and it can both promote overtreatment in FFS and deter undertreatment in managed care (see Table 41–3). State and federal regulations, and future legislation, are also having an impact on MCO incentives and policies.[49] Finally, if health plan subscribers are educated and involved in their health care, they may be less likely to accept inadequate care and more likely to understand the financial trade-offs involved in every health care decision.

THE ETHICAL HMO

Enumerating ethical principles and good practices is not enough to help us identify those organizations that are best suited to promote the provision of health care in an atmosphere relatively untainted by financial conflicts of interest. Many authors have developed important and useful guidelines and principles for MCOs,[50] but I would like to summarize from the above discussion the structural features of health care organizations that nurture and reinforce the best principles of medical practice. MCO structure determines in large part the nature of the conflicts providers within it have to face, and can also impact the quality of the care delivered.[51] For example, preauthorization requirements for hospitalization or emergency care are a structural barrier to good patient care.[52] A direct financial incentive to reduce hospital admissions is an ethical hurdle the physician must overcome to keep the patient's welfare foremost.

What would an MCO look like were it structured to buffer or neutralize the incentive to undertreat patients and to maximize the incentives to provide quality medical care? What features should we look for in evaluating the degree of ethical stress a physician experiences in providing health care in different practice settings?

- The organization should be nonprofit.[53] This removes the shareholder and profit maximization as the bottom line, which theoretically puts less pressure on the physician to meet financial goals (as opposed to patient outcome goals).
- To remove the cash register from the examination room, physician income should primarily come from a salary.[54] Divorcing the individual patient encounter from the physician's immediate income helps to focus the encounter on meeting the patient's

Table 41–3 Forces That Balance the Negative Consequences of Managed Care Incentives

Principles of Practice
Desire to prevent harm from undertreatment (beneficence)
Professionalism/self-respect (integrity)
Desire for the respect of one's peers

External Forces
Treatment guidelines
Peer review
Fear of malpractice
Patient/member involvement
Regulation and legislation

needs and frees the physician to practice according to his or her professional principles. Group model and staff model HMOs both meet this ideal.

- Sharing the risk of capitation among a large group of physicians dilutes the temptation to cut corners inappropriately.[55] The manner in which capitated funds are distributed varies and influences the degree of conflict of interest that the physician experiences. Direct or individual capitation and linking financial incentives directly to cost-containment targets should be avoided.
- Clinical practice should be managed by physicians. Physicians should be centrally involved with utilization review, quality management, and the development and implementation of clinical practice guidelines. Utilization review should not serve as a barrier to providing health care services, and should focus on undertreatment as well as overtreatment.
- The patients or members of the MCO should have a role in the operations of the organization, at a number of levels.[56] First, subscribers should receive full disclosure from the health plan about any incentives to limit treatment and any restrictions on coverage. Second, MCOs need to find a mechanism to include health plan members in discussions of benefit coverage and conflict-resolution procedures. Third, community members should be involved in the ethics committees of managed care hospitals and organizational ethics committees of the health plans, where these committees exist.[57] Fourth, vigorous efforts at patient/member health education should be ongoing, both to improve the health of members and to improve their understanding of the financial trade-offs involved in treatment and benefit decisions. An educated member may be more likely to challenge unfair limits to treatment.

CONCLUSION

Managed care is not one entity but a broad category that includes a variety of health care delivery structures and practices, relationships with physicians, and physician incentives. While all managed care forms face the challenge of avoiding conflicts of interest leading to undertreatment, some are more challenged than others. Whether an MCO minimizes conflict of interest for physicians depends on the way it is organized and financed, the degree of physician involvement in managing patient care quality, and the nature of the incentives used to control costs. The form of managed care that currently works best to prevent undertreatment is one that is nonprofit and has a large salaried physician group that manages the clinical aspects of the provision of health care services.

Having drawn these distinctions, it is clear that managed care as a subject of study is a rapidly moving target. Nonprofit HMOs themselves are sorely challenged to compete with the for-profit entities.[58] All are taking measures to cut costs, and, in many instances, are adopting the methods of the for-profit HMOs.[59] If this trend continues, it is possible that the distinction between for-profit and nonprofit MCOs will blur. Moreover, for-profit organizations are rearranging themselves into new and unique forms at a rapid rate. Thus, as these new structures evolve, we must encourage the growth of those that foster the highest quality of patient care and physician satisfaction.

ACKNOWLEDGMENTS

I thank the following people for their generous contribution of ideas and comments: Robert Klein, M.D.; William Andereck, M.D.; Jim Rose; Francis J. Crosson, M.D.; Robert Erickson; Lawrence Schneiderman, M.D.; Bruce Merl, M.D.; Cecilia Runkle, Ph.D.; Art Rosenfeld, J.D.; Bernard Lo, M.D. The author is the Regional Ethics Coordinator and an internist with The Permanente Medical Group in Northern California.

The original article was based on a presentation given at "Managed Care Systems: Emerging Health Issues from an Ethics Perspective," sponsored by the Allina Foundation and the American Society of Law, Medicine & Ethics, Minneapolis, Minnesota, June 1995.

NOTES

1. M. A. Rodwin, *Medicine, Money & Morals: Physicians' Conflicts of Interest* (New York: Oxford, 1993), 17; J. Fletcher and C. Engelhard, "Ethical Issues in Managed Care," *Virginia Medicine Quarterly,* 122, no. 3 (1995): 162–67; M. Quint, "Health Plans Force Changes in the Way Doctors Are Paid," *New York Times,* 9 February 1995, sec. A1; A. S. Relman, "Medical Practice under the Clinton Reforms—Avoiding Domination by Business," *N. Engl. J. Med.*, 329, no. 21 (1993): 1574–76; M. Mitka, "HMOs See Steady Growth, Some Market Shifts," *American Medical News,* 1 May 1995, 9; V. Tabbush and G. Swanson, "Changing Paradigms in Medical Payment," *Arch. Int. Med.,* 156 (1996): 357–60.
2. M. Freudenheim, "Medicare, Jot This Down: Employers Offer Valuable Lessons on Saving Money with Managed Care," *New York Times,* 31 May 1995, sec. C1; J. Johnsson, "Medicare's Bumpy Ride into Private Sector," *American Medical News,* 12 June 1995, 1; A. Clymer, "An Accidental Overhaul: Major Revamping of Health Care System Could Be Byproduct of Steep Budget Cuts," *New York Times,* 26 June 1995, sec. A1; M. Freudenheim, "Corporations Step up Efforts To Get Retirees into H.M.O.'s," *New York Times,* 13 June 1995, sec. C1.
3. A. Relman, "The Impact of Market Forces on the Physician-Patient Relationship," *Journal of the Royal Society of Medicine,* 87 (supp. 22) (1994): 22–25; A. Relman, "Medical Insurance and Health: What about Managed Care?" *N. Engl. J. Med.* 331, no. 7 (1994): 471–72; E. Pellegrino, "Ethics," *JAMA* 271, no. 21 (1994): 1668–70.
4. J. Johnsson, "Megamerger of Two Public Plans Spurs New Interest in Stock Offering," *American Medical News,* 24 April 1995, 1; M. Freudenheim, "Penny-Pinching H.M.O.'s Showed Their Generosity in Executive Paychecks," *New York Times,* 11 April 1995, sec. C1.
5. California Code for Non-Profit Corporations, section 5130-B.
6. See Freudenheim, *supra* note 4; M. Rodwin, "Conflicts in Managed Care," *N. Engl. J. Med.* 332, no. 9 (1995): 604–7; J. Kassirer, "Mergers and Acquisitions—Who Benefits? Who Loses?" *N. Engl. J. Med.* 334, no. 11 (1996): 722–23.
7. S. Thompson and Z. Valentine, "The Profiteering of HMOs," *California Physician* (July 1994): 28–32, based on a California Department of Corporations report for 1992.
8. Alameda-Contra Costa Medical Association, "Latest CMA Study Shows Rise in HMO Costs and Profits," *ACCMA Bulletin* (February 1995): 14; M. Freudenheim, "A Bitter Pill for the HMO's," *New York Times,* 28 April 1995, sec. C1.
9. L. Kreiger, "Study Finds HMOs Less Efficient If For-profit," *San Francisco Examiner*, 13 February 1996, A8.
10. See Freudenheim, *supra* note 6; M. Hiltzik and D. Olmos, "Are Executives at HMOs Paid Too Much Money?" *Los Angeles Times,* 30 August 1995, sec. A13.
11. See Fletcher and Engelhard, *supra* note 1.
12. "How Good Is Your Health Plan?" *Consumer Reports* (August 1996): 28–42.
13. For an interesting discussion of the pros and cons of for-profit HMOs, see M. Hasan, "Let's End the Nonprofit Charade," *N. Engl. J. Med.* 334, no. 16 (1996): 1055–57, and P. Nudelman and L. Andrews, "The 'Value Added' of Not-for-Profit Health Plans," *N. Engl. J. Med.* 334, no. 16 (1996): 1057–59.
14. J. M. Eisenberg, "Economics," *JAMA* 273, no. 21 (1995): 1670–71.
15. A. Hillman, "Financial Incentives for Physicians in HMOs: Is There a Conflict of Interest?" *N. Engl. J. Med.* 317, no. 27 (1987): 1743–48; see Rodwin, *supra* note 6, p. 152–56.
16. L. Prager, "State Licensing Boards Consider Curbing Financial Incentives," *American Medical News,* 16 October 1995, 1, 74.
17. E. Emanuel, "Preserving the Physician-Patient Relationship in the Era of Managed Care," *JAMA* 273, no 4 (1995): 323–29; see Rodwin, *supra* note 1, 98.
18. L. Kreiger, "Family Doctors Are Disappearing," *San Francisco Examiner*, 18 June 1995, sec. A1.
19. M. Gold et al., "A National Survey of the Arrangements Managed Care Plans Make with Physicians," *N. Engl. J. Med.* 333, no. 25 (1996): 1678–83.
20. D. Olmos, "Some Doctors Head to Idaho, a State without Managed Care," *Los Angeles Times,* 29 August 1995, sec. A11.
21. S. Herschberg, "Potential Conflicts of Interest in the Delivery of Medical Services: An Analysis of the Situation and a Proposal," *Quality Assurance and Utilization Review* 7, no. 2 (1992): 54–58.
22. B. Shenkin, "The Independent Practice Association in Theory and Practice," *JAMA* 273, no. 24 (1995): 1937–42.
23. J. Robinson and L. Casalino, "The Growth of Medical Groups Paid through Capitation in California," *N Engl. J. Med.* 333, no. 25 (1995): 1684–87.
24. E. Friedman, "Changing the System: Implications for Physicians," *JAMA* 269, no. 18 (1993): 2437–42.
25. Council on Ethical and Judicial Affairs, American Medical Association, "Ethical Issues in Managed Care," *JAMA* 273, no. 4 (1995): 330–35.
26. See Rodwin, *supra* note 1, 138–44.
27. See Relman, *supra* note 1; Vincent Cangello, "The Real Issue," *ACCMA Bulletin* (January 1995): 18.

28. M. Hiltzik, "Emergency Rooms, HMOs Clash over Treatments and Payments," *Los Angeles Times,* 30 August 1995, sec. A12.
29. W. Phillips, "Hassle Hypertension: A Risk of Managed Care," *JAMA* 274, no. 10 (1995) (letter to editor): 795–76.
30. See Rodwin, *supra* note 1, 135.
31. One study of IPAs and physician groups with capitated contracts shows that physicians in the study tend to employ the same type of barriers to care, such as preauthorization requirements, as health plans. The study did not include the largest group practice HMO in California, Kaiser Permanente, which does not use preauthorization requirements to control costs. E. Kerr et al., "Managed Care and Capitation in California: How Do Physicians at Financial Risk Control Their Own Utilization?" *Annals of Internal Medicine* 123, no. 7 (1995): 500–504.
32. F. J. Crosson, "Why Outcomes Measurement Must Be the Basis for the Development of Clinical Guidelines," *Managed Care Quarterly* 3, no. 2 (1995): 6–11; D. Eddy, "Broadening the Responsibilities of Practitioners: The Team Approach," *JAMA* 268, no. 14 (1993): 1849–55; L. Zendle, "Controlling Costs: The Case of Kaiser," *JAMA* 274, no. 14 (1995): 1135; J. LaPuma, D. Schiedermayer, M. Siegler, "Ethical Issues in Managed Care," *Trends in Health Care, Law & Ethics* 10, no. 1/2 (1995): 73–77.
33. See Friedman, *supra* note 24.
34. See Crosson, *supra* note 32.
35. A. Hillman, "Health Maintenance Organizations, Financial Incentives, and Physicians' Judgments," *Annals of Internal Medicine* 112, no. 12 (1990): 891–93.
36. Rodwin, *supra* note 1, 139–41.
37. N. S. Jecker, "Managed Competition and Managed Care," *Clinics in Geriatric Medicine* 10, no. 3 (1994): 527–40; see Emanuel, *supra* note 17; Council on Ethical and Judicial Affairs, *supra* note 25.
38. D. Clement et al., "Access and Outcomes for Elderly Patients Enrolled in Managed Care," *JAMA* 271, no. 19 (1994): 1487–92.
39. See Council on Ethical and Judicial Affairs, *supra* note 25; D. Sulmasy, "Managed Care and Managed Death," *Archives of Internal Medicine* 155 (1995): 133–36; M. Hiltzik and D. Olmos, "A Mixed Diagnosis for HMO's," *Los Angeles Times,* 27 August 1995, sec. A1.
40. J. Richmond, "The Health Care Mess," *JAMA* 273, no. 1 (1995): 69–71; E. Rosenthal, "Managed Care Has Trouble Treating AIDS, Patients Say," *New York Times,* 15 January 1996, sec. A1.
41. S. Miles, "End-of-Life Treatment in Managed Care: The Potential and the Peril," *Western Journal of Medicine* 163, no. 3 (1995): 302–5.
42. See Eisenberg, *supra* note 14; "Study: Managed Care Lowers Hospital Costs, Improves Quality," *American Medical News,* 19 June 1995, 6.
43. J. Meisel, "Quality of Care in HMOs: A Review of the Literature," September 1994, CAHMO, Sacramento, California; California Cooperative HEDIS Reporting Initiative, Report on Quality of Care Measures (San Francisco: CCHRI, February 1995); National Committee for Quality Assurance, *Report Card Pilot Project/ Technical Report* (New York: NCQA 1994).
44. J. Somerville, "CMA Study: High HMO Administrative Costs for Medicaid," *American Medical News,* 15 May 1995, 12.
45. See Hillman, *supra* note 15.
46. Woodstock Theological Center, *Ethical Considerations in the Business Aspects of Health Care* (Washington, D.C.: Georgetown University Press, 1995), 9–14.
47. Woodstock Theological Center, *supra* note 46, 20–22.
48. Board of Directors of Kaiser Foundation Hospitals and Kaiser Foundation Health Plan, "Principles of Responsibility," 1984.
49. Forces external to managed care are exerting a growing pressure against undertreatment; for example, the 1990 Medicare amendment restricts prepaid plans contracting with the Health Care Financing Administration (HCFA) from creating an "incentive plan as an inducement to reduce or limit medically necessary services to a specific individual"; see Medicare law in 42 USC § 1395 mm (1)(8)(A); legislation pending in several states would put limits on the type of cost-control measures that MCOs can employ: E. Ogrod, "The Many Faces of Managed Care," *California Physician* (August 1995): 10; J. Johnsson, "State Laws on Managed Care Spur New Battles," *American Medical News,* 24 July 1995, 3, 51.
50. J. D Biblo et al., *Ethical Issues in Managed Care: Guidelines for Clinicians and Recommendations to Accrediting Organizations* (Kansas City. Mo.: Midwest Bioethics Center, 1995); S. M. Wolf, "Health Care Reform and the Future of Physician Ethics," *Hastings Center Report* (March–April 1994): 28–41; see Council on Ethical and Judicial Affairs, *supra* note 25; H. T. Engelhardt and M. A. Rie, "Morality for Medical-Industrial Complex: A Code of Ethics for the Mass Marketing of Health Care," *N. Engl. J. Med.* 319, no. 16 (1988): 1086–89.
51. D. Barr, "The Effects of Organizational Structure on Primary Care Outcomes under Managed Care," *Annals of Internal Medicine* 122, no. 5 (1995): 353–59.
52. L. Johnson and R. Derlet, "Conflicts between Managed Care Organizations and Emergency Departments in California," *West. J. Med.* 164 (1996): 137–42.
53. See Relman, *supra* note 1; M. Angell, "The Beginning of Health Care Reform: The Clinton Plan," *N. Engl. J. Med.* 329, no. 21 (1993): 1569–70; Cardinal J. Bernadin,

"Making the Case for Not-for-Profit Healthcare" (speech by Cardinal Joseph Bernadin, The Harvard Business School Club of Chicago, 12 January 1995).

54. See Rodwin, *supra* note 1, 136.
55. See Council on Ethical and Judicial Affairs, *supra* note 25.
56. E. Emanuel, "Managed Competition and the Patient-Physician Relationship," *N. Engl. J. Med.* 329, no. 12 (1993): 879–82.
57. J. Harding, "The Role of Organizational Ethics Committees," *Physician Executive* 20, no. 2 (1994): 19–24; see Emanuel, *supra* note 17.
58. D. Azevedo, "Can the World's Largest Integrated Health System Learn To Feel Small?" *Medical Economics,* 23 January 1995, 82–103.
59. D. Azevedo, "What You Can Bargain for When HMO's Compete," *Business & Health* (June 1995): 44–56.

CHAPTER 42

Outcomes Research: The Answer to All Our Health Care Questions or the Question to All Our Health Care Answers?

Cory Franklin

It is probably not an exaggeration to say that more changes occurred in health care delivery in America during the still-to-be completed decade of the 1990s than in any other decade in the history of our republic. Spiraling health care costs that threatened to reach the $1 trillion mark pressured the government, large corporations, and small businesses to demand changes in the system of health care delivery, which was primarily practiced under the traditional fee-for-service system at the outset of the decade.

In 1992, when the Democrats won control of the White House for only the second time since 1968, one of the centerpieces of Bill Clinton's campaign was health care reform. Liberal reformers stepped up their campaign for a single-payer national health care system with Canada as the operative model. It became clear that the single-payer model, which had been proposed in one form or another since before World War II, simply did not have sufficient support among the American populace for adoption. Consequently in 1993, a health care team assembled by President Clinton, cochaired by his wife, Hilary, and aide Ira Magaziner, proposed a hybrid plan that was essentially part national health care and part private sector managed care. The compromise that emerged did not satisfy critics in Congress, and the plan was defeated and shelved.

During the time that the Clinton health care plan was being forged, private corporations were exploring the use of managed care plans in conjunction with, or in lieu of, traditional insurance plans. The vacuum left by the failure of the Clinton health care plan was rapidly filled by managed care plans marketed by health maintenance organizations (HMOs), preferred provider organizations (PPOs), and point of service plans (POSs) whose goal was to sell those plans to both large and small companies that provided benefits packages to employees. By the end of 1996, these managed care plans had made major penetrations into many of the largest markets in the United States (most notably in California), in many cases offering alternatives to the fee-for-service system. The plans were also introduced into the public sector as several states employed them for citizens without private insurance.

The jury remains out on whether the shift to managed care will benefit the American health care system and patients. Early indications suggest that while managed care has had some success in moderating cost increases and has substantial public support, enough examples of abuse have surfaced to raise serious concerns. To add to these concerns, as of this writing the Medicare trust fund is projected to be operating at a deficit by the year 2001 and it is unclear what impact this potentially devastating development could have on the private sector.[1]

In the traditional health delivery model, patients required physicians' services and physicians evaluated patients' needs for those services. The operative ethic was the Hippocratic Oath—physicians determined what the patients' best interests were and acted accordingly. One of the profound changes wrought by managed care in this decade has been to cast the health care system's traditional players in new roles. Corporate control has diminished the influence (and not coincidentally the salary) of bedside physicians. Perhaps most important, physicians' allegiance to the corporate structure has placed a potential barrier between them and their patients, with the prospect of compromising the Hippocratic ethic.

As part of the management aspect of managed care, a new class of professionals—gatekeepers—has emerged. Armed with teams of data and computer software, their function is to identify which medical interventions are necessary and which are not. Referrals, payment approval, and ultimately the delivery of care are subsequently based on the information that such data provides. Both physicians and nonphysicians have assumed roles as gatekeepers, essentially creating a quasimedical "mandarin" class of information analysts. The ethical questions this raises, while not new to medicine, are certainly more prominent than ever before. The central question becomes: Is the role of this mandarin class to protect the corporate bottom line, as cynics claim, or to optimize patient outcomes, as the managed care industry claims?[2]

The answer to this question lies in the examination of the developing field known as "outcomes research."[3] Pared to its essentials, outcomes research is simply the tabulation of what happens to patients—who lives, who dies, whose surgery is successful, how well patients' blood sugars are controlled, how long patients stay in the hospital, and so forth. This type of data, ignored by the medical community for far too long, is now being pursued avidly by the health care industry and has become part of the core strategy of managed care.[4] If all that were involved in outcomes research was simply to track what happens to patients, the ethical questions involved would not be very complicated. Not surprisingly, though, when issues of reimbursement and patient referral are involved, outcomes research takes on a far more complex role.

Outcomes research involves three steps: defining what an outcome is, measuring and adjusting that outcome for severity, and ultimately evaluating the results of that outcome. All three steps involve human values, uncertainties, and assumptions—the fountains from which the ethical questions of outcomes research spring.

At the outset there is subjectivity in the definition of an outcome. When the term *outcome* is used, it is important to know what that means. Anytime one observes large numbers of patients in different care settings in different places over a long period of time, variability is bound to creep in.[5] The ideal outcome would be one where the variability among observers would be minimal. Uniformity is what is sought in outcomes research, but unfortunately uniformity is hard to come by.[6]

Certain outcomes, hospital survival and mortality for instance, are uniform; i.e., they are measured the same way in every hospital and there is no discrepancy between hospitals as to what constitutes being discharged alive or dead. Yet, even ostensibly uniform variables such as life and death take on subjectivity when a time element is introduced—some patients die shortly after being discharged from the hospital. For years, Medicare statistics reflected this in the publication of 30-day mortality figures—whether patients died within the month after hospital discharge. Not surprisingly, the statistics indicated that the hospitals with the highest mortalities were chronic care facilities, a fact that made it hard to evaluate hospital care based on mortality.[7]

Consider the implications for the outcome analysis of 30-day mortality. Some posthospital discharge deaths are to be expected (and actually may be planned to occur in the home setting) and thus indicate appropriate discharge. Other deaths reflect premature discharge from the hospital or some other form of medical mismanagement (errors in diagnosis and/or treatment). Obviously, these two situations are at diametrically opposite ends of the spectrum of the quality of medical care. Without more data and a deeper understanding of how *outcome* is defined, one can easily draw the wrong conclusion from what would seem to be a straightforward variable. A hospital with a high postdischarge mortality may be stigmatized for sending terminally ill patients home appropriately. Conversely, a hospital may cover up an inappropriate postdischarge mortality by claiming that patients who died were terminally ill when in fact the patients did not receive good medical management. This inherent variability in a defined outcome means that the results can be tailored to the agenda of those collecting the information. In many cases, the gatekeepers will have broad discretion over the information that they are responsible for.

Many outcomes are even less well-defined and subject to the same sort of interpretation. Consider as an example the functional outcome after vascular surgery for arterial insufficiency of the leg. Outcomes for this type of surgery include survival or death, length of hospital stay, whether patients return to pain-free ambulation or how many patients progress to amputation. This is the type of information most managed care companies want to know in evaluating a specific surgical procedure or a specific surgeon's performance. This appears to be a simple process, but there is a key assumption behind the definition of *postoperative outcome.* Some patients invariably refuse surgery and opt for medical therapy, even if surgery offers the promise of better functional outcome. How does the defined outcome account for those patients in evaluating the surgical procedure or the surgeon's performance? Put simply, a sufficient number of patients who decide not to undergo surgery can radically alter the conclusions about the surgeon or surgery itself. This subject bias means that if patients who refuse surgery are older and sicker, the surgical procedure will appear to be better for an individual patient than it actually may be (the outcomes will occur on healthier patients). If younger and healthier patients refuse surgery, the procedure may appear to be less successful than it actually is (with sicker patients more likely to suffer complications). While it may be possible to incorporate patient autonomy in this assessment of vascular surgery outcomes, it is certainly no small task. This is simply one example of how outcomes research is not a strictly objective process and how human values color the definition of an outcome. Anyone attempting to understand this outcome study must be aware of this and other similar biases.

Along these lines, another important factor is the actual adjustment of outcome for severity of illness.[8] Simple outcomes—life, death, length of stay, frequency of postoperative infections—have little intrinsic meaning unless they are adjusted for severity of illness; i.e., how sick the patients are. A crude postoperative mortality rate of 5 percent means quite different things depending on whether the surgical candidates are healthy, moderately ill, or desperately ill. Creating models that measure severity of illness involves some degree of assumption and uncertainty so that terms such as *healthy, moderately ill,* and *desperately ill* themselves become subjective.

In the field of outcomes research, severity of illness models have been employed in three major ways: in performing clinical studies, in predicting the future course of patients, and in preparing report cards.[9] From these, a number of related offshoots have been developed, some of which have profound implications to patients and the health care system. In each area, severity of illness modeling has demonstrated specific strengths and limitations that dictate how it should and should not be used.

As part of outcomes research programs, large clinical studies are being performed more frequently than ever before to test new and existing treatments. This information is being used to develop clinical guidelines and practice parameters in an attempt to standardize medical treatment. Standardizing medical treatment is a development eagerly sought by managed care companies (and gatekeepers) because it facilitates the evaluation of care being delivered.[10] (This proceeds on the assumption, proven or not, that minimizing variability in the type of care delivered is better, or at least cheaper). Most, if not all, clinical studies would be impossible to perform without severity of illness adjustments.[11]

The evaluation of a particular medication or surgical procedure demands some measure of how sick the observed patients are. Any patient-randomization method must include severity of illness as a measured variable to ensure that the randomization process is valid. While a number of different models have been developed to measure severity of illness for different diseases, no model has been proven to apply across broad populations. This means that different models must be developed and validated for different diseases and patient populations, a cumbersome and expensive undertaking. Of necessity, this inability of models to apply across different cohorts means that broad (e.g., nationwide) conclusions about treatment (and the resulting practice parameters and clinical guidelines) must be viewed with caution. (Some of the originally developed practice parameters have been a source of controversy within the medical community.) Even though every scoring model has recognized limitations, few managed care organizations have opted to devote significant resources to validating practice-parameter results derived from them.

Severity-of-illness models have also been instrumental in attempting to predict the future course of patients. This has obvious value to anyone overseeing care because it allows one to make decisions regarding triage and resource allocation (the essence of the gatekeeper function).[12] If it can be confidently predicted that a particular patient group will not suffer complications even if it does not receive a specific treatment, that treatment can be withheld from those in the group with scientific justification. The cost implications are obvious. In this respect the experience of scoring systems for the purpose of intensive-care triage deserves examination.

For the past two decades there has been an effort to evaluate better the impact of intensive-care units (ICUs) on patient survival. ICUs are limited resource areas that are labor-intensive and consequently extremely expensive. It would be desirable to know whether patients benefit from the services delivered there; i.e., the patients using them are neither too healthy (because they require ICU care) nor too sick (because they are likely to die in spite of ICU care). To evaluate this question, numerous studies have been performed.[13] Unfortunately, the ideal test, the randomized controlled trial, is precluded by the nature of the question. It would not be ethical to simply randomize most groups of patients to ICU or non-ICU care.[14] Consequently, these studies have traditionally used an alternative format—assessing patients by using a scoring system, giving each patient a score, observing the outcomes of groups of patients with similar scores, and then attempting to predict how future groups of patients with those scores will do.

What has been the result of these efforts at predicting the future? While some small subgroups of patients have been characterized with a high degree of accuracy, in most situations scoring systems have performed in the range of 80–95 percent correct predictions, essentially no better than experienced clinicians. In general, the systems have done better at predicting group outcomes than outcomes of individual patients.[15] This is an important distinction because the inability to accurately predict individual outcomes drastically limits the widespread applicability of the models in allocating (and denying) ICU care to individual patients. Most experts believe that scoring systems should not be used without corroboration by expert judgment (essentially a manual override). Even the most sophisticated systems should be used only in conjunction with clinical judgment exercised by practitioners. Interestingly, no study or analysis has been performed to assess the practical implications when computerized scoring models predict one outcome and an experienced clinician decides differently.

Some observers claim this is simply a matter of lack of refinement of the computer models.[16] They claim that future models will be able to tell administrators whether a patient will benefit from ICU care. No one can be certain, but it is fair to say that prognostic systems with acceptably low error rates for individual patients are not on the immediate horizon. Moreover, an intellectually honest appraisal of the field makes it clear that a prognostic system that predicts outcome with 100 percent accuracy is impossible. A high severity score will never be indicative of the absolute irreversibility of disease or the impossibility of survival. Likewise, a low score will never guarantee against unforeseen complications or chance mortality. Despite this, several companies have been created with the goal of selling scoring models to hospitals and managed care companies for gatekeepers to use. The vendors for these companies market their software by promising huge savings through improved allocation of resources (e.g., does this patient benefit by receiving ICU care?). One measure of managed care will be how the industry responds to such claims that currently have little substantiation in peer-reviewed medical literature. This may become the litmus test of improved profit margins at the expense of patient outcomes.[17]

A final area where severity of illness modeling has found utility is in the generation of "report cards."[18] A specific type of severity of illness measurement using multiple regression modeling has been widely used to evaluate the performance of physicians and hospitals. The theory is simple: Observe outcomes for groups of patients and adjust those outcomes for severity of illness. The conclusions should flow smoothly on who is doing a good job and who is not. The approach seeks to identify "outliers," situations or performers that fall outside a certain confidence level. These outliers are usually defined as falling at two or three standard deviations from average, although that decision itself is often subjective since it makes an arbitrary definition of what constitutes "chance" in complex situations. The implications for quality-assurance activities, staff credentialing, and granting privileges are obvious. Unfortunately, the efforts in this regard have been less than unqualified successes.

New York State has used mortality-prediction models to rate every cardiac surgeon in the state. An initial uproar was followed by grudging acceptance of the methodology. After several years, surgical mortality did indeed go down. Unfortunately, it was later suggested that some surgeons turned down high-risk cases and others learned to report risk factors in ways that enhanced their results (e.g., making their patients who had successful operations appear sicker). In addition, some data turned out to be misleading because some postoperative deaths were unrelated to surgery.[19]

States such as Pennsylvania and Iowa employed severity scoring to rate hospitals, but they found that the benefits of improved care were difficult to document even as millions of dollars were being spent to monitor severity information. In some cases the costs of monitoring care were being passed on to patients. The experience with report cards in Ohio and California has been similar, with expensive databases often yielding results that were either confusing or contradictory.[20]

This experience suggests there are a number of legitimate concerns over severity modeling and outcomes research for the purpose of generating report cards affecting decisions about patient care. In some cases, methodology is questionable or the software systems may not work, and if they do it is unclear what the data show (what is it exactly that constitutes quality?).[21] The premature release of raw data may mislead the public. All too often these systems have not been reviewed in peer-review publications, and in some instances the information is proprietary, i.e., the models and the logic they use cannot be independently verified because they are not in the public domain. In virtually all systems used to date the costs are high—they are labor-intensive and paperwork heavy. This generates pressures for the systems to justify their own costs, a situation that vendors often take advantage of through promotional campaigns geared to purchasers rather than to users. Cost considerations may have moved large-scale purchasers (businesses and government agencies) through their gatekeepers to adopt a less skeptical attitude than physicians about severity and/or outcome report cards, leaving patients caught in the middle. The degree of due diligence assumed by gatekeepers in assessing and utilizing outcomes research information will ultimately determine whether they are simply protecting corporate financial interests or optimizing patient outcomes.

One final point about the ethical implications of outcomes research deserves mention. It was perhaps inevitable that with hundreds of billions of dollars at stake the health care industry would ultimately find itself answering to Wall Street. A growing fear is that decisions will be made with the interests of stockholders placed ahead of those of patients. The developers of one of the best known and most widely employed severity scoring systems used in outcomes research have created a private corporation and taken it public, hoping to market their experience and data analysis to managed care companies. Along the way they will have the chance to realize millions of dollars while still keeping their information proprietary. Clearly, an important issue is the potential conflict of interest generated by the huge profits in the sale of a product that could affect the medical care of thousands of patients.

In this respect it should not be surprising to find that the topic of outcomes research has found its way to the stockholders' bible, the *Wall Street Journal.* A widely circulated opinion piece, written in August 1995 by the nonphysician director of a health care data analysis and research firm, extolled the virtues of outcomes research:

> a truism that rankles physicians most: a healthy patient is a unit of production and for all units of production there is an optimal production function which can be calculated . . . in the end there emerges a simple truth about a singular patient's situation: one clinical approach is clearly better, more cost-effective, and less risky than a competing approach. While a doctor may have seen 100 patients with an unusual clinical condition and have a fair idea as to how those patients respond . . . a cutting edge data base has a good idea how 100,000 of those patients did respond . . . more pointedly the data base knows which providers did the best job on their share of those 100,000 patients.[22]

On the surface, these words seem innocent enough, portraying medicine in terms of management science. However, those who practice and understand medicine are wary of such sentiments, believing as Hippocrates did several millennia ago that there is an art to the practice of medicine that distinguishes it from widget making.[23] While the article calls attention to the large number of patients in a database, it fails to mention that the number of variables influencing such a database is nearly infinite and has the potential to render invalid broad conclusions about care. Physicians learned long ago that simply amassing large numbers does not always provide the answers to the questions of diagnosis and treatment.

Closer examination and deconstruction of the article in the *Wall Street Journal* reveals an ominous ethic and suggests another hidden danger of outcomes research—the potential for depersonalization on a vast scale. While physicians are continually berated for not treating patients as people (often with good reason, given those "Dantesque" waiting rooms), imagine the reaction if a physician had authored an opinion piece (in the *Wall Street Journal,* no less) referring to patients as "units of production" and their care as "an optimal production function." Not only would the public be justifiably outraged but such Orwellian depersonalization would make the author a pariah both within and outside the medical community. Because the sentiments emanated from the business sector, no such opprobrium was forthcoming. The lessons should be clear.

Outcomes research will be an important aspect of restructured health care in the twenty-first century. Nevertheless, one must be wary of the new commercial attitude toward health care if the sentiment is that all problems can be solved with more (though not necessarily better) data. Not only is such an opinion factually incorrect, it brings with it the prospect of a depersonalized environment that could ultimately pave the way for widespread abuse, mistreatment, and misery in the pursuit of quick profit.

One looks for metaphors to anticipate such a situation. "Units of production" to describe patients sounds Orwellian. But 1984 has passed and the fears of Big Brother failed to materialize, so perhaps another metaphor is needed. We must look at what a blind devotion to outcomes research could mean for patients and summon the image of another popular icon whose reference base coincides with the turn of the millennium. Remember Kubrick's classic film *2001* and its central character, the computer HAL 9000, which was programmed never to make a mistake but wound up destroying all those it was built to help? This is what can happen when we fail to appreciate that there is a critical difference between what is collected as data and what is appreciated as wisdom.

NOTES

1. R. Pear, "New Medicare Trust Fund Data Show Unusually Large Shortfall: Program Is Solvent, But Gap Shows a Weakness," *New York Times,* 23 April 1996, 1.
2. R. L. Perkel, "Ethics and Managed Care," *Med. Clin. North Am.* 80 (1996): 263–78; A. S. Relman, "Controlling Costs by Managed Competition: Would It Work?" *N. Engl. J. Med.* 328 (1993): 133–35.
3. P. Ellwood, "Shattuck Lecture—Outcomes Management: A Technology of Patient Experience," *N. Engl. J. Med.* 318 (1988): 1549–56; A. S. Relman, "Assessment and Accountability: The Third Revolution in Medical Care." *N. Engl. J. Med.* 319 (1988): 1220–22.
4. E. A. Codman, *A Study in Hospital Efficiency as Demonstrated by the Case Report of the First Five Years of a Private Hospital* (Boston: Thomas Todd Company, 1917); A. G. Mulley Jr., "E. A. Codman and the End Results Idea: A Commentary," *The Milbank Quarterly* 67 (1989): 257–61.
5. S. D. Horn, et al., "Interhospital Differences in Severity of Illness: Problems for Prospective Payment Based on Diagnosis-Related Groups (DRGs)," *N. Engl. J. Med.* 313 (1985): 20–24.
6. J. P. Kassirer, "The Use and Abuse of Practice Profiles," *N. Engl. J. Med.* 330 (1994): 634–36.
7. J. Brinkley, "U.S. Releasing Lists of Hospitals with Abnormal Mortality Rates," *New York Times,* 12 March 1986, 1.
8. L. I. Iezzoni et al., "Predicting Who Dies Depends on How Severity Is Measured: Implications for Evaluating Patient Outcomes," *Ann. Intern. Med.* 123 (1995): 763–70; L. I. Iezzoni et al., "The Role of Severity Information in Health Policy Debates: A Survey of State and Regional Concerns," *Inquiry* 28 (1991): 117–28.
9. W. A. Knaus et al., "Variations in Mortality and Length of Stay in Intensive Care Units," *Ann. Intern. Med.* 118 (1993): 753–61; D. P. Schuster, "Predicting Outcome after ICU Admission: The Art and Science of Assessing Risk," *Chest* 102 (1992): 1861–70; United States General Accounting Office, *Health Care Reform: Report Cards Are Useful But Significant Issues Need To Be Addressed,* Report to the Chairman, Committee on Labor and Human Resources, U.S. Senate (Washington, D.C.: U.S. General Accounting Office, 1994), GAO/HEHS-94-219.
10. Kassirer, "The Use and Abuse of Practice Profiles."
11. Q. E. Whiting-O'Keefe et al., "Choosing the Correct Unit of Analysis in Medical Care Experiments," *Med. Care.* 22 (1984): 1101–14.
12. C. Franklin et al., "Triage Considerations in Medical Intensive Care," *Arch. Intern. Med.* 150 (1990): 1455–59.
13. Knaus et al., "Variations in Mortality"; Franklin, "Triage Considerations"; R. W. S. Chang et al., "Predicting Outcome among Intensive Care Unit Patients Using Computerized Trend Analysis of Daily APACHE II Scores Corrected for Organ System Failure," *Intensive Care Med.* 14 (1988): 558–66; S. Lemeshow et al., "A Comparison of Methods To Predict Mortality of Intensive Care Unit Patients," *Crit. Care Med.* 15 (1987): 715–22.
14. S. Hellman and D. S. Hellman, "Of Mice and Men: Problems of the Randomized Clinical Trial," *N. Engl. J. Med.* 324 (1991): 1585–89.
15. D. K. McClish et al., "Profile of Medical ICU vs. Ward Patients in an Acute Care Hospital," *Crit. Care Med.* 13 (1985): 381–86; A. L. Brannen et al., "Prediction of Outcome from Critical Illness: A Comparison of Clinical Judgment with a Prediction Rule," *Arch. Intern. Med.* 149 (1989): 1083–86; J. A. Kruse et al., "Comparison of Clinical Assessment with APACHE II for Predicting Mortality Risk in Patients Admitted to a Medical Intensive Care Unit," *JAMA* 260 (1988): 1739–42.
16. W. A. Knaus et al., "Short-Term Mortality Prediction for Critically Ill Hospitalized Adults: Science and Ethics," *Science* 254 (1991): 389–94.

17. R. Winslow, "In Health Care, Low Costs Beats High Quality," *Wall Street Journal,* 18 January 1994, B1.
18. Kassirer, "The Use and Abuse of Practice Profiles"; United States General Accounting Office, *Health Care Reform.*
19. J. Green and N. Wintfeld, "Report Card on Cardiac Surgeons: Assessing New York State's Approach," *N. Engl. J. Med.* 332 (1995): 1229–32.
20. L. I. Iezzoni and L. G. Greenberg, "Risk Adjustment and Current Health Policy Debates," in *Risk Adjustment for Measuring Health Care Outcomes,* ed. L. I. Iezzoni (Ann Arbor, Mich.: Health Administration Press, 1994), 347–408.
21. A. Epstein, "Performance Reports on Quality: Prototypes, Problems, and Prospects," *N. Engl. J. Med.* 333 (1995): 57–61.
22. J. D. Kleinke, "Medicine's Industrial Revolution," *Wall Street Journal,* 21 August 1995, A8.
23. J. P. Kassirer, "Managed Care and the Morality of the Marketplace," *N. Engl. J. Med.* 333 (1995): 50–52.

Chapter 43

Hospital Ethics Committees: Roles, Memberships, Structure, and Difficulties

David C. Thomasma and John F. Monagle

It has become commonplace for technological growth to outstrip society's methods of dealing with it.* Nowhere is this more true than in medical care. Life-saving equipment and techniques at times work only to preserve a semblance of life. These tragic results are becoming increasingly common. Physicians, when unable to predict what treatment will achieve in an individual case, must apply the best treatment available in emergency situations.

But after a patient is stabilized, the prognosis often becomes clear, and the patient's family and physician may have to confront difficult questions: Is it ethical to discontinue treatment? Is it ethical to continue? Having to make hard decisions is becoming more frequent, producing in recent years a number of highly publicized, emotionally charged court actions over the ethical approach to withdrawal of treatment.

When two southern California physicians agreed with a patient's family that they should remove life support systems, including medical feeding and hydration, from a hopelessly brain-damaged patient, they were accused of murder, although the charges were eventually dismissed.[1] Baby Doe cases are proliferating, with some families and physicians deciding to treat and others refusing to treat children born with serious birth defects. What is society's ethical position? Is there any consensus toward resolution?

BASIC ROLES OF THE ETHICS COMMITTEE**

The idea that ethics committees can form a consensus toward resolution and assist in bioethical decision making has now become widespread. Enough has been written about the ideal scope of such committees to allow their intended roles to be summarized as follows:

- *Education:* educating hospital staff about issues in ethical decision making and about how to use the hospital ethics committee[2]
- *Multidisciplinary Discussion:* providing a locus for interdisciplinary participation in value clarification and prioritization leading to conflict resolution[3]

**Source:* The following material is reprinted from *CHA Insight,* Vol. 8, No. 26, pp. 1–4, with permission of California Hospital Association, © June 1984.

***Source:* © *Quality Review Bulletin.* Oakbrook Terrace, IL: Joint Commission on Accreditation of Healthcare Organizations, 1985, pp. 204–208. Reprinted with permission.

†Reprinted with permission from *CHA Insight,* Vol. 8, No. 26, pp. 1–4, © 1984, California Hospital Association.

‡‡*Source:* © *Quality Review Bulletin.* Oakbrook Terrace, IL: Joint Commission on Accreditation of Healthcare Organizations, 1985, pp. 204–208. Reprinted with permission.

Note: This chapter was updated July 1997.

- *Resource Allocation:* recommending in-hospital allocation policies to maintain quality of care in the face of cost-containment measures.[4]
- *Institutional Commitments:* expressing the spirit of the hospital regarding its stated mission, philosophy, image, and identity (most often applicable to religious or private hospitals)[5]
- *Policy Formulation:* developing policies and guidelines regarding ethical issues
- *Consultation:* assisting attending physicians regarding difficult decisions

Education

Even if a hospital ethics committee cannot function, because of its large membership, as the ethical decision maker or directly in a consulting or policy-formulating capacity, nevertheless it can become the backbone of an institution's effort to educate its staff about ethics, ethical principles, and ethical issues. Initially, what is needed is a process for conducting interdisciplinary discussions about specific ethical issues. Later, as the issues become more clearly defined, a process should be established whereby ideas and guidelines about specific hospital policies can be directed to the hospital's ethical policy subcommittees for their consideration and for policy formulation. In this way, although it may function mainly to recommend guideline policies for further review and formulation, the hospital ethics committee remains deeply involved in ethical issues and is never cut off from the clashes of fundamental values experienced by clinical staff and administration.

But what kinds of activities are appropriate? Many hospital staff members are interested in discussing ethical issues but feel their training in ethics to be inadequate. They may also see formal education in ethics as too esoteric and remote from real-life problems. Given this common intimidation about ethics education, it is best to concentrate on case discussions in the context of a formal plan and under the leadership of an educator or medical ethicist. Most university medical centers employ such professionals,[6] as do many other hospitals and hospital systems.[7] Also, as existing hospital ethics committees have discovered, the faculty of nearby colleges may include professionals interested in discussing ethical problems in health care.

A necessary activity for the hospital ethics committee is to provide bioethical education for patients, their families, and the larger community in order to promote an understanding of ethical problems and an awareness of the desire and responsibility of physicians and hospitals to respond in an ethical manner. Hospital ethics committees, given the specific charge to analyze the community's ethical concerns, issues, and dilemmas and the authority to develop (through ethical policy subcommittees) policies for the care of severely handicapped infants and terminally ill patients, can be a source of great help to families and physicians directly involved in difficult decisions. Properly structured, an ethics committee thereby demonstrates the hospital's and the medical staff's commitment to protecting patients' rights and community values.

Multidisciplinary Discussion

An interdisciplinary approach both to the makeup of hospital ethics committees and to proposed ethics discussions in hospitals is essential for several reasons. Ethical dilemmas are not confined to the physician-patient relationship alone; they occur in regard to many other health care professionals, institutional demands, and social factors. The increased specialization of health care demands "defragmentation" of staff during attempts to resolve ethical issues. Communication across disciplines regarding difficult emotional issues (often involved in ethically complex cases) tends to minimize disruptions that could damage health care delivery.

For example, when a patient's wife and children request that the father be taken off a respirator, does the request represent the wishes of the father or of the family? Sometimes the nurses or the significant attending nurse know the answer better than the attending physicians, who in many hospital situations may not know the family well. In such cases, a sound decision cannot be reached without involving the nursing staff (or the significant nurse) and other relatives who know the patient's lifestyle, desires, and requests.

A second consideration is the effect that the decision will have on the caregivers. Staff members often form emotional bonds with patients, especially when the patient is so helpless as to need ventilator support. A physician's order to "wean" the patient off the respirator when this action may result in death requires at the very least some discussion with the attending nurses and respiratory specialists who have been providing the care (see the section "Consultation: Ethics Advisory Groups" later in this chapter). Nurses often ask hospital ethicists to approach physicians about such determinations—not in a spirit of rebellion but with a simple request that the decision be discussed with them. Any attempt to avoid such interdisciplinary discussion at the specific case level not only ignores the emotional dimensions of ethical issues but also causes new ethical issues to arise for those who must carry out the orders. As one nurse stated privately years ago, the most fundamental ethical issue for nurses concerns the expectations that they will remain silent and "get used to" being excluded from the decision-making process.

Multidisciplinary discussion does not merely address the emotional aspects of ethical issues; it is required by the inherently multidisciplinary nature of the ethical dilemmas that occur today. The federal government is directly involved in promulgating guidelines on research and on the care of defective newborns. State authorities are involved in executing prospective payment policies that may cause some persons not to receive the care they need. Insurance companies are involved, especially through preferred provider organizations (PPOs) and health maintenance organizations (HMOs), since they reward physicians who keep their patients away from expensive care. Hospital administrators are involved in determining who will receive expensive care that will not be reimbursed. And, of course, physicians and consultants are involved in day-to-day decisions to which they bring legal, moral, and professional standards. It becomes impossible to resolve some clinical ethical problems without considering the involvement of all these participants.

Resource Allocation

One of the least discussed of the possible functions of a hospital ethics committee is assisting the hospital governing body to develop policies for resource allocation.[8] As the trend toward cost containment continues, more difficult allocation issues will arise in every institution. For example, can the hospital ethically limit the number of certain types of expensive cases it accepts should reimbursement fail to meet its actual costs? Should certain services no longer be offered at the hospital? Has the community been represented in these decisions?

A study at Rush–Presbyterian–St. Luke's Medical Center in Chicago revealed the loss of approximately $20,000 per elderly patient receiving care in an intensive-care unit, despite reimbursement under Medicare's prospective payment system. The researchers expressed a concern that if costs cannot be recovered elsewhere, critical care for the aged will dwindle and patients will not receive the quality of care to which they have become accustomed.[9] Their concern rests on a profound ethical principle of medicine: Physicians must act in the best interests of their patients, no matter the cost. Fortunately, at Rush as elsewhere, costs for some services have been recovered through reimbursement for other more cost-effective services. But this momentary respite from hard choices is just that—momentary. The national plan, of course, is to equalize the payment for each procedure throughout the country. When this is fully accomplished, cost shifting will no longer be possible, and resource allocation decisions will become all the more difficult.

The luxury of individual cases for which payments can be received will almost completely cease, replaced by the hardship of no longer being able to provide expensive services for which little or no payment will be received. Cost will become an essential ingredient in the ethical decisions regarding allocation of scarce resources unless the necessary finances are made available. The claim to necessary but expensive health care is to be weighed in the balance (of resource allocation).

As outside entities establish even greater control over reimbursement for specific diseases, each institution will face a major ethical question: How can cost containment and institutional survival be balanced with quality of care? If it is the responsibility of a hospital to fulfill its stated mission, philosophy, identity, and image, then particular judgments regarding allocation should be appropriate discussion matter for relevant administrators, staff, and community members. Each hospital employee ostensibly commits himself or herself to the aims of the institution, and individual determinations and actions should further these aims. When the achievement of these aims is in jeopardy, a consensus should be sought on how to maintain the best possible balance of values. This balance can then be conveyed to the community that the hospital serves. The hospital ethics committee can be central to this effort to renew and communicate the hospital's aims and the community's values and choices.

Institutional Commitment

The hospital ethics committee can begin to develop (or, in private and religious facilities, continue to develop) an ethical tradition for the hospital. By recommending policies—after consideration by the ethical policy subcommittees—on such issues as the care of newborns, cardiopulmonary resuscitation, do not resuscitate (DNR) orders, resource allocation, and procedures that will not be performed, the ethics committee itself in effect becomes the conscience of the institution, linking the institutional philosophy with practical judgments about how to proceed in the best interests of the patient and the larger community.

Because of the extraordinary pressures currently brought to bear on hospitals as social institutions, they face the same kind of crisis regarding goals that universities faced in the 1960s. The social good traditionally offered—the highest quality of care—is called into question not only by "bureaucratic parsimony"[10] but also by alternative forms of delivery ranging from HMOs to surgical-, emergency-, and ambulatory-care centers. Hospitals are responding to the challenge by altering their characters, becoming less social institutions than businesses. Departments become product lines and services become ciphers in computer printouts of cost analyses.

However, one fact that often becomes lost in the jumble remains essential: Hospitals provide a good that people cannot obtain on their own using their own resources.[11] This good is not like most consumer products, which in some sense are luxuries. To reduce it to mathematical or economic analysis alone is to diminish its vast importance.

To preserve its aims in the thicket of economics and bureaucracy, the hospital must have at its disposal a realistic but firm vision of its nature and purpose. Siegler has suggested that if we are to ration health care, perhaps we should begin by withholding it from the wealthy and articulate and giving it to the poor and downtrodden.[12] Less dramatically, a hospital ethics committee might suggest a policy that would involve donating several hours a week to care for the poor. Further, it might consider practical measures to foster cooperation among competing hospitals so that needed care can be provided to all who seek it. Philanthropy, charitable giving, marketing, and fund-raising must be encouraged to ensure survival. Diversified business endeavors should be explored and implemented.

Policy Formulation: Ethical Policy Subcommittees[13]

Every hospital governing body has the duty to ensure that the institution reflects the mission and philosophy stated in its charter and developed in its traditions.[14] Staff turnover and a natural tendency, especially in institutions, for ideals to decay over time make it desirable to establish perdurable policies regarding ethical decision making. In effect, such policies are a form of prescriptive or directive ethics.

Yet one of the most astonishing features of hospitals to outsiders is precisely the lack of such directive ethics. Although most hospitals have numerous policies directing health care practice within their walls, few have attempted, until recently, to establish ethics guidelines. Religious hospitals have long had "mission and philosophy" committees, which have offered guidelines about procedures such as abortion and elective sterilization. Many other hospitals have developed guidelines for DNR orders as well. Apart from these exceptions, however, little attention has been given to policies regarding the significant ethical problems that challenge daily practice in the hospital, e.g., stopping certain forms of therapy for terminally ill patients, interprofessional conflicts, informed consent, and decision making for incompetent patients.

Resistance to policies governing such ethical problems stems from several sources. Inertia is certainly one; distractions and the pressures of time are two others. Some people think decisions by committee do not represent a sufficient advancement over individual decisions to warrant the effort. Still others are concerned that guidelines about care will adversely affect physician-patient relationships. Resistance also almost certainly results from the wrongheaded philosophy of medicine that views the one-on-one relationship of the physician and patient as sacred and exempt from outside interference.[15] Evidence exists that traditional Hippocratic ethics have been welded to an entrepreneurial concept of health care.[16] In a traditional fee-for-service system, emphasis on the almost "sacred" quality of the physician-patient relationship is not entirely altruistic. Keeping other interests out of the relationship could be seen, at least in part, as a protectionist rather than a beneficent action. Traditional ethics and entrepreneurship can be decoupled without damage to the important ethical dimensions of the physician-patient relationship.

The hospital ethics committee's preliminary work serves as a starting point for more detailed analysis by ethical policy subcommittees appointed to study and recommend policy on specific areas of ethical uncertainty. The subcommittees, composed of physicians, some members of the hospital's ethics committee, and other health professionals with expertise in the subject area, forward the results of their analyses to the hospital ethics committee, which then can send them on to the appropriate authority for adoption as hospital policy.

Consultation: Ethics Advisory Groups†

These hospital policies are then available as guidance for ethics advisory groups, which are formed ad hoc when a specific case involving ethical issues arises. At this level there is direct involvement of the attending physician and the patient and/or family.

The composition and membership of an ethics advisory group might include the following:

- attending physician
- patient and/or family members
- significant nurse in the case
- clergy or bioethicist
- physician or other member of the ethical policy subcommittee of the subject area

In cases where there seem to be unresolved civil or criminal liabilities, an attorney for the hospital should be included. In certain cases, upon request of the patient or family, the attorney for the patient may also be invited to participate.

Perhaps the most important and most problematic role of the ethics-advisory group is consultation.** Should the consultation on cases be, strictly speaking, an offering of advice to the physician or, alternatively, an actual decision-making process? Physicians often resist interpolations of decision-making bodies between themselves and their patients.[17] In part, this resistance stems from the view that the physician-patient relationship is the moral center of medicine.[18] But it may also derive from a failure to recognize that medical ethics is no longer the private domain of physicians, if it ever was. The issues almost always involve public perceptions, social and political presuppositions, legal standards, and ethical traditions.[19]

It is not yet clear which of the two options should predominate. At present, the group should function at least as an advisory body. Successful optional consultation by the ethics advisory group requires support from the board members, administrators, and medical executive committee, along with continuing educational activities for the staff. Since, ethically and legally, society has placed the burden of medical decisions on the attending physician, the final treatment decision remains with the physician and the patient or family.

A hospital's bioethics committee (High Desert Hospital, Lancaster, California, operated by the Department of Health Services, County of Los Angeles) was the first to be named in a malpractice suit. The plaintiff was Elizabeth Bouvia. Her attorney was Richard S. Scott. Elizabeth Bouvia, 30 years old, suffered since birth from cerebral palsy and was a spastic quadraplegic, immobile and entirely dependent on others. She alleged that a nasogastric tube for forced feeding was inserted, against her will and without her consent, on January 16, 1986. On April 16, 1986, the Court of Appeals, Second Appellate District, Division Two, ordered the tube removed. In an amended complaint filed on July 23, 1986, in the Superior Court of the State of California for the County of Los Angeles, Elizabeth Bouvia named the hospital's bioethics committee and individual members as defendants. (Case No. C583828). Bouvia's attending physicians were free to disregard the advice of the bioethics committee. The physicians are legally responsible for the actions taken, but was the bioethics committee? The suit against the bioethics committee and the individual members should not chill or intimidate members of bioethics committees who act in good faith in the interest of the patient. Bioethics committees reduce, not increase, legal exposure.

Ethics Committees: Membership[†]

The membership of hospital ethics committees should represent a broad range of value perspectives, professional expertise, and community representation. The committee should include[20]

- Medical staff—staff from specialty areas such as obstetrics, neurosurgery, neurology, nephrology, oncology, psychiatry, and so forth.
- Nursing staff—the director of nursing, operating room supervising nurse, emergency department supervising nurse, etc.
- An administrator—a high-level qualified administrative person who is interested in ethical issues, sensitive to medical staff responsibilities, patient and employee rights, financial realities, and community concerns.
- A social services representative—a person knowledgeable about what the hospital, as well as the larger community, can provide in the way of care for patients.
- Clergy or bioethicists—having at least one such person is essential for the multidisciplinary discussions. Candidates should have training not only in moral theology but also in the formal discipline of philosophical ethics in order to present the ethical theories and principles that can be applied to the individual case. Some clergy do not have these credentials. Although they can bring important and essential insight to the committee, it cannot replace the formal discipline in ethics that is also needed.
- A member of the hospital board—since the hospital board represents the community, the person selected should be knowledgeable about the larger community's concerns as to the kinds of medical procedures and treatments that are needed in the demographic area that the hospital serves. And since all of the hospital's services are ultimately the responsibility of the hospital board, the governing-body representative should participate in and have knowledge of the hospital ethics committee's discussions and decisions.

STRUCTURES: THREE MODELS*

There are at least three possible structures for an ethics committee, each determined by the part of the hospital that has authority over its operations. The three organizational diagrams presented in Figure 43–1 show an ethics committee as a committee of the hospital's governing board, as a committee reporting to the hospital's chief executive officer, and as a committee responsible to the hospital medical staff executive committee.

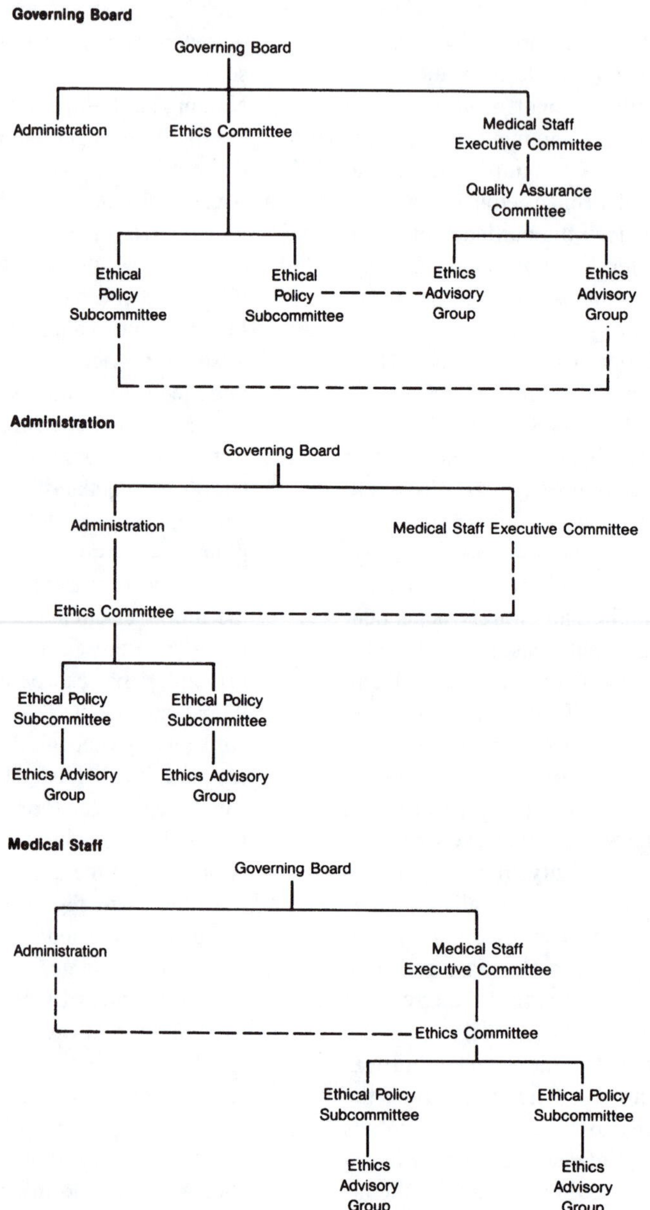

Figure 43–1 Three Hospital Ethics Committee Structures. *Source:* Reprinted with permission from *CHA Insight,* Vol. 8, No. 20, p. 3, © 1984, California Hospital Association.

Each structure has its advantages and disadvantages. The committee's structure and membership, its authority and responsibility, its charge and scope of activity, and its limits of purpose and authority should be clearly defined according to the particular needs of each hospital.

Under the governing-board model, the ethics committee uncovers, discusses, and clarifies ethical concerns or problems and, in consultation with the medical staff executive committee and the hospital administration, forms an ethical policy subcommittee to analyze the available information on the subject.

The subcommittee's policy recommendations are reviewed by the ethics committee and forwarded for adoption by the governing board as hospital policy. When a case involving those issues arises, those policies serve as guidelines to ethics advisory groups formed to help the family and physician understand the ethical choices involved. The flow of information and development of hospital policies is similar in the other two models, but in those models the hospital's administration or the medical staff executive committee has more or less direct authority for final review and approval of the policies.

One of the differences among the governing board, administration, and medical staff organizational models is in the level of public disclosure each affords. Because the ethics committee's primary focus is on patients' rights and hospital and community education in bioethical issues, it may not be advisable to seek the protection from discovery in legal action that state law gives to the deliberations of medical staff quality-care review committees.[21]

To the extent that the discussions and recommendations about or solutions to ethical concerns, issues, and dilemmas are shared openly, the medical staff's and the institution's assumption of ethical responsibility for policies and actions will be visible and recognized. Furthermore, if a hospital's ethical practices are challenged through civil or criminal suit, summary documentation of the ethics committee's proceedings may well serve as a defense for the physicians and the hospital.

Under the medical staff organizational model, the ethics committee may seek protection from discovery for the records and proceedings of its ethical policy subcommittees, since these report to the ethics committee of the medical staff. Likewise, protection from discovery may be sought for the ethics advisory groups under either the medical staff or governing board organizational models. The governing board structure may be the most amenable to openness of information, discussion, and recommendations, while at the same time protecting records and proceedings related to individual case discussions of the ethics advisory groups.

The administration model, while unable to seek protection from discovery under quality-assurance confidentiality statutes, may be more responsive to management control of cost-effectiveness and to evaluating risk management and professional liability implications of hospital ethical policies. The medical staff model, while fully protected from disclosure of discussions, has to guard against domination by physicians and lack of interaction with the community.

DIFFICULTIES AND NEEDS: ETHICS COMMITTEES AND ETHICISTS

1. The necessary money by which we can fund and allocate time in order to discuss and resolve present and evolving ethical issues, "soft money," is now difficult to acquire.[22] It takes time and expert personnel to develop and implement a single ethical policy. If a committee has only one or two hours a month to discuss, formulate, and prepare to implement an ethical policy, only one or two policies can be produced in a year. The issues are many but the policies are few.[23] A national network of health care committees that have formulated and are willing to share policies does not exist. One unified national organization of bioethicists, to educate and share, is necessary, yet it still does not exist.[24]

2. At present, bioethicists are not recognized as "certified" in their discipline, profession, or field.[25] A certification standard needs to be developed and implemented, so that bioethics can be recognized in academic and clinical arenas.

The Society for Bioethics Consultation has a panel that will make recommendations in the future.

3. Some money-strapped health care institutions find difficulty in justifying expenditures on "ethicists" or ethics committees, since they are not seen as clinically necessary to direct patient care.

4. Issues such as abortion, sterilization, surrogate motherhood, transplantations, euthanasia, assisted suicide, and other issues regarding death and dying[26] have not been resolved successfully by any universally applicable solutions to benefit the care of patients. Furthermore, ethicists and ethics committees in general are not able to offer practical discussion and resolution of evolving issues, such as the relationship of high technology to possibilities for cloning and all other forms of genetic manipulation and engineering. The academic discussions are presented, but clinical resolutions to the problems are not discussed.

5. Pass-through costs for academic or clinical services are under scrutiny. Managed care, curtailed by cost, has led to severe limitations on the consultative care to be offered. Physician survival has forced professionals into managed care organizations. Less money spent by managing care is the dominant goal of these organizations. In fact, because of these organizations' rules and regulations, the quality of patient care is a secondary consideration. The prime directive is reduction of managed care costs. This is the reality.[27]

6. Most ethicists and ethics committees are not trained in business or managed care ethics. Ethicists have come more readily from the humanities background and are not corporate business practitioners. They do not easily deal with enforced government rationing as demonstrated by Medicare and Medicaid. Not all demands can or will be met by a corporate business mentality into which health care institutions and professionals have been forced. Ethicists in general are not financially experienced in the cost of personnel staffing requirements. They have not been trained in business marketing and health service plans. In addition, most ethicists are not able to contribute to the ethical and financial issues involved in health care mergers, joint ventures, corporate restructuring, and the financial limitations of institutions in providing uncompensated care. Ethical demands are consequently not realistically or fully understood in the context of financially-based insurance policies limiting or denying certain options of coverage.

7. Comparatively few ethicists have entered into public discussion and initial proposals reflecting public desires related to the financial problems of the health care industry. Only recently have several states conducted educational public inquiries addressing public demands and preferences for health care treatments and procedures. Examples include the Health Care Decision Making Surveys conducted in California, Colorado, Oregon, and Massachusetts.[28] Ethicists need to establish and participate in similar statewide activities involving decision making and policy planning related to bioethical and financial interests. Furthermore, they should increasingly become part of the organizations that raise the "soft money" that finances public studies of patients' viewpoints, priorities, preferences, and desires regarding health care. Eventually, state legislatures may modify and mandate publicly acceptable solutions, based on the activities of these statewide organizations.

8. Thus, bioethics has reached a crisis in its young adulthood as to: (a) who its practitioners are, what their qualifications are, and what their training and experience should be; (b) what problems and issues they can professionally and skillfully handle; (c) in what areas they need to educate themselves and contextualize their views; and (d) to what extent they need to adopt a financial or "Wall Street" approach to managed care.

9. Most of the bioethicists who will survive and progress in the new millennium will be those who become involved in the administrative, financial, and clinical functions of managed care organizations, health care facilities, and socially responsible entities that deal with more comprehensive ethical issues, such as environmental concerns including hazardous waste, and issues involving the homeless, disabled, home care, and hospice efforts. A focus on these efforts will be necessary if

bioethicists are to be considered necessary and valued to the administrative and public views of the health care system.

10. There has been a reluctance in the past, as there undoubtedly will be in the future, by some bioethicists to become involved in "the dirty business of finance." Unless he or she is so fortunate as to have an endowed academic or clinical chair, an ethicist will quickly realize the necessity that he or she become involved in the financial concerns pervading the health care industry, since these concerns influence ethical issues and decisions constantly. Otherwise, there is a danger that bioethicists and ethics committees will be considered parasitic to the financial efficiency of health care entities. They cannot afford to be marginalized in this way.

CONCLUSION‡‡

To retain the ethical dimension of health care delivery, hospitals interested in ethics committees can select from the roles discussed in this chapter. The needs of each institution are different, as is each institution's capacity to establish such committees firmly. Some of the roles are more problematic than others. In many hospitals, several of the roles are already carried out by other committees—allocation decisions by the quality-assurance committee, institutional commitments by the mission and philosophy committee, and so on. None of the functions, however, will be successfully integrated within the hospital unless the ethics committee is part of an educational effort that involves both the primary disciplines responsible for patient care and the personnel responsible for hospital govemance.

Ethical issues are not going to diminish in frequency or complexity.** The individual treatment dilemmas raised by new technology are difficult enough. But even more agonizing dilemmas have surfaced, with the introduction of PPOs, HMOs, diagnosis-related groups and the other responses to limited resources.

In *Securing Access to Health Care,*[29] the President's Commission for the Study of Ethical Problems in Medicine and Biomedical and Behavioral Research concluded that society is obligated to provide "equitable" access to "adequate" health care.[30] But as new technology redefines what care is adequate, its cost restricts access to its benefits. The inequity of limited access—first to the poor, but eventually to everyone—may become society's thorniest bioethical dilemma, one that will necessitate more hospitals to establish and support ethics committees.

BIBLIOGRAPHY

American Hospital Association. *Hospital Committees on Biomedical Ethics.* Chicago: American Hospital Association, 1984.

Chinn, P. L. *Ethical Issues in Nursing.* Rockville, Md.: Aspen, 1986.

Craig, Robert P. *Ethics Committees: A Practical Approach.* St. Louis, Mo.: The Catholic Health Association, 1986.

Hosford, B. *Bioethics Committees.* Rockville, Md.: Aspen, 1986.

NOTES

1. 47 Cal. App. 3d 1006 (1983). See J. F. Monagle, "A Question of Ethics on Murder," *CHA Insight* 13 April 1984, 1–4.
2. A. R. Fleischman and T. H. Murray, "Ethics Committees for Infants Doe?" *Hastings Center Report* 13 (December 1983): 5–9; J. A. Robertson, "Ethics Committees in Hospitals: Alternative Structures and Responsibilities," *Quality Review Bulletin* 10 (January 1984): 6–10; R. J. Rooney, "Ethics from the Bottom Up: A Participative Approach to Health Care Ethics," *Bioethics Reporter* 3 (1984): 970.
3. J. Curtis, "Multidisciplinary Input on Institutional Ethics Committees: A Nursing Perspective," *Quality Review Bulletin* 10 (July 1984): 199–208; D. Ozar, "The

Challenge of Multiple Professional Perspectives in Institutional Ethics Committees," *Bioethics Reporter* 1 (1984): 153.

4. A. Griffin and D. Thomasma, "Health Care Distribution and Hospital Impartial Panels," *Bioethics Reporter* 1 (1984): 124.
5. B. Bader, "Medical Moral Committees: Guarding Values in an Ambivalent Society," *Hospital Progress* 63 (October 1982): 80; E. Lisson, "Active Medical Morals Committee: Valuable Resource for Health Care," *Hospital Progress* 63 (October 1982): 36.
6. T. K. McElhenny and E. D. Pellegrino, *Teaching Ethics, the Humanities, and Human Values in Medical Schools: A Ten-Year Overview* (Washington, D.C.: Institute on Human Values in Medicine, Society for Health and Human Values, 1981).
7. M. M. McDonnell, "Holy Cross Health System: Medical Ethics Program," *Bioethics Reporter* 3 (1984): 960; G. Graber, "One Philosopher's History in His Work with Hospital Ethics Committees," *Bioethics Reporter* 3 (1984): 956.
8. Griffin and Thomasma, "Health Care Distribution."
9. P. W. Butler et al., "Technology under Medicare Diagnosis-Related Group Prospective Payment: Implications for Medical Intensive Care," *Chest* 87 (February 1985): 229–34.
10. M. Siegler, "Should Age Be a Criterion in Health Care?" *Hastings Center Report* 14 (October 1984): 24–27.
11. D. Ozar, "Justice and a Universal Right to Basic Health Care," *Social Science and Medicine (Ethics)* 15 F (March 1981): 135–41.
12. Siegler, "Should Age Be a Criterion in Health Care?"
13. J. F. Monagle, "Blueprints for Hospital Ethics Committees," *CHA Insight* 8, no. 20 (26 June 1984); see note 23.
14. D. Thomasma, "Hospitals' Ethical Responsibilities as Technology, Regulation Grow," *Hospital Progress* 63 (December 1982): 74–79.
15. D. Ozar, "Social Ethics in the Philosophy of Medicine, and Professional Responsibility," *Theoretical Medicine* 6 (1985): 281–294.
16. W. B. Schwartz and H. J. Aaron, "Rationing Hospital Care: Lessons from Britain," *New England Journal of Medicine* 310 (1984): 52–56.
17. Robertson, "Ethics Committees in Hospitals."
18. E. D. Pellegrino and D. C. Thomasma, *A Philosophical Basis of Medical Practice* (New York: Oxford University Press, 1981).
19. D. Thomasma, "Medical Ethics Committees Find New Roles," *Quality Assurance—Risk Management Bulletin* 5 (January–February 1985): 1–3; D. Callahan, "Shattuck Lecture: Contemporary Biomedical Ethic," *New England Journal of Medicine* 302 (1980): 1228–33.
20. Monagle, "Blueprints."
21. Forty-five states protect medical staff committee records under the state's evidence code or peer-review statute.
22. *Hospital Ethics* 11, no. 5 (1995): 1.
23. J. F. Monagle and D. C. Thomasma, eds., *Medical Ethics: Policies, Procedures, Guidelines, and Programs* (Gaithersburg, Md.: Aspen Publishers, 1997).
24. *Hospital Ethics,* 5
25. *Hospital Ethics,* 4.
26. *Hospital Ethics,* 6, 11, 13.
27. "To Confess Role in Man's Death," *San Francisco Chronicle,* 15 April 1997, A13, A15. A Kentucky physician for the Humana HMO allegedly saved $500,000 for the HMO, an allegation that the HMO denies.
28. *Hospital Ethics,* 15ff.
29. President's Commission for the Study of Ethical Problems in Medicine and Biomedical and Behavioral Research, *Securing Access to Health Care,* vol. 1 (Washington, D.C.: U.S. Government Printing Office, 1983). For a review of its conclusions, see Allen Toon, "Equitable Access to Adequate Care," *CHA Insight,* 19 October 1983, 9.
30. Bader, "Medical Moral Committees."

CHAPTER 44

Clinical Ethics Consultants: Survey and Practice

Martha Jurchak

INTRODUCTION

The work of ethics consultants is born from the difficult and complicated task that decision making in modern health care has become. Until relatively recently in history, saving a person's life was the unanimous goal of patients and their health care providers. When this was not possible, alleviating suffering until death was the best available alternative[1] and the physician alone made the decision about which goal was most appropriate. However, advancements in modern medicine have produced a multitude of life-sustaining technologies, and questions on the appropriateness of their use have often come as an afterthought.[2] In addition, changes have occurred in the sociopolitical climate that encouraged the declaration of patients' rights[3] and strengthened patient self-determination in health care decision making.[4] Together, these changes have provoked a multitude of questions for health care providers and their patients. The highly publicized cases of Karen Quinlan, Baby Doe, and Nancy Cruzan represent many less famous but no less compelling stories.

Providers of health care and recipients of that care faced questions of values, of justice, and of conscience. In a pluralistic society, the answers to these questions are many and varied. A forum for discussion and decision making about a best course of action became needed. Also needed was someone or a group of people to share the burden of angst, someone who could provide wise and helpful counsel as well as support in the moral dilemmas that were confronting clinicians and their patients and families.[5]

These needs—for support, for thoughtful weighing of benefits and burdens of various alternatives, for facilitation in clinical decision making among all the parties involved—have been met in a variety of ways.[6] These have included committees that would provide education and consultation,[7] individual consultants,[8] or small interdisciplinary groups of two to four whose expertise would be the facilitation of moral discourse in clinical settings.[9]

There have been recommendations on how ethics consultation should be accomplished,[10] warnings about potential problems with various forms of ethics consultation,[11] and reports of particular approaches to ethics consultation.[12] Yet, it is difficult to assess what is being practiced as ethics consultation. Is there a predominate model for ethics consultation? What is it? Is there consistency of a process across different models of ethics consultation? Who can request an ethics consultation? How multidisciplinary are the committees that provide consultation? An attempt at beginning to answer these questions was made through a nationwide study reported here.

METHODOLOGY

The purpose of the study was to describe ethics consultants themselves as well as the process they used when involved in end-of-life ethics case consultations. The study design was a descriptive retrospective survey. Investigation was limited to end-of-life consultations in an effort to control for variation in the experiences and approaches of ethics consultants.

A survey questionnaire, developed for the study, included 58 items identified in the literature to be aspects of the process of ethics case consultation. These process items reflected a model of ethics case consultation that combined elements of both philosophical case analysis[13] and elements of group process and mediation.[14] The philosophical model asks questions such as, "What are the benefits and burdens of a particular course of action?" and "What are the ethical principles reflected in the case?" Elements of the mediation and group process model include issues such as, "All participants' perspectives were encouraged in the discussion" and "The leader identified common points of interest in the claims of each party." The elements from both philosophical case analysis and group process and mediation were combined in this study to create the Integrated Model of ethics case consultation. The Integrated Model reflects the complex nature of clinical ethics consultations. The problems presented for consultation are of an ethical nature (requiring consideration of philosophical analysis) and are also interpersonal and conflict-driven (requiring attention to issues of group process and conflict resolution).

The following is a list of the elements of the combined Integrated Model of ethics case consultation that were included in the survey questionnaire:

1. Elements from Philosophical Case Analysis
   - gathering facts
   - identifying reasons for a claim
   - identifying benefits and burdens
   - identifying best interests
   - identifying patient's wishes
   - patient-centered discussion
   - identifying moral principles
   - inclusiveness in discussion of all involved parties
   - follow-up
2. Elements from Mediation
   - third-party facilitation of discussion
   - investigating and presenting facts
   - summarizing
   - exploring mutual perspectives
   - identifying common points of interest
   - generating new ideas/option building
   - facilitating mutual respect among parties
   - perspective taking/reframing
   - joint problem solving
   - neutrality
   - planning for implementation of agreement

Using a four-point Likert scale, respondents estimated the frequency of occurrence of the process items in their practice of ethics consultation. The response categories were 1 = never, 2 = occasionally, 3 = frequently, 4 = always, and NA = not applicable. Seven of the 58 items were negatively worded and a priori coded negatively. The process items were presented as occurring in three phases: an intake phase, a discussion phase, and a follow-up phase.[15] Respondents were also asked demographic questions and questions about the institutional ethics committee. The sample consisted of members of the Society for Bioethics Consultation who had been involved in ethics case consultation during the past year at the time of the survey.

ESTABLISHMENT OF RELIABILITY AND VALIDITY

The content and construct validity were assessed by a review of the survey questionnaire by experts in survey design and health care ethics. Four experts in ethics case consultation were sent the questionnaire and asked to evaluate it. In addition to these reviews, the questionnaire was also reviewed and completed by members of a multidisciplinary ethics consultation service actively involved in ethics case consultation. Positive responses from all these reviews affirmed the construct and content validity of the questionnaire.

Further reliability testing in the form of Chronbach's alpha reliability score was calculated for the responses in the implementation phase of the study; this was necessary because the population of the study is relatively small and difficult to access. The Chronbach's alpha reliability scores were calculated after a factor analysis of the 58 process items. These analyses indicated six factors with eigenvalues of 2.0 or greater and the individual alpha reliability scores for these six factors ranged from .92 to .68. Together these six factors accounted for 48.4 percent of the variance in responses.

After four mailings sent over an eight-week period, the response rate for completed surveys was 74 percent ($n = 289$).

DEMOGRAPHIC DESCRIPTION OF THE SAMPLE

Description of Ethics Consultants

Those ethics consultants responding to the survey reported a range of 1 to 41 years of experience in ethics case consultation and a mean of 8.2 years (with a standard deviation of 5.35 years). The professional affiliation of respondents is displayed in Table 44–1. Physicians and PhDs together represented 69.3 percent of the respondents, a percentage that is consistent with the membership of the Society for Bioethics Consultation as reported at the 1994 Annual Meeting. Nurses represented 15 percent of respondents. The "Others" category included those with the following degrees: JD, MPH, MBA, and Master's degrees in philosophy and theology. The total is more than 100 percent because respondents were asked to choose all the categories that applied.

Sixty-one percent of respondents were male and 37.1 percent were female. This total percentage is less than 100 percent because not all respondents answered this question.

Description of Institutional Setting

The vast majority of respondents (94 percent) reported working in a hospital setting. The distribution of institutional settings for respondents is displayed in Table 44–2. Total percentages are greater than 100 percent because respondents were asked to include all the sites in which they provided consultation. "Other" types of health care facilities identified by respondents and reported in Table 44–2 included hospices, health maintenance organizations, academic health services systems, and rehabilitation centers.

The size of the hospitals in which respondents worked varied from under 100 to over 1,000 beds, with the median being a hospital with 251–500 beds. The distribution of hospital size among respondents is illustrated in Table 44–3.

Most of the hospitals (88.4 percent) with which respondents were affiliated were teaching hospitals associated with a medical school or hosting medical residents. Sixty-nine percent of respondents reported working in private nonprofit institutions, 27.7 percent in public institutions, and 2.2 percent in private for-profit institutions.

Table 44–1 Professional Affiliation of Study Sample Respondents

Professional Affiliation	*Percentage of Respondents*
Physicians	37.5%
PhDs	31.8%
RNs	15%
Divinity	17.1%
MSWs	1.1%
Others	17.9%

$n = 277$

Table 44–2 Type of Institutional Setting Where Study Consultations Were Conducted

Type of Institution	*Respondents*
Hospital	94%
Long-term care facility	3.2%
Home care agency/ visiting nurse association	1.8%
Other	8.9%

$n = 278$

Table 44–3 Hospital Size among Study Sample Respondents

Number of Beds	*Percentage of Respondents*
1–100	1.5%
101–250	13.7%
251–500	39.3%
501–800	28.1%
801–1,000	11.5%
1,001+	5.9%

n = 270

Respondent Relationship to the Institutional Ethics Committee

Respondents reported a surprising variety of relationships with the institutional ethics committee. The majority of respondents were members of the ethics committee (85.7 percent). Many, however, were not and their relationship to the institution's Ethics Committee is reported in Table 44–4. The "Other" category included several variations:

- membership on an ethics consultation service, which in some cases was part of the ethics committee and in other cases was not
- membership in a department of bioethics that was distinct from the ethics committee
- being a fellow or an advisor to the ethics committee
- being an ex-officio member of the ethics committee

Table 44–4 Relationship of Respondent to Institution's Ethics Committee

Description of Respondent's Relationship to Institution's Ethics Committee	*Percentage of Respondents*
Member of ethics committee	85.7%
Functions independently from the ethics committee	8.9%
Institution does not have an ethics committee	7.4%
Provides reports but not an ethics committee member	3.9%
Other	13.2%

n = 279

The percentages reported in Table 44–4 total more than 100 percent because respondents were asked to choose all the answers that described their situation.

Approaches to Ethics Consultation

Many approaches to ethics consultation were used by the respondents. The most frequently used approach, chosen by 61.8 percent of respondents, was several members of the ethics committee together responding to the case consultation. The least-chosen approach was that of a consultant who functioned independently from the ethics committee. Other variations and their distribution among respondents are found in Table 44–5. Percentages total more than 100

Table 44–5 Approaches to Ethics Case Consultation within Study Sample

Description of Approach	*Percentage of Respondents Who Chose Description*
Several members of the ethics committee together respond as consultants	61.8%
Whole ethics committee acts together as consultants	30.4%
One member of the ethics committee is the consultant	26.1%
Several ethics committee members are consultants, but they respond as single consultants	17.5%
Consultation is provided by someone independent of the ethics committee	12.1%
Other	16.1%

n = 277

percent because respondents were asked to choose all the responses that applied. The predominant description of "Other" types of approaches was that of a consultation team, often referred to as the "Ethics Consultation Service." This team was distinct from the ethics committee.

Respondents were asked to identify *all* the ways in which ethics case consultation was accomplished. One-third of the respondents indicated that they used more than one approach to providing consultation. When more than one approach was used, the one most frequently used was that of several members of the committee responding together. The least frequently used approach was that of an individual, independent of the ethics committee, providing consultation. The distribution of the most frequently used approach for ethics case consultation intervention when more than one is used is illustrated in Table 44–6.

Access to Ethics Consultation

Respondents were also asked who in their institution could *request* an ethics consultation. Table 44–7 shows the respondents' answers to this question, identifying the percentage of respondents who indicated that the corresponding group could request ethics consultation. For example, 98.3 percent of respondents indicated that attending physicians could request ethics consultation. Responses are listed in the table in descending order of percentage, and it is interesting to note that the nurses are the second most frequently identified group who could request ethics case consultation.

Approximately one-third of respondents indicated choices in the "Other" category. Seventy percent of respondents choosing this Other category identified "anyone" or "anyone with an interest in the case" as those others who could request an ethics consultation, which indicates a fairly open access to the request for ethics case consultation. For a small percentage of these respondents (approximately 9 percent), the request for consultation must be agreed to by the attending physician.

Ethics Committees

Respondents who were members of the institution's ethics committee (EC) were asked

Table 44–6 Most Frequent Approach to Ethics Case Consultation When More Than One Approach Is Used

Consultation Approach	*Percent of Respondents*
Several members of the ethics committee together respond as consultants	32.6%
One member of the ethics committee is the consultant	28.4%
Whole ethics committee acts together as consultants	15.8%
Several ethics committee members are consultants, but they respond as single consultants	15.8%
Consultation is provided by someone independent of the ethics committee	3.2%
Other	5.3%

n = 95

Table 44–7 Identification of Who Can Request Ethics Case Consultation within the Study Sample

Professional/ Lay Group	*Percentage of Respondents Indicating This Group Can Request Consultation*
Attending physicians	98.3%
Nurses	92.1%
Patients/families	91.1%
Social workers	87.1%
Chaplains	86.2%
Medical residents	85.7%
Administrators	82.5%
Other clinical staff	78.6%
Others	32.5%

n = 278

several questions about the EC itself. Respondents who were members of ECs indicated that the committees themselves ranged in age from 1 year to 24 years, with a mean of 8.78 years and a standard deviation of 4.22 years. Respondents were also asked to describe the EC membership by indicating the number of people in each category who were members of the EC during the past year. For the 245 respondents answering this question, results are reported in Table 44–8 in terms of the minimum, maximum, and mean number (and standard deviation) of people in each category, listed in decreasing frequency. In the "Others" category, there were 37 different roles or professional representatives identified in written responses. The most frequently identified groups (in decreasing order of frequency) were a patient representative or ombudsperson, board representative or trustee, medical resident or intern, psychologist or psychiatrist, risk manager, respiratory therapist, lawyer, academic professor, and medical student. In general, these results seem to indicate that ECs on average have a fairly multidisciplinary membership.

Respondents were also asked who were the chair or cochairpersons of the EC. Responses to this question are reported in Table 44–9. The most frequent group serving as the chair or cochair was physicians, followed by nurses, ethicists, clergy, hospital administrators, "Others," social workers, community representatives, and lawyers. The "Others" included a vice-president for nursing, hospital board member, and quality assurance representative.

Reporting Structure of Ethics Committee

Respondents were also asked about the reporting structure of the EC, that is, "to whom in the organizational structure does the EC report?" The results showed a diverse reporting structure among ECs and are summarized in Table 44–10. Half of the ECs reported to the medical branch of the institution (including the department of medicine, the medical executive committee, or the chief of staff) and slightly more than one-quarter reported to the board of directors. Less than 2 percent reported to the department of nursing. One-quarter reported to other entities in the organizations including the chief executive officer, the administration, hospital patient care review committee, president, clinical practice committee, executive committee, medical policy council, and the director of patient services. The percentages total more than 100 percent because some ECs reported to more than one organizational area.

Ethics Committees' Functions

Respondents were asked about the proportion of time the EC spends performing its functions.

Table 44–8 Ethics Committee Membership within Study Sample

Category	*Mean (± S.D.)*	*Minimum*	*Maximum*
Physicians	6.29 (3.5)	1.0	28
Nurses	4.03 (2.1)	0	14
Clergy/spiritual advisors	1.45 (.86)	0	6
Hospital administrators	1.37 (1.8)	0	10
Social workers	1.34 (.88)	0	7
Community representatives	1.32 (1.2)	0	7
Ethicists	1.20 (.90)	0	5
Lawyers	1.01 (.67)	0	4
Others	.81 (1.1)	0	4

n = 245

Table 44–9 Chair or Cochairperson of Ethics Committee within Study Sample

Professional/ Lay Group	*Percentage of Respondents Identifying Them as EC Chair/Cochair*
Physicians	79.7%
Nurses	16.2%
Ethicists	14%
Clergy/spiritual advisors	10.9%
Hospital administrators	4.1%
Others	2.7%
Social workers	1.4%
Community representatives	1.4%
Lawyers	.9%

$n = 222$

For each of four identified functions and two "write-in" options, respondents were asked to estimate the time spent on a scale of 1 to 5, where 1 = none, 2 = very little, 3 = some, 4 = most, and 5 = all. The mean of these responses is reported in Table 44–11. It is interesting to note that on average, EC time was fairly evenly divided among the pursuits of education, policy development, case consultation, and case review. Only a small number of respondents (n = 46) indicated work on "Other" activities and these were predominately identified as research, evaluation, community education, work on specific ad-hoc projects (e.g., preparing for Joint Commission on Accreditation of Healthcare Organizations accreditation), and involvement in regional and national organizations.

Table 44–10 Ethics Committee Reporting Structure as Identified by Study Respondents

Organizational Area	*Percentage of Respondents*
Medical Branch	50.2%
Board of Directors	29.1%
Department of Nursing	1.6%
Other	25.9%

$n = 242$

Table 44–11 Identified Mean Time Ethics Committees in Study Sample Spend in Various Functions

Function	*Mean*
Education	3.18
Consultation	2.95
Policy development	3.03
Case review	3.07
Other	3.27

$n = 250$

FINDINGS ON ETHICS CASE CONSULTATION PROCESS

Description of Consultation Process

In order to answer the question of whether the ethics consultants surveyed consistently used a process of ethics case consultation that was based on the Integrated Model of ethics case consultation, the frequency distributions of the 58 process items were examined. For each item, a mean score of 2.5 indicated that the item was reported by respondents to be more than occasionally part of end-of-life consultations (based on the questionnaire scale: 1 = never, 2 = occasionally, 3 = frequently, 4 = always). The data analysis showed that of the 58 items, 47 items had mean scores of 2.5 or greater. Only 11 had a mean score of less than 2.5, and of these 11, seven were negatively worded and expected *not* to be part of the process of ethics case consultation. These items are discussed in more detail later in this section.

Considering first the 47 items with mean scores of 2.5 or greater, they represent, in general, a process that includes both characteristics of philosophical case analysis and mediation. Taken together, the ethics case consultation elements and the mediation elements provide an outline for a process that incorporates the philosophical approach of ethics case analysis with the approach to interpersonal conflict resolution provided by mediation—the Integrated Model of ethics case consultation. There was support in the results for three phases of consultation.

In the intake phase, information is gathered from the many parties involved in the case, including the attending physician, the nurses, the family, and the social worker as well as by seeing or interviewing the patient and reviewing the patient's chart. The discussion phase reflects a facilitated, mediation-based discussion that is fact based, inclusive, patient centered, and morally reflective and in which conclusions are nonbinding recommendations reached by consensus. The follow-up phase often includes contact with the consultee, patient, family, and an assessment of the usefulness of the consultation by the parties involved. The case is often presented retrospectively to the ethics committee. Recommendations are often carried out.

The 11 items that had mean scores less than 2.5 represented three themes: infrequent intake, unlikely discussion, and informal follow-up. The first three items were all part of the intake phase of the consultation and represented the theme of infrequent intake. They refer to professionals with whom the ethics consultant *less* frequently discussed the concerns of the case and were the institution attorney, respiratory therapist, and dietitian.

The second theme, reflected in seven items that were all part of the discussion phase of the consultation, addressed group-process issues. These were all negatively worded process items that were not expected to be part of the process of ethics case consultation. Taken together, they described a leaderless discussion with a threatening or domineering tone in which the patient's point of view was subordinate to others and in which final recommendations were reached by voting. It is reassuring that these items are infrequently reported to be part of the process of ethics case consultation, and therefore represent an unlikely discussion in ethics case consultation.

The third theme, informal follow-up, was reflected in a single item. The low mean score of this item indicated that a *formal* meeting to discuss the outcomes of the case consultation was not often reported by respondents.

In general, these results support the argument that, by their own report, ethics consultants do consistently use a process of ethics consultation that combines elements of philosophical case analysis and interpersonal conflict resolution when intervening in end-of-life consultations. The results also support the argument that this process seems to have three phases—intake, case discussion, and follow-up.

Demographic Findings

The sample closely resembled the membership of the study group, the Society for Bioethics Consultation, in terms of professional affiliation. Physicians and PhDs represented 69 percent of respondents and nurses represented 15 percent. The representativeness of this sample to the population of ethics consultants is difficult to estimate. As discussed earlier, it is not known how many ethics consultants there are in the United States. This newly developing area of expertise is without widely accepted standards for training[16] or a system for certification or recognition.[17] The Society for Bioethics Consultation is the only organization among several national and international bioethics organizations whose focus is solely the activity of ethics consultation. Estimates of the number of ethics consultants currently practicing range from 1,000 (Christine Mitchell, personal communication, August 1994) to over 2,000 according to La Puma and Schiedermayer in their 1994 book on ethics consultation.[18] Because of the nascent state of development of this field, this study offers an exploratory description of those individuals practicing in this field.

Though there are no recent data on ethics consultants in the United States available for comparison, a recent study of Canadian ethics consultants provides some international comparison. Coughlin and Watts[19] report on a survey of Canadian ethics consultants, carried out in conjunction with a larger Canadian project looking at the issue of credentialing ethics consultants. Of 350 questionnaires sent out to ethics consultants, ethics committee networks, and hospitals, the authors reported a 72 percent response rate with 161 completed questionnaires returned. Though limited to Canada, Coughlin and Watts state that it is "reasonable to believe that the findings . . . may be applicable to ethics consultants throughout North America,"[20] and a limited comparative analysis of both surveys would seem to support this. The Canadian study found that 70 percent of ethics consultants were male and 28 percent were female, compared to the findings of this study that found 61 percent of ethics consultants were male and 37 percent were female. Canadian results indicated that 79 percent of ethics consultants were members of ethics committees, compared to 86 percent of the U.S. respondents of this study. Both surveys found ethics consultants had heterogeneous professional backgrounds, and these are reported in Table 44–12. It is interesting to note that in general, not only are the backgrounds of ethics consultants in both countries multidisciplinary, but they are so in very similar proportions.

Though the authors of the Canadian study stated that most respondents worked in acute-care hospitals, data were not given to support this. In this study, 94 percent of respondents reported working in acute-care settings. Unfortunately, the Canadian survey as reported lacked any information regarding the process of ethics case consultation.

Table 44–12 Comparison of Canadian and United States Ethics Consultants' Professional Affiliation

Professional Affiliation	*Canada*	*United States*
MD	33%	38%
RN	12%	15%
Theology/divinity	26%	17%
PhD/philosophy	31%	32%

Source: Data from M. D. Coughlin and J. L. Watts, What Does a Health Care Ethics Consultant Look Like?: Results of a Canadian Study, in *The Health Care Ethics Consultant,* F. E. Baylis, ed., pp. 163–188, © 1994, Humana Press.

The Use of a Consistent Process in End-of-Life Ethics Case Consultations

The findings of the study supported the position that ethics consultants do consistently use a process of ethics case consultation when intervening in end-of-life consultations. The process is based on an Integrated Model that combines elements of philosophical case analysis with elements of group process and mediation. However, it is important to appreciate the fact that there is not "one way" of doing ethics consultation for which there is agreement in the literature.

Ross and colleagues identify three general models for case consultation: the medical model, the legal model, and the educational model.[21] Briefly, the medical model is akin to medical consultation in which one or two consultants personally interview the individuals involved in the case. The medical model emphasizes expertise of the consultants while the emphasis on a multidisciplinary perspective is diminished. The legal model is based on thinking of case consultation as a kind of "hearing," with a focus on gathering "evidence" from all the parties and attending to issues of due process. This model emphasizes legal precedent and assumes that a dispute involves two conflicting sides that require a separate individual or group to decide which side has the "better argument" and should therefore "win."

The educational model suggests an egalitarian perspective that downplays characterizing cases as "conflicts" and emphasizes the importance of multidisciplinary input. This model assumes that problems can be resolved if individuals sit down together and talk about their different perspectives, knowledge, and thoughts. Emphasis is on "process, active listening, and careful articulation of the issues."[22] Of these types, the educational model is most similar to the model used in the survey instrument.

Ross et al. acknowledge that in practice, more than one model or a hybrid of two or three may be used.[23] The point they emphasize is that there should be clarity by those consulting as to the model they are using, which would include making its perspective (and assumptions) clear to those requesting consultation. While the results of this study do not address the consultee's perspective, they do indicate that consultants use an identifiable process when intervening in ethics case consultations. Some of the written comments from respondents indicated that they employed more than one model when intervening in consultations and that the decision on how to intervene was based on the nature of the request.

Emphasis on the importance of an identifiable and consistent process is made by several authors.[24] Walker notes that in the literature from the mid-1970s to the mid-1980s, articles about ethics consultants focused on what ethicists knew, figuring them to be "moral engineers" who upheld standards for rigorous argument and logic.[25] Since the mid-1980s, the focus shifted to the ethicists' role as facilitator of a process of moral decision making within a community. The ethics consultant was neither a "virtuoso of moral theory nor a moral virtuoso."[26] The unique role of the ethics consultant in a health care organization was to foster a collective and collaborative moral process.[27]

In writing about practical aspects of ethics case consultation, La Puma and Schiedermayer also emphasize the importance of attention to process in this endeavor.

> Whether consultations can be considered successful will . . . depend not just on the empiric measurement of satisfaction and cost-effectiveness, but also on the value of the consultation process. What is meant by a good "process" of ethics consultation? The consultative process is formed by the various elements of information gathering, case analysis, and interpersonal communication.[28]

Some details of the process that these authors identify are different from the one described in this survey (e.g., it includes the consultant's performing a thorough physical examination and mental-status examination of the patient). However, their emphasis on process lends credibility to the focus of this study.

In recent years there has been increasing concern about the need for standards and evaluation in ethics consultation.[29] This has been driven, at least in part, by the accrediting agency's standards that require a mechanism for addressing ethical issues that arise within the health care institution.[30] Recently initiated work to evaluate ethics case consultation, funded by the Agency for Health Care Policy Research,[31] has begun with the need to develop a consensus statement on the goals of ethics consultation.[32] After pointing out the paucity of published studies on the process and outcomes of ethics case consultation, these authors point out several important basic questions that need to be studied in order to establish the credibility of this newly developing field. Among them is the question "Do ethics consultants follow a particular process in performing ethics consultations, or are their practices highly variable?"[33] The findings of this study are an important beginning step to addressing that question.

Limitations of the Study

There are several limitations of the study related to the research design. First, there are the limitations on the generalizability of the results because of the nonrandom sampling technique employed. The decision to sample the entire membership of the only professional group specifically for ethics consultants was justified for two reasons. The first was the exploratory nature of the study and the second was the uncertainty as to the size of the total population and difficulty gaining access to them. As noted earlier, estimates of the number of ethics consultants in the United States range from 1,000 to over 2,000. The latter estimate comes from La Puma and Schiedermayer, though they offer no references or justification for how they arrived at this number, except to say that "in 1985, only 51 consultants attended a NIH/UCSF exploratory meeting. . . ."[34]

The second limitation of the study relates to the survey design, which asked respondents to report retrospectively on their own or other ethics consultants' observed behavior. Problems of eliciting a social desirability response set given the content of the survey, despite careful attention to the wording of the survey items, remains a limitation.[35] Another limitation related to the respondent self-report design is that of perspective. Respondents were asked how frequently on average a process item was part of the ethic case consultations in which they were involved. A limitation of this study design is that different parties participating in the consultation may have had different answers to how frequently an event occurred and consequently their perspective is not captured in the survey.

A third limitation was the decision to limit the ethics consultation cases to those involving end-of-life decisions. Though these decisions are often a source of conflict for health care providers,[36] this limits interpretation of the results to these kinds of cases and raises the question of whether the process of case consultation is different for other types of cases.

SUMMARY

At a time when there is both increasing encouragement and scrutiny of ethics case consultation, this study was undertaken to describe the process of ethics case consultation and ethics consultants themselves. The response rate for the study was 74 percent and the results indicated that the ethics consultants responding to the survey reported a range of 1 to 41 years of experience in ethics case consultation and a mean of 8.2 years (with a standard deviation of 5.35 years). Physicians and PhDs represented 69 percent of respondents and nurses represented 15 percent. Approximately two-thirds of the sample were male. The institutional setting for 94 percent of respondents was the hospital, with a median size of 251–500 beds. Most of the hospitals (88 percent) were teaching hospitals and 69 percent of them were private, nonprofit institutions. Two percent were private, for-profit.

The majority of ethics consultant respondents were members of the institution's ethics committee (86 percent), though respondents reported a number of relationships to the EC, as well as a variety of approaches to ethics consultation. The predominant approach chosen by 62 percent of respondents was several members of the EC together responding to the case consultation. Requests for ethics consultation were generally open. Over 90 percent of the sample indicated that attending physicians, nurses, patients, and families could request an ethics consultation. Over 80 percent of respondents indicated that social workers, chaplains, and administrators could request consultation.

In responding to questions about ECs, those respondents who were members indicated that the committees had a mean age of almost nine years. On average, committees had a diverse multidisciplinary membership that was dominated by physicians and nurses, with three-fourths having a chair or cochair who was a physician. Over three-fourths of these ECs reported to either the medical branch of the institution or to the board of directors. The committees' time was reported to be nearly evenly divided among the pursuits of education, policy development, consultation, and case review.

The survey results indicated that the ethics consultants responding to the study use a consistent and identifiable consultation process when intervening in end-of-life consultations. The process has three phases and is based on an Integrated Model of ethics consultation that incorporates elements of philosophical case analysis and a mediation approach to conflict resolution. In the intake phase, information is gathered from the parties involved in the case. The discussion phase reflects a facilitated, mediation-oriented discussion that is fact based, inclusive, patient centered, and morally reflective. Conclusions in the discussion are nonbinding recommendations reached by consensus. The follow-up phase of the consultation includes contact with many of the parties involved and assessment of the consultation by them.

Limitations of the study exist related to the nonrandom sampling techniques, respondent self-report, and limitation to end-of-life case consultations. However, the strong factor analysis and Chronbach's alpha scores enhance the argument that the results of the study make a useful contribution to the empirical study of ethics case consultation.

NOTES

1. The Hastings Center, *Guidelines on the Termination of Treatment and the Care of the Dying* (Bloomington, Ind.: Indiana University Press, 1987).
2. L. Blackhall, "Must We Always Use CPR?" *New England Journal of Medicine* 317, no. 20 (1987): 1281–84.
3. American Hospital Association, "Hospitals" in *Ethics in Medicine,* ed. S. J. Reiser et al. (Cambridge, Mass.: MIT Press, 1985), 148–49.
4. President's Commission for the Study of Ethical Problems in Medicine and Biomedical and Behavioral Research, *Making Health Care Decisions* (Washington, D.C.: U.S. Government Printing Office, 1982).
5. K. Teel, "The Physicians' Dilemma: A Doctor's View. What Should the Law Be?" *Baylor Law Review* 27 (1975): 109–15.
6. J. C. Fletcher and M. Siegler, "What Are the Goals of Ethics Consultation? A Consensus Statement." *Journal of Clinical Ethics* 7, no. 2 (1996): 122–26.
7. B. Freedman, "One Philosopher's Experience on an Ethics Committee," *Hastings Center Report* 11, no. 2 (1981): 20–22; R. E. Cranford and A. E. Doudera, "The Emergency of Institutional Ethics Committee," in *Institutional Ethics Committees and Health Care Decision Making,* ed. R. Cranford and A. Doudera (Ann Arbor, Mich.: Health Administration Press, 1984); M. D. Swensen and R. B. Miller, "Ethics Case Review in Health Care Institutions," *Archives of Internal Medicine* 152 (April 1992): 694–97.
8. J. La Puma and E. R. Priest, "Medical Staff Privileges for Ethics Consultants: An Institutional Model," *Quality Review Bulletin* 18, no. 1 (1992): 17–20; J. La Puma and D. Schiedermayer, *Ethics Consultation* (Boston: Jones and Bartlett, 1994).
9. M. Siegler, "Ethics Committees: Decisions by Bureaucracy," *Hastings Center Report* (June 1986): 22–24; J. E. Fleetwood et al., "Giving Answers or Raising Questions: The Problematic Role of Institutional Ethics Committees," *Journal of Medical Ethics* 15 (1989): 137–42.
10. La Puma and Schiedermayer, *Ethics Consultation*; A. R. Jonsen, *Clinical Ethics,* 3d ed. (New York: McGraw-Hill, 1992).
11. B. Lo, "Behind Closed Doors: Promises and Pitfalls of Ethics Committees," *New England Journal of Medicine* 317, no. 1 (1987): 46–50; M. B. Mahowald, "Hospital Ethics Committees: Diverse and Problematic," *Hospital Ethics Committee Forum* 1 (1989): 237–46; J. A. Tulsky and B. Lo, "Evaluating Ethics Consultation: Framing the Question," *American Journal of Medicine* 92 (1992): 343–45.
12. J. C. Fletcher, "Needed: A Broader View of Ethics Consultation," *Quality Review Bulletin* 18 (1992): 12–14; J. La Puma et al., "Community Hospital Ethics Consultation: Evaluation and Comparison with a University Hospital Service," *American Journal of Medicine* 92 (1992): 346–51.
13. M. Gordon et al., "Clinical Judgment: An Integrated Model," *Advances in Nursing Science* 16, no. 4 (1994): 55–70; A. R. Jonson, "Case Analysis in Clinical Ethics," *Journal of Clinical Ethics* 1, no. 1 (1990): 63–65.
14. M. B. West and J. M. Gibson, "Facilitating Medical Ethics Case Review: What Ethics Committees Can Learn from Mediation and Facilitation Techniques," *Cambridge Quarterly of Healthcare Ethics* 1 (1992): 63–74.
15. West and Gibson, "Facilitating Medical Ethics Case Review."
16. La Puma and Schiedermayer, *Ethics Consultation.*
17. F. E. Baylis, "A Profile of the Health Care Ethics Consultant," in *The Health Care Ethics Consultant,* ed. F. E. Baylis (Totowa, N.J.: Humana Press, 1994), 25–44.
18. La Puma and Schiedermayer, *Ethics Consultation.*
19. M. D. Coughlin and J. L. Watts, "What Does a Health Care Ethics Consultant Look Like? Results of a Canadian Study," in *The Health Care Ethics Consultant,* ed. F. E. Baylis (Totowa, N.J.: Humana Press, 1994), 163–88.
20. Coughlin and Watts, "What Does a Health Care Ethics Consultant Look Like?" 164.
21. J. W. Ross et al., *Health Care Ethics Committees: The Next Generation* (Chicago: American Hospital Publishing, 1993).
22. Ross et al., *Health Care Ethics Committees,* 93.
23. Ross et al., *Health Care Ethics Committees.*
24. Fleetwood et al., "Giving Answers or Raising Questions"; D. C. Blake, "The Hospital Ethics Committee," *Hastings Center Report* 22, no. 1 (1992): 6–11.
25. M. U. Walker, "Keeping Moral Spaces Open: New Images of Ethics Consulting," *Hastings Center Report* 23, no. 2 (1993): 33–40.
26. Ibid., 38.
27. Walker, "Keeping Moral Spaces Open."
28. La Puma and Schiedermayer, *Ethics Consultation,* 32.
29. J. C. Fletcher and D. E. Hoffmann, "Ethics Committees: Time to Experiment with Standards," *Annals of Internal Medicine* 120, no. 4 (1994): 335–38; R. M. Arnold and S. J. Youngner, "Task Force on Standards for Ethics Consultation," *Cambridge Quarterly of Healthcare Ethics* 5, no. 2 (1996), 284.
30. Joint Commission on Accreditation of Hospitals, *Accreditation Manual for Hospitals* (Chicago: Joint Commission on the Accreditation of Hospitals, 1993).

31. J. A. Tulsky and E. Fox, "Evaluating Ethics Consultation: Framing the Question," *Journal of Clinical Ethics* 7, no. 2 (1996): 109–15.

32. Fletcher and Siegler, "What Are the Goals of Ethics Consultation?"

33. Ibid., 124.

34. La Puma and Schiedermayer, *Ethics Consultation,* 43.

35. D. F. Polit and B. P. Hungler, *Nursing Research* (Philadelphia: J. B. Lippincott, 1991).

36. M. Z. Solomon et al., "Decisions Near the End of Life: Professional Views on Life-Sustaining Treatments," *American Journal of Public Health* 83, no. 1 (1993): 14–23.

Chapter 45

Can There Be Educational and Training Standards for Those Conducting Health Care Ethics Consultation?

Mark P. Aulisio, Robert M. Arnold, and Stuart J. Youngner

INTRODUCTION: MOTIVATING THE QUESTION

The question of educational and training standards for those conducting health care ethics consultation (HCEC) has been raised with increasing frequency in the last few years.[1] Indeed, the Society for Health and Human Values and the Society for Bioethics Consultation have recently convened a joint task force to study this issue. Though it is viewed with cynicism by some, we think that the concern with standards is motivated primarily by the complexity of the issues involved in HCEC; its increasing prevalence; its practical impact on patients, families, and health care providers; and, therefore, the inevitable demand for accountability.[2] Ultimately, the concern with educational and training standards for those performing HCEC should be a call for quality assurance.

In contemporary health care settings, ethics consultation often involves highly complex ethical issues that also have medical, legal, and psychosocial dimensions. Health care professionals face difficult issues ranging from abortion, euthanasia, and assisted suicide to organ donation and transplantation, genetic testing, and the spread of sexually transmitted diseases. In addition to their obvious medical dimensions, these issues raise moral and legal questions about, among other things, patient autonomy, informed consent, health care provider rights of conscience, medical futility, resource allocation, and confidentiality. Furthermore, the types of issues listed above usually emerge in actual cases inextricably bound up with complex interpersonal and affective aspects such as guilt over a loved one's death, disagreement between different health care providers, conflicts of interest, and distrust of the medical system. Due to the complexity of these ethical issues, health care providers, patients, or families may request assistance to help think through the issue in question or resolve conflicts that may be present.

Given the plethora of complex moral questions raised by the delivery of health care in contemporary society, it is not difficult to understand HCEC's increasing prevalence. The development of HCEC has been indirectly sup-

---

Please Note: Though the authors are leading the SHHV-SBC Task Force on Standards for Bioethics Consultation, the views expressed by them in this chapter do not represent those of the Task Force. Furthermore, the chapter is meant to raise, not answer, questions that will need to be addressed before standards for the education and training of those who do ethics consultation could be adopted. Lastly, the authors want to be clear at the outset that in this chapter they are neither endorsing nor rejecting the setting of educational and training standards for those conducting ethics consultation.

ported by the courts and endorsed by the 1983 President's Commission for the Study of Ethical Problems in Medicine and Biomedical and Behavioral Research as a mechanism for dispute resolution outside of litigation.[3] Indeed, the Joint Commission on Accreditation of Healthcare Organizations (Joint Commission) now requires that each institution have a "process to address ethical issues" that may emerge in patient care and organizational issues that affect it.[4] It is estimated that 80 to 90 percent of all United States hospitals now have an ethics committee.[5] Other health care institutions, such as home health agencies and nursing homes, are rapidly developing ethics services as well.[6]

It is not surprising that as ethics consultation becomes increasingly prevalent, concerns with accountability grow. To date, there have been at least six legal cases in which ethics committees or consultants were named or negatively implicated.[7] Consider, for example, the famous case of Elizabeth Bouvia:

> *Elizabeth Bouvia v. Superior Court of the State of California of the County of Los Angeles (Glenchur).* In 1983, Ms. Bouvia, a 25-year-old quadriplegic suffering from cerebral palsy and crippling arthritis, sought the right to be cared for in a public hospital in Riverside, California, while she carried out her intention to starve herself to death. She was denied this right by a county court. After dropping her appeal, Ms. Bouvia eventually transferred to several different facilities, ending up at Los Angeles County High Desert Hospital in 1985. In order to eat, Ms. Bouvia had to be spoon-fed. Ms. Bouvia would take in only very small amounts of food, complaining that she could not swallow more without nausea and vomiting. She insisted that she was eating as much as she could. Fearing that she was attempting to starve herself to death the medical staff had her fed by nasogastric tube against her explicit written wishes. Before doing this the medical staff sought the backing of the ethics committee, which, in spite of the fact that Ms. Bouvia was found to be a competent decision maker by a psychiatrist, apparently supported the decision to force-feed her. In 1986, the California Court of Appeals ruled in her favor and overturned a lower court's decision supporting the action of the medical staff. Once the nasogastric tube was removed, Ms. Bouvia sued the hospital and medical staff for damages. Upon learning that her physicians had acted with the support of the ethics committee (which they claimed was as responsible as they for the decision), Ms. Bouvia filed an amended complaint which named each member of the ethics committee. Ms. Bouvia eventually voluntarily dropped the suit to avoid further publicity.[8]

For our purposes, the Bouvia case serves to underscore the complexity of HCEC; its real impact on patients, families, and health care providers; and the demand for accountability.

First, the case raises a number of interconnected medical, psychosocial, legal, and moral questions. Those offering ethics consultation would need to have a basic understanding of the medical facts of the case, the implications of the law for various courses of action, and relevant psychosocial data (for example, why Ms. Bouvia considered her life not to be worth living or whether there might be ways of giving her more control over her life). With an understanding of these dimensions of the case, those offering ethics consultation might need to be prepared to consider any or all of the following moral issues:

- provider duties of beneficence especially regarding the provision of hydration and nutrition
- rights to patient autonomy
- the difference between requests for and refusals of treatment

- the notion of competence
- the concept of suicide
- relevance of particular value structures for determinations of quality of life
- the difference between assisting and allowing (or not interfering)
- the implications of deep societal values, such as a right to privacy or self-determination, for any of the above

Second, the case illustrates HCEC's real impact on patients and providers and the inevitable demand for accountability. According to Ms. Bouvia's physicians, consultation with the ethics committee strongly influenced the course of action adopted by the medical staff. Indeed, her physicians argued that because they acted with its support, the ethics committee should share responsibility for the coercive feeding. It is interesting to note here that implicit in the physicians' claim that the ethics committee should be held accountable before the law are at least two other domains of accountability. The claim of Ms. Bouvia's physicians suggests that (1) those conducting HCEC need to be accountable to health care providers, patients, and families and to the institutions that authorize them to offer it, and (2) the institution needs to be accountable to health care providers, patients, and families in authorizing those who offer HCEC to do so.

Though the case of Ms. Bouvia reached litigation, those who engage in HCEC know that it can influence patient care, for better or for worse, and raise questions of accountability in much less dramatic cases. All of this leads to concerns about quality assurance in HCEC. Fear of *legal* accountability alone might suffice for some to be concerned with quality assurance in HCEC.[9] The most compelling reasons to be so concerned, however, stem from the other two domains of accountability identified above. Patients, families, and health care providers *deserve* assurance of competence when they seek HCEC. Likewise, institutions need to be reasonably sure that those they authorize to conduct HCEC are qualified to do so. How can patients, families, and providers be reasonably sure that those from whom they seek ethics consultation are qualified to speak to the range of difficult issues that may come up? How can institutions be reasonably sure that those whom they authorize to offer HCEC are competent to do so? Is it enough that those conducting HCEC merely have an interest in ethics or are well-intentioned? If quality assurance is important for HCEC—if goodwill is not enough to make one competent to offer HCEC—then standards for the education and training of those involved in it may have to be set. In this chapter, we will explore some of the issues that would need to be addressed before such standards could be adopted. We will start by discussing three background questions that have implications for any attempt to set standards for HCEC.

BACKGROUND QUESTIONS

Is HCEC Justifiable in Our Society?

One of the deepest and most difficult issues facing any attempt to set standards for the education and training of ethics consultants is to show whether HCEC itself is consistent with the deep societal values of our liberal constitutional democracy. Indeed, some critics of ethics consultation have argued that the practice of HCEC is *contrary* to such values.[10] Though it *may* be a mistake to think that all forms of HCEC are at odds with the fundamental values of our society, these values, at least, set limits on the types of models for HCEC that will be acceptable. This is because such deep societal values form part of the context within which HCEC must be understood and practiced. What does this mean for HCEC?

The feature of our society's political values that is most relevant to the discussion here is that they afford individuals and communities the right to pursue divergent concepts of the good life, i.e., different moralities or value hierarchies.[11] Furthermore, pluralism in our society is an obvious social fact. We are, among others, widely diverse atheists, agnostics, and theists. We are Catholic, Protestant, Jewish, and Islamic. We are egoists, utilitarians, Kantians, natural lawyers, contractarians, and virtue theorists. We are risk-takers, risk avoiders, optimists, and pessimists. The social fact of pluralism remains true in any contemporary health care setting. Similarly, the right to pursue divergent substantive concepts of morality does not disappear simply because one takes up the practice of various medical professions or falls ill and becomes a patient. HCEC, therefore, may not be understood in such a way that it threatens to undermine this right. This means that, *ceteris paribus*, in a nonsectarian health care setting, HCEC may not be understood and practiced in a way that *privileges* any particular substantive view of morality over this right.[12] Any set of educational and training standards for those conducting HCEC in our society must reflect this requirement, i.e., they must embody and respect our liberal constitutional values. However, if HCEC turns out to be inconsistent with those values, then not only should no set of educational and training standards for HCEC be adopted, but the practice of HCEC itself should be abandoned.

Is the Push for Standards Merely a Veiled Power Play?

Another important background question is the extent to which standard setting amounts to being merely a political exercise by which some groups carve out domains of power at the expense of other groups.[13] In this view, far from being a call for quality assurance, the push for standards is really a push for economic and social privilege. Those who win the battle over the *content* of educational and training standards take the spoils. For example, some might consider a requirement that ethics consultants have a highly specialized knowledge of moral theory to be motivated by the desire of philosophers to establish a domain of power in health care. Or, to take another example, some might consider a requirement that those conducting HCEC be able to complete a physical exam of the patient to be nothing more than a thinly veiled attempt by physician ethics consultants to ensure that the field of HCEC becomes their exclusive province. On this view, standard setting ultimately serves only to promote the social and economic interests of those who set and then satisfy the standards. Anyone attempting to set educational and training standards for those performing HCEC must not be naive about the political dimensions of this endeavor.

Should HCEC Maintain Disciplinary Diversity?

An important related issue is the extent to which standard setting will affect disciplinary diversity. One of the more unique features of the developing field of ethics consultation is its multidisciplinary nature. We, along with many others, believe that this disciplinary diversity is a strength that should be preserved. It is not only the *content* of educational and training standards (as suggested above), but also the *implementation* of those standards that may affect this diversity in different ways. For example, the *implementation* of educational and training standards through national *certification* or *licensing* of individuals to conduct HCEC could easily lead to the development of a new profession that required disciplinary homogeneity rather than diversity.[14] If disciplinary diversity is a strength of the field that should be preserved, then the content and, especially, implementation of educational and training standards for HCEC will have to be assessed for their impact on it.

CENTRAL QUESTIONS

What Is Ethics Consultation and What Are Its Goals?

Against this backdrop, we are now ready to consider some of the more central questions that will have to be addressed before standards can be set. First, if standards are to be set for a given activity, it will be important to identify what the activity is supposed to be and, further, what it is supposed to achieve. Without at least a rough characterization of HCEC there will be no way to identify appropriate education and training for those who will conduct it. Indeed, it is doubtful that HCEC should go on at all if those of us who endorse it are unable to even say what it is and what it aims to achieve. The question of the nature and goals of HCEC itself raises a question about the relation between them.

Is the Setting of Goals Prior To Characterizing the Nature of HCEC?

There are a variety of goals for HCEC that have been suggested in the literature.[15] For example, some have suggested that they are:

- [T]o improve patient outcomes
- [T]o assist the primary physician, the patient, and the family to reach a right and good clinical decision[16]

or:

- To maximize benefit and minimize harm to patients, families, healthcare professionals, and institutions by fostering a fair and inclusive decision-making process that honors patients'/proxy preferences and individual and cultural value differences among all parties to the consultation
- To facilitate resolution of conflicts in a respectful atmosphere with attention to the interests, rights, and responsibilities of those involved
- To inform institutional efforts at policy development, quality improvement, and appropriate utilization of resources by identifying the causes of ethical problems and to promote practices consistent with ethical norms and standards
- To assist individuals in handling current and future ethical problems by providing education in healthcare ethics[17]

To these, in the absence of a concept of the nature of HCEC, we might arbitrarily add:

- To build consensus among the concerned parties
- To lower health care costs
- To increase patient satisfaction
- To protect health care providers and institutions against lawsuits
- To return patients to normal functioning
- To promote patient's rights
- To morally police medical practice

Some of the above goals are so general that they can be promoted by many activities. For example, increasing patient satisfaction or improving patient outcomes can be promoted by medical practice, nursing, dietetics, and many other clinical services. Other goals are very specific, but they, too, may be served by several different activities. For example, the goal of protecting health care providers and institutions against lawsuits could be served by legal services, patient advocacy, or ethics consultation. Though many would recognize the realization of this goal as a possible side effect of ethics consultation, few, if any, would suggest that it is one of its central goals. How does one identify which goals are central, or even relevant, to HCEC? Intuitively, most of us would probably identify similar goals for HCEC, but what drives this intuition?

Underlying any intuition one might have regarding the proper goals of an activity is, at the very least, an implicit concept of the nature of that activity. It is that concept of what the activity is *supposed* to be that allows one to identify certain goals as *appropriate* to it. To use a humorous example, imagine that your colleague professed that one of his goals in going to the dentist was to have a bunion removed from his foot. With the possible exception of a colleague who was constantly, and quite literally, putting his foot in his mouth, we would be sure that your colleague was confused about the nature of dentistry. To be sure, any characterization of the nature of a purposeful activity will have built into it certain goals. This follows directly from the purposefulness of the activity. Indeed, it is precisely because a characterization of the nature of an activity includes certain proximate goals that it allows one to identify other possible goals as appropriate or inappropriate for the activity. What is important for our purposes is that the nature and goals of HCEC are integrally related, and, if standards are to be adopted for HCEC, how its nature and goals are characterized will be of paramount importance.

How Shall the Nature of HCEC and Its Goals Be Characterized?

There are at least two ways that one could attempt to arrive at a characterization of HCEC. One way is to conduct empirical research to determine what actually goes on in the name of HCEC. Here one's characterization would amount to a description of the current practice of HCEC. At present, this empirical data has not been adequately gathered.[18] Though useful for various purposes, the gathering of empirical data regarding what *is* going on in the name of HCEC would be of only limited relevance for setting standards. This is because standard setting is an intrinsically *normative* endeavor. The attempt to derive standards from empirical data alone would amount to an attempt to derive an *ought* from an *is*. What is needed before standards for the education and training of ethics consultants can be set is a *normative* characterization of the nature and goals of HCEC, i.e., a characterization of what HCEC *ought* to be and aim to achieve. As we shall see in a moment, different *normative* characterizations of the nature and goals of HCEC will have important implications for educational and training standards for those conducting it.

What Is the Proper Scope of HCEC?

Another question that will affect the setting of educational and training standards for those conducting HCEC concerns its proper scope. Standards for education and training might be quite different depending on whether HCEC is supposed to extend only to case consultation or whether its scope is expanded to include, for example, policy consultation. Matters of policy about which HCEC might be sought could range from those that are directly relevant to patient care (e.g., development of a do not resuscitate (DNR) policy) to those that will indirectly affect patient care. The latter might include, among other things, issues of organizational ethics such as marketing (e.g., targeting populations, creating "needs," and so forth), institutional resource allocation (e.g., the purchase of expensive technologies, etc.), and the acceptance of donor funds from suspect sources (e.g., tobacco companies, and so forth). It is clear that standards for the education of those who may conduct HCEC regarding, for example, institutional resource allocation issues may be quite different from standards for those who will conduct case-oriented HCEC. This is because important knowledge bases would differ for the two areas.

In Light of a Normative Characterization of HCEC, Its Goals, and Scope, What Kinds of Skills, Knowledge, or Character Traits Might Be Required for HCEC?

If the daunting task of characterizing the nature, goals, and scope of HCEC can be surmounted, the setting of educational and training standards would require that the kinds of skills, knowledge, and character traits necessary for HCEC be identified.[19] The core features of the characterization of HCEC will help to pick out the elements necessary to engage in it. To illustrate this, we will consider, in turn, caricatures of three models of ethics consultation that can be elicited from the literature.[20] We want to emphasize at the outset that these models are caricatures. *Certain features of these models will be exaggerated so that we can clearly show how these models, which capture different views of the nature and goals of ethics consultation, have different implications for the skills, knowledge, and character traits that would be necessary for conducting it.*

The first model for HCEC we will term the secular-priest model. Let us suppose that a defining characteristic of this model is that those conducting HCEC are thought to be substantive moral experts. That is to say that, on this caricatured model, ethics consultants are akin to *mahatma* who have special access, partly because of their wisdom, to the proper concept of the good life and its instantiation in everyday life. Those who seek consultation from them do so much as one would seek the counsel of a spiritual director. Like a wise sage, the secular priest ethics consultant will seek to instruct parties to the consultation in the ways of moral truth and guide them to the "right" answer. Let us say that ultimately, on the secular-priest model, the goal of ethics consultation is to get parties to the consultation to do the right thing. Right here is in reference to the ethics consultant's particular approach to morality whatever that might be (orthodox Catholicism, utilitarianism, Kantianism, virtue theory, etc.).[21]

For our purposes, the caricatured secular-priest model for HCEC can be contrasted with what we will term the pure-facilitator model. On our caricature of the facilitator model, let us suppose that those conducting HCEC *merely* attempt to facilitate agreement among all concerned parties. Indeed, for the sake of contrast, let us stipulate that the pure-facilitator model presumes no form of ethical expertise whatsoever. The goal of the pure-facilitator model is to get parties to the consultation to form a consensus, whatever that consensus might be.[22]

Lastly, either the caricatured secular-priest model or the pure-facilitator model could be supplemented with a third caricatured model, the medical model. The medical model, though compatible with either of the above, would add core features to the nature and goals of HCEC that are not found in those models. For our caricature, the key feature of the medical model is that those conducting HCEC would need to be able to do a complete medical assessment of the patient. Thus, one of the goals of the medical model of HCEC would be to *evaluate* the medical assessment of the patient made by the medical staff.[23]

It is easy to see how, in each of these exaggerated models for HCEC, different views of its nature and goals will have implications for the skills and knowledge that will be necessary for conducting it. Thus, on the secular-priest model, ethics consultants would need to have detailed knowledge of a particular moral framework and skill in seeing the implications of that framework for individual cases or policy questions. Ethics consultants would have to be skilled in justifying the right course of action or policy. That justification would be a function of each ethics consultant's approach to morality (i.e., value structure or concept of the good life). In this caricature, the ethics consultants would also need to be effective in educating and persuading parties to the dispute to adopt the right course of action or policy, i.e., that which reflects the consultants' substantive moral views. To the extent to which wisdom or any other virtues might be required to understand and apply the moral framework in question, the ethics consultant would need to embody these virtues.

In contrast, on the pure-facilitator model, the only skills and knowledge required would be those that are necessary to build consensus among the parties to the consult. Good interpersonal skills would be critical for the pure facilitator, i.e., the ability to communicate clearly and persuasively, listen well, and facilitate group processes. To the extent that these skills presupposed knowledge of various theories of communication or group dynamics, such knowledge would be required. Likewise, if certain character traits, such as honesty or openness, were identified as critical to consensus building, these might also be required by the model. Since building consensus is the sole aim of the pure-facilitator model as we have caricatured it, a knowledge of ethical theory, skills in ethical analysis or conceptual clarification, or even the ability to identify a problem as moral in nature will not necessarily be requisite.

Last, if the medical model for HCEC is adopted in conjunction with either of the above models, ethics consultants will also need to have the skills and knowledge base of medical specialists. These include, among other things, the skills and knowledge required for medical diagnosis, treatment, and follow-up. Those conducting HCEC would need to be able to do a physical exam of the patient, read lab data, and so forth. Thus, the core features of the medical model impose additional skill and knowledge requirements on the above models.

If the Skills, Knowledge, and Character Traits Required for HCEC Can Be Identified, What Educational and Training Standards Might Be Set for Those Who Will Conduct HCEC To Ensure Competence?

It is clear from the preceding discussion that the type of model adopted for HCEC will have important ramifications for the skills, knowledge, and character traits required to conduct it. Presumably there will be strong correlation among skills, knowledge, and character requirements for conducting HCEC and any educational and training standards that might be set. Thus, the type of model adopted for HCEC will likewise have important ramifications for educational and training standards.

For the secular-priest model, education and training in ethics would be required only insofar as it was training in a particular substantive moral framework. One might also need education and training that would make one an effective communicator and educator. To the extent that certain virtues might be critical for understanding and discerning a particular approach to morality, an intense socialization, possibly through a clinical practicum with an accomplished consultant, might be necessary. In contrast, for the pure-facilitator model, education and training in interpersonal communications, group dynamics, and facilitation or mediation theory and technique might be necessary. Finally, the medical model, if merged with either of the above, would obviously impose additional educational and training requirements similar to that of medical specialists, especially that of physicians.

In discussing educational and training requirements, it may be important to distinguish among those who will do HCEC in different capacities, e.g., as part of a full ethics committee, small consultation group, or individual consultants. Since the scope of HCEC will impact knowledge and skills requirements (and, therefore, educational and training requirements), it might also be important to leave open two tracks, case and policy. We will focus on the different capacities in which HCEC *case* consultation might be conducted.

Educational and Training Standards for Conducting HCEC as Part of the Full Ethics Committee

For the sake of discussion, suppose that the model for HCEC that is adopted required a certain knowledge of the medical, legal, and ethical dimensions of a specified range of issues. Suppose that the model also required skill in ethical analysis and interpersonal communication.[24] Since educational and training standards presuppose certain knowledge and skill requirements, the standards will presumably be far less rigorous for those who do HCEC as part of the full ethics committee than for those who do HCEC individually or as part of a small group. This is because the committee as a whole, rather than individuals or a small group of individuals, will have to embody the requisite skills and knowledge. Thus, if the committee as a whole included physicians and social workers, important elements of the skills and knowledge base supposed above would be satisfied. Indeed, depending on the skills and knowledge base that are required for conducting HCEC, it might be appropriate to set standards regarding the *composition* of the ethics committee.

The fact that HCEC will be done by a full ethics committee, as opposed to individuals or small groups, raises other questions that may have to be addressed to ensure quality. One question that will have to be addressed is whether the whole committee is more than the sum of its parts. To take an extreme example, suppose that one person on the committee had highly specialized knowledge of ethics and skill in analysis, while other members lacked such knowledge and skills altogether. If a group is more than the sum of its parts, a well-functioning group may need to have each member satisfy certain basic requirements. This is particularly important if one wants different viewpoints to be actively represented in ethics committee discussion. For example, to have a certain level of discussion of a complex case, a full ethics committee may need each member to have a basic knowledge of typical issues in bioethics, some skills of ethical analysis, and certain interpersonal skills. One way to help to ensure that each committee member has this might be to require that each HCEC member participate in certain continuing education programs.

Educational and Training Standards for Conducting HCEC as Part of an Ethics Committee Subgroup or Independent HCEC Team

If HCEC is done by an ethics committee subgroup or an independent HCEC team, then the requisite skill and knowledge will have to be contained in the team. Nearly all of the remarks that we made above, regarding the full ethics committee, are applicable here. The main difference is that the skills and knowledge that are required for ethics consultation will have to be concentrated in fewer people. Thus, the educational and training requirements for those who will do HCEC in this capacity might be much more demanding than for those who will do HCEC with a full ethics committee.

There is another interesting difference between doing ethics consultation as part of a small group and doing it as part of the full ethics committee. Full ethics committees will rarely do bedside consultation, but small consultation teams will. This means that not only the degree but also the type of certain skills or knowledge may have to appropriately altered. For example, the sensitive nature of bedside consultation may require a knowledge of small-group dynamics and the ability to communicate support and empathy in a way that consultation with a full ethics committee does not.

Educational and Training Standards for Conducting HCEC as an Individual "Consultant"

If HCEC is conducted by an individual, then that individual will have to embody whatever skills, knowledge, and character traits HCEC requires. This clearly means that individuals who conduct HCEC by themselves will have to satisfy a more rigorous education and training program than those who conduct HCEC in either of the above capacities. In setting educational and training standards for individual consultants, it will be important to distinguish between two senses of *consultant* that have come to be common in the literature. *Consultant* is sometimes used in its literal sense, i.e., those who will conduct consultation. However, *consultant* in some recent bioethics literature has come to have a much broader meaning, i.e., it has come to be synonymous with the term *ethicist.*[25] In this latter sense, there may be many different services offered by ethicists in the clinical setting. These range from case and policy consultation to education and research. Presumably, these areas will place added demands on the appropriate education and training for such individuals by adding knowledge and skill requirements. It may turn out, however, that since individual consultants, in the narrow sense, have to embody whatever knowledge and skills are required for HCEC, they may be very close to being qualified as consultants, in the broad ethicists sense.[26]

If They Are Arrived at, How Shall Educational and Training Standards Be Implemented: Recommending, Credentialing, Accrediting, Certifying, Licensing?

In a very real sense, once educational and training standards have been identified for those who will do ethics consultation in various capacities, the question of standards will have been answered. Questions about recommending, credentialing, accrediting, certifying, and licensing are really questions about how best to *implement* educational and training standards. In answering these questions, the strengths and weaknesses of each form of implementation will have to be considered. Questions of recommending, credentialing, accrediting, certifying, and licensing are very difficult to address in the abstract, that is, without knowing the content of the educational and training standards for those who will do HCEC in various capacities. Before concluding, we will briefly consider a few possible alternatives for implementing educational and training standards.

First, educational and training standards for those who will conduct HCEC in various capacities could be issued as a set of *recommendations* to be taken into account by (1) individuals in planning their own educational/training programs, (2) programs designed for the education and training of those who will conduct HCEC in various capacities, (3) committees or teams in seeing to it that each member along with the collective group is adequately prepared for HCEC, or (4) institutions trying to ensure that those who offer HCEC are competent to do so. Though this approach has much to be said for it, one of its weaknesses is the danger that educational and training standards for HCEC may not achieve the end goal of quality assurance because they may not be widely followed.

Second, educational and training standards could be implemented through the *credentialing*, *certifying*, or *licensing* of individuals or groups who do ethics consultation. Credentialing, certifying, or licensing could be done either by the state or an organization (such as one or all of the major bioethics societies). Sorting out the differences among each of these options and their relative strengths and weaknesses would take us far beyond the purview of this chapter.[27] Indeed, these questions themselves merit a full essay. Furthermore, as mentioned above, it is very difficult to do this without a knowledge of the *content* of the educational and training requirements stipulated.

In spite of this, we think that several points should be underscored. First, initial attempts to set educational and training standards should be modest and flexible since the links between certain types of education and training; certain skills, knowledge, and character traits; and quality consultation must be empirically tested. This suggests that more rigid standards such as certifying or licensing individuals or groups may not be appropriate. Second, as one goes from voluntary standards or guidelines to those that have the state's power (for example, licensing), one increases the exclusionary power of the standards. This increases the probability that certain approaches to consultation will be deemed illegitimate and increases the likelihood that disciplinary homogeneity will result. Third, it is important to remain cognizant of the bureaucratic downside of state-driven approaches. This is particularly true for group methods of HCEC, which are most prevalent in the United States, because members of such groups frequently change. One can imagine the difficulty of having to recertify or license an ethics committee every time there was a turnover in membership.

Last, educational and training standards for those who will do HCEC in various capacities could be directed to *certifying* or *accrediting* educational and training *programs*. Educational programs could be developed for training individuals to do HCEC with the full ethics committee, as part of a small consultation team, or as individual consultants. The curriculum could be tailored to ensure that graduates would have the skills, knowledge, and character traits needed to conduct HCEC in the relevant capacity. One could imagine, for example, continuing-education programs for those who will do consultation with a full ethics committee and more intensive programs for those who will perform HCEC as part of a small team or as individual consultants. The programs could then be accredited by one of the major bioethics organizations or some other accrediting body (the Joint Commission, North Central, and so forth). This tactic might serve to ensure quality in HCEC better than issuing standards as mere recommendations that might be accepted or rejected while avoiding the abovementioned problems of certifying individuals or groups.

CONCLUSION

We have now reached our terminus. Our focus in this chapter has been on the broad question of whether there can be educational and training standards for those who conduct health care ethics consultation. We have suggested that concern with such standards should ultimately be a concern for quality assurance. The need for quality assurance, we argued, stems from the complexity of the issues involved in HCEC; its increasing prevalence, its practical impact on patients, families, and health care providers; and, therefore, the inevitable demand for accountability.

Herein, we have explored some of the issues that would need to be addressed before educational and training standards for those conducting HCEC could be adopted. These issues include three background questions regarding (1) the justifiability of HCEC in our society, (2) the extent to which standard setting amounts to a mere political exercise of power, and (3) the impact of standard setting on disciplinary diversity in the field. These background questions, we suggested, have implications for any attempt to set educational and training standards for those conducting HCEC.

Against this backdrop, we then argued that before standards for the education and training of those conducting HCEC could be adopted, a series of central questions would have to be addressed. Educational and training standards presuppose an idea of the skills, knowledge, and character traits that such standards should engender. However, the skills, knowledge, and character traits necessary for conducting HCEC cannot be nonarbitrarily identified without a notion of what HCEC is supposed to be, what it is supposed to achieve, and the types of issues to which it is supposed to extend, i.e., a normative concept of its nature, goals, and scope. Thus, a critical issue for any attempt to set educational and training standards for those conducting HCEC involves the nature, goals, and scope of ethics consultation. We looked at how different models for HCEC—different concepts of its nature and goals—have different implications for the skills, knowledge, and character traits that might be necessary to conduct it and, therefore, for the content of educational and training standards. Along the way, we also considered how educational and training standards might differ for those who will conduct HCEC in various capacities, e.g., as part of a full ethics committee, as a small consultation group, or as individual consultants. This difference stems especially from how skills and knowledge will be differently instantiated in large groups, small groups, and individuals.

Finally, we looked at several possible alternatives for *implementing* educational and training standards for those conducting HCEC, e.g., recommending, accrediting, credentialing, certifying, and licensing. If the types of questions above can be addressed and educational and training standards for HCEC are adopted, the strengths and weaknesses of different ways of implementing such standards will have to be assessed. Ultimately, the question of the best way to implement educational and training standards, though important in itself, is secondary to the question of whether such standards can be set at all. The latter has been our focus. We are well-aware that it is one thing to raise the types of questions that would have to be addressed before educational and training standards for those conducting HCEC could be set and quite another to answer those questions. It is the answer to the kinds of questions we have raised herein that will determine not only whether such standards *can* be set, but more important, whether they *should* be set. Though *ought* implies *can*, *can* does not imply *ought*, and it is the latter, we think, that *ought* to settle the issue.

NOTES

1. P. A. Singer et al., "Ethics Committees and Consultants," *Journal of Clinical Ethics* 1, no. 4 (1990): 263–67; E. D. Pellegrino et al., "Future Directions in Clinical Ethics," *Journal of Clinical Ethics* 2, no. 1 (1991): 5–9; J. La Puma and D. Schiedermayer, *Ethics Consultation: A Practical Guide* (Boston: Jones and Bartlett, 1994); F. E. Baylis, ed., *The Health Care Ethics Consultant* (Totowa, N.J.: Humana Press, 1994); and J. C. Fletcher and D. E. Hoffmann, "Ethics Committees: Time to Experiment with Standards," *Annals of Internal Medicine.* 120, no. 4 (1994): 335–38.
2. J. W. Ross, "Why Clinical Ethics Consultants Might Not Want To Be Educators. [Commentary]," *Cambridge Quarterly of Healthcare Ethics* 2, no. 4 (1993): 445–48; *id.,* "Response to Jonathan Moreno [on ethics consultation]," *HEC (HealthCare Ethics Committee) Forum* 8, no. 1 (1996): 22–28; G. R. Scofield, "Here Come the Ethicists!" *Trends in Health Care, Law and Ethics* 8, no. 4 (1993): 19–22.
3. President's Commission for the Study of Ethical Problems in Medicine and Biomedical and Behavioral Research, *Decisions To Forgo Life Sustaining Treatment* (Washington, D.C.: U.S. Government Printing Office, 1983), 153–160.
4. Joint Commission on Accreditation of Healthcare Organizations, *Comprehensive Accreditation Manual For*

Hospitals: Patients' Rights and Organizational Ethics (Chicago, Ill.: 1995), 66; see also the 1997 manual, *Patients' Rights and Organization Ethics,* RI–1 to RI–32.

5. J. C. Fletcher and E. M. Spencer, "Ethics Services in Healthcare Organizations," in *Introduction to Clinical Ethics*, ed. J. C. Fletcher et al. (Frederick, Md.: University Publishing Group, 1995), 7–8.
6. Ibid.; A. M. Burger et al., "Factors Influencing Ethical Decision Making in the Home Setting," *Home Healthcare Nurse* 10, no. 2 (1992): 16–20; P. E. Abel, "Ethics Committees in Home Health Agencies," *Public Health Nursing* 7, no. 4 (1990): 256–59.
7. J. C. Fletcher and E. M. Spencer, "Ethics Services in Healthcare Organizations," typescript, 22–30, offer a very fine discussion of these cases.
8. We have fashioned this description from the following sources: Ibid.; also *Elizabeth Bouvia v. Superior Court of the State of California of the County of Los Angeles (Glenchur),* 225 *California Reporter* 297 (Cal. App. 2 Dist.), April 16, 1986; G. E. Pence, *Classic Cases in Medical Ethics*, 2d ed. (New York: McGraw-Hill, 1995); L. J. Nelson, "Legal Liability of Institutional Ethics Committees to Patients," *Clinical Ethics Report* 6, no. 4 (1992): 1–8.
9. S. Fry-Revere, *The Accountability of Bioethics Committees and Consultants* (Frederick, Md.: University Publishing Group, 1992); *id,* "Ethics Consultation: An Update on Accountability Issues," *Pediatric Nursing* 20, no. 1 (1994): 95–98; S. M. Wolf, "Quality Assessment of Ethics in Health Care: The Accountability Revolution," *American Journal of Law and Medicine* 20 (1994): 105–28; J. Fleetwood and S. S. Unger, "Institutional Ethics Committees and the Shield of Immunity," *Annals of Internal Medicine* 120, no. 4 (1994): 320–25.
10. G. R. Scofield, "Here Come the Ethicists!" 19–22; G. R. Scofield, "Ethics Consultation: The Least Dangerous Profession?" *Cambridge Quarterly of Healthcare Ethics* 2, no. 4 (1993): 417–26; *id,* "Ethics Consultants, Architects, and Moral Enclosures," *Trends in Health Care, Law and Ethics* 9, no. 4 (1994): 7–12; *id,* "Ethics Consultation: The Most Dangerous Profession: A Reply to Critics," *Cambridge Quarterly of Healthcare Ethics* 4, no. 2 (1995): 225–28.
11. H. T. Engelhardt Jr. *The Foundations of Bioethics*, 2d ed. (New York: Oxford University Press, 1996). Chapter one has an excellent discussion about why moral diversity is not only a matter of fact but also a matter of principle. Regarding the latter, Engelhardt emphasizes our inability to rationally establish a single contentful morality. Though his discussion is quite penetrating, where Engelhardt himself goes wrong is that he too fails to take seriously this contextual dimension of HCEC, i.e., in part, that it must be understood within the liberal constitutional framework of our society. For a fuller discussion of this point see M. P. Aulisio's review of Engelhardt's work in the *Journal of General Internal Medicine* (April 1997).
12. Sectarian institutions, on the other hand, may privilege particular moral views in keeping with the nature of their institutions. For example, it would be appropriate for a Catholic hospital to employ an ethicist to help health care providers in the institution sort through the implications of the Catholic identity of the hospital for the provision of health care. There are still limits on this in light of the rights of individuals to pursue their own substantive concept of morality. This, of course, can get very complicated, and it is well beyond the purview of this essay. For our purposes here, it will suffice to note that there is an important difference between sectarian and nonsectarian institutions in this regard.
13. This is perhaps nowhere better demonstrated than in E. Friedson's seminal work *The Profession of Medicine: A Study in the Sociology of Applied Knowledge* (New York: Harper and Row, 1970).
14. S. Sherwin, "Certification of Health Care Ethics Consultants: Advantages and Disadvantages," in *The Health Care Ethics Consultant*, ed. F. E. Baylis (Totowa, N.J.: Humana Press, 1994), 11–24.
15. Singer et al., "Ethics Committees and Consultants"; M. Siegler, "Defining the Goals of Ethics Consultations: A Necessary Step for Improving Quality. [Editorial]," *QRB/Quality Review Bulletin* 18, no. 1 (1992): 15–16; M. Siegler et al., "Clinical Medical Ethics," *Journal of Clinical Ethics* 1, no. 1 (1990): 5–9; J. Fletcher and M. Siegler, "What Are the Goals of Ethics Consultation? A Consensus Statement," *The Journal of Clinical Ethics* 7, no. 2 (1996): 122–26; J. C. Fletcher, "Goals and Process of Ethics Consultation in Health Care," *BioLaw* 2 (1986): S:37–S:47; T. F. Ackerman, "Moral Problems, Moral Inquiry, and Consultation in Clinical Ethics," in *Clinical Ethics: Theory and Practice*, ed. B. Hoffmaster et al. (Clifton, N.J.: Humana Press, 1989), 141–60.
16. Singer et al., "Ethics Committees and Consultants."
17. J. Fletcher and M. Siegler, "What Are the Goals of Ethics Consultation?"
18. J. A. Tulsky and E. Fox, "Evaluating Ethics Consultation: Framing the Questions," *The Journal of Clinical Ethics* 7, no. 2 (1996): 109–15.
19. In this tripartite categorization, we follow the Strategic Research Network on "Health Care Ethics Consultation" as in F. E. Baylis, "A Profile of the Health Care Ethics Consultant," in *The Health Care Ethics Consultant*, ed. F. E. Baylis (Totowa, N.J.: Humana Press, 1994), 25–44.
20. Various classifications of broad approaches to HCEC have been offered in the literature. For two of these see R. M. Zaner, "Voices and Time: The Venture of Clinical Ethics," *Journal of Medicine and Philosophy* 18, no. 1 (1993): 9–31; and B-J. Crigger, "Negotiating the Moral Order: Paradoxes of Ethics Consultation," *Kennedy Institute of Ethics Journal* 5, no. 2 (1995): 89–112.

21. We again want to emphasize that we are *exaggerating* features of views that can be found in the literature because the caricatures make clearer how different models for HCEC have different implications for skills, knowledge, and so forth. As described, the secular-priest model is a good example of how HCEC could be understood and practiced in a way that is at odds with the fundamental political values of our society as discussed. For strands of this view see B. D. Weinstein, "The Possibility of Ethical Expertise," *Theoretical Medicine* 15, no. 1 (1994): 61–75; and D. J. Self, "Is Ethics Consultation Dangerous? [Commentary]," *Cambridge Quarterly of Healthcare Ethics* 2, no. 4 (1993): 442–45.

22. The following emphasize a facilitator approach to HCEC: U. Walker, "Keeping Moral Spaces Open: New Images of Ethics Consulting," *Hastings Center Report* 23, no. 2 (1993): 33–40; B-J. Crigger, "Negotiating the Moral Order"; A. Lynch, ". . . Has Knowledge of [interpersonal] Facilitation Techniques and Theory; Has the Ability to Facilitate [interpersonally] . . .: Fact or Fiction?," in *The Health Care Ethics Consultant,* ed. F. E. Baylis (Totowa, N.J.: Humana Press, 1994), 45–62; and R. M. Zaner, "Voices and Time: The Venture of Clinical Ethics," *Journal of Medicine and Philosophy.* 18, no. 1 (1993): 9–31. Though all of the above emphasize a facilitator model for HCEC, none of them endorse a *pure* facilitation model. We again want to underscore that we are intentionally exaggerating the facilitation feature of the model to emphasize how different models will have different implications for the matter under discussion.

23. Strands of this view can be seen in J. La Puma and D. L. Schiedermayer, "Ethics Consultation: Skills, Roles and Training," *Annals of Internal Medicine* 114, no. 2 (1991): 158, where they assert that "ideal" candidates to train as ethics consultants are "clinicians who are expert in their own medical discipline and who have or wish to gain the skills and play the roles of consultant . . . such candidates include physicians who are completing a primary care residency or who are the ethics committee chairperson"; also, *id., Ethics Consultation: A Practical Guide* (Boston: Jones and Bartlett, 1994), 45–46, where they reassert this: "Physicians and nurses . . . are probably best suited to train as ethics consultants"; and, M. Siegler et al., "Clinical Medical Ethics," *Journal of Clinical Ethics* 1, no. 1 (1990): 7–8 echo this view: "The physician who is competent as a clinician and has been trained in medical ethics is particularly effective as a consultant."

24. For the sake of brevity and clarity, we are limiting our discussion in the next three sections to knowledge and skills. Regarding character traits, it should be noted that, aside from cultivating certain character traits through training, one way to put character requirements into standards might be through the development of a code of ethics for ethics consultants.

25. For example, Singer et al., "Ethics Committees and Consultants," 263, employ the term *consultant* in the broader sense as referring to those who offer education, policy development, and case consultation services.

26. Since we have focused on educational and training standards from the outset, we have deliberately not addressed the question of practice standards for HCEC. It should be noted, however, that even a discussion of practice standards will require a normative characterization of HCEC and its goals. This is because there will be no way to evaluate which methods of doing HCEC will achieve its goals unless the goals themselves have first been identified. Furthermore, as we suggested above, these goals cannot be nonarbitrarily identified without at least an implicit concept of the nature of HCEC. For preliminary work on evaluating methods for HCEC, see E. Fox and J. A. Tulsky, "Evaluation Research and the Future of Ethics Consultation," *The Journal of Clinical Ethics* 7, no. 2 (1996): 146–49.

27. Indeed, one of the tasks for a complete assessment of various ways to implement a set of educational and training standards will be to give a detailed definition of each of these terms and to clarify the differences between them. Because we don't want to get into disputes about the proper understanding of "certifying," "licensing," "credentialing," "accrediting," etc., we will not attempt to define these terms beyond their ordinary language meanings.

Chapter 46

Health Care Institutional Ethics: Broader Than Clinical Ethics

Dennis Brodeur

Bioethical problems have dominated the ethical concerns of hospitals and other health care institutions for the past 25 years. The termination of treatment, autonomy, informed consent, advance directives, and issues of reproduction have occupied center stage. In the late 1980s, many institutions began to recognize and address many other ethical issues that focused on business practices, corporate ethics, and managed care concerns.

In the first years of the 1990s, still other complex developments took place. Institutional focus in clinical, business, and ethical matters began to give way to network concerns. Networks comprised institutions, physician organizations, financing mechanisms, other health businesses, and relationships or partnerships with community organizations to promote community health status. This change resulted in new and organizationally complex ethical dilemmas that demanded difficult analytical frameworks and broader ethical analysis.

Today, health care networks and their various institutions are complex, interdependent systems of patients, families, professionals, payers, processes, communities, and businesses. These multiple players interact in intricate ways. Their daily activities, a network and an institution's mission, and their impact on the community and the community's health status are sources of ethical concern. The bioethical principles of autonomy, beneficence, nonmalificence, and justice as traditionally formulated are not sufficient to address the ethical issues that arise. Although these principles have their place, justice questions demand greater attention and the principles of business ethics are more prevalent.

There is, of course, still a need to address bioethical issues. Because patients and their needs are still the focus of much of an institution's activity, clinical ethical issues do arise and require attention. Other chapters in this book analyze these issues. This chapter focuses on the ethical issues that network and institutional administrators (and sometimes trustees) need to address from a personal, institutional, and communal perspective. These include issues of justice (social, distributive, and commutative), the promotion of the common good, the role of the "community" in emerging networks, the meaning of work, the definition of health, the role of government, and the allocation of resources, to name a few. This chapter will not outline a comprehensive theory of justice, argue for a process of allocating or rationing resources, define the concept of health, or argue for a particular philosophical understanding of work. It will attempt to describe areas of concern in the value or ethical conflicts that arise in health care networks and institutions.

Health care networks and institutions play a significant public role in their communities. They provide medical services and education and are often one of the largest employers. The trustees and the managers of health care networks and institutions confront ethical issues that involve clinical matters, corporate and institutional structure, strategic direction, personal and personnel commitments, and the public nature of health care.

CLINICAL CONCERNS

Institutions have been asked by external groups to play a role in clinical and patient-family ethical issues. A few examples are the patient self-determination act, required community education for Medicaid recipients, organ donation request laws, and regulations for medical experimentation involving human subjects. The Joint Commission on Accreditation of Healthcare Organizations, in the patient-rights section of its accreditation manual for hospitals, requires that "the patient or the patient's designated representative participate in the consideration of ethical issues that arise in the care of the patient."[1] Institutions must develop processes to allow the patient or the patient's proxy access to ethics consultants, an ethics committee, or a defined process to address ethical questions.

These clinical issues are typically dealt with using traditional ethical principles such as autonomy, beneficence, and justice.[2] The limits of these principles (e.g., the limits of an institution's or professional's obligation to treat a patient who requests "everything") force health care institutions into other arenas of ethical concern than those represented by the clinical setting. Clinical issues often wind up involving questions of community need,[3] government regulation,[4] and organizational structure.[5]

Trustees and managers must ensure that mechanisms are established to address clinical ethical concerns. New clinical ethical issues will arise as medicine and technology continue to develop. New financial structures that link hospitals, physicians, and financial concerns raise questions about appropriate medical care; advocacy for the patient in the patient/physician relationship; self-interest in referral patterns by physicians to institutions in which they have a financial interest; and the benefit of services to the community as a whole when preventive or primary health care services are offered by an institution but where the institution is not reimbursed for these services. It is more likely that consensus will be achieved in response to some of these clinical concerns than in the group of issues that involve the network or institution's work life, its sense of justice, the concept of health, or the definition of a socially accountable health care network.

HUMAN RESOURCES

Usually agreement exists about the organization's ethical commitments to human resources and personnel issues. Most people would state that an organization's greatest resources are its human resources and that the inappropriate or unethical treatment of the work force leads to a collapse of the institution's mission and its ability to serve the public. A list of ethical principles and rules could be developed that, prima facie, seem to be normative: Treat people as an end not as a means; pay personnel justly; do not lie to or manipulate individuals in the work force; institute mechanisms for participatory decision making; ensure that personnel policies are just and do not discriminate; treat all with dignity and respect; ensure fair disciplinary policies; do not allow physical or sexual harassment in the workplace.

Surveys of human-resource professionals reveal that there are issues underneath this normative agreement about what is ethical in the workplace. A survey of human-resource management personnel indicates that the 10 most serious ethical situations are as follows:[6]

1. hiring, training, or promotion based on favoritism
2. allowing differences in pay, discipline, promotion, and so on, because of friendships with top management
3. permitting sexual harassment
4. yielding to sexual discrimination in promotion
5. using discipline for managerial and nonmanagerial personnel inconsistently
6. not maintaining confidentiality
7. tolerating sex discrimination in compensation

8. using nonperformance factors in appraisals
9. arranging with vendors or consulting agencies situations leading to personal gain
10. acquiescing to sex discrimination in recruitment and hiring

For example, 22.6 percent of the personnel managers who responded indicated that sex discrimination in recruitment and hiring was an ethical issue they confronted in 1991, and nearly 31 percent indicated that the hiring, training, or promotion of personnel based on favoritism was an issue.

Clearly, the prima facie agreement on normative ethical principles among human-resource managers does not ensure that all people in the workplace act in accordance with ethical standards. The temptation might be to dismiss unethical practices as aberrant behaviors of unethical managers. Yet, one suspects that most managers would identify themselves as behaving ethically in most if not all situations. The root cause of some of these ethical problems lies in the culture of the organization or in the inability of the organization to hold accountable the unethical practices of its managers.

Boards of trustees who establish ethical parameters for personnel policies and managers who implement these policies in the workplace must be attentive to the policies, practices, processes, and other factors that contribute to unethical behavior. For example, they need to give careful consideration to the writing of policy manuals, the designing of disciplinary procedures, and other activities that reflect the ethical commitment of the organization. This attention to ethical matters in personnel policies has to be deliberate, ongoing, and public.

Emerging health care networks raise additional concerns. Key among these is a change in an institution's commitment to its work force. There once existed an unwritten, perhaps mythical quid pro quo, where loyalty to the organization by an employee resulted in or was matched by the loyalty of the organization to the employee for lifetime employment. In today's health care, this has changed. Now the ethical questions are not about loyalty but about commitment to human resources that allows workers to learn new skills, to respond to changed work environments, and not to be treated as a temporary means to create a particular good or service. Conversely, employees need to be open to change, to constant learning and to new challenges.

WORK AND HUMAN RESOURCES

There are philosophical and ethical assumptions about work and the nature of the workplace that undergird the human-resource commitments of all institutions. Primary among them is an understanding of the nature of work. Philosophical,[7] religious,[8] and management-science[9] writings explore these issues.

What is the relationship among work processes, products or goods, and human life? Is work a drudgery for human beings, something to be done for a shift or work week or to scrape out a living? Are the products and services that are developed the most important focus, taking precedence over the people who produce them? Or, is the worker the primary focus?

Work is a means through which human beings express significant aspects of personal life, support the development of family, build community, and create a culture. Human beings are not made for work; rather, work is the expression of the dignity, specialness, and creativity of human beings. The ethical demand is to create a work environment in which all people are allowed to express their personal dignity and realize their creative possibilities. Health care institutions employ a great number of individuals who view their work as a vocation, a calling, or a ministry. Even those workers who perform more routine tasks, when discussing their jobs, often characterize their activity and work processes as contributing to a greater end—the care of those in need. The ethical challenge to managers is to create a work environment that is expressive of human dignity, filled with joy, and personally fulfilling.

Authors who focus on the question of work, including management-science authors, describe a number of other "normative" principles that help create a meaningful work environment. First, there is the principle of subsidiarity, which entails that decisions should be made at the level where they have the greatest impact and that the owners of work processes should be involved in the decision-making process.

The second principle is that decisions, whenever possible, should be based on consensus. This does not preclude decisiveness or quick decision making in certain settings. Rather, it suggests that groups who work together, examine the root causes of problems, and seek functional and crossfunctional solutions are more likely to find effective solutions and to create a work environment that is respectful of human dignity. Autocratic, nonconsensus processes give the impression that the most important things about work are the products or services and not the people doing the work.

Third, organizational assistance must be provided to workers to ensure that they are able to assert their rights. The means of such assistance can take different forms: Unions as understood in European social, political, and economic life; associations of workers and employees; and councils or governing bodies of workers within an institution.

The creation of labor law in the United States was spurred on by the discrepancy in power between the owners of capital and the workers. Although legal experts, philosophers, and theologians would acknowledge this historical fact, their exploration of the meaning of worker rights does not result in the same conceptual framework. For example, worker and manager groups could be developed that protect workers' rights without any third-party intervention. Two groups of rights holders exist—the owner/managers and the worker—and structures are necessary to address any power imbalance between the two that would result in the exploitation of the worker. Labor law, however, sees three rights holders—owner/managers, workers, and the union. This creates a different pattern of rights holders and needed protections among the various groups. In the last decade, this is evident when one examines how unions claim that quality-management teams of workers and managers are a mechanism that undercuts union rights, even if such arrangements respect and promote the dignity and rights of the workers.[10]

Managers and trustees—sometimes quick to seek an "operations" solution to these issues—need to think about the rights of workers and the power and responsibilities of ownership. Ethical commitments need to be worked out in the workplace. Owners/managers need to make a commitment to the assurance of employee rights and to the inclusion of workers in the process of creating, nurturing, and sustaining the work environment.

Finally, although perhaps not purely an ethical commitment, managers need to ask what management style, technique, or process best helps to build the work environment that respects the dignity of each worker. Management style will have a direct impact on the type of managers recruited and hired. Ultimately, management style is a means to achieve an ethical end—a workplace where employees are not subordinated to goods and services and where their human dignity is given due regard.

ORGANIZATIONAL IDENTITY AND STRATEGIC DIRECTION

Another area for ethical reflection for trustees and managers is the mission of the health care network and institution and the means it uses to accomplish this mission. The latter part of the 1980s and the early part of the 1990s saw issues related to organizational mission come to the forefront because many health care institutions saw their nonprofit tax status challenged in state and federal courts.[11] The early 1990s saw this issue raised to new heights as proprietary organizations, such as Columbia/HCA, questioned the tax status of community nonprofit organizations.

What are the ethical commitments that an institution has to the community it serves? In part, the ethical commitments of health care institutions arise out of the value commitments of the community, the community's identified needs, and the institution's resources available to meet these needs. Ideally, managers lead health care institutions in an analysis of community needs to develop the organization's strategic directions that are designed to meet these needs.

For the purpose of this discussion, the focus will be on nonprofit health care organizations. Nonprofit institutions must be financially sound, act as appropriate stewards of resources, and generate excess revenues over expenses. Questions about how a manager behaves in business activities as a responsible steward of resources or how the organization acts justly in the "business community" are particular questions of business ethics. Ethical business practices are the subject matter of a particular line of ethical inquiry. The more specific question to be addressed here is, What are the organizational ethical concerns of nonprofit health care institutions as they provide goods and services to the community?

Paul Starr and Rosemary Stevens both trace the growth of the voluntary health care sector.[12] According to Stevens' analysis, this growth also involved a shift from voluntary hospitals whose purpose was to mobilize resources at the local level to a range of disparate institutions that successfully fought government intervention and organized medicine. By the late 1930s, voluntary hospitals exemplified (in ideal cases) "public responsibility without government compulsion" and "private initiatives untainted by selfish gain."[13]

In time, voluntary or nonprofit institutions lost touch with the principles of that earlier era. Medicine was increasingly more organized, health care institutions depended on federal and state government for a large part of their revenues, and the government had an increasingly larger role in designing both health care financing and health care delivery systems, especially with the growth of Medicare and Medicaid. Health care institutions adjusted their practices to survive and grow in that environment. As a result, some people looking at health care did not see public charitable corporations but rather, big business.

In the most recent times, this has again changed as the focus of care shifted from hospitals and illness to communitywide networks, financing institutions, and community health. Traditional nonprofit "hospitals" are now part of networks that include proprietary insurance companies or products, physician networks with equity incentives, as well as more traditional nonprofit organizations. The values of the "health system" as described by Stevens and Starr seem to be long gone.

Municipalities, pressed for tax dollars to maintain other community services, ask questions about the appropriateness of the tax status of health care institutions and emerging networks in light of their "charity" care and community benefit. If things have changed so much, and if the organizations look more like a business, then perhaps they need to pay their fair share of community support through taxes and municipal fees.

But there is a schizophrenic attitude in American society regarding its health care institutions. On the one hand, communities expect that health care institutions will be close to home; be filled with the latest high technology; abound in expertise; be efficient, quality, full-service providers; take care of the poor; not be worried about insurance or payment arrangements; and not be very expensive. The costs of providing these services should be mostly covered by income derived from the overall activities of the institutions, which should not overly depend on public monies from towns, cities, counties, or states. And while health care institutions do all of the things demanded of them, questions of global health care budgets or the rationing of resources should not be necessary. On the other hand, health care institutions should not be involved in projects that raise money through non–health-related activities (except for philanthropic fund-raising), should be wary of joint ventures and other business practices, and should compete openly in the marketplace while not looking like a business. Obviously there needs to be some resolution of these conflicting requirements.

This is not to suggest that there are not appropriate limits to a nonprofit institution's excess revenue, capitalization of proprietary projects, inurement, or executive compensation. However, at the root of these issues are questions about whether health care services are public or private goods, whether competition and the marketplace help or hinder the provision of these goods, and how many tiers of health care services society really wants.

There is no clear policy that will resolve every issue. In the absence of a national health plan (and even if there were a national health plan), managers and trustees of voluntary institutions must do their best to create institutions that respond to the needs of the communities they serve. This will not be easy, and strategies may differ depending on regulations, court decisions, and laws. Managers and trustees need to develop strategic directions that guide their institutions through this maze while meeting the needs of as many as possible. This is not only sound business strategy, it is at the root the ethical imperative if one understands health care as a social good.

The ethical components of strategy are definitional and procedural (stated differently, they involve both ends and means). Definitional concerns include the defining of health. What is health? Is it the optimal functioning of the whole person? Is the definition, from a health care institution's perspective, individual-focused or does it need to include a broader community perspective? What end is the institution aiming for? Which services are for patients individually and which are for the community's health benefit? Increasingly, the health benefit is measured in terms of both community gain and individual gain. Consequently, preventive services, community-education programs, primary health care, advocacy programs, and other activities become part of the institution's mission in the community.[14]

The means that are used require managers to define the process of the allocation and rationing of health care resources. No global budget for health care in the United States exists at this time. Yet each health care institution has a general sense of an "annual total budget" available to it through implementation of the strategic- and financial-planning process, its cash reserves, its charitable funds, and its debt capacity. After determining the health needs of the community, managers must match the human and fiscal resources necessary to meet these needs. If all health needs cannot be met, the institution must ration services based on the revenues it has.

The institution must devise a definition of rationing—the denial of certain possible beneficial resources to some or all people—that is publicly defensible, socially accountable, quantitative, and clear.[15] Often this is not done. Rationing is surreptitious and secret, leveled only against the poor and not publicly recognized. Or in certain circumstances an institution will fall into fiscal difficulty because rationing was not done and services were provided without appropriate reimbursement.

Not all people agree that rationing is necessary, and some believe that the elimination of inefficiencies and waste could go a long way toward ensuring universal access to cost-effective and quality health care services. The ethical challenge for those who believe that rationing is not necessary is to define appropriate outcomes and cost-efficient practices and then build a system that allows sound stewardship of available resources.

Procedural concerns include ensuring that managers exhibit integrity and behave ethically. For example, financial managers must be honest and must establish financial mechanisms that are not illegal or unscrupulous, are respectful of persons, and so on. Planners must honestly assess the needs of the community when developing health care services and match available financial resources with the institution's commitment to serve those in need. Operations personnel must make decisions about services and personnel that are aligned with these strategic directions, and the chief executive officer must integrate these activities within the institution and revise them accordingly as he or she interacts with the external environment.

THE PUBLIC NATURE OF THE CORPORATION

A health care organization's commitment to service is a kind of public statement. Such a statement has ethical importance because it can contribute to the building of a community.

Trustees must ask a basic question: How will this network or institution make a difference to the community that is served in the future? The fiduciary responsibility of trustees can cause them to look backward: What *was* the financial performance of the organization last month (or last year)? How many goals *were* achieved last year? How well *did* the people manage debt? But their ethical responsibility is mainly a forward-looking responsibility: How *will* this network make a difference in the world tomorrow? Planning how the ethical obligations of the organization will be met is the work of the board.[16]

Creating tomorrow's vision demands ethical sensitivity to the public nature and service orientation of the organization. Generally, this includes a special concern for the disenfranchised and the poor. Both types of concern will influence the trustees. The managers will need to respond to community, state, or national demands for a more just social order, to address personal and communal factors that contribute to poor health, and to use their considerable financial and institutional power to help shape the community's future. These ethical concerns are often addressed through networking; building partnerships among business people, educators, and payers; and working with public and elected officials to achieve improvements in the health status of the community.

The preferential tax treatment of most health care organizations, their public trust, and their mission to serve obligate trustees and managers to work for the public good, creating a social order that allows for the fuller development of all members of their communities. At times, this requires an institution to challenge the medicalization of social problems—to point to, for example, the causes of lead poisoning; the prevalence of malnutrition; the abusive treatment of children, the vulnerable, and the elderly; the lack of vaccinations; and the inaccessibility of health services. If these issues are not addressed in the community, in part through health care organizational leadership, costs will rise, people will continue to be harmed, and the health status of the community will deteriorate.

Very often, health care institutions in smaller communities and groups of health care institutions in suburban and urban communities constitute a leading economic and political force. Structuring an institution's powerful economic position for community gain and not just self-interest is an ethical requirement flowing from the mission of the institution. Moral persuasion may be the tool most often employed in these situations, but a community's trust in and dependence upon an institution or a network gives tremendous ethical power to trustees and managers.

The ethical commitment to the common good has implications for other institutional practices as well. Why would a health care institution not be sensitive to environmental issues? In the wake of the increasing costs of cure and care, can health care organizations be indifferent to returning people to a polluted or harmful environment? Environmental awareness will lead institutions to consider more closely the appropriate disposal of their wastes and toxins and the use of environmentally harmful products. Addressing environmental issues impacts on daily operations and public-policy stances.

Networks also need to develop self-critical perspectives. They need to ask how their location, clinics, and policies affect access to care for the poor. Suburban institutions that share a community concern may ask where to place the newest clinic or professional office building or where to advertise and market their products. How do institutions contribute to the geographical isolation of the sick? What policies or regulations should institutions advocate to increase access, equitable reimbursement, and community support? There is a tendency in health care institutions only to advocate policies that will ensure their own continued existence. The ethical question of tomorrow is whether health care institutions can advocate changes that are consonant with increased outpatient services, lower reimbursement, and different delivery structures. Can there be a redistribution of public dollar commitments to address preventive health needs and decrease institutional and technological use? What improvement of the social structures will prevent illness and increase the health status of the community? There will always be a need for health care institutions, but perhaps the most equitable health care structure will consist of a new and different alignment of institutions, payers, and providers.

CONCLUSION

Institutions are powerful forces in public and political life. Health care networks are no exception. The ethical concerns of health care are broader than the practice of clinical medicine. Managers and trustees of a health care system, if faithful to their mission, identity, and public commitment, must systematically address the network's role to promote the welfare of the public it serves, to protect the good of its employees, to create a better environment for healthy living, to influence the politics and economics of its community, and to help develop a just public order. Trustees and managers should focus on distinct but complementary objectives to achieve these general goals. Neither group will be able to accomplish much, however, if there is not a deliberate and systematic approach to address the ethical commitments of the network.

NOTES

1. Joint Commission on Accreditation of Healthcare Organizations, *Accreditation Manual for Hospitals,* vol. 1 (Oakbrook Terrace, Ill.: Joint Commission on Accreditation of Healthcare Organizations, 1993), 106.
2. See. T. L. Beauchamp and J. Childress, *Principles of Biomedical Ethics* (New York: Oxford University Press, 1983), 59–220.
3. See D. Seay and R. Sigmond, "The Future of Tax Exempt Status for Hospitals," *Frontiers of Health Services Management* 5, no. 3 (1989): 3–39.
4. C. Mackelvie and B. Sandborn, "Mooring in Safe Harbours," *Health Progress* 70 (1989): 32–36; J. Inglehart, "The Recommendations of the Physician Payment Review Committee," *New England Journal of Medicine* 320 (1989): 1156–60; D. Kinzer, "The Decline and Fall of Deregulation," *New England Journal of Medicine* 318 (1988): 112–16.
5. See, for example, A. Enthoven and R. Kronick, "A Consumer-Choice Health Plan for the 1990s," *New England Journal of Medicine* 320 (1989): 29–37; U. Reinhardt, "Whither Private Health Insurance? Self Destruction or Rebirth?" *Frontiers of Health Services Management* 9, no. 1 (1992): 5–31.
6. Human Resources Management: 1991 SRHM-CCH Survey (Commerce Clearing House, Chicago, June 26, 1991), 1–12.
7. See, for example, H. Arendt, *The Human Condition* (Chicago: University of Chicago Press, 1958), 79–174.
8. J. Coleman, ed., *100 Years of Catholic Social Thought: Celebration and Challenge* (Marynoll, N.Y.: Orbis Books, 1991), 201–69.
9. E. Marszalek-Gaucher and R. Coffey, *Transforming Health Care Organizations: How To Achieve and Sustain Organizational Excellence* (San Francisco: Jossey-Bass, 1990), 148–71; L. Dobyns and C. Crawford-Mason, *Quality or Else: The Revolution and World Business* (Boston: Houghton-Mifflin, 1991), 52–126.
10. K. Jenero and C. Lyons, "Employee Participation Programs: Prudent or Prohibited?" *Employee Relations Labor Journal* 17 (1992): 535–66.
11. Seay and Sigmond, "The Future of Tax Exempt Status for Hospitals"; D. Pellegrini, "Hospital Tax Exemption: A Municipal Perspective," *Frontiers of Health Services Management* 5, no. 2 (1989): 44–46.
12. P. Starr, *The Social Transformation of American Medicine* (New York: Basic Books, 1982); R. Stevens, *In Sickness and in Wealth: American Hospital in the Twentieth Century* (New York: Basic Books, 1989).
13. Stevens, *In Sickness and in Wealth,* 141.
14. See the American Hospital Association, *Community Benefit and Tax Exempt Status: A Self-Assessment Guide for Hospitals* (Chicago: American Hospital Association, 1988); Catholic Health Association, *Social Accountability Budget: A Process for Planning and Reporting Community Service in a Time of Fiscal Constraint* (St. Louis, Mo.: Catholic Health Association, 1989).
15. One suggested approach is presented in Catholic Health Association, *With Justice for All? The Ethics of Health Care Rationing* (St. Louis, Mo.: Catholic Health Association, 1991).
16. See J. Carver, *Boards That Make a Difference: A New Design for Leadership in Non-Profit and Public Organizations* (San Francisco: Jossey-Bass, 1991), 1–23, 40–55.

CHAPTER 47

The Ethics of Health Care as a Business

Patricia H. Werhane

The crisis in health care about which we read and worry is real. Fully 12 percent of our gross national product is spent on health care, and costs are rising. Even so we are not providing even minimum access to health care for at least 37 million citizens. Yet few Americans want to relinquish their ability to choose their health care specialist and place of treatment. With improved technology the vague claim to a right to health care has been translated into the demand for good health care. Indeed, a demand for the best available treatment is considered by many to be an entitlement. Along with these increased costs and development of rights claims, malpractice suits proliferate by those who find their rights have been abrogated.

The blame for the crisis in health care often falls to the alleged exploitation and commodification of health care by the market. In what follows I am going to suggest that this is too simple a description of the problem. I shall argue that we have misread the market model as the self-regulating glorification of economic egoism and that therefore the market paradigm adopted by health care is a faulty one. Further, I shall argue, no one model or paradigm can deal with the complexity of health care nor its difficulties. However, I shall claim that a careful rereading of Adam Smith, the eighteenth-century economist and philosopher to whom is often erroneously attributed an egoistic market model, might be helpful in setting out a framework for dealing with many of these issues.

According to Charles Dougherty,

> general features of the pervasive hold of commercialism in medicine include an increase in competition and decline in professionalism among physicians, a view of health care as a commodity and patients as consumers, and a general depersonalization of doctor-patient relationship including dilution of the tradition of physician as patient advocate.[1]

According to this view, a form of economic egoism has corrupted the health care system, replacing the caring and professional models with that of competing self-interests, encouraging greed, confusing professional interests with profit, depersonalizing patient relationships, diluting benevolence and charity with a concern for economic viability, and thus excluding those who cannot afford health care from the system.

These serious accusations and many of the problems Dougherty and others cite have arisen because of the commodification of health care. Without contesting that, I shall argue that the fault for these difficulties lies not in commodification per se but in the kind of market model we have projected on the health care

Source: Reprinted from *Business & Professional Ethics Journal,* Vol. 9, Nos. 3 & 4, pp. 7–20, University of Florida, Center for Applied Philosophy, with permission of Patricia H. Werhane, © 1991.

system and in our assumption that such a complex system or set of systems can be subsumed under one paradigm.

To begin, let us review briefly the theory of the market that is said to dominate health care. Such a view is often attributed to Adam Smith, and it defends a sort of nineteenth-century radical individualism, linking it with self-interest. Summarily put, the model seems to presuppose that

> economic man, self-interested and fundamentally asocial, motivated by an insatiable desire to improve his material condition, is the model that explains human motivation and action.[2]

In his well-known book, the *Wealth of Nations*, Adam Smith is read as having promulgated this egoistic picture of human motivation and as having solved the problem of the dichotomy between one's alleged natural selfish passions and the public interests. When human beings are granted what Smith calls the "natural liberty" to pursue their own interests, Smith is then interpreted as having concluded that self-interested economic actors in competition with each other create a market through which its famous invisible hand functions both to regulate self-interests and to produce economic growth and well-being such that no individual or group of individuals is allowed to take advantage or to take advantage for very long.[3] So, more crudely put, in the marketplace, at least, under optimal competitive conditions, the relentless pursuit of self-interest or at least disinterest in the well-being of others (within specified conditions such as the law) is both self-regulating and contributes to the public good.

Given this sort of moral psychology and philosophy of economics, it is no wonder that when this paradigm becomes the modus operandi for health care, or even for business, there are difficulties. How is it we have allowed ourselves to become enamored with this paradigm, and what else is at issue?

As background to answer these sorts of questions I want to suggest, all too briefly, an obvious point. It is this. "Our conceptual scheme mediates even our most basic perceptual experiences."[4] To state the point simply, we each operate our own "camera" of the world, projecting intentions, interests, desires, points of view, and biases that work as selective filters or censors on experience.[5]

This phenomenon accounts for our pluralism—the variety of ways we conceive the world and the variety of disparate social structures we create. The latter, noticed by Michael Walzer, explains the fact that sometimes individuals, social groups, institutions, or even whole societies are able to organize their concerns, institutions, and social goods into overlapping but distinct spheres of analysis and interest. Walzer focuses on what he calls "spheres of justice," arguing that each social sphere generates its own set of social goods, and each set of social goods commands distinct principles of distribution. These spheres may conflict or even contradict each other, but our ability to run several projectors on our experience at the same time and to distinguish and compartmentalize our foci allows these spheres to function simultaneously. Conversely, the projectival organization of experience also explains another phenomenon noticed and criticized by Walzer, namely, the disconcerting fact that sometimes individuals, groups, institutions, or even whole societies attempt to bring all their concerns, activities, organizations, social structures, and social goods under the framework of one paradigm, or one theory, or one principle of distribution. Specifically, Walzer contends that the dominance of the market model, or what he calls "market imperialism," skews the distribution of a variety of social goods, obstructs distributions based on need and desert, and commodifies political power.[6] In health care, we shall see how this alleged market imperialism has led to such difficulties. But, I shall argue, these difficulties arise as much from an unjustifiable concept of the market as from the misapplication of that concept in regard to the health care system.

How does the fact that we either project a number of different paradigms on the world or try to unify experience under one framework apply to health care? Until recently, I would suggest, there were at least six overlapping health care scenarios operating in our society, each of which had its distinct domain of influence. Because they overlapped, in some cases they were contrary to each other, but somehow these conflicts did not always precipitate serious dilemmas.

First there was an ideal of the profession, the notion that health care providers and specialists are autonomous, self-regulating individuals whose primary professional commitment is to medicine, and more specifically to the health care and healing of patients. Second, part of that ideal included the view that these professionals are caring, benevolent, even self-sacrificing in pursuit of their professional goals—a sort of Albert Schweitzer or Mother Teresa picture of medical professionals.

Third, hospitals and nursing homes were by and large nonprofit institutions. It was thought that their first concern, too, was the care and healing of patients. Fourth, for those who could not pay, there were thought to be benevolent health care specialists, organizations, and institutions, in particular, local community hospitals, who would provide for their needs.

Fifth and sixth, two other social phenomena existed as adjuncts to the health care system, the judicial system to protect constitutional rights, and the market, which provided material goods and services. These two spheres were thought to be peripheral to the health care system. By and large, issues of health care, e.g., malpractice, poor provision of nursing care, etc., were seldom brought to the attention of the courts. And while there certainly was commercialization of health care, that is, for-profit institutions and physicians and other health care specialists who made money as well as treated patients, these phenomena were thought to be relatively secondary to the motivation of health care specialists and to the operation of health care institutions.

These scenarios each captured some of what in fact was true while highlighting some concerns and neglecting other data. These spheres seemed to operate simultaneously without causing much friction despite obvious problems, e.g., that some physicians were involved in entrepreneurial ventures that conflicted with patients' interests, that not all hospitals or nursing homes were unprofitable nor was their care always adequate, that malpractice was going on, that not every indigent patient was treated or treated adequately, and that not everyone in our society had access even to minimum health care.

Part of the present crisis in health care originates in the fact that at one time we imagined these scenarios represented reality, and because they overlapped, altogether by and large they did. But seldom did we try to make sense of all six spheres in terms of one paradigm, nor did we subject these spheres to one set of evaluative criteria. More recently, however, we have created or were led by changing circumstances to new models. At the same time we have sometimes imagined that there is *a* system of health care conflating these distinct spheres of operation and thereby subjected the whole system to one evaluative perspective, attempting to apply a single set of principles for evaluation or distribution for quite different social phenomena.

At least three models now dominate our way of thinking about health care. First, and not on my previous list of paradigms, the technology model. There have been enormous advances in medical technology and with them a sort of "invincible" or Robocop notion that technology will make possible widespread advances in healing coupled with a sort of *Cocoon* view of immortality. Second, along with technological growth and the escalating costs partly due to the use of technology, we have developed an "entitlement theory" of rights. Briefly put, this is the thesis that as citizens of a constitutional democracy under our Bill or Rights, each one of us has extended basic entitlements: rights to minimum basic health care, rights to good health care or even a right to the best technology can provide, rights to choose our provider, and rights to be protected from malpractice, poor treatment, or neglect. We have tried to empower our legislatures to grant these entitlements and the courts to protect them without regard to costs nor with attention to reciprocal duties to ensure equal entitlements for everyone.

Third, in the last 20 years, commercialization of medicine has become a dominant trend in health care. Physicians have become entrepreneurs; for-profit hospitals, nursing homes, and health maintenance organizations (HMOs) have proliferated; insurance policies have quantified treatment with diagnosis-related groups (DRGs); health care specialists and health care organizations have begun advertising; and there is a trend toward the commodification of blood, organs, and, if Richard Posner has his way, even babies.

Accompanying this rising market orientation of health care is another confusing phenomenon. Where formerly there were overlapping but distinct spheres of concern in health care, we now sometimes superimpose one model or one methodology for analysis on another. For example, using the methodology from economics, one sometimes analyzes crucial dilemmas in medicine only in terms of markets, costs, and benefits, sometimes imagining that markets will both create benefits and regulate abuses. Or we conflate all cases under a rights model and wonder why we have problems with cost containment or even with providing equal minimum care. Or, appealing to the advances of technology, we treat patients as objects of experimentation rather than as human beings.

At the same time, we are reminded of "the good old days" of the caring model and try to keep it alive. One remembers the country doctors and the visiting nurses, benevolent, kindly, caring souls, and one wonders why our present health care specialists no longer emulate these ideals.

We have, then, mixed up our paradigms. We are at best unclear as to how to analyze conflicting claims, resorting often to the temptation to conflate issues and paradigms in an attempt to come up with solutions to growing health care dilemmas. Worse, having allowed an egoistic market paradigm to play a central role, we then blame the commercialization of medicine for the crisis in health care.

How, then, are we to deal with these issues? I do not have a solution for the problems in health care. But I want to argue that the kinds of paradigms one uses as frameworks for dealing with these issues both create dilemmas *and* determine the kinds of solutions available to solve these dilemmas. Since part of the crisis in health care is the adoption of an egoistic market model as I have depicted it, to get at the roots of the issues, let us reexamine that model. To do so I shall return to the philosophy of Adam Smith. Interestingly, this egoistic model is not an accurate reflection of the philosophy of Adam Smith. More important, Smith's moral psychology and the kind of framework Smith actually sets out for a viable political economy are useful not merely to bring into question economic egoism, but can serve as a metaframework for the analysis of complex social, ethical, and economic issues such as those introduced by health care. Let me outline briefly some salient features of Smith's moral psychology and then turn to his philosophy of economics to see why this is the case.

In his book on moral psychology, *Theory of Moral Sentiments*, Smith attacks radical individualism, recognizing that each of us is dependent on each other and on society. At the same time he defends the value of autonomy, advancing a more moderate individualism that claims that each of us is best able to care for himself or herself. But Smith does not identify individualism with egoism. While he clearly states that acting in one's own self-interest is not always bad, and indeed may produce benefits, Smith also carefully differentiates prudence from greed and avarice. More important, Smith argues that each of us is motivated by a variety of selfish, social, and unsocial passions of equal strength, each of which develops its particular interests and thus its virtues and vices. Self-interest or self-love is derived from the selfish passions, but self-love is not identified with selfishness, because self-love, like the other interests, can be virtuous (the virtue of prudence) or evil (greed or avarice).[7] Our interests in others, including empathy, the desire for approval, and the desire to emulate what society finds to be virtuous are motivated by the social passions that have equal weight with the selfish ones. Again these interests can be virtuous (the virtues of benevolence and justice) or evil.

Smith uses his moral psychology as a groundwork for his philosophy of economics in the *Wealth of Nations*. There Smith argues that self-interest is not the sole motivating force even in economic activities and that the social passions play three essential roles in economic activities. First, part of our pursuit of wealth, Smith notices, is not greed but is due to the desire for the approval of others. Second, economic exchanges are not based merely on competition but on mutual cooperation and coordination in which such competition takes place. Smith writes that "it is not from the benevolence of the butcher, the brewer, or the baker, that we expect our dinner, but from their regard to their own interest"[8] to illustrate the point that while our self-interests appear to dominate in the economy, cooperation is both natural and essential. None of these tradespeople acts benevolently, yet each depends on our approval for his or her self-interest. Moreover, in the small-town atmosphere implied in the example, these tradespeople depend on mutual cooperation to stay in business. Although the butcher, brewer, and baker are not necessarily benevolent, they not only are *not* malevolent but in the "corner grocery store" economy Smith depicts these shopkeepers cannot function without mutual cooperation. The fact that we "never talk to them of our own necessities but of their advantages" illustrates that some sort of fellow-understanding underpins economic relationships and in particular competition. Third, the virtue of justice, the "consciousness of ill-desert,"[9] is externalized in the legal system of jurisprudence that is an essential part of any societal framework and a necessary condition for the functioning of any viable economy. Indeed, in defending economic liberty Smith argues that every man, *as long as he does not violate the laws of justice*, is left perfectly free to pursue his own interest"[10] (emphasis added).

It is true that Smith argued that "nobody but a beggar chooses to depend chiefly upon the benevolence of his fellow-citizens."[11] Despite this, Smith clearly distinguishes between acting in one's self-interest and greed and argues that avarice prevents good economic performance.[12] Thus, whereas benevolence may not play a role in economic exchanges, greed is antithetical to a well-run system and is to be prevented or discouraged. Moreover, neither prudent self-interest nor benevolence is the most basic virtue in economic affairs, justice is. Although both benevolence and justice derive from the social passions, Smith distinguishes them. Benevolence is not universally applicable nor enforceable, because one is not obliged to be benevolent. Justice, on the other hand, is limited to the protection of citizens from harms, safeguarding basic rights, and the guarantee of contracts and other forms of fair play. So defined, justice embraces only those principles that are always immoral to violate. Since, Smith continues, one has perfect duties not to cause harm, to protect rights, and, as consciousness of ill-desert, to safeguard fair play, those duties are universally applicable or enforceable.[13] This is the reason why benevolence or charity should not play a role in economic exchanges. Fair play in competition can be enforced; benevolence cannot. So, while the beggar cannot expect kindness, he or she *can* expect and require justice.

But what about the market itself, the famous invisible hand? Here Smith is most cautious and least understood. First, he argues, the market is most efficient and most fair when there is competition between similarly matched parties—a level playing field.[14] Second, the famous invisible hand, the market itself, is not an independent or autonomous regulator of economic behavior. Rather, the character of the market is created by economic activities. How and to what extent the market regulates economic behavior is a direct outcome of the kind of behaviors that create various market conditions. So greed, unfair competition, lack of enforcement of justice, and/or the absence of economic cooperation produce different market conditions and thus give the market a different personality than when those factors are not operative. The market, then, is a complex set of outcomes created by and changing as a result of economic activities. So it functions as a regulator only to the extent that economic actors are self-restrained, that there is not unfair competition, in a climate of judicial enforcement.

Finally, an ideal political economy is one that emulates justice as well as utility. A free market for commerce is the best sort of economy, but Smith limits the scope of economic activities to those appropriate for commerce and competition. Markets deal with goods and services, not with persons. Nor is it ever the case that any economic consideration overrides those of rights and justice. Smith is critical of economic regulations, and he is worried that most of us do not have the capability of understanding what is good for society. But government does have positive functions, specifically to provide universal education and public works, those works that are in no one's particular interest to provide.

Smith's analysis, then, far from defending an egoistic laissez-faire model for economic behavior, develops a highly qualified version of economic liberty in which economic liberty can function effectively and beneficially only where one is also prudent and cooperative in a system of law and justice and a climate of equal economic opportunity.

Despite Smith's arguments, however, we have by and large adopted the paradigm of economic egoism, assuming, wrongly, that the supposed invisible hand of the market will adjust our imprudent behavior despite our efforts to the contrary. How, then, is Smith's analysis helpful? Smith would argue that what is wrong with the market model in health care is the exploitation of the market on the basis of self-interest, and the extension of the market paradigm to inappropriate areas of concern. So Smith would question many of the "customs" currently operating that have developed from the commercialization of health care. The misreading of economic liberty as license to maximize one's interests, the misguided reliance on the market as an alleged autonomous regulator of greed, skews prudence, self-restraint, and coordination of market activities. Moreover, the misappropriation of economic egoism in areas where it is inappropriate, in particular, in dealing with human beings and their needs and rights, has led to many of the difficulties and dilemmas in health care we now face. Smith's five criteria for viable competition, economic liberty, prudence, cooperation, justice, and equal economic opportunity should set guidelines for evaluating market-driven phenomena.

In addition to questioning the egoistic model of markets, Smith would place other important caveats on the commercialization of health care. First, the market is a limited sphere applying only to those goods and services that can be commodified. Economic models, and thus commercialization, can never include commodification of persons, their bodies, or their rights. Second, Smith would admire technology but be wary of the technology mode, a Robocop caricature of human beings, because technology, like industrialization, is a means to well-being, not an end to itself. Third, the rights model has been both overextended and misconceived. Smith limits basic or natural rights to rights to life, to reputation, and to personal liberty, and rights are not entitlements. Rather, they are equal claims for which there are concomitant and reciprocal duties. Any claim to a right to health care, then, is an entitlement only to the extent that others have realizable equal entitlements, where one has concomitant responsibilities first for the care of oneself and second to honor equally the rights claims of others. The realization of these entitlements equally, Smith would admit, does in part depend on the economic well-being of a particular society. Interestingly, Smith argues that universal mandatory public education must be provided by government in any society, for without that most of us "become as stupid and ignorant as it is possible for a human being to become."[15] Given this view and Smith's theory of rights, if medicine had been in a more advanced state in Smith's day, one wonders if he might have made the same arguments for universal basic health care as part of government's duty to prevent harms to one's rights to life and liberty.

Nevertheless Smith would be critical of the caring model. Smith would argue that caring is a virtue just as benevolence is. But as a model for dealing with problems in health care, it is not comprehensive for a number of reasons. First, one need not be benevolent, caring, or charitable, and being benevolent does not preclude being arbitrary or unfair to those one does not include in the circle of benevolence. Therefore the impartial norms of justice should underlie this model. Second, caring does not preclude noncooperation or greed. Third, however, the notion of caring can be accommodated with Smith's notion of justice. What justice demands is not the absence of caring, but its equal application. What a just caring model demands, and also what the rights model demands, in the context of Smith's idea of public works, is a provision for equal minimum basic health care needs for all of society.

Smith writes little about professionalism, but it is obvious that the spheres of commerce, technology, and rights do not encompass a fourth sphere, that of the health care specialist as a professional. Each of these is a different social sphere with particular and distinct goals. While any professional is expected to be prudent, cooperative, and just, the moral guidelines for a professional are not identical with the guidelines for those engaged in commerce. However, profitability does not exclude nor preclude the ideals of a profession that set standards for the behavior of health care specialists. The confusion lies either in the conflating of commerce with professionalism, which can lead to a commodification of patient-specialist relationships, or in the absolute division of professionalism and commerce such that a professional imagines that his or her entrepreneurial endeavors in the health care field have no spillover effect on his or her patients or professional ideals.[16] But again, it is the misinterpretation of the market model, the dominance of an Ayn Rand version of egoism, and a confusion of professional and commercial interests, not commerce itself, that has led to the decline of professionalism in health care.

Given Smith's caveats or provisos, there is no reason to condemn commercialization of certain aspects of health care when they meet Smith's five criteria (economic liberty, prudence, cooperation, justice, and a level playing field). What needs to be changed, then, is the *Wall Street* movie of markets and the trend toward market imperialism that illicitly extends the scope of its application. Moreover, a limited and revised market model is not antithetical to a more equal distribution of health care benefits. There is one interesting idea to be gleaned from the market model, an idea traceable to Milton Friedman.[17] Some years ago, during one of its public education crises, the city of Chicago proposed a voucher system for public education wherein schools would be privatized and parents would be given vouchers for the education of their children, vouchers to be redeemable at the school of their choice. A form of this system had been adopted by Milwaukee and is in the process of being instituted in that school system. Similarly, one could reallocate the distribution of health care benefits by issuing vouchers for each person in an amount necessary to cover annual basic health care needs. Smith would likely approve of this model since it minimizes paternalism and places the responsibility for one's health on the individual while attempting to equalize the protection of some of our most basic rights. Like mandatory universal education, however, Smith might include mandatory minimal provisions so that one could not use one's vouchers totally frivolously. Again, however, even if this idea is worth considering, it is only one step in the direction of taking care of our society's health care, since it does not address problems of increased costs, technology, or the decline of professionalism.

Finally, Smith's precepts of justice, while limited to preventing harms, safeguarding basic rights, and ensuring fair play, are useful in setting minimum criteria for developing and evaluating health care policies, particularly those proposals that attempt to apply a single set of rules, benefits, or distributative criteria to all health care phenomena. For surely it is the case that at a minimum (1) no policy should improve the situation of some if it worsens the situation of others or in general increases harms; (2) no policy should be unfair either to individuals, to groups of individuals, or to those who would be affected by similar decisions, or minimally it should not contribute to increasing biases, unequal opportunities, or favoritism; and (3) no policy should be adopted or enforced that violates basic rights, those rights to which every person unquestionably has claim, or again, at the least, it should not violate more rights than the status quo.[18]

What is to be learned from Smith is that it is not commercialization that is evil but its exploitation. Yet without being a misanthrope, one must be cautious about the virtues of caring and benevolence. Commodification of some aspects of health care, the abandonment of the caring model, and the development of national health care policies do not imply either the end of good health care nor exclude provisions for the poor provided that justice, not self-interest, prevails.[19]

NOTES

1. C. Dougherty, "The Costs of Commercial Medicine," *Theoretical Medicine* 11, no. 4 (1991): 275–86.
2. C. Venning, "The World of Adam Smith Revisited," *Studies in Burke and His Time* 19 (1978): 61. It should be noted that Professor Venning disputes this reading of Smith in her article.
3. For versions of this interpretation of Smith, see, for example, G. Shack, "Self-Interest and Social Value," *Journal of Value Inquiry* 18 (1984): 123–37; A. O. Hirschman, *The Passions and the Interests* (Princeton, N.J.: Princeton University Press, 1977); R. H. Frank, *Passions within Reason* (New York: Norton, 1988); A. Etzioni, *The Moral Dimension* (New York: The Free Press, 1988); M. Myers, *The Soul of Modern Economic Man* (Chicago: University of Chicago Press, 1983).
4. P. Railton, "Moral Realism," *Philosophical Review* 95 (1986): 172.
5. See P. H. Werhane, "Introducing Morality to Thrift Decision Making," *Stanford Law and Policy Review* 2 (1990): 126.
6. See M. Walzer, *Spheres of Justice* (New York: Basic Books, 1983), esp. chaps. 1, 4.
7. Smith notes, "How selfish soever man may be supposed, there are evidently some principles in his nature, which interest him in the fortune of others, and render their happiness necessary to him, though he derives nothing from it except the pleasure of seeing it. . . . The greatest ruffian, the most hardened violator of the laws of society, is not altogether without it" (A. Smith, *The Theory of Moral Sentiments*, ed. L. Macfie and D. D. Raphael [Indianapolis, Ind.: Liberty Classics, 1976], I.i.1.1).
8. A. Smith, *The Wealth of Nations*, ed. R. H. Campbell and A. S. Skinner (Oxford, England: Oxford University Press, 1976), I.ii.2.
9. Smith, *The Theory of Moral Sentiments*, II.ii.3.4.
10. Smith, *The Wealth of Nations*, IV.ix.51.
11. Ibid., I.ii.2
12. Ibid., II.iii.25–26.
13. A. Smith, *Lectures on Jurisprudence*, ed. R. L. Meek et al. (Indianapolis, Ind.: Liberty Classics, 1978), i.14, v.142.
14. This is because, Smith argues, "the whole of the advantages and disadvantages of the different employments of labour and stock . . . be either perfectly equal or continually tending to equality" (*The Wealth of Nations*, I.x.a.1).
15. Ibid., V.i.f.50.
16. See R. Green, "Physicians as Businesspeople and the Problem of Conflict of Interest," *Theoretical Medicine* 11, no. 4 (February 1990): 276–300.
17. See M. Friedman, *Capitalism and Freedom* (Chicago: University of Chicago Press, 1962).
18. See Smith, *The Theory of Moral Sentiments*, II.ii; Smith, *Lectures on Jurisprudence*, i.9–15.
19. See G. Agich, "Medicine As Business and Profession," *Theoretical Medicine* 11, no. 4 (February 1990): 311–24.

Part VI

Methodology

CHAPTER 48

Basic Theories in Medical Ethics

Glenn C. Graber

MORAL DECISIONS

In straightforward situations, we all know right from wrong. Stealing, murder, and lying are morally *wrong* and thus the right thing to do is to avoid these.

Other situations are less straightforward, and here it is sometimes not easy to know the right thing to do. It is wrong to lie, but suppose you lived in Holland during the Nazi regime and knew the hiding place of Anne Frank and her family? If a Nazi official detained you for questioning and asked insistently whether you knew the whereabouts of any Jews, should you tell him the truth or should you lie? Stealing is wrong, but suppose that the money you have access to is destined for some evil purpose. (To take an extreme example, suppose you learned that it was to be used to hire a hit man to assassinate Mother Theresa.) Is it clear that it would be wrong to steal the money if this were the only way to prevent the person from accomplishing this evil purpose?

Ethical theory has two tasks: (1) for those situations in which we already know what is right and what is wrong, it should help us *explain why* the one choice is right and the other wrong; (2) for those situations in which it is not obvious what is right and what is wrong, it should guide us to discover what is the right thing to do.

It is popular nowadays to eschew ethical theory—especially those forms described in terms of epithets such as "principlism"—as abstract and clumsy. These critics favor instead more situational approaches to ethical choice. In response, I contend that any approach that offers explanation and/or guidance (as appropriate) qualifies as "ethical theory" in the sense in which I am using the term here. As we go along, we will look at the place of "antitheories" in the typology of ethical theories that I set out.

The first step we must take in developing an ethical theory is to distinguish different sorts of judgments that are made in connection with ethical issues.[1]

ETHICAL JUDGMENTS

Evaluative judgments are concerned with what it is worthwhile or valuable to have or to do. For example, one might say, "That is a good car because it gets excellent gas mileage" (or "because it is comfortable to drive" or "because it goes fast"). Or, one might say, "A career in medicine is worthwhile to pursue because you have the satisfaction of helping people" (or "because this sort of work is absorbing"). In more general terms, one might judge, "The only thing that really matters is how much pleasure you get out of life. Even if you learned all there could be to know, your life would not be very satisfying unless you had lots of enjoyment from your knowledge."

All these are evaluative judgments. They state the goals that people set out to reach in their lives (i.e., career), or they furnish the basis for choices that we make along the way (i.e., car). Some things are rated as valuable in themselves (intrinsic values); others are good because of what they lead to or produce (instrumental values). Among the latter are included technical judgments—"This is the best suture material to use for this surgical procedure because it will hold securely and not give trouble to the patient."

Judgments of moral obligation are the sorts of judgments that first come to mind when one thinks of ethics. They concern the choice of the action to be performed or avoided in a given situation. One might say, "You have an obligation to write him a letter. He has written you several times, and you promised to reply if he wrote." Or, one might say, "You should not spend that money. It does not belong to you." Or, one might speak of "obligations," "rights," "the right thing to do," "what one ought to do (or ought *not* to do)," and so forth.

All these are obligation judgments. They embody insights about the proper choice and basis of choice of actions.

One set of obligation judgments is often singled out for special attention: claims of *rights*. Rights claims have some special features. For one thing, the demand for action falls, not on the person who *possesses* the right but on the party or parties *against* whom the right is possessed. For example, if I have a right to be paid $5 by you on Friday (because I loaned $5 to you yesterday and you promised to pay me back on Friday), then the duty involved (i.e., to repay me) falls on you, although I am the one who possesses the right. However, in spite of these distinctive features, it is most plausible to treat rights as a subclass of obligation judgments since their focus is on the proper choice of actions to do or refrain from doing.

Character judgments or judgments of moral evaluation concern evaluation of *persons* in their capacity as moral agents and consider the applicability of praise and blame to them for what they have done (or have failed to do). Evaluations of agents' motives and character are central to these judgments. One might say, "I think he is reprehensible for having done that." Or, one might say, "I admire her for having the courage to do a thing like that." Notions of praise and blame, respect and condemnation, good and bad motives or reasons for acting are central here.

Character judgments embody insights about the kind of person one ought to try to become, the kinds of motives one ought to try to develop, and the kind of character one ought to cultivate.

One way of showing the distinction among these different sorts of judgments is to recognize that one sort of judgment could be made about a given issue at the same time as an opposite judgment of another of these types. One might say that a certain action was *the best thing you could do* (evaluative judgment), and perhaps it was even *the right thing to do* (obligation judgment) but it was *not the admirable thing to do* (character judgment). Suppose, for example, that a scientist works hard for several years doing research on a dread disease and achieves a dramatic breakthrough. We would undoubtedly judge that this use of her energy and skill was the right thing to do. Furthermore, given the amount of suffering that will be relieved as a result of this breakthrough, it is probable that this was the best thing she could have done with her time. But now suppose that you probe the scientist's motivations for undertaking this research and you find out that she did not care at all about the people whose lives were improved by her research, or even about the knowledge that was gained through it. Instead, you find that her *sole* reason for undertaking the research was *spite*—she knew a rival was working in this area and she wanted to "scoop" him in reaching results. If we concluded that this was her sole motivation, we would not be likely to *admire* the scientist for what she did, though it is still true that it was a right and good thing to do.

Or, one might say that a certain action was *the right thing to do* (obligation judgment) and *an admirable thing to do* (character judgment), but it was *not the best thing to do* (evaluative judgment). This might apply to some of the tragic choices faced daily in medical care. A patient with a terminal illness requests to be kept alive as long as possible; and the health providers comply. The suffering of the patient, family, friends, and caregivers may lead one to say that it would have been best for all concerned if the patient had not lingered so long; but to honor the patient's request in this matter seems to be the right thing to do, and the respect for the patient that this embodies prompts admiration of the character of the caregivers.

THEORIES OF MORAL OBLIGATION

Why is it wrong to tell a lie?

One sort of answer that is commonly given focuses on the *consequences* of the deed. The person to whom you lie may act on the basis of the misinformation you gave her and this may lead to harm to herself and others. A simple example: A child breaks her mother's favorite vase and falsely pins the blame on her brother. Her mother punishes the brother for the act—which causes pain to him (the more so since he cannot understand *why* he is being punished). Later, the mother learns the truth and experiences regret—more pain—at what she has done. She also punishes her daughter all the more severely—still more pain—since she is angry for being made to feel guilty toward her son. We must look at the long-term consequences, as well. Thus, in the example above, the daughter is likely to find people disbelieving other things she tells them in the future once they discover she has lied to them in the past. (The classic example of this is the fable of the shepherd boy who cried, "Wolf!") This is likely to be a source of frustration—still more pain—to her, and perhaps a danger to others—still more pain—if what she has to tell them is important—as it was, finally, with the shepherd boy when a wolf actually appeared.

This sort of account of right and wrong is called a "consequentialist," "goal-based," or "teleological" theory. The latter term is derived from the Greek term for outcome or goal (*telos*) and the Greek term for theory (*logos*). We will look at this sort of account more fully in the next section.

For situations in which the right thing to do is unclear, teleological theories would have us choose the alternative that can be predicted to produce the most good and the least harm.* For example, it would be morally right to lie to the Nazi official—certainly as long as you could be pretty sure that you would be successful in deceiving him (so that you and your family would not be punished). By lying, you would save the lives of Anne Frank, her family, and their friends; and the only harm you would cause is to frustrate the zealous Nazis in their search for Jews to victimize.

Some cases suggest a different explanation of the wrongness of lying. For example, informing a patient that he has an untreatable fatal disease causes such anguish for everybody concerned that it is sometimes accurate to say that it does more harm than good. And yet, surely the patient has a *right* to this information, even if the consequences of his being given it are predominantly negative. Instead of giving primacy to evaluative judgments, as teleologists do, this sort of explanation focuses directly on features of *duty*. Hence, theories that include this general sort of explanation are given the name "deontological," derived from *deontos,* the Greek term for "duty." A variety of duty-oriented elements may be focused on. Some would speak in general of a "right to know," which is violated when someone is told a lie. Other deontologists would give primacy to the notion of "respect for persons" (or, more properly, lack of it, or disrespect) embodied in the act. To tell a lie to a patient is to fail to respect her capacity to deal with the information and to make her own decisions based on it concerning her life. Similarly, to deceive a scientific rival about the progress of one's research is a personal affront to him, aside from any harm it might do by leading him astray in his own research.

Thus, on this view, it would be wrong for the child who broke the vase to tell her mother a lie about the event even if she could arrange things so her brother would not be punished and so that the mother would never find out the truth. No *harm* is done in this situation (in contrast to the

*The technical term for an act with this character is the "optimific" action.

version we first imagined), yet the daughter has shown disrespect for her mother by the lie. If she really respected her mother as a person, she would tell her the truth and trust in her compassion and reasonableness not to make the punishment greater than she deserves. (Furthermore, she should be willing to face *just* punishment for her misdeed.)

The foregoing has been a quick sketch of two general types of theories of moral obligation: teleological and deontological. The point was to communicate the "flavor" of each kind of theory. Now let us look further at some of the details of, and varieties of, each type of theory.

Utilitarianism and Other Teleological Theories

On this view, the main task of the moral life is to produce as much good as we can through our actions, while at the same time avoiding and eliminating harm or bad to the extent possible.

More formally, the basic guiding principle of teleologism can be stated as follows:

> The Principle of Teleologism: Of all the alternatives open to a given agent at a given time, the one he or she *ought* to perform is the one that produces the greatest balance of good over evil for the members of the moral reference group. If two or more alternatives are equally optimific, then the agent *ought* to perform one or the other of these and it would be equally *right* to perform any of them.

There are at least three important questions that this guiding principle of teleologism leaves unanswered: (1) Who is to be included in the moral reference group? (2) What is to count as good and bad? (3) What *sort* of alternative is to be considered? Is the standard to be applied to specific actions, one at a time, or can it be used to formulate rules or policies for actions of certain *kinds*?

The answers to these three questions are what distinguish different forms of teleological or goal-based theories. In the next several sections, we will be looking at some different answers that have been given to each of these questions.

The Moral Reference Group

Who counts, morally? Whose welfare do we, as moral agents, have a responsibility to promote? The answer to these questions determines the moral reference group.

A full spectrum of answers to these questions has been given in the history of Western philosophy and theology. (1) At one extreme is the view, known as *egoism,* that the only person toward whom each agent has any moral responsibility is himself or herself.

(2) Intermediate positions will limit membership of one's moral reference group to some identifiable set of individuals. For example, one form of *racism* is the view that only persons with a certain racial heritage count as members of the moral reference group. One form of *sexism* says the same about members of one gender. A form of *nationalism* counts only fellow-citizens of one's nation as members of the moral reference group.

(3) One intermediate group for whom these claims might perhaps be justified is the class of *one's patients.* The act that establishes a professional-patient relationship might be sufficient to single out this group for special (or even exclusive) attention to their welfare.

(4) The doctrine of the moral reference group that has been most widely held in Western thought does not close the circle as narrowly as sexism, and so forth. Known as *utilitarianism,* this view holds that the moral reference group includes *all* sentient beings or, at least, all human beings.*

Theories of Value

The second question left open by the guiding principle of teleologism deals with evaluative

*I will not go into the animal-rights implications of this difference, except to point out that a position championing animals based on a utilitarian foundation would be more appropriately called an animal-welfare position than an animal-rights one.

issues: What counts as good (and thus to be promoted), and what counts as bad (and thus to be avoided or minimized)? Without an answer to these questions, the teleological approach cannot give us guidance in particular choices we must make. We would not know what aspect of the consequences counts for and against the alternative.

Suppose, for example, that you were invited to take part in a certain activity and were told only that it would have the effect of causing certain body tissues to increase in size and quantity. No reasonable judgment can be made about whether the activity is worth the effort until we know *what* tissue is being referred to and whether an enlargement would be valuable or disvaluable. Is it muscle tissue, so that the result would be a healthier, more robust appearance? If so, then it might be worthwhile to pursue. Or is it fatty deposits, so that the result would be an obese appearance? Or, is it the tissue of a tumor so that the result would be suffering and death? Obviously, the *value* of the consequences makes all the difference.

In general philosophical ethics, at least three different kinds of answers have been given to this question of what things have value.

Subjective Preference. Many people would contend that it is at once both futile and presumptuous to attempt to develop a general theory of value, because value judgments are regarded as totally subjective and individualistic.

The only sound alternative, then, would be to make subjective preference the standard of value and to orient teleological theories toward maximizing the satisfaction of preferences and minimizing their frustration. This is the approach that many contemporary economists, sociologists, and psychologists take in their analyses of values, especially as applied in social planning.

Hedonism. The theory of value most discussed in the history of Western philosophy is the view known as *hedonism,* which holds that the one and only thing intrinsically good is pleasure and the one and only thing intrinsically bad is pain.

This view may appear initially to be just as subjective as leaving values a matter of individual preferences, but it can be shown to bring at least some improvement. For example, a hedonist view provides a basis for criticizing some specific goals as mistaken. Individual preferences would, on this view, be regarded as involving predictions about what would bring the person pleasure (or the avoidance of pain);* and any goal could be criticized on the basis of being an incorrect prediction.

The disvalue of pain is especially well-recognized in the health care setting, where enormous efforts are directed at palliation. And the value of pleasurable states seems to require no defense. To experience them is ipso facto to recognize their value as goals worth pursuing.

It is notoriously difficult to establish objective standards for measuring these parameters. The measure that is especially difficult is intensity. It is extremely difficult for one to compare two different pains or pleasures of one's own with respect to intensity (Is the pain of today more or less intense than the one I experienced yesterday?); but the difficulty is even greater for interpersonal comparisons (Is my pain of today more or less intense than your pain of yesterday?). Anyone who has ever worked with patients in pain knows how difficult it can be to judge the intensity of the pain. The health sciences have developed some descriptive terms that may help in classifying degrees of pain, but these are still far from precise and objective.

Pluralism. Another possibility is suggested by standard criticisms of hedonism—that certain things (such as knowledge) are intrinsically good independent of their relation to pleasure or pain. Since theorists who take this approach almost always identify more than one such intrinsic good, the position is usually called *pluralism.*

Sir David Ross, for example, whose theory of obligation we shall examine later, maintains that

---

*In other words, every preference except the desire to experience pleasure and avoid pain is regarded as an instrumental value.

at least four things are fundamental intrinsic goods:

- pleasure
- knowledge
- virtue
- justice

William Frankena[2] offers a comprehensive list of things that have been claimed to be intrinsic goods:

- life, consciousness, and activity
- health and strength
- pleasures and satisfactions of all or certain kinds
- happiness, beatitude, contentment, and so forth
- truth
- knowledge and true opinion of various kinds, understanding, wisdom
- beauty, harmony, proportion in objects contemplated
- aesthetic experience
- morally good dispositions or virtues
- mutual affection, love, friendship, cooperation
- just distribution of goods and evils
- harmony and proportion in one's own life
- power and experiences of achievement
- self-expression
- freedom
- peace, security
- adventure and novelty
- good reputation, honor, esteem, and so forth

Values in Medicine. Beauchamp & McCullough[3] offer the listing of goods (and corresponding harms) in Table 48–1 that are especially relevant to the health care context.

Table 48–2 is a list of goals of medical intervention that is, in effect, a list of fundamental values in medicine.

At least one additional basic value that should be added to these is the intrinsic value of the professional-patient relationship. This sort of intimate, trust-filled, human-to-human tie is itself an important value, above and beyond the beneficial results that may be achieved through such a relationship.[4]

Maintaining Relationships as a Value. Carol Gilligan[5] observed that, whereas little boys at play quarrel about the rules of the game and who is in the right (typical deontological considerations), little girls are more likely to compromise when misunderstandings arise in order to maintain the relationships among the disputants. Furthermore, she argues that these gender differences in approach persist in the ethical thinking of adult men and women. I suggest that one helpful way of interpreting the feminine approach here is as a form of teleologism with the key value being the maintenance of relationships. The point of feminine choices is not how to satisfy some abstract ethical norm or another

Table 48–1 Values in Medicine

Goods	*Harms*
Health	Illness
Prevention, elimination, or control of disease (morbidity) and injury	Disease (morbidity) and injury
Relief from unnecessary pain and suffering	Unnecessary pain and suffering
Amelioration of handicapping conditions	Handicapping conditions
Prolonged life	Premature death

Source: Reprinted with permission from T. L. Beauchamp and L. B. McCullough, *Medical Ethics: The Moral Responsibilities of Physicians,* p. 37, © 1984, Prentice-Hall.

Table 48–2 Goals of Medical Intervention

1. Promotion of health and prevention of disease
2. Relief of symptoms, pain and suffering
3. Cure of disease
4. Prevention of untimely death
5. Improvement of functional status or maintenance of compromised status
6. Education and counseling of patients regarding their conditions and prognoses
7. Avoidance of harm to the patient in the course of care[6]

Source: Reprinted with permission from T. L. Beauchamp and L. B. McCullough, *Medical Ethics: The Moral Responsibilities of Physicians,* p. 37, © 1984, Prentice-Hall.

action-guiding consideration but how to promote and maintain a value that is cherished.

Conclusion. Differences in one's theory of value can make dramatic differences in one's choices, even if the theory of obligation remains constant. For example, a request for assistance in ending his life by a terminally ill patient who is in remitting pain will be categorically rejected by a physician who ranks life as a supreme value, whereas the request is likely to be given very serious consideration by a physician who is a hedonist in her theory of value, even if both are utilitarians in their theory of obligation.

Act versus Rule Approach

The third general question to be answered by a teleological or goal-based theory is whether the standard is to be applied to individual concrete actions or more generally in formulating policies for action in all situations of a certain type. A policy or rule approach offers the advantage of promoting consistency of action but at the expense of lack of sensitivity to the particularities of the situation at hand. An act approach is parallel to the process of clinical reasoning, attempting to take into account all the details of the specific case. The cost of this is added complexity of decision making and the necessity to repeat the process with each new situation.

Much of the critique of principlism that is heard in applied-ethics circles nowadays is actually a reaction against rule theories—especially in their most simplified versions. An act approach that pays careful attention to the context of action would avoid virtually all of the criticisms lodged against ethical theory by those who describe themselves as clinical or contextual ethicists.

The characteristic flavor of teleological theories of moral obligation is that of an ethics of production. Once the fundamental values are determined, the task of ethical decision making is to predict what values and disvalues will be brought into being by the alternatives open to one. The option is to choose the one that is likely to maximize good and minimize harm.

Deontological Theories

As we saw earlier, this approach proposes a very different way of making moral decisions from the process we have just examined. Instead of weighing and balancing the values in the situation, a duty-based theory examines the situation for moral factors of a different order.

Kant's Deontological Theory

Immanuel Kant is often taken to be the classic deontologist. He maintains that it is absolutely and always wrong to treat persons "merely as a means and not at the same time as an end in themselves."[7] To treat someone as an end is to respect the ends or goals that she has set for herself. Thus, Kant is maintaining that we should never impose anything on a person against her will. We may even have a positive obligation to do what we can to help her further her goals.

In other words, moral factors serve as "side constraints" on our goal-based calculations. They restrict our freedom to choose to serve our own interests as well as restrict our attempt to maximize the balance of good over evil for others.

Absolute Duties

According to Kant and some other deontological theories, these side constraints (or, at least, certain ones of them) cannot be overridden by *any sort of consideration whatever.* This claim has a certain initial plausibility, for example, in connection with very serious moral principles such as the following:

1. It is wrong to kill an innocent person.
2. It is wrong to tell a lie.
3. It is wrong to do physical harm to an innocent person.

Charles Fried expresses his view of the absolute or categorical character of these norms in the following:

> It is part of the idea that lying or murder are wrong, not just bad, that these are things you must not do—no matter what. They are not mere negatives that enter into a calculus to be outweighed by the good you might do or the greater harm you might avoid. Thus the norms which express deontological judgments—for example, Do not commit murder—may be said to be absolute. They do not say: "Avoid lying, other things being equal" but "Do not lie, period." This absoluteness is an expression of how deontological norms or judgments differ from those of consequentialism.[8]

Prima Facie Duties

One serious problem with the absolutist view is that moral rules may conflict with one another. If one holds that it is absolutely and always wrong to tell a lie and also to do physical harm to an innocent person, what is one to do if a situation arises in which the only way to *prevent* physical injury to an innocent person is through telling a lie, as in the Anne Frank example above?

One way of dealing with this sort of problem is to deny that moral rules are absolute. Instead, they may be taken to hold prima facie or "other things being equal." This means that nothing *other than* another moral rule could override them. It would not be justified to ignore a moral duty because I found it *inconvenient,* or because I did not *want* to do what it dictates. However, when two moral rules conflict with each other (such as in the example above where the only way to avoid bringing physical injury to an innocent person is to tell a lie), then the weight or stringency of the conflicting rules must be determined and the weightier or more stringent rule takes precedence.

Ross's List of Prima Facie Duties

Sir David Ross[9] sets out a list of seven fundamental prima facie duties:

- *Fidelity*—We ought to keep promises we have made.
- *Reparation*—We ought to make restitution for wrongful acts we have done in the past.
- *Gratitude*—We owe a debt to others who have benefitted us in the past.
- *Justice*—We ought to do what we can to ensure that pleasure or happiness are distributed in accordance with merit of the persons concerned.
- *Beneficence*—Whenever we can improve the condition of others with respect to virtue, intelligence, or pleasure, we ought to do so.
- *Self-Improvement*—Whenever we can improve our own condition with respect to virtue or intelligence, we ought to do so.
- *Nonmaleficence*—We ought not to do anything that would injure another.

This list incorporates some teleological elements (especially in the principle of beneficence), but it also includes some deontological side constraints. The verdict with the greatest weight of duty behind it is the final or "actual" duty.

Prima Facie Principles in Medical Ethics

A number of medical-ethics theorists offer a listing of prima facie principles as the foundations of their approach to ethical decision making in health care situations.

The *Belmont Report*[10] argues for regarding three principles as the basis of ethical decision making in medicine.

1. Respect for Persons
2. Beneficence
3. Justice

Beauchamp and Childress[11] present four basic principles:

1. The Principle of Autonomy
2. The Principle of Nonmaleficence
3. The Principle of Beneficence
4. The Principle of Justice

The bulk of their highly regarded book is occupied with exploring the meaning of these principles and their application to medical decisions.

Robert M. Veatch[12] develops his ethical theory with greater attention to formal conditions of its justification than to substantive principles per se. In his view, what is most important about a theory of obligation is that it can be justified as the set of principles that would be agreed to in a (hypothetical) situation of a social contract or (as he prefers to call it) "covenant." However, as a part of his "Draft Medical Ethical Covenant," he sets out the following substantive principles (for which I have supplied the names):

1. *Principle of Fidelity:* We acknowledge the moral necessity of keeping promises and commitments to one another, including the commitment of this covenant.
2. *Principle of Autonomy:* We acknowledge the moral necessity of treating one another as autonomous members of the moral community free to make choices that do not violate other basic ethical requirements.
3. *Principle of Honesty:* We acknowledge the moral necessity of dealing honestly with one another.
4. *Principle of Respect for Life:* We acknowledge the moral necessity of avoiding actively and knowingly the taking of morally protected life.
5. *Principle of Justice/Equality:* We acknowledge the moral necessity of striving for equality in individual welfare and equality in the right of access to health care necessary to provide an opportunity for health equal insofar as possible to the health of others.
6. *Principle of Respect for Persons:* We acknowledge the moral importance of producing good for one another and treating one another with respect, dignity, and compassion insofar as this is compatible with the other basic principles to which we are bound.

Jonsen, Siegler, and Winslade[13] develop their ethical theory in terms of four "topics that designate the essential features of clinical care":

1. medical indications
2. patient preferences
3. quality of life
4. the contextual features surrounding the case, such as social, economic, legal, and administrative features

This is particularly interesting in that one of the authors of this book (i.e., Jonsen) is also an author of a highly regarded exploration of casuistry[14] and the approach of casuistry is widely assumed to be an alternative to principlism. However, Jonsen emphatically repudiates this assumption:

> Neither classical nor modern casusistry repudiates principles. Casuistry is not merely another name for situationism or contextualism. Rather, principles are seen to be relevant to cases in varying degrees. In some cases, principles will rule unequivocally; in others, exceptions and qualifiers will be appropriate[15]

Even the recent political debate about access to health care is formulated in terms of prima facie principles of obligation. The Clinton health reform plan included a set of 28 prima facie principles that were to serve as the "ethical foundations of health reform."[16]

Conclusion

In general, a deontological theory of obligation offers decisive side constraints on choices.

Instead of the flavor of production and of balancing values and disvalues, deontologism establishes firm limits to action, things that one *must not* do.

THEORIES OF CHARACTER

Another point of focus in ethical theory is, not merely what things it would be good to achieve through action (evaluative judgments) or what one ought to do (moral obligation judgments), but what sort of person one ought to strive to *become.* This may be an important supplement to judgments of the other sorts, with attention paid to one's motives and patterns of action as well as to the "externals" of action. This is the approach suggested by Beauchamp and Childress[17] in Table 48–3 parallel to the principles listed above.

Other authors argue that virtues can and/or should be the primary focus of the moral life. For example, Gregory Pence develops an ethical theory in which moral virtues form the core of the moral life.

> Certain core virtues are always necessary for any decent society—the cardinal virtues of courage, justice, temperance, and *phronesis.* I would also add friendship (from Aristotle) and honesty and love (from Christianity). . . . physicians need additional virtues, such as humility (the opposite of arrogance), compassion, and respect for good science (integrity).[18]

Pellegrino and Thomasma focus more on virtues that arise in the physician-patient relationship:

> the virtues that interest us in this book are those that arise from the caring bond (which includes healing, caring, and curing) and the public trust implied by the commitment to care for another—faith and healing, trust, hope, compassion, courage, fidelity, and the like.[19]

NARRATIVE APPROACHES

Another basis for the critique of principlism nowadays is from the perspective of narrative. These theorists maintain that abstract principles are too lean a basis for communicating moral guidance and (especially) motivating moral action. Instead of a list of rules, they contend that moral discourse is better communicated in the

Table 48–3 Table of Virtues

Fundamental Principles	**Primary Virtues**
Respect for Autonomy	Respectfulness
Nonmaleficence	Nonmalevolence
Beneficence	Benevolence
Justice	Justice or Fairness
Rules	**Secondary Virtues**
Veracity	Truthfulness
Confidentiality	Confidentiality
Privacy	Respect for Privacy
Fidelity	Faithfulness
Ideals of Action	**Ideals of Virtue**
Exceptional Forgiveness	Exceptional Forgiveness
Exceptional Generosity	Exceptional Generosity
Exceptional Compassion	Exceptional Compassion
Exceptional Kindness	Exceptional Kindness

form of stories or narrative scenarios.

To see this as an alternative to principlism, however, is to take too narrow a view of the forms that a principle may take. There is no reason to believe that a moral principle needs to be stated in 25 words or less. If a narrative offers determinate guidance for situations of a certain sort, then it embodies a moral principle. The richness of the story may be necessary to convey (1) the nuances of the principle itself, if it is a very complex one, (2) the underlying rationale for accepting the principle, and/or (3) a sketch of the way of life embodied in following this principle of action. Element three is an exercise in character judgment; element two is a sketch of a theory of moral obligation and, depending on whether the wider narrative focuses on the consequences of acting in a certain way or on nonconsequential moral considerations, it could be classified teleological or deontological respectively. Thus, I continue to maintain that most allegedly antiprinciplist approaches are actually merely attempted refinements of the classic theories introduced above.

CONCLUSION

We have examined the several aspects of an ethical theory and have sketched different theories. These can be most helpful if used to identify which of these ways of thinking about moral issues most closely matches one's own approach to moral decisions. Then each theory can be applied to some problematic cases to see which yields the answer that seems most plausible. By establishing what has been called a "reflective equilibrium"[20] between concrete insights and the implications of theory, one can begin to determine which approach to use in his or her own critical thinking about moral issues.

NOTES

1. For this tripartite distinction, as for much else in this typology, I am indebted to W. K. Frankena, *Ethics,* 2d ed. (Englewood Cliffs, N.J.: Prentice-Hall, 1973).
2. Ibid., 87–88.
3. T. L. Beauchamp and L. B. McCullough, *Medical Ethics: The Moral Responsibilities of Physicians* (Englewood Cliffs, N.J.: Prentice-Hall, 1984), 37.
4. See C. Fried on "the good of personal care" in *Medical Experimentation: Personal Integrity and Social Policy* (New York: American Elsevier, 1974), 67–78.
5. C. Gilligan, *In a Different Voice: Psychological Theory and Women's Development* (Cambridge, Mass.: Harvard University Press, 1982).
6. A. R. Jonsen et al., *Clinical Ethics: A Practical Approach to Ethical Decisions in Clinical Medicine,* 3d ed. (New York: McGraw-Hill, 1992), 17.
7. See I. Kant, *Foundations of the Metaphysics of Morals,* trans. Lewis White Beck (Indianapolis, Ind.: Bobbs-Merrill, 1959).
8. C. Fried, *Right and Wrong* (Cambridge, Mass.: Harvard University Press, 1978), 9–10.
9. W. D. Ross, *The Right and the Good* (Oxford: Clarendon Press, 1930). The names for the duties are Ross's. I have supplied the summary descriptions.
10. National Commission for the Protection of Human Subjects of Biomedical and Behavioral Research, *Belmont Report*—Ethical Principles and Guidelines for the Protection of Human Subjects of Research. 44 FEDERAL REGISTER 76 (Wednesday, April 18, 1979), 23192–197.
11. T. L. Beauchamp and J. F. Childress, *Principles of Biomedical Ethics,* 4th ed. (New York: Oxford University Press, 1994).
12. R. M. Veatch, *A Theory of Medical Ethics* (New York: Basic Books, 1981), 327–30.
13. Jonsen et al., *Clinical Ethics,* 2.
14. A. R. Jonsen and S. E. Toulmin, *The Abuse of Casuistry: A History of Moral Reasoning* (Berkeley and Los Angeles: University of California Press, 1988).
15. A. R. Jonsen, "Casuistry," in *Encyclopedia of Bioethics,* rev. ed. (New York: Macmillan Library Reference, 1995), 349.
16. The White House Domestic Policy Council, *The President's Health Security Plan: The Clinton Blueprint* (New York: Times Books, 1993), 11–13; see also D. W. Brock and N. Daniels, "Ethical Foundations of the Clinton Administration's Proposed Health Care System," *Journal of the American Medical Association* 271, no. 15 (20 April 1994): 1189–96.

17. Beauchamp and Childress, *Principles of Biomedical Ethics,* 67–68, see also 466–74 on "four focal virtues."
18. G. E. Pence, *Ethical Options in Medicine* (Oradell, N.J.: Medical Economics Company, 1980), 49–50.
19. E. D. Pellegrino and D. C. Thomasma, *The Virtues in Medical Practice* (New York: Oxford University Press, 1993), xii. See also J. F. Drane, *Becoming a Good Doctor: The Place of Virtue and Character in Medical Ethics* (Kansas City, Mo.: Sheed & Ward, 1988), and E. E. Shelp, *Virtue and Medicine: Explorations in the Character of Medicine* (Dordrecht, Netherlands: D. Reidel, 1985).
20. J. Rawls, *A Theory of Justice* (Cambridge: Harvard University Press, 1971), 20.

ADDITIONAL REFERENCES

The Encyclopedia of Bioethics, Revised Edition, Warren T. Reich, Editor-in-Chief (New York: Macmillan Library Reference, 1995).

Beneficence, Larry R. Churchill Vol. 1, 243–47.

Bioethics, Daniel Callahan Vol. 1, 247–56.

Casuistry, Albert R. Jonsen Vol. 1, 344–50.

CLINICAL ETHICS: I. Elements and Methodologies, John C. Fletcher, and Howard Brody Vol. 1, 399–404.

Conscience, Martin Benjamin Vol. 1, 469–73.

Double Effect, Jorge L. A. Garcia Vol. 2, 636–41.

ETHICS: I. Task of Ethics, Michael Slote Vol. 2, 720–27.

ETHICS: II. Moral Epistemology, Michael J. Quirk Vol. 2, 727–36.

ETHICS: III. Normative Ethical Theories, W. David Solomon Vol. 2, 736–48.

ETHICS: IV. Social and Political Theories, Jean Bethke Elshtain Vol. 2, 748–58.

ETHICS: V. Religion and Morality, Robin W. Lovin Vol. 2, 758–65.

Feminism, Karen Lebacqz Vol. 2, 808–18.

Fidelity and Loyalty, David H. Smith Vol. 2, 864–68.

Future Generations, Obligations to, Bryan G. Norton Vol. 2, 892–99.

Harm, Bettina Schöne-Seifert Vol. 2, 1021–26.

Justice, James P. Sterba Vol. 3, 1308–15.

Natural Law, Russell Hittinger Vol. 4, 1805–12.

Obligation and Supererogation, David Heyd Vol. 4, 1833–38.

Pain and Suffering, Eric J. Cassell Vol. 4, 1897–1905.

Paternalism, Tom L. Beauchamp Vol. 4, 1914–20.

Responsibility, Thomas W. Ogletree Vol. 4, 2300–5.

RIGHTS: I. Systematic Analysis, Carl Wellman Vol. 4, 2305–10.

Risk, Bettina Schöne-Seifert Vol. 4, 2316–21.

Trust, Caroline Whitbeck Vol. 5, 2499–2504.

Utility, Courtney S. Campbell Vol. 5, 2509–13.

Value and Valuation, Thomas W. Ogletree Vol. 5, 2515–20.

Virtue and Character, Stanley Hauerwas Vol. 5, 2525–32.

Joseph Fletcher, *Morals and Medicine* (Boston: Beacon Press, 1954). [A teleological approach to a variety of ethical issues in medicine. Fletcher is the author who coined the term "Situation Ethics" in an earlier book with that title.]

Glenn C. Graber, Alfred D. Beasley, and John A. Eaddy, *Ethical Analysis of Clinical Medicine* (Baltimore and Munich, Germany: Urban & Schwarzenberg, 1985), especially pp. 98–112, 255–78.

Glenn C. Graber and David C. Thomasma, *Theory and Practice in Medical Ethics* (New York: Continuum, 1989).

CHAPTER 49

A Method of Ethical Decision Making

Edmund L. Erde

A person has a dilemma when, caring to do a good job, he or she believes that serious losses are at risk or gains at stake in a situation no matter what is done. In health care, moral dilemmas can arise in several ways. They can arise when determining what is permissible in trying to correct a patient's medical problem. They can arise when what is medically indicated conflicts with other loyalties, for example, concern about society's limited resources. Finally, they can arise when what is indicated for a patient conflicts with one's own well-being—one's health, income, and relations with partners or legal authorities. To resolve a dilemma, one must be clear about what is involved and have a method for generating options and choosing from among them. This chapter sketches such a method.

Although we do encounter tough cases about which it could be said there is no right answer, this is not restricted to ethics. The same is true of many kinds of practical problems. Diagnosing, investing, and deciding where to live are subject to this kind of uncertainty. Thus, we must take to heart Aristotle's warning not to seek answers that are more precise than a field of inquiry allows.[1] So perhaps the most this chapter can provide is a way of asking better questions, both about cases and about underlying ethical theories, concepts, rules, and principles.

The gist of the method is this. First, characterize the dilemma as fully as possible: Analyze its constituents by gathering all of the relevant facts and identifying the ideas and values in conflict. (This is no easy feat—there can be controversies about how to characterize a case.)

Second, keeping the nature of morality in mind, discard those constituents that arise as a result of inclinations and prejudices.

Third, if the second step does not suffice to solve the problem, consider the fully characterized case in the light of the available moral theories. This should increase one's grasp of what is at issue in each option.

The method presupposes that moral decision making has a logic. To be sure, the logic is not as mechanical as, say, the rules of arithmetic. A moral decision has to be assembled more like a bridge than a chain. Assembling takes imagination. We should not expect the method to produce incontestable resolutions.

SOME KEY CONCEPTS AND THEIR BEARINGS ON DILEMMAS

To clarify the nature of one's dilemma (and reassess it frequently) the following notions are helpful: (1) welfare, (2) interests, (3) the moral status of the patient, and (4) social ties (which primarily involves reference to approaches to morality and to social roles). In elaborating upon these, I first discuss each concept and then explain its application.

Welfare

Welfare is the *general* condition enabling any relatively independent person of any age, in any era, culture, or circumstance to function well and happily. Many separate elements of welfare are necessary for it to be realized. None alone is sufficient. Trying to specify welfare's elements produces platitudes: "It is better to be alive, sane, pain-free (and comfortable in other ways), strong, healthy, whole (including having good hearing, sight, all limbs working, etc.), free, wealthy, attractive, well liked, and smart than the opposites." Fine-grained specifications such as "It is better not to have blood pressure above 135 over 90" or "It is good to have investments in IBM" do not describe welfare. Rather they state markers, predictors, or indicators of it.

Medicine is the science that specifies the fine-grained markers of bodily welfare. It also concerns ways of bringing abnormal values into normal range and even defines tests of being alive and dead.

Application

Sometimes reminding oneself about the logic of the concept *welfare* will resolve problems by showing that an upsetting situation is a pseudodilemma. One may, for example, feel trapped in a dilemma because certain test values imply that an intervention is appropriate but other features of the situation speak against using it. If a patient's white count is high, typically one should try to determine the cause of infection and treat it. However, attempting to bring a value into line may not be required if the patient is fine or if other indicators of welfare are grim and cannot be corrected. Consider the sense of conflict that arises over the issue of feeding an anencephalic baby or adjusting the blood gases of someone about to die. To refrain in these situations is not to refrain from pursuing welfare. It is to refrain from pursuing a marker of welfare. Treating the marker when welfare is not expected to be served is "treating the numbers," not "treating the person."

Interests

Interests are variable, relative, and subjective values. They may appear arbitrary, in that those who hold them just subscribe to or adopt them.[2] In general, they appear as (1) ideals and goals (investments of meaningfulness, aspirations), (2) practical interests (a sense of the worth of various ingredients in a trade-off), and (3) dispositions (gut-level or experienced values, including preferences, prejudices, and tastes, which might be called one's "preset").

Interests can be fleeting or lifelong, common or unusual, legitimate or illegitimate (that an interest is illegitimate does not mean that anyone may intervene to stop its pursuit). Interests make life worth living for the person who lives it. When understood in the richest way, interests are essential constituents of one's personality. We hold them (1) as individuals, (2) as members of groups (e.g., the professions), or (3) as products of socialization.[3] Typically a person is interested in his own welfare (as discussed above). Consider one possible distribution of interests regarding abortion (Table 49–1).

Application

In a conflict situation, use the kind of grid shown in Table 49–1 to understand the sources of the positions of all concerned— patient, caregivers, and others.

Regarding patients, use a grid to see what is at stake for an individual. Is her or his interest an ideal, a sense of the worth of risks, or a disposition? All have moral significance. For example, a demented patient's enjoyment of meals or visits from friends is a personal, gut-level interest, and it carries moral weight.

Regarding caregivers, use a grid to identify prejudices. For example, it is often alleged that caregivers have been conditioned to act rather than wait. If so, they may be inclined to rush a patient and take his or her delay as irrational and as creating a dilemma. Is anyone holding unachievably high goals as standards of

Table 49–1 A Sample Distribution of Interests regarding the Issue of Abortion; Many Others Are Possible

	Personal	*Professional*	*Social*
Ideals, goals, and aspirations	Treasure life	Care for individual women	Prize big families
Practicality	Make money by performing them	Lie low on the issue; avoid mortality and morbidity	Respect self-determination
Gut-level dispositions (preset)	Guilt, disgust	Detached concern	Repulsion

success? Ageism may incline some to neglect an elderly patient. The grid can help identify what one should note about oneself and perhaps disclose as prejudices to patients or patients' spokespersons.[4]

A grid can show how a patient's decision to refrain from pursuing his or her own welfare may not be irrational. We should define *irrational* in such a way as to provide individuals maximum freedom to pursue interests.[5] Consider something irrational if and only if it is destructive and serves no interest.[6]

The Patient's Moral Status

Concepts of the moral status of the patient structure dilemmas. Frequently the question is cast in terms of whether the patient should be considered a person or a human. The difference is momentous. Being human is being a member of a biological species. Being a person is having certain mental abilities, specifically those needed to process one's interests.

We see humans as makers (self-determiners) of much of their own lives. However, given that there is so much about human beings' welfare that they cannot know or, knowing, cannot manipulate on their own, we also see them as less than masters of their own lives. Further, as creatures who slowly emerge from the oblivion of infancy through interacting with others, humans develop ideas, ideals, feelings, and preferences. Sometimes these are driving passions. Not infrequently we find individuals who are rash and self-destructive.

Application

Not all humans achieve personhood. And having once achieved it, no one retains it forever. That is the point behind the concept of *brain death.* It recognizes that the human part is still alive, i.e., alive in the biological sense (metabolizing). But it also recognizes that the person is dead—has permanently and irreversibly lost the power to experience, act, think, remember, and communicate.

There seems to be a general assumption that we are most clearly immoral when we act against a person's welfare, especially without his or her permission.[7] Such actions we treat as the most criminal. The model of criminal law, however, is a misleading one for ethics. Many actions that fail to respect someone's ideals are not criminal but are clearly immoral.[8]

Taking all actions against someone's welfare to be morally wrong is an error. It is an error because an action contrary to welfare might conform to the person's expressed interests. Forcing conformity to the prescriptions of welfare inflicts moral wrong by treating persons as mere biologic entities and by giving no weight to their (other) interests. If we overcome the bias toward welfare, we are most likely to give recognition to a person's ideals. We generally think that to fail to respect a person's ideals is a serious wrong. Self-determination regarding one's ideals is central to the autonomy that is constitutive of personhood. Acting against a person's ideals can be construed as making a mockery of those ideals. That is why the refusal of Jehovah's Witnesses to accept life-saving blood transfusions is so poignant. Thus, in deciding whether to override a patient's choice, one should know whether the choice is based on an ideal or a lesser value.

But a person's sense of what is practical can be just as worthy of respect, just as authentic as his or her ideals, and just as rational as those of caregivers. Moreover, a person's preference may be very ingrained. A hospitalized patient's constipation might be disregarded because the teams comanaging him or her might be absorbed by their interest in the fine-grained aspects of the patient's welfare. But ignoring the patient's values and preferences is very disrespectful even if all of his or her ideals are acknowledged. This wrong can be characterized as treating a rational individual with interests as a creature subject to assessment in regard to welfare alone.

The mirror image of this wrong is to treat humans as persons. Giving in to the unsafe preferences of young children or retarded, confused, intoxicated, or psychotic individuals *may* be wrong. I emphasize "may," because there seems to be a concept that negotiates the gap between personhood and mere humanhood. This is the concept of the *self.* Its nature is a vast topic. To put the point intuitively, note that there can be a self even in the case of individuals who may not yet have reached rational personhood or have declined from it due to dementia, intoxication, or mental illness. The enduring self has a sense of continuity with its past and future, a sense of having a story it is living.[9] Selves can suffer great harm if action is taken on behalf of their welfare when their values strongly dispose them another way.

A methodological advantage to using the concept of the self is that the concept personhood, through its connection to rationality, sets a very high standard for humans. Furthermore, personhood is probably associated with more prescriptive cultural assumptions than is the concept of the self. Personhood suggests individuality. But to talk of a patient as a self may allow ready recognition that the patient does not see his or her own individuality as central, but rather sees him- or herself as a member of a family or tribe. To talk of the self allows ready recognition of the patient's preset (perhaps ethnically derived) notions about the body and expectations about the doctor-patient relationship (expectations that may not involve informed consent or confidentiality). One way of looking at the matter is that a person is a *kind* of self—the kind for whom individuality and what attaches to it is central.

Some dilemmas arise because some patients—newborns, severely demented individuals, profoundly retarded individuals—are neither persons nor selves. Other patients are selves but not rational persons. Others are marginally able to weigh risks and benefits. They have values and think in ways that tempt caregivers to consider them incompetent, perhaps partly because caregivers are welfare-oriented, while patients are not.

These variations have moral implications. To care for patients as humans inclines one to treat them as *objects* of value—their existence counts most. To care for them as persons inclines one to respect their zone of autonomous decision making (what caregivers value is thus irrelevant). To care for patients as selves is to refrain from transgressing their interests (such as the joy they get from having their hair combed). When the patient has no interests at all and is incapable of regaining the capacity to have them, moral respect for the patient can only be minimal. All of this helps show the contrast between the two rival approaches to morality that I turn to now: those that direct dilemma resolving.

Social Ties

Because we can affect one another's welfare and interests for good, we benefit from social ties. Because we have the means to communicate, we can create such ties, including authority, roles, shared values, ideals, ideas, language, moral theory, science, myths, economic cooperation, and prejudices. Not all of these are wonderful, however. Some socially created expectations can be dangerous. For example, society has idealized the family. We should not expect people to be good to each other just because they share a family. Thus, we should not turn control of a patient's health care over to people just because they are members of the same family. Other nonwonderful ties include social prejudices such as racism, ageism, and sexism. Social ties both help and cause havoc. In this chapter, roles and morality are the two most important ties that will be explored.

MORAL THEORIES

Moral theories come in several variants. Consider three prominent ones: (1) those emphasizing consequences, (2) those emphasizing compliance to rules, and (3) those emphasizing dispositions to behave (what used to be called *character*). Each variant provides insights but also runs into difficulties.

Consequentialism

The consequentialist approach (sometimes called *teleological* or *utilitarian*) has us focus on effects of actions in deciding a dilemma. The best decision is taken to be the one that produces the greatest happiness (or least unhappiness). Medicine would have us understand this approach as welfare-centered, which tends to engender paternalism. This is because humans are not perfectly rational and patients cannot foresee how they will react or adjust to their condition, whereas an experienced professional can make fairly accurate predictions.

Aside from the problems with paternalism, difficulties of consequentialism include questions about whose experiences should be taken into consideration (those of society? caregivers? family members?). Also, how much weight should be accorded to each person? How shall the consequences be weighed? How far into the future should we project? How shall levels of certainty influence such judgments? (Many of these questions can only be answered by having made assumptions about the third approach to morality discussed below.)

Application

To take advantage of consequentialism's strengths, be willing to live with its implications, even the less felicitous ones. Imposing treatment over protestations becomes much more morally hazardous if those who impose it cannot recreate the state of the patient at the time of imposition and follow the patient's choice the second time around. Sometimes the recreation is easy. Forcing continuation of dialysis for a time is not very morally risky, since it can be discontinued if the patient's predictions about his or her quality of life are correct. Sometimes, however, recreating the state is difficult. For example, a patient who was forced onto a ventilator may cease to need it to live, but find his or her life unacceptable anyway. Those who were willing to force the patient onto the machine might now rectify the error only by killing the patient. The logic of consequentialism seems to require such killing. Finally, sometimes recreating the state is impossible. The bad consequences for a Jehovah's Witness from a forced blood transfusion cannot be undone (e.g., the sense that her soul is irreparable). But these consequences should not be ignored. Perhaps they justify refraining from the transfusing.

Note, too, that different individuals live with the consequences differently. A physician might not be able to sleep a wink the night after performing elective sterilization for a young woman. Even so, that sleeplessness is slight in contrast with what the woman would suffer from an unwanted pregnancy.

Deontological Theories

The deontological approach to moral decision making has us focus on obligations and duties that are specified independently of consequences. The commanding duty is to respect persons. This does *not* mean that one should esteem or value persons. Rather, it means that one should respect the person's rights and the boundaries within which the person can exercise self-rule (autonomy). Rights are entitlements to protection, courses of action, goods, and control over information.

Rights are taken to belong to persons not merely as matters of social convention. Rival justifications for them exist, but we need not choose among these for most purposes of method.[10] Rights are often the basis of claims that persons can make against evildoers, such as those who compromise their welfare against their will (e.g., by raping or stabbing them), *and* against do-gooders, such as those who want to force them to adopt a religion or remain fertile. Within the limits of equal protection for all, rights protect a person's control over the holding and pursuing of the person's interests (at the personal, professional, and social levels). They protect a person from other individuals and from the all-powerful state itself.

Many rights relevant to medical ethics are well-known. They include rights to the truth about diagnosis and prognosis, to confidentiality, to helpful information about the risks and potential benefits of the various tests and interventions available, and to the opportunity to freely choose among such interventions. Less well-known are rights to information about the hospital's quality of care or the professional competency of consultants.

That persons possess a sphere of decision making that no one is entitled to infringe is one of the principle insights of deontological theories. This acknowledges the moral equality of persons. However, deontological theories have several important problems. Who should get which rights? What should be done when rights conflict? How shall one handle a case in which respecting a right seems likely to produce an easily avoided disaster? How far does a right extend? Controversies over what constitutes a person and issues about duties to nonpersons also present complications. These problems suggest that among the social ties an authoritative source of answers will be needed. In a functional society, someone (or some group) will have to voice stipulative answers on behalf of the people when logic fails.

Application

This approach to morality suggests a way to distinguish the bad, the sad, and the wrong. *Bad* connotes negative consequences regarding welfare or interests. *Sad* connotes negative feelings. *Wrong* connotes actions that violate boundaries of moral conduct. Rights to privacy and to informed consent are boundaries.

The moral applications of this approach begin with an instruction. Do not cross a person's boundary without authorization from (1) the person, (2) society, when it produces the authorization in a fair and publicly accepted fashion, or (3) ourselves, when a reasonable understanding of what is explicitly authorized strongly implies that if there were a process for consulting it, a fair society would allow crossing the boundary in that kind of case.[11] Not getting one of these kinds of authorization and usurping autonomy on one's own is the height of presumptuousness. It presumes that one has authority over the most private sphere of a moral equal. But be aware that going to society for permission to override a right—that is, going to court—can lead to the stipulation of rules that undermine autonomy and can cost the patient money. Respecting autonomy in such cases may lead to a sad outcome but leave us free from the encumbrances of unwise legal decisions.

Although sometimes those who resolve controversies of meaning (courts or legislatures) do provide help (e.g., in stipulating *brain death*), sometimes their answers are disastrous. For example, the law's language and ideas regarding death and dying are terribly confusing and generate moral dilemmas. Desperate attempts have been made to retain the traditional repugnance to killing, to endorse letting die, and to declare withholding and withdrawing life-prolonging interventions to be acceptable equivalents.[12] Part of the error depends on ignoring the function of social roles, which is dealt with below. Note here that if one is in a role that makes one responsible for a patient, then action and omission are moral equivalents. They do not divide in such a way that letting die is permissible and killing is not.[13] They are both morally acceptable options in some cases and both unacceptable in others, depending on what the patient chooses.

Having recognized the muddle, one might still have a dilemma about acting morally versus complying with stipulations (especially when it is the law that is stipulating). But that is not a purely moral matter. It involves one's own practical interests. The moral dimension shifts to whether there is a moral way to refuse to comply with laws that draw illogical distinctions that force great injury. If one considers the general system moral (government by consent, due process of law, law subject to public review and alteration), then disobedience is most justified when one disagrees with a particular law (not just its application to a particular case) and violates it openly, seeking a public hearing in order to alter it. Approving of the system and the particular law but disregarding both in a given case without putting oneself on the line is very self-indulgent at best. It seems to happen often, especially in "no coding" patients without authorization from an appropriate source or, even worse, "slow coding" patients.

The Role of Character

Many dilemmas arise from conflicts between the two approaches to ethics described above. In short, they shape the controversy over the nature of morality itself. The two approaches clash when, for example, caregivers feel that telling a patient the truth will discourage the patient from accepting a "needed" intervention (at least on the physician's timetable) or when a patient declines all interventions. In cases like these, the exercise of the patient's rights is thought to conflict with the patient's pursuit of his or her welfare. So when, if at all, may caregivers disregard rights?[14] Before answering, I shall discuss the third approach to morality. Perhaps it will be helpful in dissolving the sense that there is a dilemma in many situations that otherwise beckon caregivers to override patient's rights.

This approach focuses on character or integrity. It brings us back to the fact that roles are social ties. The point is that persons will reliably know and fulfill the duties attached to a specific role only if they themselves are defined by performing its fundamental actions well.

Roles establish expectations about behavior. There are, of course, many roles: sex roles, family roles, etc. Each role forms relationships with the complementary roles with which the role holders interact. These relationships create ill-defined strata in society, along with duties and rights for each holder.

Professionals have their places in the strata and among the relationships. Through licensing and through funding education and research, society directs what the institutions and practitioners may do. What they do relates to both society at large and to patients. Until recently, patients occupied what has been called "the sick role."[15] To enter it, one needs certification from an expert (professional) that one falls below certain norms of welfare determined by science. That is part of the professional's role. While in the sick role, patients may receive official benefits (insurance, prescriptions) and unofficial ones (attention from family members). A principal official benefit is being excused from ordinary responsibilities, but one is obliged to try to recover and leave the role.[16] Assisting in the patient's recovery in ways that untrained persons could not is another part of the professional's role. This requires patients to comply with the professional's advice.

Application

Under this approach to morality, physicians who take their role as complementary to the sick role should be conditioned to do the following: (1) certify honestly, and (2) do anything to get patients out of the sick role. Dilemmas frequently arise because such built-in imperatives conflict with patients' interests and rights to choose freely. Realizing that a conflict has arisen because original aspects of the social role have been transported inappropriately to new kinds of cases should be very helpful. For example, if society creates and sustains a role for acute and unexpected conditions from which patients could recover, the role may not fit those suffering from a horrible chronic disease. To force them to conform would be an error.

One problem with the character approach to morality is the rival formulations of a role. Often a formulation is too vague to help with a problem (e.g., "The physician is a teacher"). Or what sounded fine in the abstract may seem heartless, rigid, and morally wrong when we get to cases (e.g., "The physician fights disease").[17]

Many dilemmas arise from professionals' sense of their enterprise—the "proper ideals of the profession." If society creates and sustains medicine to prolong life and restore health, letting persons die will be difficult or impossible to accept. If the purpose is to provide an effective work force, caring for a dying or unemployable person will be very difficult. If the purpose is to reduce suffering in ways consistent with patients' wishes, forcing treatment on patients will be nearly unthinkable.

The ideals define what could be called the profession's "ultimate logic," its reason for being. Ultimate logic contrasts with domestic logic—the practical structures of conduct. Many such practical structures are compromises with the physical and human environment, but they eventually become norms of behavior. For example, if a policy requires cardiopulmonary resuscitation (CPR) on *all* patients suffering cardiac arrest, it may be a compromise to avoid the emotional difficulties involved in discussing death with patients, and it may also give rise to that great hypocrisy "the slow code." Having to economize leads to rooms in which "privacy" is "provided" by curtains. Compromises with limited salaries, space, time to gather information, etc., do shape day-to-day functioning.

Subscribing to the correct ultimate logic is important. The correct ultimate logic will help avoid the inspired or conscientious wronging of others. And it will help avoid making a sham of the calling to which one is dedicated. Shamming occurs if one is driven to violate fundamentals of the profession because of commitments to incidentals, such as protecting a partnership instead of a patient.

Two rival ultimate logics for health care should be assessed.

One contends that medicine exists to foster welfare. The imperative in every case, then, is to bring tests, values, etc., into line with what is scientifically indicated unless welfare itself will not be served by doing so. The domestic logic of this encourages caregivers to treat even when the prospects of success are extremely unlikely and even when patients decline treatment. It encourages a plan of tests that starts with the least invasive, even if that test is the least reliable and even if the patient would accept some risk to welfare for a faster diagnosis. It inclines caregivers to get court orders if patients are acting against their own welfare.[18] Thus, how the ultimate logic is defined and, once defined, how efficiency and emotional frailty affect the domestic logic raise important moral questions.

The second rival for the ultimate logic of medicine contends that health care exists to help persons pursue those interests that involve their having a human body. This includes the persons' particular interests in their own welfare. To be sure, there must be stipulations about the bounds of permissible help. (One may not help a patient hurt another person; however, one may be obliged, owing to confidentiality, to allow such injury, for example, by not disclosing to a woman that her prospective husband is a homosexual.) The domestic logic of this view would include ways to discover and honor the preferences of patients, for example, through effective advance directives, patient advocates, and revised ways of history taking (so that each patient's "value history" is documented).

The rivalry between the two ultimate logics is in the background of many dilemmas. How could there be professional dilemmas unless professionals have made assumptions about or commitments to the purpose of their profession? Without a goal, no sense of seriousness could attach to making a choice. This approach leads us to distinguish those who make good surgeons because they enjoy cutting and sewing from those who like to solve medical problems and are good at cutting and sewing.

The resolution to the conflict between ultimate logics appears to be in a third option. Assume that the role of caregivers is to help selves with the problems arising from their bodily nature. This is consistent with the idea that medicine exists to help selves as valuable entities, and it gives caregivers license to foster a patient's welfare. Consequences for that welfare would then be nearly decisive for medical decision making.[19]

Taking selves to be the object of medicine incorporates insights from the view that directs us to help persons with the problems arising from the nature of the body. This offers several advantages. When appropriate, it acknowledges the self as a person with rights. Second, it avoids the presumptuousness of approaching individuals as though they are not persons and treating them as something of value rather than respecting their rights. Third, it suggests the moral necessity of helping patients toward personhood, for example, by teaching children to think about risks, benefits, confidentiality, etc.

THE METHOD

1. By means of the above concepts, state the dilemma as fully as possible.
2. Assess how much of it is driven by the personal and professional biases of the caregivers (e.g., inclinations to foster patients' welfare, professionals' finances, etc.).
3. Eliminate all of the biases except those of the patient (except where allocation of resources and duties to third parties is the dilemma).
4. Consider the case and options in light of the ethical theories. Take the option most strongly indicated by that process. If two are very close, discuss the dilemma with several reasonable persons playing the devil's advocate. If the issue still seems too close to call, flip a coin.

That's it—that's the method.

But before closing, I must elaborate a bit more and then make some theoretical remarks on the nature and limits of method.

Medical Dilemmas and Decision Making

Competent Patients

In dealing with a competent patient, use respect for autonomy and the ultimate logic of helping persons with their interests. Remember the difference between sad and bad. If the patient is exercising a fundamental right—especially in ways that do not violate the rights of others—consider the right a moral trump (i.e., as decisive).[20] Resist paternalism and appeal to consequences unless (1) you are sure (and I do not see how one could be) that informing the patient will cause his or her becoming incompetent and you can find a trustworthy representative of the patient's interests; (2) the patient's ideals, practical interests, or notions about the quality of experience are known and the patient seems to be speaking inauthentically (this should not be just an excuse for professionals to have their way, and the evidence should be very compelling, since none of us is a mind reader); (3) the protesting patient is unwilling to give reasons and the caregiver can undo what would be forced upon the patient; or (4) the protesting patient is basing his or her refusal on a completely and incontrovertibly false premise, not just playing a long shot.

Assuming that there is time, one should go to court to test one's judgment that society would accept overriding the right.[21] Be very careful about doing this, though. If the ultimate logic of medicine is to help persons, caregivers should be very reluctant to create legal precedents that undermine the autonomy of persons.[22]

Short of being able to get to court, one should try to test one's thinking on someone functioning as an ethics consultant. This person should work in two stages. First, from as objective a presentation of the case as possible, the person should reach his or her own decision. Second, after being told the caregivers' inclinations, the person should play the devil's advocate. An ethics committee might be able to do this as well or better than a solo consultant. And if one decides not to risk violating the law and being heard in court, perhaps one should agitate for reform.

Incompetent Patients

If the patient is not competent but had a self that might be restored, try to determine what the patient would want in the situation. Comply with that, not with the preferences of others (the family, caregivers, or hospital administrators). Advance directives and "value history" should help here.

If nothing about the patient's value history is known, use *welfare* broadly considered. If a self can be restored, try to restore it. Be sure social prejudices are not operating to dilute the pursuit of welfare. Having a guardian appointed is the ideal solution, and inconvenience to caregivers is not morally relevant. What is relevant is how well the guardians would do their job. There is no requirement to comply with mere ritual.[23] One really is thrown back on custom here, except that one should minimize suffering.

Newborns

Regarding newborns, society's stipulations (e.g., through law) can have acceptable moral goals. Thus, society may wish to protect newborn babies for the symbolic value of doing so. However, those that will never even develop a self (much less personhood) can hardly serve that moral purpose. If society forces parents and caregivers to sustain such newborns, society should pay all monetary costs. Humans lacking a self should receive attention regarding their welfare. Usually this means they should not suffer. But there is no direct moral duty to sustain them. Morally, *parents* ought to be free to decide whether and how to treat them. One would not want the *state* managing or directing mercy killing in this context.

Nondilemmatic Decision Making

Consider two kinds of cases. First, consider persons who endanger the welfare or interests of others. Can they so abuse their liberty that they alienate themselves from some of their rights to health care? Second, consider persons in serious situations beyond their control (indeed, even barely involving them) that may threaten the welfare and interests of many others. May we override the rights of such persons in trying to defeat the threat?

Above, rights were considered to be a moral trump. However, perhaps they should not always be decisive. It seems that persons are entitled to have their rights respected unless they have done or will do something so bad that they destroy their entitlement to the right *or* unless the world is such that complying is impossible. Rarely is a caregiver able to decide on his or her own whether either of these situations obtains. Furthermore, one should have criteria to justify overriding rights or to justify claims that persons have alienated themselves from their rights. For example, one should be sure that overriding will not undermine the point of society's having established the right in the first place or that a thoughtful, consistent ethic would accept the override for all persons equally.

Using the misbehavior of others and the serious needs of third parties can sometimes justify too much. If misdeeds or needs are taken vaguely, one might find any previous infraction by the patient or any shortage of resources sufficient to justify depriving individuals of their rights. Strong social safeguards are supposed to protect individuals from such abuse. Primary among these is the due process of law. It provides that governmental powers must be passed into law in an elaborate way that includes being open to public scrutiny. So, too, the exercise of power must be open to review. In law, individuals can ask for judicial review both of the rules that are being used against them and of the trials in which they are litigants. Ideally such due process should protect people from the overly zealous. There should be no less protection in health care.

Deontological theories, as well as the role society has constructed for caregivers, imply that it is not up to caregivers to decide how to allocate resources. A caregiver should not decide that using a workable treatment is wasteful because the patient does not contribute to society or because he or she offends caregivers in some way. This does not mean that allocation cannot be controlled in some ways. But it does mean that the criteria or policies should not be set by a patient's caregivers. The hospital door should not be a trap for uninformed patients. Yet the application of policy on a case-by-case basis will demand discretion on the part of practitioners.

Policy must be publicly made and be subject to revision, and the consequences of its applications must be subject to review.

The best examples of this are the laws requiring caregivers to report certain conditions and situations to specific authorities. That such laws are "on the books" is a mark in favor of taking them as justifying certain exceptions to the right of confidentiality. But it is just a mark in favor. The right answer can be murky. We do not know whether confidentiality should be an absolute right. If medicine is a social creation, perhaps society can experiment with varying approaches to problems, collect data, and see what is the best policy.[24] Society should be able to test what is best regarding child abuse or impairment and addiction.

Cases like these draw caregivers away from the ideal of helping selves with the problems they have that are derived from possessing a human body. Singleness of purpose may be more than we can hope for. But surely if we remember the difference between a role that binds professionals to patients deontologically and a role that makes one responsible for consequences, we will recognize that one cannot have the duty to prevent all sad and bad things.

CONCLUSION

It should be part of methodology—underlying ideas about how to devise a method—to acknowledge that if a situation poses a true moral dilemma, losses should be expected no matter which option is taken. Further, it should be part of methodology to recognize that one situation can embody different dilemmas for different parties. Patients, friends, family members, medical students, physicians, nurses, and janitors will likely face different dilemmas in their roles. Perhaps each needs a different method for deciding. An analysis of welfare, interests, and social ties may help all of them. Should rights be further in the background for some than others? Are friends bound to the same duties and limited by the same patients' rights as professionals?[25] Is the language of political morality more applicable to strangers taking care of strangers?[26]

Sometimes the method offered above implies that taking a situation as a dilemma is a mistake. For example, it may depend on conflating the sad and the bad. Those who disagree in a given case will find the method shallow or worse. Sometimes the method implies that there are moral problems that practitioners fail to notice. To those who disagree, the method might appear picky or worse. Sometimes it implies resolutions that individuals will find morally offensive. They will want to work through the justifications of the method (the methodology) to critique the method. For example, they will want to know how to recognize a principle invoked to justify a choice. I wish there were enough methodology to do them the honor, but space forbids anything more than the incidental attention that has been paid to it. The most I can say about this is that I have found the method useful in teaching and consultation.

Sometimes, no doubt, the method will not generate a resolution. We may feel then that we need both more method and more methodology, or even more factual information. This, however, may be naive. In many fields, methods have led to the discovery of limits to and difficulties about themselves. This holds even in former paradigms of potentially complete and absolutely certain systems of knowledge, such as advanced mathematics or advanced physics. But this does not reduce the field of study or the problem solving to insignificance, subjectivity, or relativism. "There are no right answers" cannot be used in a flip way to dismiss either cases that can be compellingly resolved after hard analysis or cases that cannot be so resolved. Regarding the former, society has made progress in its method of deciding. Regarding the latter, there is a morally appropriate way of dealing with pure, true dilemmas: Share them as dilemmas with those involved. Face the fact that serious matters are at issue. Do not allow the secondary inference that there is no right answer to detract from the seriousness of the situation.[27]

NOTES

1. Aristotle, *Nicomachean Ethics,* 2.2.1104a5–7.
2. This contrasts with the values specified about welfare; they seem objective, universal, rational, etc.
3. A discussion of the particulars of (2) will be offered later. A discussion of (3) belongs in the next section. I omit it from the chapter in the hope that the meaning is evident enough. For a general discussion of values see E. L. Erde, "On Peeling, Slicing and Dicing an Onion: The Complexity of Taxonomies, Values and Medicine," *Theoretical Medicine* 4 (1983): 7–26.
4. This could be a threatening prescription. It bears on the issue of how few dilemmas are purely moral and absent of any self-serving considerations. It also requires one to know a patient's prejudices. "Poor quality of life" may represent one thing to young, healthy, energetic, resident physicians and another to older patients or in regard to the retarded. See J. A. Robertson, "Dilemma in Danville," *Hastings Center Report* 11 (October 1981): 5–8.
5. Accordingly, the term *best interests* should be avoided. It is pretentious in implying some connection with noble interests. It is presumptuous in implying that some stranger is an expert about what should interest a person. *Welfare* is much less likely to mislead. But neither *best interests* nor *welfare* does the work necessary for moral communication with patients. Both are general terms with many individual ingredients. Furthermore, neither political science nor the science of medicine provides knowledge of an ideal type. The most they can do is inform about trends within populations. We live in a pluralistic world with few certainties about how one should live or define oneself.
6. See C. M. Culver and B. Gert, *Philosophy in Medicine* (Oxford, England: Oxford University Press, 1982). Culver and Gert distinguish irrational ideas and desires from incompetence in a helpful way.
7. Entering competition, e.g., sports, is a form of risking one's welfare. Many forms of competition risk welfare in many ways. Some people thrill to the risk. There is nothing patently immoral about such competition. And though competitors do not consent to losing, they consent to risking loss.
8. To baptize a baby known not to be Christian but brought to an emergency ward with critical injuries is wrong, but not criminally wrong.
9. See S. Hauerwas, "Self as Story," in *Vision and Virtue: Essays in Christian Ethical Reflection* (Notre Dame, Ind.: Fides Press, 1974).
10. But it is worth identifying them. One bases rights in the kind of beings we are—persons. Rights are options to which persons are entitled. They are social ties, both because they specify the moral grounds of peaceful coexistence among persons and because social cooperation is necessary for their realization. Another account bases rights in the value of allowing persons to look out for themselves given the shortcomings of existing social arrangements.

    Their approaches to the right to abortion will exemplify the differences between the two accounts of rights. The first acknowledges women's inviolate right to privacy and bodily self-determination. The second creates a right as an "out" in a society that stigmatizes illegitimate and adopted children, has not created or made accessible safe and effective contraception, and does not decently supplement the costs of raising children.
11. See R. Dworkin, *Taking Rights Seriously* (Cambridge, Mass.: Harvard University Press, 1977), especially chap. 7.
12. Two opinions of the Supreme Court of New Jersey are worth reading critically in this regard: In re Quinlan, 355 A 2d 647 (N.J. 1976) and In re Conroy, 98 N.J. 321 (1985). The process laid out in Conroy has been challenged as seriously flawed. However, some of the decision's analyses are excellent. The flaws probably arise from a concern to be politically tactful or a lack of courage by the justices to face pressure groups.
13. J. Rachels, *The End of Life: Euthanasia and Morality* (New York: Oxford University Press, 1986).
14. Actually not many dilemmas arise from this sphere, for patients have been found to want more information than caregivers tend to give them. (Many studies show this. See, for example, W. M. Strull et al., "Do Patients Want To Participate in Medical Decision Making?" *Journal of the American Medical Association* 252 [1984]: 2990–94.) Also, paperwork (i.e., the informed consent form, terrible as it is) is often taken as a substitute for true consent. Rarely is a patient told all that the moral (and legal) model requires. The moral model requires offering the patient all the options so that informed choosing occurs rather than mere consenting to the physician's choice. For example, consider that physicians' professional values may incline them to offer the least risky test procedure of several available ones, even though it is least likely to yield useful information. However, the patient may, for personal reasons, wish not to climb the ladder of increasingly risky procedures, but take the riskiest one first to get answers as quickly as possible. But see H. Brody *The Healer's Power* (New Haven, Conn.: Yale University Press, 1992), Chapters 6 and 7.
15. T. Parsons, *The Social System* (New York: The Free Press, 1951).
16. That compliance is built into the patient role is in part the triumph of medicine's power play over the last century and a half. Compare J. L. Berlant, *Profession and Monopoly: A Study of Medicine in the United States and Great Britain* (Berkeley, Calif.: University of California Press, 1975) and P. Starr, *The Social Transformation of American Medicine* (New York: Basic Books, 1982).

17. For an excellent discussion of some rival characterizations of the physician's role, see W. F. May, *The Physician's Covenant: Images of the Healer in Medical Ethics* (Philadelphia: Westminster Press, 1983). Part of the reason that the character approach to morality does not work fully is that wc are unavoidably in the grip of history. Perhaps society's reasons for sustaining an institution are different from the reasons for having created it or sustained it in the past. Perhaps there were several values involved in creating or sustaining an institution, and some of them conflict from time to time. It is possible that we have brought forward and feel bound to ideals that are now inappropriate.
18. One problem with the account thus far, though, is that professionals who subscribe to this view seem to have evolved their own focus on bodily welfare and leave a great deal out that would seem to belong in. For example, if caregivers were attuned to all aspects of bodily welfare, they would note and take action about such mundane considerations as whether a patient is uncomfortably warm or cold or needs a hearing aid, eyeglasses and/or podiatric care, even though the patient is being seen for a completely different problem. This pattern of attending only to long-term welfare tends to cause neglect of the patient who is at the end of life and suffering a great deal.
19. The consequences for welfare could not be completely decisive, because caregivers might be tempted to certify about a patient's health in the way the patient prefers, and this could become quite dangerous, for example, if the patient is a pilot.
20. I cannot say exactly what makes a right fundamental. It is connected with rules that all should agree to live by—rules that respect moral equality. But consider the difference in invasiveness between forcing a parent to live with and take care of a child on the one hand and forcing a parent to contribute economically to the support of a child on the other. The first is reminiscent of slavery. The second is simply holding a person economically accountable. To force someone to accept a live-saving intervention because he or she has dependent children violates the fundamental rights of the parent. Children do not have a right to be raised by their biological parents.
21. Do not consider the time qualification lightly. Economics cannot side with those who want to deprive persons of their rights. We have to keep lawyers and courts available, astute, and fair.
22. According to this ethic, it is proper (but might be sad) to help someone—even someone who is not terminally ill—die. And awful as the case may be, we should not compromise the fundamental freedom of persons to determine what happens in their own private sphere of control. We should not invade that sphere, e.g., for the sake of a fetus or even the person a fetus may become. If a law were to be made prohibiting a woman carrying a fetus from endangering it, the law would be terribly invasive. Both deontological theories and the approach to character ethics that conforms to them produce morally binding social ties between caregivers and patients that require caregivers to allow many sad and harmful events to occur. They probably will not happen often. See G. Annas, "Forced Cesareans: The Most Unkind Cut," *Hastings Center Report* 12 (June 1982): 16–17, 45.
23. A few studies and analyses show how this has dilemmatic dimensions. See J. W. Warren et al., "Informed Consent by Proxy: An Issue in Research with Elderly Patients," *New England Journal of Medicine* 315 (1986): 1124–28; also, the companion editorial by G. J. Annas and L. Glantz, "Rules for Research in Nursing Homes," *Ibid.* Also see G. H. Morris, "Conservatorship for the 'Gravely Disabled': California's Nondeclaration of Nonindependence," *San Diego Law Review* 15 (1978): 201–37, esp. 225–37.
24. M. W. Wartofsky, "Medical Knowledge as a Social Product: Rights, Risks and Responsibilities," in *New Knowledge in the Biomedical Sciences,* ed. W. B. Bondeson et al. (Boston: Kluwer, 1982).
25. E. L. Erde and A. H. Jones, "Diminished Capacity, Friendship, and Medical Paternalism: Two Case Studies from Fiction," *Theoretical Medicine* 4 (1983): 303–22.
26. R. A. Burt, *Taking Care of Strangers: Rule of Law in Doctor-Patient Relations* (New York: The Free Press, 1979).
27. I would like to thank Professors Nancy Moore and Jay Yanoff for their help with early drafts of this chapter.

BIBLIOGRAPHY

Bedell, Susanna E., and Thomas L. Delbanco. "Choices about Cardiopulmonary Resuscitation in the Hospital." *New England Journal of Medicine* 310 (1984): 1089–93. This is worth reading to get a grasp of how poor is decision making and communicating regarding do not resuscitate (DNR) status decisions. Almost three-quarters of the patients suffering an arrest did so unexpectedly. Physicians and residents had different ideas about who did not want to be code status. Only 30 percent of the patients and half the patients' "families" were consulted about code status in advance. Fifteen percent of those receiving the code were alive a year later. A third of those would have refused the code and were still sorry to have been put through it. If the physicians were consequentialists, they do not have a record of which to be proud.

Brody, Howard. *Ethical Decisions in Medicine,* 2d ed. Boston: Little, Brown, and Co., 1981. An early attempt to put ethical theory into a decision-making format. Flow chart-like instructions are incorporated. The author is a physician and holds a Ph.D. in philosophy.

Buchanan, Allen. "Medical Paternalism," *Philosophy and Public Affairs* 7 (Summer 1978): 370–90. This is a masterful critique of paternalism, both when the patient is put in the child's role and when the family is. The argument is very reminiscent of some by John Stuart Mill, who is considered a consequentialist in the sense defined in this chapter. On this view, paternalism should be rejected, because only the person who is living a life can know what fits into it best when the choices are grim. The distinction between ordinary and extraordinary is convincingly rejected as nonsensical or question begging.

———. "Medical Paternalism or Legal Imperialism: Not the Only Alternatives for Handling Saikewicz-type Cases." *American Journal of Law and Medicine* 5 (1979): 97–118. As the title suggests, this essay attempts to negotiate between two opposing positions on the role of the courts in deciding not to treat terminal conditions. The rival options were articulated by Charles Baron, a professor of law who favors legal oversight, and Arnold Relman, now editor of *The New England Journal of Medicine,* who recoils from the intrusiveness of the court. Buchanan suggests ethics committees as a way of getting the best of both sides. He does not explore well enough the shortcomings of these committees, but represents the public policy dilemmas very well.

Childress, James F. *Who Should Decide?* Oxford, England: Oxford University Press, 1982. This detailed analysis of paternalism and the issues surrounding it is very well written and well thought out. Many kinds of paternalism are distinguished. Paternalism of most sorts requires both minimizing harm to the patient and that the patient be mentally incapable of deciding. Cases are provided and referred to as the argument develops.

Clements, Colleen D. "Bioethical Essentialism and Scientific Population Thinking," *Perspectives in Biology and Medicine* 28 (Winter 1985): 188–207. This essay offers a powerful critique of attempts to devise a formal moral theory. The critique is based on the idea that just as science gave up ideal types and began to build its study on populations and variations, so too ethics should do the same. Clements does not even sketch how the scientific paradigm should be applied to ethics. Nevertheless, I believe I have used her view in writing this chapter, especially in stressing the role of the concept of *self* over any other notion of the patient. Perhaps her view could be furthered by combining my approach and that of Jonsen, Siegler, and Winslade, which is discussed below.

Clouser, K. Danner. "The Sanctity of Life: An Analysis of a Concept." *Annals of Internal Medicine* 78 (January 1973): 119–25.

Englehardt, H. T., Jr. *The Foundations of Bioethics,* 2d ed. New York: Oxford University Press, 1996. This is an exploration of the fundamental concepts and principles in bioethics. Englehardt is a thoroughgoing deontologist. He grants government very little authority in medical matters, and holds that competency establishes very strong rights. The book is very scholarly. The author holds both an M.D. and Ph.D. in philosophy.

Englehardt, H. T., Jr., and Edmund L. Erde. "Philosophy of Medicine." In *A Guide to the Culture of Science, Technology, and Medicine,* edited by Paul T. Durbin, 2 vols. New York: The Free Press, 1982, 1984. This is a comprehensive review of both medical ethics and philosophical issues in medicine, such as the analyses of concepts of health and disease. The volume in which the cited chapter is contained provides a survey of the issues and literature in the history, sociology, and philosophy of science, technology, and health care. Extensive bibliographies accompany each chapter.

Jonsen, Albert, Mark Siegler, and William J. Winslade. *Clinical Ethics,* 2d ed. New York: Macmillan, 1986. This has been referred to as a "Merck Manual" for ethics. The authors are highly accomplished writers on ethics who are trained in philosophy, theological ethics, medicine, and law. They categorize medical conditions according to how the condition should direct moral thinking. Chronic conditions allow patients time to think, adjust, etc.; acute onset serious diseases or injuries may require more impulsive decisions. The method they offer adjusts to kinds of medical conditions.

McCullough, Laurence B. "Methodological Concerns in Bioethics." *Journal of Medicine and Philosophy* 11 (February 1986): 17–39. This is a very keen overview of the issues concerning theories or methodologies that could give rise to methods, public policies, and medical education.

The President's Commission for the Study of Ethical Problems in Medicine and Biomedical and Behavioral Research produced several volumes in its series of reports and appendixes that are relevant to this chapter. They are major public policy statements. One volume is *Deciding to Forgo Life-Sustaining Treatment. Making Health Care Decisions* is a set of volumes. Volume 1 is the *Report*; volumes 2 and 3 include studies (e.g., on informed consent and on medical education) commissioned for preparing the report and materials submitted to the Commission. Readers should remember that the *Report* is the product of a political process.

Shelp, Earl E. *Virtue and Medicine: Explorations in the Character of Medicine.* Dordrecht, Holland: D. Reidel, 1985.

Veatch, Robert M. *A Theory of Medical Ethics.* New York: Basic Books, 1981. The author gives compelling arguments for why professions may not develop their own ethics independent of those whom they serve. He attempts to provide a three-way contrast among practitioners, patients, and society to justify governmental intervention into the doctor-patient relationship when, for example, doctors learn of dangers to third parties. This book is a classic, but see the critique by John Kultgen, "Veatch's New Foundation for Medical Ethics," *Journal of Medicine and Philosophy* 10 (November 1985): 339–69.

White, W. D. "Informed Consent: Ambiguity in Theory and Practice," *Journal of Health Politics, Policy and Law* 8 (Spring 1983): 99–119. This is one of the best criticisms of the legal doctrine of informed consent.

CHAPTER 50

Getting Down to Cases: The Revival of Casuistry in Bioethics

John D. Arras

THE REVIVAL OF CASUISTRY

Developed in the early Middle Ages as a method of bringing abstract and universal ethico-religious precepts to bear on particular moral situations, casuistry has had a checkered history.[1] In the hands of expert practitioners during its salad days in the sixteenth and seventeenth centuries, casuistry generated a rich and morally sensitive literature devoted to numerous real-life ethical problems, such as truth telling, usury, and the limits of revenge. By the late seventeenth century, however, casuistical reasoning had degenerated into a notoriously sordid form of logic chopping in the service of personal expediency.[2] To this day, the very term *casuistry* conjures up pejorative images of disingenuous argument and moral laxity.

In spite of its tarnished reputation, some philosophers have claimed that casuistry, shorn of its unfortunate excesses, has much to teach us about the resolution of moral problems in medicine. Indeed, through the work of Albert Jonsen[3] and Stephen Toulmin,[4] this "new casuistry" has emerged as a definite alternative to the hegemony of the so-called "applied ethics" method of moral analysis that has dominated most bioethical scholarship and teaching since the early 1970s.[5] In stark contrast to methods that begin from "on high" with the working out of a moral theory and culminate in the deductivistic application of norms to particular factual situations, this new casuistry works from the "bottom up," emphasizing practical problem solving by means of nuanced interpretations of individual cases.

This chapter will assess the promise of this reborn casuistry for bioethics education. In order to do that, however, it will be necessary to say quite a bit in general about the nature of this form of moral analysis and its strengths and weaknesses as a method of practical thinking. Indeed, a general catalogue of the promise and potential pitfalls of the casuistical method should be directly applicable to the assessment of casuistry in educational settings.

Before we can exhibit the salient features of this rival bioethical methodology, we must first confront an initial ambiguity in the definition of casuistry. As Jonsen describes it, "casuistry" is the art or skill of applying abstract or general principles to particular cases.[6] In this context, Jonsen notes that the major monotheistic religions were likely sources for casuistic ethics, since they all combined a strong sense of duty

---

Source: Reprinted with permission from J. D. Arras, Getting Down to Cases: The Revival of Casuistry in Bioethics, *The Journal of Medicine and Philosophy*, Vol. 16, No. 1, pp. 29–51, © 1991, with kind permission of Kluwer Academic Publishers.

This article is based upon a presentation at a conference on "Bioethics as an Intellectual Field," sponsored by the University of Texas Medical Branch, Galveston, Texas. The author would like to thank Ronald Carson and Thomas Murray for their encouragement.

with a definite set of moral precepts couched in universal terms. The preeminent task for devout Christians, Jews, and Muslims was thus to learn how to apply these universal precepts to particular situations, where their stringency or applicability might well be affected by particular factual conditions.

Defined as the art of applying abstract principles to particular cases, the new casuistry could appropriately be viewed, not so much as a rival to the applied ethics model, but rather as a necessary complement to any and all moral theories that would guide our conduct in specific situations. So long as we take some general principles or maxims to be ethically binding, no matter what their source, we must learn through the casuist's art to fit them to particular cases. But on this gloss of "casuistry," even the most hidebound adherent of the applied ethics model, someone who held that answers to particular moral dilemmas can be deduced from universal theories and principles, would have to count as a casuist. So defined, casuistry might appear to be little more than the handmaiden of applied ethics.

There is, however, another interpretation of casuistry in the writings of Jonsen and Toulmin that provides a distinct alternative to the applied ethics model. Instead of focusing on the need to fit principles to cases, this interpretation stresses the particular nature, derivation, and function of the principles manipulated by the new casuists. Through this alternative theory of principles, we begin to discern a morality that develops, not from the top down, as in most interpretations of Roman law, but rather from case to case (or from the bottom up), as in the common law. What differentiates the new casuistry from applied ethics, then, is not the mere recognition that principles must eventually be applied, but rather a particular account of the logic and derivation of the principles that we deploy in moral discourse.

A "CASE-DRIVEN" METHOD

Contrary to "theory-driven" methodologies, which approach particular situations already equipped with a full complement of moral principles, the new casuistry insists that our moral knowledge must develop incrementally through the analysis of concrete cases. From this perspective, the very notion of "applied ethics" embodies a redundancy, while the correlative notion of "theoretical ethics" conveys an illusory and counterproductive ideal for ethical thought.

If ethics is done properly, the new casuists imply, it will already have been immersed in concrete cases from the very start. To be sure, one can always apply the results of previous ethical inquiries to fresh problems, but to the casuists good ethics is always "applied" in the sense that it grows out of the analysis of individual cases. It's not as though one could or should first develop a pristine ethical theory planing above the world of moral particulars and then, having put the finishing touches on the theory, point it in the direction of particular cases. Rejecting the idea that there are such things as "essences" in the domain of ethics, Toulmin,[7] citing Aristotle and Dewey, argues that this pursuit of rigorous theory is unhinged from the realities of the moral life and animated by an illusory quest for moral certainty. Thus, whereas many academic philosophers scorn "applied ethics" as a pale shadow of the real thing (i.e., ethical theory), the new casuists insist that good ethics is always immersed in the messy reality of cases and that the philosophers' penchant for abstract and rigorous theory is a misleading fetish.

According to both Jonsen and Toulmin, the work of the National Commission for the Protection of Human Subjects of Biomedical and Behavioral Research provides an excellent example of this case-driven method in bioethics.[8] Although the various commissioners represented different academic, religious, and philosophical perspectives, Jonsen and Toulmin (who served, respectively, as commissioner and consultant to the commission) attest that the commissioners could still reach consensus by discussing the issues "taxonomically." Bracketing their differences on "matters of principle," the commissioners would begin with an analysis of paradigmatic cases of harm, cruelty, fairness, and generosity and then branch out to more complex and difficult cases posed by biomedical research. The commissioners thus "triangulate[d] their way across the complex terrain of moral life,"[9] gradually extending their analysis of relatively straightforward problems to issues requiring a much more delicate balancing of competing values.

Thus, instead of looking for ethical progress in the theoretical equivalent of the Second Coming—i.e., the establishment of *the* correct ethical theory—Jonsen and Toulmin contend that a more realistic and attainable notion of progress is afforded by this notion of moral "triangulation," an incremental approach to problems whose model can be found in the history of our common law. Just as English-speaking peoples have developed highly complex and sophisticated legal frameworks for thinking about tort liability and criminal guilt without the benefit of preestablished legal principles, so (Jonsen and Toulmin argue) ought we to develop a "common morality" or "morisprudence" on the basis of case analysis—without recourse to some preestablished moral theory or moral principles.

THE ROLE OF PRINCIPLES IN THE NEW CASUISTRY

Contrary to common interpretations of Roman law and to deductivist ethical theories, wherein principles are said to preexist the actual cases to which they apply, the new casuistry contends that ethical principles are "discovered" in the cases themselves, just as common law legal principles are developed in and through judicial decisions on particular legal cases.[10] To be sure, common law and "common law morality" (or "morisprudence") contain a body of principles too, but the way these principles are derived, articulated, used, and taught is very different from the Roman law and deductivist ethical approach.[11]

The Derivation and Meaning of Principles

Jonsen and Toulmin have sent mixed messages regarding their views of the derivation of moral maxims and principles. In some places they appear to incline toward a weaker interpretation of casuistry as the art of applying whatever moral maxims happen to be lying around at hand in one's culture. At other places, however, Jonsen and Toulmin suggest a much stronger and more controversial view, according to which moral principles of "common law morality" are entirely derived from (or abstracted out of) particular cases. Rather than stemming originally from some ethical theory, such as utilitarianism or Rawls's theory of justice, these principles are said to emerge gradually from reflection upon our responses to particular cases.

Whichever view of the derivation of principles modern casuistry ultimately embraces, both are fully compatible with the casuistical thesis that the full articulation of those principles cannot be determined in isolation from particular factual contexts. In order to fully understand any principle or maxim, one has to ask, through a process of interpretation, how it might apply to a variety of situations. Thus, whereas "privacy" might simply mean an undifferentiated interest in "liberty" to a theorist unfamiliar with the cases, to the casuist the meaning and scope of personal privacy is delimited and shaped by the features of the cases that have called for a public response. Thus, whether or not consensual sodomy is protected by a moral right of privacy will depend upon how the casuist interprets the features of previous controversial cases dealing with such issues as family life, contraception, and abortion.

The Priority of Practice

In the applied ethics model, principles not only "come before" our practices in the sense of being antecedently derived from theory before being applied to cases, they also have priority over practices in the sense that their function is to justify (or criticize) practices. Indeed, it is precisely through this logical priority of principles over practice that the applied ethics model derives its critical edge. It is just the reverse for the new casuists, who sometimes imply that ethical principles are nothing more than mere *summaries* of meanings already embedded in our actual practices.[12] Rather than serving as a justification for certain practices, principles within the new casuistry often merely seem to *report* in summary fashion what we have already decided.

This logical priority of practice to principles is clearly evident in Jonsen's and Toulmin's ruminations on the experience of the National Commission for the Protection of Human Subjects. In attempting to carry out the mandate of Congress to develop principles for the ethical conduct of research on humans, the commissioners could have straightforwardly drafted a set of principles and then applied them to problematic cases. Instead, note Jonsen and Toulmin, the commissioners acted like good casuists, plunging immediately into nuanced discussions of cases. Progress in these discussions was achieved, not by applying agreed-upon principles, but rather by seeking agreement on responses to particular cases. Indeed, according to this account, the *Belmont Report*, which articulated the commission's moral principles and serves to this day as a major source of the "applied ethics" approach to moral reasoning, was written at the end of the commission's deliberations, long after its members had already reached consensus on the issues.[13]

The Open Texture of Principles

In contrast to the deductivist method, whose principles glide unsullied over the facts, the principles of the new casuistry are always subject to further revision and articulation in light of new cases. This is true not only because casuistical principles are inextricably enmeshed in their factual surroundings, but also because the determination of the decisive or morally relevant features of this factual web is often a highly uncertain and controversial business.

By way of example, consider the question of withdrawing artificial feeding as presented in the case of Claire Conroy.[14] One of the crucial precedents for this case, both legally and morally, was the *Quinlan* decision.[15] What were the morally relevant features of Karen Quinlan's situation, and what might they teach us about our responsibilities to Claire Conroy? Was it crucial that Ms. Quinlan was described as being in a persistent vegetative state? Or that she was being maintained by a mechanical respirator? If so, then one might well conclude that Claire Conroy's situation—i.e., that of a patient with severe dementia being maintained by a plastic, nasogastric feeding tube—is sufficiently disanalogous to Quinlan's to compel continued treatment. On the other hand, a rereading of *Quinlan* might reveal other features of that case that tell in favor of withdrawing Conroy's feeding tube, such as the unlikelihood of Karen ever recovering sapient life, the bleakness of her prognosis, and the questionable proportion of benefits to burdens derived from the treatment.

Although the *Quinlan* case may have begun by standing for the patient's right to refuse treatment, subsequent readings of that case in light of later cases have fastened on other aspects of the case, thereby giving rise to modifications of the original principle, or perhaps even to the wholesale substitution of new principles for the old. The principles of casuistic analysis might thus be said to exhibit an "open texture."[16] Somewhat in the manner of Thomas Kuhn's "paradigms" of scientific research,[17] each significant case in bioethics stands as an object for further articulation and specification under new or more complex conditions. Viewed this way, casuistical analysis might be summarized as a form of reasoning by means of examples that always point beyond themselves. Both the examples and the principles derived from them are always subject to reinterpretation and gradual modification in light of subsequent examples.

Teaching and Learning

In contrast to legal systems derived from Roman law, where jurors are governed by a systematic legal code, common-law systems derive from the particular judicial decisions of particular judges. As a result of these radically differing approaches to the nature and derivation of law, common law and Roman law are taught and learned in correspondingly different ways. Students of Roman law need only refer to the code itself, and perhaps to the scholarly literature explicating the meaning of the code's various provisions, whereas students of common law must refer directly to prior judicial opinions. Consequently, the so-called "case method" of legal study is naturally suited to common-law jurisdictions, for it is only through a study of the cases that one can learn the concrete meaning of legal principles and learn to apply them correctly to future cases.[18]

What is true of the common law is equally true of "common-law morality." According to the casuists, bioethical principles are best learned by the case method, not by appeals to abstract theoretical notions. Indeed, anyone at all experienced in teaching bioethics in clinical settings must know (often by means of painful experience) that physicians, nurses, and other health care providers learn best by means of case discussions. (The best way to put them to sleep, in fact, is to begin one's talk with a recitation of the "principles of bioethics.") This is explained not simply by the fact that case presentations are intrinsically more gripping than abstract discussions of the moral philosophies of Mill, Kant, and Rawls; they are, in addition, the best vehicle for conveying the concrete meaning and scope of whatever principles and maxims one wishes to teach. Contrary to ethical deductivism and Roman law, whose principles could conceivably be taught in a practical vacuum, casuistry demands a case-driven method of instruction. For casuists, cases are much more than mere illustrated rules or handy mnemonic devices for the "abstracting impaired." They are, as Jonsen and Toulmin argue, the very locus of moral meaning and moral certainty.

Although Jonsen and Toulmin have yet to consider the concrete pedagogical implications of their casuistical method, we can venture a few suggestions. First, it would appear that a casuistical approach would encourage the use, whenever possible, of real as opposed to hypothetical cases. This is because hypothetical cases, so beloved of academic philosophers, tend to be theory driven; that is, they are usually designed to advance some explicitly theoretical point. Real cases, on the other hand, are more likely to display the sort of moral complexity and untidiness that demand the (nondeductive) weighing and balancing of competing moral considerations and the casuistical virtues of discernment and practical judgment (*phronesis*).

Second, a casuistical pedagogy would call for lengthy and richly detailed case studies. If the purpose of moral education is to prepare one for action in the real world, the cases discussed should reflect the degree of complexity, uncertainty, and ambiguity encountered there. If for casuistry moral truth resides "in the details," if the meaning and scope of moral principles is determined contextually through an interpretation of factual situations in their relationship to paradigm cases, then cases must be presented in rich detail. It won't do, as is so often done in our textbooks and anthologies, to cram the rich moral fabric of cases into a couple of paragraphs.

Third, a casuistical pedagogy would encourage the use, not simply of the occasional isolated case study, but rather of whole sequences of cases bearing on a related principle or theme. Thus, instead of simply "illustrating" the debate over the termination of life-sustaining treatments with, say, the single case of Karen Quinlan, teachers and students should read and interpret a sequence of cases (including, e.g., the cases of Quinlan, Saikewicz, Spring, Conroy, and Cruzan) in order to see just how reasoning by paradigm and analogy takes place and how the so-called "principles of bioethics" are actually shaped in their effective meaning by the details of successive cases.

Fourth, a casuistically driven pedagogy will give much more emphasis than currently allotted to what might be called the problem of "moral diagnosis." Given any particular controversy, exactly what kind of issues does it raise? What, in other words, is the case really about? As opposed to the anthologies, where each case comes neatly labelled under a discrete rubric, real life does not announce the nature of problems in advance. It requires interpretation, imagination, and discernment to figure out what is going on, especially when (as is usually the case) a number of discussable issues are usually extractable from any given controversy.

PROBLEMS WITH THE CASUISTICAL METHOD

Since the new casuistry attempts to define itself by turning applied ethics on its head, working from cases to principles rather than vice versa, it should come as no surprise to find that its strengths correlate perfectly with the weaknesses of applied ethics. Thus, whereas applied ethics, and especially deductivism, are often criticized for their remoteness from clinical realities and for their consequent irrelevance,[19] casuistry prides itself on its concreteness and on its ability to render useful advice to caregivers in the medical trenches. Likewise, if the applied ethics model appears rather narrow in its single-minded emphasis on the application of principles and in its corresponding neglect of moral interpretation and practical discernment, the new casuistry can be viewed as a defense of the Aristotelian virtue of *phronesis* (or sound practice judgment).

Conversely, it should not be surprising to find certain problems with the casuistical method that correspond to strengths of the applied ethics model. I shall devote the second half of this essay to an inventory of some of these problems. It should be stressed, however, that not all of these problems are unique to casuistry, nor does applied ethics fare much better with regard to some of them.

What Is "a Case"?

For all of their emphasis upon the interpretation of particular cases, casuists have not said much, if anything, about how to select problems for moral interpretation. What, in other words, gets placed on the "moral agenda" in the first place, and why? This is a problem because it is quite possible that the current method of selecting agenda items, whatever that may be, systematically ignores genuine issues equally worthy of discussion and debate.[20]

I think it safe to say that problems currently make it onto the bioethical agenda largely because health practitioners and policy makers put them there. While there is usually nothing problematic in this, and while it always pays to be scrupulously attentive to the expressed concerns of people working in the trenches, practitioners may be bound to conventional ways of thinking and of conceiving problems that tend to filter out other, equally valid experiences and problems. As feminists have recently argued, for example, much of the current bioethics agenda reflects an excessively narrow, professionally driven, and male outlook on the nature of ethics.[21] As a result, a whole range of important ethical problems—including the unequal treatment of women in health care settings, sexist occupational roles, personal relationships, and strategies of *avoiding* crisis situations—have been either downplayed or ignored completely.[22] It is not enough, then, for casuistry to tell us *how* to interpret cases; rather than simply carrying out the agenda dictated by health professionals, all of us (casuists and ethicists alike) must begin to think more about the problem of *which* cases ought to be selected for moral scrutiny.

An additional problem, which I can only flag here, concerns not the identification of "a case"—i.e., what gets placed on the public agenda—but rather the specification of "the case"—i.e., what description of a case shall count as an adequate and sufficiently complete account of the issues, the participants, and the context. One of the problems with many case presentations, especially in the clinical context, is their relative neglect of alternative perspectives on the case held by other participants. Quite often, we get the attending's (or the house officer's) point of view on what constitutes "the case" while missing out on the perspectives of nurses, social workers, and others. Since most cases are complicated and enriched by such alternative medical, psychological, and social interpretations, our casuistical analyses will remain incomplete without them. Thus, in addition to being long, the cases that we employ should reflect the usually complementary (but often conflicting) perspectives of all the involved participants.

Is Casuistry Really Theory Free?

The casuists claim that they make moral progress by moving from one class of cases to another without the benefit of any ethical principles or theoretical apparatus. Solutions generated for obvious or easy categories of cases adumbrate solutions for the more difficult cases. In a manner somewhat reminiscent of pre-Kuhnian philosophers of science clinging to the possibility of "theory free" factual observations, to a belief in a kind of epistemological "immaculate perception," the casuists appear to be claiming that the cases simply speak for themselves.

As we have seen, one problem with this suggestion is that it does not acknowledge or account for the way in which different theoretical preconceptions help determine which cases and problems get selected for study in the first place. Another problem is that it does not explain what allows us to group different cases into distinct categories or to proceed from one category to another. In other words, the casuists' account of case analysis fails to supply us with principles of relevance that explain what binds the cases together and how the meaning of one case points beyond itself toward the resolution of subsequent cases. The casuists obviously cannot do without such principles of relevance; they are a necessary condition of any kind of moral taxonomy. Without principles of relevance, the cases would fly apart in all directions, rendering coherent speech, thought, and action about them impossible.

But if the casuists rise to this challenge and convert their implicit principles of relevance into explicit principles, it is certainly reasonable to expect that these will be heavily "theory laden." Take, for example, the novel suggestion that anencephalic infants should be used as organ donors for children born with fatal heart defects. What is the relevant line of cases in our developed "morisprudence" for analyzing this problem? To the proponents of this suggestion, the brain death debates provide the appropriate context of discussion. According to this line of argument, anencephalic infants most closely resemble the brain dead; and since we already harvest vital organs from the latter category, we have a moral warrant for harvesting organs from anencephalics.[23] But to some of those opposed to any change in the status quo, the most relevant line of cases is provided by the literature on fetal experimentation. Our treatment of the anencephalic newborn should, they claim, reflect our practices regarding nonviable fetuses. If we agree with the judgment of the National Commission that research that would shorten the already doomed child's life should not be permitted, then we should oppose the use of equally doomed anencephalic infants as heart donors.[24]

How ought the casuist to triangulate the moral problem of the anencephalic newborn as organ donor? What principles of relevance will lead him or her to opt for one line of cases instead of another? Whatever principles he or she might eventually articulate, they will undoubtedly have something definite to say about such matters as the concept of death, the moral status of fetuses, the meaning and scope of respect, the nature of personhood, and the relative importance of achieving good consequences in the world versus treating other human beings as ends in themselves. Although one's position on such issues perhaps need not implicate any full-blown ethical theory in the strictest sense of the term, they are sufficiently theory laden to cast grave doubt on the new casuists' ability to move from case to case without recourse to mediating ethical principles or other theoretical notions.

Although the early work of Jonsen and Toulmin can easily be read as advocating a theory-free methodology composed of mere "summary principles," their recent work appears to acknowledge the point of the above criticism. Indeed, it would be fair to say that they now seek to articulate a method that is, if not "theory free," then at least "theory modest." Drawing on the approach of the classical casuists, they now concede an indisputably normative role for principles and maxims drawn from a variety of sources, including theology, common law, historical tradition, and ethical theories. Rather than viewing ethical theories as mutually exclusive, reductionistic attempts to provide an apodictic *foundation* for ethical thought, Jonsen and Toulmin now view theories as limited and complementary *perspectives* that might enrich a more pragmatic and pluralistic approach to the ethical life.[25] They thus appear reconciled to the usefulness, both in research and education, of a severely chastened concept of moral principles and theories.

One lesson of all this for bioethics education is that casuistry, for all its usefulness as a method, is nothing more (and nothing less) than an "engine of thought" that must receive *direction* from values, concepts, and theories outside of itself. Given the important role such "external" sources of moral direction must play even in the most casebound approaches, teachers and students need to be self-conscious about which traditions and theories are in effect driving their casuistical interpretations. This means that they need to devote time and energy to studying and criticizing the values, concepts, and rank orderings implicitly or explicitly conveyed by the various traditions and theories from which they derive their overall direction and tools of moral analysis. In short, it means that adopting the casuistical method will not absolve teachers and students from studying and evaluating either ethical theories or the history of ethics.

Indeterminacy and Consensus

One need not believe in the existence of uniquely correct answers to all moral questions to be concerned about the casuistical method's capacity to yield determinate answers to problematical moral questions. Indeed, anyone familiar with Alastair MacIntyre's disturbing diagnosis of our contemporary moral culture[26] might well tend to greet the casuists' announcement of moral consensus with a good deal of skepticism. According to MacIntyre, our moral culture is in a grave state of disorder: Lacking any comprehensive and coherent understanding of morality and human nature, we subsist on scattered shards and remnants of past moral frameworks. It is no wonder, then, according to MacIntyre, that our moral debates and disagreements are often marked by the clash of incommensurable premises derived from disparate moral cultures. Nor is it any wonder that our debates over highly controversial issues such as abortion and affirmative action take the form of a tedious, interminable cycle of assertion and counterassertion. In this disordered and contentious moral setting, which MacIntyre claims is *our* moral predicament, the casuists' goal of consensus based upon intuitive responses to cases might well appear to be a Panglossian dream.

One need not endorse MacIntyre's pessimistic diagnosis in its entirety to notice that many of our moral practices and policies bear a multiplicity of meanings; they often embody a variety of different, and sometimes conflicting, values. An ethical methodology based exclusively on the casuistical analysis of these practices can reasonably be expected to express these different values in the form of conflicting ethical conclusions.

Political theorist Michael Walzer's remarks on health care in the United States provide an illuminating case in point. Although Walzer might not recognize himself as a modern day casuist, his vigorous antitheoretical stance and reliance upon established social meanings and norms certainly make him an ally of the methodological approach espoused by Jonsen and Toulmin.[27] According to Walzer, if we look carefully at our current values and practices regarding health care and its distribution—if we look, in other words, at the choices we as a people have already made, at the programs we have already put into place, etc.—we will conclude that health care services are a crucially important social good, that they should be allocated solely on the basis of need, and that they must be made equally available to all citizens, presumably through something like a national health service.[28]

One could argue, however, that current disparities—both in access to care and in quality of care—among the poor, the middle class, and the rich reflect equally "deep" (or even deeper) political choices that we have made regarding the relative importance of individual freedom, social security, and the health needs of the "nondeserving" poor. In this vein, one could claim that our collective decisions bearing on Medicaid, Medicare, and access to emergency rooms—the same decisions that Walzer uses to argue for a national health service—are more accurately interpreted as grudging aberrations from our free market ideology. According to this opposing view, our stratified health care system pretty well reflects our values and commitments in this area: a "decent minimum" (read "understaffed, ill-equipped, impersonal urban clinics") for the medically indigent, decent health insurance and health maintenance organizations (HMOs) for the working middle-class, and first-cabin care for the well-to-do.[29]

Viewed in the light of Walzer's democratic socialist commitments, which I happen to share, this arrangement may indeed look like an "indefensible triage," but placed in the context of American history and culture, it could just as easily be viewed as business as usual. Thus, on one reading our current practices point toward the establishment of a thoroughly egalitarian health care system; viewed from a different angle, however, these same "choices we have already made" justify pervasive inequalities in access to care and quality of care. The problem for the casuistical method is that, barring any and all appeals to abstract principles of justice, it cannot decisively adjudicate between such competing interpretations of our common practices.[30] When these do not convey a univocal message, or when they carry conflicting messages of more or less equal plausibility, casuistry cannot help us to develop a uniquely correct interpretation upon which a widespread social consensus might be based. Contrary to the assurances of Jonsen and Toulmin, the new casuistry is an unlikely instrument for generating consensus in a moral world fractured by conflicting values and intuitions.

In Jonsen and Toulmin's defense, it should be noted that abstract theories of justice divorced from the conventions of our society are equally unlikely sources of uniquely correct answers. If philosophers cannot agree among themselves upon the true nature of abstract justice—indeed, if criticizing our foremost theoretician of justice, John Rawls, has become something of a philosophical national pastime[31]—it is unclear how their theorizing could decisively resolve the ongoing debate among competing interpretations of our common social practices.

It might also be noted in passing that even Rawls has become increasingly loath in his recent writings to appeal to an abstract, timeless, and deracinated notion of justice as the ultimate court of appeal from conflicting social interpretations. Eschewing any pretense of having established a theory of justice "sub specie aeternitatis," Rawls now claims that his theory of "justice as fairness" is only applicable in modern democracies like our own.[32] He claims, moreover, that the justification of his theory is derived, not from neutral data, but from its "congruence with our deeper understanding of ourselves and our aspirations, and our realization that, given our history and the traditions embedded in our public life, it is the most reasonable doctrine for us."[33] Notwithstanding the many differences that distinguish their respective views, it thus appears that Rawls, Walzer, and Jonsen and Toulmin could all agree that there is no escape from the task of interpreting the meanings embedded in our social practices, institutions, and history. Given the complexity and tensions that characterize this moral "data," the search for uniquely correct interpretations must be seen as misguided. The best we can do, it seems, is to argue for our own determinate but contestable interpretations of who we are as a people and who we want to become. Neither theory nor casuistry is a guarantor of consensus.

Conventionalism and Critique

The stronger, more controversial version of casuistry and its "summary view" of ethical principles gives rise to worries about the nature of moral truth and justification. Eschewing any theoretical derivation of principles and insisting that the locus of moral certainty is the particular, the casuist asks, "What principles best organize and account for what we have already decided?" Viewed from this angle, the casuistic project amounts to nothing more than an elaborate refinement of our intuitions regarding cases. As such, it begins to resemble the kind of relativistic conventionalism recently articulated by Richard Rorty.[34]

Obviously, one problem with this is that our intuitions have often been shown to be wildly wrong, if not downright prejudicial and superstitious. To the extent that this is true of *our own* intuitions about ethical matters, then casuistry will merely refine our prejudices. Any casuistry that modestly restricts itself to interpreting and cataloguing the flickering shadows on the cave wall can easily be accused of lacking a critical edge. If applied ethics might rightly be said to have purchased critical leverage at the expense of the concrete moral situation, then casuistry might be charged with having purchased concreteness and relevance at the expense of philosophical criticism. This charge might take either of two forms. First, one could claim that the casuist is a mere expositor of *established* social meanings and thus lacks the requisite critical distance to formulate telling critiques of regnant social understandings. Second, casuistry could be accused of ignoring the power relations that shape and inform the social meanings that its practitioners interpret.

In response to the issue of critical distance, Jonsen and Toulmin could point out that the social world of established meanings is by no means monolithic and usually harbors alternative values that offer plenty of critical leverage against the regnant social consensus. As Michael Walzer has recently argued, even such thundering social critics as the prophet Amos have usually been fully committed to their societies rather than "objective" and detached, and the values to which they appeal are often fundamental to the self-understanding of a people or group.[35] (How else could they accuse their fellows of hypocrisy?) The lesson for casuists here is not to become so identified with the point of view of health care professionals that they lose sight of other important values in our culture.

The second claim, while not necessarily fatal to the casuistical enterprise, is harder to rebut. As Habermas has contended in his longstanding debate with Gadamer, interpretive approaches to ethics (such as casuistry) can articulate our shared social meanings but ignore the economic and power relations that shape social consensus. His point is that the very conversation through which cases, social practices, and institutions are interpreted is itself subject to what he calls "systematically distorted communication."[36] In order to avoid merely legitimizing social understandings conditioned on power and domination—for example, our concept of the appropriate relationship between nurses and physicians—casuistry will have to supplement its interpretations with a critical theory of social relationships, or with what Paul Ricoeur has called a "hermeneutics of suspicion."[37]

Reinforcing the Individualism of Bioethics

Analytical philosophers working as applied ethicists have often been criticized for the ahistorical, reductionist, and excessively individualistic character of their work in bioethics.[38] While the casuistical method cannot thus be justly accused of importing a shortsighted individualism into the field of bioethics—that honor already belonging to analytical philosophy—it cannot be said either that casuistry offers anything like a promising remedy for this deficiency. On the contrary, it seems that the casuists' method of reasoning by analogy only promises to exacerbate the individualism and reductionism already characteristic of much bioethical scholarship.

Consider, for example, how a casuist might address the problem of heart transplants. He or she might reason like this: Our society is already deeply committed to paying for all kinds of "halfway technologies" for those in need. We already pay for renal dialysis and transplantation, chronic ventilatory support for children and adults, expensive open-heart surgery, and many other "high-tech" therapies, some of which might well be even more expensive than heart transplants. Therefore, so long as heart transplants qualify medically as a proven therapy, there is no reason why Medicaid and Medicare should not fund them.[39]

Notwithstanding the evident fruitfulness of such analogical reasoning in many contexts of bioethics, and notwithstanding the possibility that these particular examples of it might well prevail against the competing arguments on heart transplantation, it remains true that such contested practices raise troubling questions that tend not to be asked, let alone illuminated, by casuistical reasoning by analogy. The extent of our willingness to fund heart transplantation has great bearing on the kind of society in which we wish to live and on our priorities for spending within (and without) the health care budget. Even if we already fund many high-technology procedures that cost as much or more than heart transplants, it is possible that this new round of transplantation could threaten other forms of care that provide greater benefits to more people, and we might therefore wish to draw the line here.[40]

The point is that, no matter where we stand on the particular issue of heart transplants, we *might* think it important to raise such "big questions," depending on the nature of the problem at hand. We might want to ask, to borrow from a recent title, "What kind of life?"[41] But the kind of reasoning by analogy championed by the new casuists tends to reduce our field of ethical vision down to the proximate moral precedents and thereby suppresses the important global questions bearing on who we are and what kind of society we want. The result is likely to be a method of moral reasoning that graciously accommodates us to any and all technological innovations, no matter what their potential long-term threat to fundamental and cherished institutions and values.

CONCLUSION

The revival of casuistry, both in practice and in Jonsen and Toulmin's recent defense,[42] is a welcome development in the field of bioethics. Its account of moral reasoning (emphasizing the pivotal role of paradigms, analogical thinking, and the prudential weighing of competing factors) is far superior, both as a description of how we actually think and as a prescription of how we ought to think, to the tiresome invocation of the applied ethics mantra (i.e., the principles of respect for autonomy, beneficence, and justice). By insisting on a *modest* role for ethical theory in a pragmatic, nondeductivist approach to ethical interpretation, Jonsen and Toulmin join an important chorus of contemporary thinkers troubled by the reductionism inherent in most analytical ethics.[43]

As for its role in bioethics education, no one needs to tell teachers about the importance of cases in the classroom. It's pretty obvious that discussing cases is fun, interesting, and certainly more memorable than any philosophical theory, which for the average student usually has a half-life of about two weeks. Moreover, a casuistical education gives students the methodological tools they are most likely to need when they later encounter bioethical problems in the "real world," whether as health care professionals, clergy, lawyers, journalists, or informed citizens. For all of the obviousness of these points, however, it remains true that all of us, as teachers, could profit from sound advice on how better to use cases, and some such advice can be extrapolated from the work of Jonsen and Toulmin.

For all its virtues vis-à-vis the sclerotic invocation of "bioethical principles," the casuistical method is not, however, without problems of its own. First, we found that the very principles of relevance that drive the casuistical method need to be made explicit, and we surmised that, once unveiled, these principles will turn out to be heavily theory laden. Second, we showed that the casuistical method is an unlikely source of uniquely correct interpretations of social meanings and therefore an unlikely source of societal consensus. Third, we have seen that, because of the casuists' view of ethical principles as mere summaries of our intuitive responses to paradigmatic cases, their method might suffer from ideological distortions and lack a critical edge. Moreover, relying so heavily on the perceptions and agenda of health care professionals, casuists might tend to ignore the existence of important issues that could be revealed by other theoretical perspectives, such as feminism. Finally, we saw that casuistry, focusing as it does on analogical resemblances, might tend to ignore certain difficult but inescapable "big questions" (e.g., "What kind of society do we want?") and thereby reinforce the individualistic tendencies already at work in contemporary bioethics.

It remains to be seen whether casuistry, as a program in practical ethics, will be able to marshal sufficient internal resources to respond to these criticisms. Whatever the outcome of that attempt, however, an equally promising approach might be to incorporate the insights and tools of casuistry into the methodological approach known as "reflective equilibrium."[44] According to this method, the casuistical interpretation of cases, on the one hand, and moral theories, principles, and maxims, on the other, exist in a symbiotic relationship. Our intuitions on cases will thus be guided, and perhaps criticized, by theory, while our theories and moral principles will themselves be shaped, and perhaps reformulated, by our responses to paradigmatic moral situations. Whether we attempt to flesh out this method of reflective equilibrium or further develop the casuistical program, it should be clear by now that the methodological issue between theory and cases is not a dichotomous "either/or" but rather an encompassing "both-and."

In closing, I gather together my various recommendations for the use of casuistry in bioethics education:

1. Use real cases rather than hypotheticals whenever possible.
2. Avoid schematic case presentations. Make them long, richly detailed, messy, and comprehensive. Make sure that the perspectives of all the major players (including nurses and social workers) are represented.
3. Present complex sequences of cases that sharpen students' analogical reasoning skills.
4. Engage students in the process of "moral diagnosis."
5. Be mindful of the limits of casuistical analysis. As a mere engine of moral argument, casuistry must be supplemented and guided by appeals to ethical theory, the history of ethics, and moral norms embedded in our traditions and social practices. It must also be supplemented by critical social analyses that unmask the power behind much social consensus and raise larger questions about the kind of society we want and the kind of people we want to be.

NOTES

1. A. R. Jonsen and S. Toulmin, *The Abuse of Casuistry* (Berkeley, Calif.: University of California Press, 1988).
2. B. Pascal, *Lettres Écrites à un Provincial*, ed. A. Adam (Paris: Flammarion, 1981).
3. A. R. Jonsen, "Can an Ethicist Be a Consultant?" in *Frontiers in Medical Ethics*, ed. V. Abernethy (Cambridge, Mass.: Ballinger, 1980); A. R. Jonsen, "Casuistry and Clinical Ethics," *Theoretical Medicine* 7 (1986): 65–74; A. R. Jonsen, "Casuistry," in *Westminster Dictionary of Christian Ethics*, edited by J. F. Childress and J. Macgvarrie (Philadelphia: Westminster Press, 1986), 78–80.
4. S. Toulmin, "The Tyranny of Principles," *Hastings Center Report* 11 (1981): 31–39; Jonsen and Toulmin, *The Abuse of Casuistry*.
5. T. L. Beauchamp and J. F. Childress, *Principles of Biomedical Ethics*, 3d ed. (New York: Oxford University Press, 1989).
6. Jonsen, "Casuistry."
7. Toulmin, "The Tyranny of Principles."
8. Jonsen and Toulmin, *The Abuse of Casuistry*, 16–19, 264, 305, 338.
9. Toulmin, "The Tyranny of Principles."
10. Jonsen, "Casuistry and Clinical Ethics."
11. H. Pitkin, *Wittgenstein and Justice* (Berkeley, Calif.: University of California Press, 1972).
12. Toulmin, "The Tyranny of Principles."
13. Jonsen, "Casuistry and Clinical Ethics," 71.

14. *Matter of Claire C. Conroy,* Supreme Court of New Jersey, 486 A.2d 1209 (1985).
15. *Matter of Quinlan,* Supreme Court of New Jersey, 355 A.2d 647 (1976).
16. H. L. A. Hart, *The Concept of Law* (Oxford, England: Oxford University Press, 1961), 120ff.
17. T. Kuhn, *The Structure of Scientific Revolutions*, 2d ed. (Chicago: University of Chicago Press, 1970).
18. E. W. Patterson, "The Case Method in American Legal Education: Its Origins and Objectives," *Journal of Legal Education* 4 (1951): 1–24.
19. R. C. Fox and J. P. Swazey, "Medical Morality Is Not Bioethics: Medical Ethics in China and the United States," *Perspectives in Biology and Medicine* 27 (1984): 336–60; C. Noble, "Ethics and Experts," *Hastings Center Report* 12 (1982): 7–9.
20. O. O'Neill, "How Can We Individuate Moral Problems?" in *Applied Ethics and Ethical Theory*, ed. D. M. Rosenthal and F. Shehadi (Salt Lake City, Utah: University of Utah Press, 1988), 84–99.
21. A. L. Carse, "The 'Voice of Care': Implications for Bioethics Education," *Journal of Philosophy and Medicine* 16 (1991): 5–28.
22. V. Warren, "Feminist Directions in Medical Ethics," *Hypatia* 4 (1989): 77–82.
23. M. R. Harrison, "The Anencephalic Newborn as Organ Donor" (Commentary), *Hastings Center Report* 16 (1986): 21–22.
24. G. Meilaender, "The Anencephalic Newborn as Organ Donor" (Commentary), *Hastings Center Report* 16 (1986): 22–23.
25. Jonsen and Toulmin, *The Abuse of Casuistry*, chap. 15.
26. A. MacIntyre, *After Virtue* (Notre Dame, Ind.: Notre Dame University Press, 1981).
27. M. Walzer, *Spheres of Justice* (New York: Basic Books, 1983); M. Walzer, *Interpretation and Social Criticism* (Cambridge, Mass.: Harvard University Press, 1987).
28. Walzer, *Spheres of Justice*, 86ff.
29. R. Dworkin, "*Spheres of Justice*: An Exchange," *New York Review of Books* 30, no. 12 (1983): 44; G. Warnke, "Social Interpretation and Political Theory: Walzer and His Critics," *Philosophical Forum* 21 (1989–1990): 204–206.
30. Dworkin, "*Spheres of Justice*: An Exchange."
31. N. Daniels, *Reading Rawls*, 2d ed. (Stanford, Calif.: Stanford University Press, 1989); R. J. Arneson, ed., "Symposium on Rawlsian Theory of Justice: Recent Developments," *Ethics* 99 (1989): 695–944.
32. J. Rawls, "Kantian Constructivism in Moral Theory: The Dewey Lectures, 1980," *Journal of Philosophy* 77 (1980): 518.
33. Ibid., 519; see also J. Rawls, "Justice as Fairness: Political Not Metaphysical," *Philosophy and Public Affairs* 14 (1985): 228.
34. R. Rorty, *Contingency, Irony, and Solidarity* (Cambridge, England: Cambridge University Press, 1989).
35. Walzer, *Interpretation and Social Criticism.*
36. J. Habermas, "The Hermeneutic Claim to Universality," in *Contemporary Hermeneutics*, ed. J. Bleicher (London: Routledge and Kegan Paul, 1980), 181–211.
37. P. Ricoeur, "Hermeneutics and the Critique of Ideology," in *Hermeneutics and Modern Philosophy*, ed. B. R. Wachterhauser (Albany, N.Y.: State University of New York Press, 1986), 300–339.
38. Fox and Swazey, "Medical Morality Is Not Bioethics"; Noble, "Ethics and Experts"; MacIntyre, *After Virtue.*
39. D. Overcast et al., "Technology Assessment, Public Policy and Transplantation," *Law, Medicine and Health Care* 13, no. 3 (1985): 106–11.
40. Report of the Massachusetts Task Force on Organ Transplantation (Massachusetts Task Force on Organ Transplantation, Boston 1984); G. Annas, "Regulating Heart and Liver Transplants in Massachusetts," *Law, Medicine and Health Care* 13, no. 1 (1985): 4–7.
41. D. Callahan, *What Kind of Life*? (New York: Simon and Schuster, 1990).
42. Jonsen and Toulmin, *The Abuse of Casuistry.*
43. B. Williams, *Ethics and the Limits of Philosophy* (Cambridge, Mass.: Harvard University Press, 1985); S. Hampshire, *Morality and Conflict* (Cambridge, Mass.: Harvard University Press, 1983); C. Taylor, "The Diversity of Goods," in *Utilitarianism and Beyond*, ed. A. Sen and B. Williams (Cambridge, England: Cambridge University Press, 1982), 129–44.
44. J. Rawls, *A Theory of Justice* (Cambridge, Mass.: Harvard University Press, 1971); N. Daniels, "Wide Reflective Equilibrium and Theory Acceptance in Ethics," *Journal of Philosophy* 76 (1979): 256–82.

Chapter 51

Literature and Medicine: Contributions to Clinical Practice

Rita Charon, Joanne Trautmann Banks, Julia Connelly, Anne Hunsaker Hawkins, Kathryn Montgomery Hunter, Anne Hudson Jones, Martha Montello, and Suzanne Poirier

Introduced to United States medical schools in 1972, the field of literature and medicine contributes methods and texts that help physicians develop skills in the human dimensions of medical practice. Five broad goals are met by including the study of literature in medical education: (1) literary accounts of illness can teach physicians concrete and powerful lessons about the lives of sick people; (2) great works of fiction about medicine enable physicians to recognize the power and implications of what they do; (3) through the study of narrative, the physician can better understand patients' stories of sickness and his or her personal stake in medical practice; (4) literary study contributes to physicians' expertise in narrative ethics; and (5) literary theory offers new perspectives on the work and the genres of medicine. Particular texts and methods have been found to be well suited to the fulfillment of each of these goals. Chosen from the traditional literary canon and from among the works of contemporary and culturally diverse writers, novels, short stories, poetry, and drama can convey both the concrete particularity and the metaphorical richness of the predicaments of sick people and the challenges and rewards offered to their physicians. In more than 20 years of teaching literature to medical students and physicians, practitioners of literature and medicine have clarified its conceptual frameworks and have identified the means by which its studies strengthen the human competencies of doctoring, which are a central feature of the art of medicine.

Sick persons rely on their physicians for skilled diagnosis, effective therapy, and human recognition of their suffering. Although medicine has made dazzling progress achieving the first two of these goals, its capacity to fulfill the third goal seems to have diminished.[1] Medicine has incorporated the knowledge and methods of scientific disciplines such as molecular biology, human genetics, and bioengineering to achieve progress in diagnosis and therapy. Physicians are now beginning to turn to the humanities, to disciplines such as literary studies, to achieve equally essential progress in comprehending their patients' suffering so that they can accompany patients through illnesses with empathy, respect, and effective care.[2]

Until the initiation of progressive educational reforms in the 1960s, medical schools expected their students to become empathic and attentive clinicians by watching skilled physicians at work. Students were supposed absorb the human competencies of doctoring—what many call "the art of medicine"—during training.[3] But just as physicians can no longer learn the scientific bases of practice in apprenticeship programs, they can no longer learn the human bases of practice without explicit and ongoing training. Such training is not meant to recapture some

Source: Reprinted with permission from Charon et al., Literature and Medicine: Contributions to Clinical Practice, *Annals of Internal Medicine,* Vol. 122, pp. 599–606, © 1995, American College of Physicians.

long-lost proficiency in compassionate doctoring from generations ago but to extend the accomplishments of the past using knowledge that was unavailable to physicians in former times.

Along with other disciplines in the humanities and along with the social and behavioral sciences, literature and literary studies contribute to this educational effort. The relation between literature and science has fueled impassioned debate since the Victorian era. Matthew Arnold defended literature—he called it "criticism of life"—when Thomas Huxley proposed to replace humane letters with natural sciences in general education.[4] C. P. Snow's 1959 suggestion that the scientific and the literary cultures were irreparably estranged and that the future belonged to the scientists elicited profound disagreement from scientists and literary scholars alike.[5] This historical conversation continues today in U.S. medical schools, in many of which, since 1972, literature has joined science in the curriculum. Using literary methods and texts, literary scholars have been teaching medical students and physicians how to listen more fully to patients' narratives of illness and how to better comprehend illness and treatment from patients' points of view.[6] These skills help physicians to interview patients, to establish therapeutic alliances with patients and their families, to arrive at accurate diagnoses, and to choose and work toward appropriate clinical goals.

The most quickly growing area of the medical humanities, the field of literature and medicine is a recognized subdiscipline of literary studies that has its own scholarly journals, professional societies, graduate school programs, federally funded training programs, and research agendas.[7] In 1994, approximately one-third of United States medical schools taught literature to their students, according to our informal surveys of members of the Society for Health and Human Values, and the number is growing quickly. Medical students in the preclinical and clinical years, house officers, and practicing physicians participate in literature courses and writing workshops. Usually cotaught by literary scholars and physicians, such courses can be either required or elective elements of the curriculum. Physicians have joined literary scholars in writing about the connections between literature and medicine and the benefits that literature provides to the physician; this confirms the clinical relevance of such teaching and scholarship.[8]

The study of literature contributes in several ways to achievement in the human dimensions of medicine: (1) literary accounts of illness can teach physicians concrete and powerful lessons about the lives of sick people; (2) great works of fiction about medicine enable physicians to recognize the power and the implications of what they do; (3) through narrative knowledge, the physician can better understand patients' stories of sickness, thereby strengthening diagnostic accuracy and therapeutic effectiveness while deepening an understanding of his or her own personal stake in medical practice; (4) literary study contributes to physicians' expertise in narrative ethics and helps physicians to perform longitudinal acts of ethical discernment; and (5) literary theory offers new perspectives on the work and the genres of medicine. Although our discussion of literature's contributions to medicine focuses on works of fiction, genres such as poetry, drama, and film are equally valuable to the physician and the medical educator.

THE PATIENT'S LIFE

What do sick people worry about? How do they live their lives around their diseases? What sense can they make of the random events of illness? How can their physicians help them to find meaning in their experiences of illness and thereby facilitate participation in treatment or acceptance of the inevitability of death? The asking and answering of such questions should permeate all aspects of diagnosis and treatment, yet medical training does not generally confer on physicians the skills that make this possible. One rich source of knowledge about the human experience of illness is literature. Illuminating patients' experiences in the full, rich, nuanced particularity seldom if ever available elsewhere, literary accounts of illness widen physician-readers' knowledge of the concrete realities of being sick and enable these readers to appreciate their own patients' stories of sickness.

By mobilizing the imagination, literary works engage the reader more fully than do clinical, sociologic, or historical descriptions, even when the same experiences are portrayed.[9] Although physicians witness countless actual people wrestling with illness, few can articulate, as could William Shakespeare or John Donne or Henry James, the universal and complex human sequelae of disease. By reading narratives of illness written by gifted writers, physicians can more precisely fathom the fears and losses of patients with serious illnesses, identifying in fictional characters and then in their own patients the inevitable conflicts and uncertainties that sickness brings.

Narrative accounts of patients' experiences of illness are regularly considered in medical school courses and in professional reflections on the patient-physician relationship, aging, death and dying, disability, and women's health.[10] Examples of such writings vary in period and in genre. Dante's epic journey in *The Inferno* parallels the journey of illness; Virgil, his guide, stands for the patient's physician.[11] Leo Tolstoy's *The Death of Ivan Ilych* brings the reader to the bedside of a middle-aged bureaucrat who is dying of cancer and who articulates, without flinching, the regrets of a selfish life and the fears of a lonely death.[12] Tillie Olsen's "Tell Me a Riddle" represents the living and dying of Eva—Russian–Jewish immigrant, revolutionary, mother, grandmother, and patient with cancer whose diagnosis is withheld from her—amid the deceptive gambits and the caring acts of her family.[13] Henry James's aging protagonist Dencombe in "The Middle Years" reviews his waning life, seeking from his physician the chance for "another go" but receiving instead a deep and healing confirmation of his worth.[14] Franz Kafka's Gregor Samsa awakens as an insect in "The Metamorphosis"; this is an allegory of the many-leveled transformations of illness for patients and their families and clinicians.[15] In his madness, the protagonist of *King Lear* finds the clarity of vision and value that many dying persons and their families crave.[16]

Besides works of fiction and imagination, pathographies—the narratives that patients write about their illnesses—offer "case histories" of illness and treatment from the patients' points of view.[17] Both biographical and fictional writings by members of particular cultural or ethnic groups help physicians by situating illness within specific cultural and spiritual understandings of the body.[18]

Reading these and other accounts of illness and death deepens the physician-reader's grasp of human need. In a time when physicians and patients are often strangers from different religious traditions and cultural backgrounds, physicians cannot rely on what they know of illness from their personal lives. Literature can supply full-bodied and profound accounts of illness and death in all places and among all peoples. Great works of literature may be unsurpassed in their ability to teach about suffering, death, and the human condition.

THE PHYSICIAN'S WORK

Literary representations of the physician's work, written by nonphysicians as well as physicians, clarify the many roles and expectations of medicine and thereby help readers to understand not only the responsibilities of physicians and the position of medicine within a culture but also the social crises to which physicians must respond. Such novels as *Middlemarch* by George Eliot, *The Magic Mountain* by Thomas Mann, and *The Plague* by Albert Camus delve into the personal, professional, and political worlds of physicians and explicitly acknowledge the nonclinical implications of the physician's work.[19] Because the creative writer is often at the forefront of a culture's awareness, literature often heralds the understanding of new crises in medicine such as the acquired immune deficiency syndrome (AIDS) or the threat of nuclear war.[20]

Physician-writers such as Anton Chekhov, William Carlos Williams, Walker Percy,

Richard Selzer, and Oliver Sacks write with great insight about medicine. Chekhov's "Ward Number Six" describes the inner conflicts of Dr. Ragin, simultaneously the paralyzed idealist and the nihilistic stoic.[21] Williams's short stories about a small-town general practitioner capture the contradictions of the physician's work with scathing accuracy.[22] Percy's *The Moviegoer* follows the course of one troubled young man on his way to deciding to become a physician; the story delineates not only the personal conflicts but also the larger cultural issues that are often involved in this choice.[23] Oliver Sacks, in *Awakenings,* describes the investment of physician and patient in a "miraculous" cure.[24] Physician-writers frame the events and emotions of medicine in ways that lead physician-readers to examine critically their own intimate and complicated relationships with their work and with their patients.

The teaching of such works to physicians and medical students achieves a critical goal in medical education: It allows physicians and students to examine what they do in medicine and what medicine has done to them. During a class on "Ward Number Six," one internist found herself agreeing with Dr. Ragin's cynicism but identifying with his patient's insistence on compassionate care, thereby showing that her own occasional pessimism did not rule out a simultaneous empathy. Reading Ernest Hemingway's "Indian Camp" as a part of medicine attending rounds allowed a medical team of housestaff to come to terms with their cavalier attitude toward a patient in pain, realizing that for them, as for the physician in the story, the patient's screams were unimportant diagnostically but conferred on them the clinical and moral responsibility to control the patient's pain. Literary accounts about medicine, then, contribute a needed ingredient to medical education and training: They give rich and accurate "case histories" of the physician's life that can stimulate important personal introspection about and examination of all that the physician is called on to do.

Narratives written by or about physicians can also teach particular medical lessons. The short stories of Arthur Conan Doyle can help readers examine the humanistic content of ordinary medical encounters as well as the hypothesis-generating and -ratifying processes that constitute diagnostic reasoning.[25] Literary representations of particular aspects of the physician's life or of specific medical events can provide a mirror for practitioners who face parallel or analogous issues in their own lives.[26] Gothic tales or surreal science fiction can help physicians to project their fears into consciousness, thereby allowing them to examine primitive but important terrors and qualms.[27] Reading medical narratives, finally, can suggest to physicians and medical students that acts of healing encompass acts of interpretation and contemplation alongside the technical and scientific aspects of medicine.[28]

NARRATIVE KNOWLEDGE

When a physician meets a patient in the office or at the bedside, the patient tells a complex and many-staged story. Using words and gestures, the patient recounts the events and sensations of the illness while his or her body "tells"—in physical findings, images, tracings, laboratory measurements, or biopsies—that which the patient may not yet know. If the patient is a hesitant or chaotic narrator, the physician has to be an especially alert listener, leaning forward to grasp the point, to fill in the blanks, to hear the story to the end, so that he or she can then group the data into testable hypotheses. Evaluating patients requires the skills that are exercised by the careful reader: to respect language, to adopt alien points of view, to integrate isolated phenomena (be they physical findings or metaphors) so that they suggest meaning, to organize events into a narrative that leads toward their conclusion, and to understand one story in the context of other stories by the same teller.[29]

To make sense of clinical information, physicians rely on skills that belong to the narrative sphere of knowledge. Unlike logico-scientific knowledge, narrative knowledge configures singular events befalling human beings or human surrogates into meaningful stories.[30] If newspaper stories, myths, folktales, and novels are examples of narratives, then the events of illness are, in a manner of speaking, narratives, as are the written and oral descriptions of these events.[31]

The humanities and the social sciences have taken a narrativist turn during the past two decades, during which scholars and practitioners of widely various disciplines (literary criticism, history, sociology, and anthropology) and professions (law, teaching, and psychoanalysis) have found in narrative theory new approaches to understanding their work in a postmodern world.[32] Drawing on the work of literary critics, historians, and philosophers, narrative methods focus attention on the storyteller's attempts to find causal or meaningful connections among events, on temporal orderings and reorderings of those events, on the ways in which the teller or author renders the story for the listener or reader, and on the complex cascade of events that unfold as the listener or reader interprets the story.[33] Although medicine may seem somewhat late in partaking of the explosive interest in narrative thinking, many researchers have long used narrative methods in the study of such medical phenomena as physician-patient interactions and patients' phenomenologic experiences of illness.[34] More recently, narrative methods have been adopted in the investigation of such medical issues as risk factors for hip replacement in elderly patients, patients' abilities to make sense of chronic illness, and cross-cultural examinations of the practice of oncology.[35] From medicine's point of view, narrative study allows the literary critic, the historian, the philosopher, and the anthropologist to work alongside the physician for the good of the patient.

Borrowed from literary studies, such narrative concepts as narratability, temporality, and plot are relevant to much of the physician's research and practice. Generating and conveying medical knowledge are, in part, narrative projects.[36] Although considered logico-scientific enterprises, both basic research and clinical research are now recognized to rely in part on narrative ways of knowing: The development and confirmation of scientific hypotheses are guided by plot and intention.[37] Much of the physician's day is spent in telling or listening to stories—not only at the bedside but at attending rounds, in grand rounds, in curbside consults, in referral letters. These presentations and re-presentations of cases allow physicians to think through the facts and then to choose, justify, and evaluate clinical actions. Devoted entirely to narrative and medical knowledge, a recent issue of the journal *Literature and Medicine* reports on narrative projects in patient care and teaching that span activities from hospice work to residency training in anesthesia to psychotherapy.[38]

Literary activities help physicians to develop and strengthen their narrative skills. Reading fiction or poetry exercises the pattern-finding and meaning-making operations that lead to apt clinical evaluation. Reading puts into play the mental and creative acts of imagination and interpretation, reinforcing subtle competencies of empathy and respect.[39] Writing in narrative genres about patients exercises the clinical imagination and taps into deep personal sources of knowledge about patients and what ails them.[40] Medical students in several schools are asked to adopt their patients' voices when writing the history of present illness as a means to experience, albeit vicariously, that which the patient is going through.[41] Experienced physicians, even those who are not professional writers, have begun to value their own writings about their practices. Such journals as *Annals of Internal Medicine, Journal of the American Medical Association, Journal of General Internal Medicine,* and *American Journal of Medicine* and many of the journals of the state medical societies publish physicians' personal reflections about their practices. In all of these ways, physicians and students have discovered that allowing their inner knowledge to achieve the status of language teaches them something of clinical value about their patients or their practices, something that might otherwise be ignored.[42]

Narrative knowledge offers physicians self-knowledge as well as knowledge of their patients. Many of the current challenges in medicine stem from physicians' inabilities to live up to their own professional goals and ideals. Disillusioned and exploited, and feeling betrayed by the profession, some physicians advise their children not to become doctors and seek ways of leaving their own practices.[43] Increasing self-knowledge through narrative can help these physicians to recapture their own satisfaction with their practices.[44] By helping physicians to recognize their own affective selves, reading and writing can reorient physicians toward the generous goals of service and dedication for which they entered the medical profession.

NARRATIVE ETHICS

The recognition of the importance of literature to medicine has contributed a new approach to the practice of ethics.[45] Physicians must know the principles of medical ethics; they must also learn to surmise the texture of a patient's life in all its moral complexity. Alone, the analytic approach to ethics reduces human conflicts to rational problems to be solved, but a narrative approach to ethics presents the individual events of illness, in all their contradictions and meaningfulness, for interpretation and understanding.[46]

Calling forth the moral as well as the clinical imagination, literature leads physicians to contextualize and particularize ethical issues in health care. The methods that are often called narrative ethics center the examination of ethical dilemmas squarely in the patient's life.[47] Narrative ethics offers the kind of knowing that the German neo-Kantians called *Verstehen*—a powerful, concrete, rich sense of the feelings, values, beliefs, and interpretations that make up the actual experience of the sick person.[48] Like casuistic and phenomenologic approaches to medical ethics, narrative ethics places moral dilemmas within the framework of a patient's culture and biography, allowing physicians to ask such questions as "In the face of this life, what constitutes a good death?"[49]

The practice of narrative ethics aims to prevent the development of ethical quandries by building into medical care a fully articulated recognition of the moral dimensions of the patient's actual life. Ethical moments occur not only in neonatal intensive care units or in heart-transplant suites but also in the ordinary, everyday events of primary care medical practices.[50] A hallmark of the practice of narrative ethics is the development of a longitudinal understanding of patients' values and beliefs that relies when necessary on home visits, extensive life histories, and detailed discussions with family members and caregivers. Narrative skills can help the clinician to be sensitive to moral questions as they occur, to integrate questions about values and beliefs into the routines of medical care, and to make contact with the conflicts, tragedy, humor, irony, and ambiguity that contribute to each human life.

Literary studies contribute both texts and methods to the practice of narrative ethics. Teachers of ethics have found literary narratives to be unequaled by other so-called ethics cases in the classroom. For example, texts from classical drama, 19th-century realist fiction, and contemporary short stories have been able to immerse students in the particularity of moral conflict, providing the compelling pull of the storyteller's verisimilitude within a fully rendered universe.[51] Richard Selzer's short story "Mercy" can stand as an example. In this tale, a physician cares for a terminally ill patient in great pain. The patient wants to die and his family even asks, directly, that he be released from his misery. When a lethal dose of morphine fails to bring about the patient's death, the physician cannot bring himself to do anything further to cause his patient to die. Reading this story brings out the emotional and professional conflicts that beset all who care for dying patients.[52] In addition to schooling students and physicians in the legal and professional limits on the termination of treatment, serious reading of such stories augments a comprehension of all that is at stake—intellectual, legal, existential, spiritual—in such situations.

Perhaps more fundamental to ethics than individual literary texts are literature's methods. Where does the moral sense reside if not in the creative faculties? Attunement to the right and the good is attained by imaginatively rendering, for oneself, the situations of others. Literary scholars writing in the tradition of ethical criticism examine the moral consequences of serious reading, and their findings speak to the medical ethicist. The relationship between a reader and a book—any book—implicates the reader's values, beliefs, and will. A book—or, in a medical context, a case—draws forth from the reader his or her capacity to be changed by an encounter with the unknown and challenges the reader to measure up to another's mode of comprehending the world.[53] Medicine and bioethics can benefit directly from literary insights into the confrontations between strangers over questions of goodness, justice, and the right things to do.

Analytic forms cannot contain the ambiguities and subtleties of meaning that arise in the moral life; literature is better able to capture the complex resonance of human choice and human desire.[54] The practice of any ethicist includes the tasks of formulating a case and interpreting it, and this requires the exercise of narrative skills and even of literary capacities.[55] As clinicians seek sustained and sensible means of arriving at fitting outcomes to the dilemmas of care, literary texts and methods can illuminate the nature of moral reasoning and can serve as valuable guides for individual and collective ethical behavior.[56]

LITERARY THEORY AND MEDICINE

In addition to the contributions of narrative theory and ethical criticism, several schools of literary theory address problems faced by physicians and can help them to understand the texts and work of medicine. Reader-response criticism, deconstructionism, feminist studies, and psychoanalytic literary criticism, among other schools of thought, have shown direct practical and theoretical benefits for the physician.

Reader-response critics examine the acts of reading to understand the complicated and often uneasy "colleagueship" between a text and its reader. No longer satisfied with the New Critics' assertion that the meaning of a text is a static feature of the words themselves, theorists such as Wolfgang Iser, Jonathan Culler, Norman Holland, and Jane Tompkins examine the role of the reader—his or her associations, memories, character traits, and life experiences—in making the meaning of a text.[57] As physicians face patients, they, too, respond as would any reader to the complexity of a presentation, filling in gaps in knowledge with highly individual surmises born of their own memories and associations.[58] Such findings about physicians' readerlike behaviors can only lead to more accurate receptions of patients' stories by turning physicians' unconscious reflexes into conscious and therefore fully available resources for deeper understanding.

Medicine turns out to be an "interesting case" for the deconstructionist scholar who studies the oral and written transactions of medicine and, by extension, the actual practices that constitute medical care. Using methods introduced by Jacques Derrida and Paul de Man, the deconstructionist looks between the lines of texts, suspicious that any external coherence hides inner chaos.[59] Sequestered in such ordinary medical texts as the hospital chart or the referral letter can be found evidence of scientistic assumptions, class and race biases, power relationships, and unforeseen consequences of medical care. For example, the clinical case history has recently been the subject of literary examination that calls attention to conflicts between the physician's and the patient's perspectives, the chorus of voices that speak in a hospital chart, the unforeseen limitations imposed by writing in the genre of the medical chart, and the similarities between case presentations and other literary forms, such as ancient bardic performances.[60] Rigorous examination of physicians' narrative practices can teach singular lessons about clinical detachment, presumed omniscience, and the performance of diagnostic, prognostic, and therapeutic tasks.[61]

The feminist methods for understanding the woman writer apply with great force to the narratives of patients, which are often told from a nondominant position.[62] Feminist studies offer thoughtful models for examining submerged stories and silences within texts; such examination is the very challenge facing physicians and linguists who study the oral transactions of medicine.[63] The application of feminist literary methods to physician-patient interactions grants the investigator proven research methods and a rich tradition of understanding of tales of suffering and celebratory joy.[64]

Although seemingly leagues apart, the practices of the psychoanalyst and the physician adopt similar methods and can be examined using similar means. Sigmund Freud's case histories have never been surpassed in their breadth of diagnostic creativity and depth of psychotherapeutic consequences, and the literary study of them has unearthed fundamental features of the sick role and the therapeutic presence.[65] The relation of analyst to analysand forms the very center of analytic therapy. Physicians are well served by attending closely to their transference and countertransference relationships with patients; doing so both increases their therapeutic effectiveness and maintains their own emotional health. Studies in psychoanalytic literary criticism highlight these therapeutic aspects of Freudian, neo-Freudian, and Lacanian theory by reflecting on literary works and clinical cases.[66] Recent interest in the autobiographical aspects of medical treatment testifies to the applicability of Freud's "talking cure" not only to neurosis and hysteria but to the treatment of somatic illness and ordinary medical disease.[67]

DISCUSSION

How do we know that teaching literature to physicians and medical students works? Outcome studies of literature and medicine courses have examined students' course evaluations, postcourse interviews and questionnaires, and faculty members' assessments and have shown that such courses improve students' understanding of patients' experiences, enrich students' capacities for dealing with ethical problems, or deepen students' self-knowledge in clinically relevant ways.[68] All of these researchers assume that literary knowledge extends beyond that which can be tested into lifelong alterations of the learner's modes of perception and understanding. Individual physicians describe these influences when they attest to the improvements that slowly accrue in their practice over a career of reading, writing, and listening to their patients.[69]

Nevertheless, longitudinal outcome research is needed. Students and physicians should be followed over prolonged periods of time to document the ways in which enhanced narrative knowledge and skills might alter and improve clinical practice. Such research will inevitably be qualitative rather than quantitative in method, for education in literature does not typically result in universal, replicable changes in behavior at generalizable points in time after an intervention. Not unlike numerous other clinical skills—for example, the abilities to assess quality of life and to express empathy—the effects of teaching literature in medical schools may defy quantitative measurement but may nonetheless be regarded as important contributions to medical effectiveness.[70] Because literary methods may help to answer rising demands for improving humanistic behavior in physicians and addressing the personal, cultural, and moral lives of both patients and their physicians, they must be evaluated along with other recent changes in medical training.

CONCLUSIONS

The study of literature accomplishes several goals for medicine and medical education. Reading literary works and writing in narrative genres allow physicians and students to better understand patients' experience and to grow in self-understanding, and literary theory contributes to an ethical, satisfying, and effective practice of medicine. We hope that the introduction of literature and of literary studies to medicine will allow physicians to more accurately render the lives of their patients and to recognize the human dimensions of all of the experiences that occur within their gaze. Together, medicine and literature can modulate the potentially alienating experiences of illness and doctoring into a richer and more mutually fulfilling human encounter that better brings about healing and alleviates suffering.

NOTES

1. A. Broyard, ed. *Intoxicated by My Illness and Other Writings on Life and Death* (New York: Clarkson Potter, 1992); A. H. Hawkins, *Reconstructing Illness: Studies in Pathology* (West Lafayette, Ind.: Purdue University Press, 1993).
2. A. Kleinman, *The Illness Narratives: Suffering, Healing, and the Human Condition* (New York: Basic Books, 1988); H. Brody, *Stories of Sickness* (New Haven: Yale University Press, 1987); R. Coles, *The Call of Stories: Teaching and the Moral Imagination* (Boston: Houghton Mifflin, 1989).
3. F. W. Peabody, *Doctor and Patient: Papers on the Relationship of the Physician to Men and Institutions* (New York: Macmillan, 1930); E. J. Cassell, *The Healer's Art* (Cambridge, Mass.: MIT Press, 1985).
4. M. Arnold, "Literature and Science," in *Discourses in America* (London: Macmillan, 1885), 72–137.
5. C. P. Snow, *The Two Cultures and the Scientific Revolution: The Rede Lecture, 1959* (Cambridge: Cambridge University Press, 1959); L. Trilling, "The Leavis-Snow Controversy," in *Beyond Culture: Essays on Literature and Learning* (New York: Harcourt Brace Jovanovich, 1965), 126–54; M. G. Bishop, "A New Cageful of Ferrets!" Medicine and the 'Two Cultures' Debate of the 1950s," [Editorial], *J. R. Soc. Med.* 84 (1991): 637–39.
6. J. Trautmann, "The Wonders of Literature in Medical Education," *Mobius* 2 (1982): 23–31; K. Rabuzzi, ed., *Toward a New Discipline: Literature and Medicine* 10 (Albany, N.Y.: State University of New York Press, 1991): 1; J. Trautmann, ed., *Healing Arts in Dialogue: Medicine and Literature* (Carbondale, Ill.: Southern Illinois University Press, 1981).
7. D. Wear et al., *Literature and Medicine: A Claim for a Discipline,* Proceedings of the Northeastern Ohio Universities College of Medicine's Literature and Medicine Conference, May 1984 (McLean, Va.: Society for Health and Human Values, 1987); A. H. Jones, ed., Tenth Anniversary Retrospective, *Literature and Medicine* 1 (Albany, N.Y.: State University of New York Press, 1991); A. H. Jones, "Literature and Medicine: Traditions and Innovations," in *The Body and the Text: Comparative Essays in Literature and Medicine,* ed. B. Clarke and W. Aycock (Lubbock, Tex.: Texas Tech University Press, 1990), 11–24.
8. N. J. Baker, "Literary Medicine," *Minn. Med.* 73, no. 11 (1990): 19–20; W. G. Porter, "Medicine and Literature," *N. C. Med. J.* 54, no. 2 (1993): 96–99; G. B. Risse, "Literature and Medicine" [Editorial], *West J. Med.* 156 (1992): 431.
9. L. Trilling, "On the Teaching of Modern Literature," in *Beyond Culture: Essays on Literature and Learning* (New York: Harcourt Brace Jovanovich, 1965), 3–27.
10. J. A. Billings, "A Seminar in 'Plain Doctoring,'" *J. Med. Educ.* 60 (1985): 855–59; C. Loughman, "Meeting the Dark: Autobiography in Hawthorne's Unfinished Tales," *Gerontologist* 32 (1992): 726–32; M. Kohn et al., eds., *Literature and Aging: An Anthology* (Kent, Ohio: Kent State University Press, 1992); I. J. Ozer, "Images of Epilepsy in Literature," *Epilepsia* 32 (1991): 798–809; D. Wear and L. L. Nixon, "Scoot Down to the Edge of the Table, Hon': Women's Medical Experiences Portrayed in Literature," *Pharos* 54, no. 1 (1991): 7–11.
11. A. H. Hawkins, "Charting Dante: The Inferno and Medical Education," *Lit. Med.* 11 (1992): 200–215.
12. R. F. Christian, "The Later Stories," in *Tolstoy: A Critical Introduction* (Cambridge, England: Cambridge University Press, 1969); J. E. Connelly, "The Whole Story," *Lit. Med.* 9 (1990): 150–61; J. T. Banks, "Death Labors," *Lit. Med.* 9 (1990): 162–71; W. J. Donnelly, "Experiencing the Death of Ivan Ilyich: Narrative Art in the Mainstream of Medical Education," *Pharos* 54, no. 2 (1991): 21–25; J. Young-Mason, "Tolstoi's 'The Death of Ivan Ilyich': A Source for Understanding Compassion," *Clinical Nurse Specialist* 2 (1988): 180–83.
13. Connelly, "The Whole Story"; Banks, "Death Labors"; C. Coiner, "'No One's Private Ground': A Bakhtinian Reading of Tillie Olsen's 'Tell Me a Riddle.'" *Feminist Studies* 18 (1992): 257–81.
14. R. P. Blackmur, "Henry James," in *Studies in Henry James,* ed. V. Makowsky (New York: New Directions, 1983), 91–124; F. Kermode, "Introduction," in *The Figure in the Carpet and Other Stories,* ed. F. Kermode (New York: Penguin Books, 1986), 7–30.
15. R. P. Preston, *The Dilemmas of Care: Social and Nursing Adaptations to the Deformed, the Disabled, and the Aged* (New York: Elsevier, 1979), 3–7; A. Flores, ed., *The Kafka Problem* (New York: Octagon Books, 1963).
16. A. Kirsch, "The Emotional Landscape of 'King Lear,'" *Shakespeare Quarterly* 39 (1988): 154–70; S. Freud, "The Theme of Three Caskets," in *The Standard Edition of the Complete Psychological Works of Sigmund Freud,* vol. 12, ed. J. Strachey (London: Hogarth Press, 1953–1974), 291–301.
17. Hawkins, *Reconstructing Illness: Studies in Pathology*; A. W. Frank, "Reclaiming an Orphan Genre: The First-person Narrative of Illness," *Lit. Med.* 13 (1994): 1–21; *id.,* "The Rhetoric of Self-Change: Illness Experience as Narrative," *Sociological Quarterly* 34 (1993): 39–52.
18. M. G. Secundy and L. L. Nixon, eds., *Trials, Tribulations, and Celebrations: African-American Perspectives on Health, Illness, Aging, and Loss* (Yarmouth, Me.: Intercultural Press, 1991); A. F. Stanford, "Mechanisms of Disease: African-American Women Writers, Social

Pathologies, and the Limits of Medicine," *NWSA Journal* 6 (1994): 28–47.

19. S. Shuttleworth, *George Eliot and Nineteenth-Century Science: The Make-Believe of a Beginning* (Cambridge, England: Cambridge University Press, 1984); H. J. Welgand, *"The Magic Mountain": A Study of Thomas Mann's Novel* Der Zeuberberg (Chapel Hill, N.C.: University of North Carolina Press, 1964); P. Gaëgan, "Notes of *The Plague*," in *Camus: A Collection of Critical Essays,* ed. G. Brée (Englewood Cliffs, N.J.: Prentice-Hall, 1962), 145–51.

20. T. F. Murphy and S. Poirier, eds. *Writing AIDS: Gay Literature, Language, and Analysis* (New York: Columbia University Press, 1993); J. Cady, "'A Common Geography of the Mind': Physicians in AIDS Literature," *Semin. Neurol.* 12 (1992): 70–74.

21. R. Wellek and N. Wellek, eds., *Chekhov: New Perspectives* (Englewood Cliffs, N.J.: Prentice-Hall, 1984); J. H. Dirckx, "Anton Chekhov's Doctors," *Pharos* 54, no. 3 (1991): 32–35.

22. J. Trautmann, "William Carlos Williams and the Poetry of Medicine," *Ethics in Science and Medicine* 2 (1975): 105–14.

23. M. W. Montello, "The Moviegoer," *Acad. Med.* 66 (1991): 332–33.

24. A. H. Hawkins, "The Myth of Cure and the Process of Accommodation: 'Awakenings' Revisited," *Medical Humanities Review* 8, no. 1 (1994): 9–21.

25. A. E. Rodin and J. D. Key, "Humanism and Values in the Medical Short Stories of Arthur Conan Doyle," *South. Med. J.* 85 (1992): 528–37; S. H. Sheldon and P. A. Noronha, "Using Classic Mystery Stories in Teaching," *Acad. Med.* 65 (1990): 234–35.

26. R. Rockney, "Life Threatening Emergencies Involving Children in the Literature of the Doctor," *Journal of Medical Humanities* 12 (1991): 153–61; S. Posen, "The Portrayal of the Physician in Nonmedical Literature: The Female Physician," *J. R. Soc. Med.* 86 (1993): 345–48; *id.,* "The Portrayal of the Physician in Nonmedical Literature: The Physician and His Family," [Editorial], *J. R. Soc. Med.* 85 (1992): 314–17.

27. J. H. Dirckx, "The Mad Doctor in Fiction," *Pharos* 55, no. 3 (1992): 27–31.

28. L. C. Epstein, "The 'Reading' of Patients," *R. I. Med.* 76 (1993): 333–35.

29. R. Charon, "Medical Interpretation: Implications of Literary Theory of Narrative for Clinical Work," *Journal of Narrative and Life History* 3 (1993): 79–97; S. L. Daniel, "The Patient as Text: A Model of Clinical Hermeneutics," *Theor. Med.* 7 (1986): 195–210; D. Leder, "Clinical Interpretation: The Hermeneutics of Medicine," *Theor. Med.* 11 (1990): 9–24; B. M. Belkin and F. A. Neelon, "The Art of Observation: William Osler and the Method of Zadig," *Ann. Intern. Med.* 116 (1992): 863–66.

30. J. Bruner, *Actual Minds, Possible Worlds* (Cambridge, Mass.: Harvard University Press, 1986).

31. P. Brooks, *Reading for the Plot: Design and Intention in Narrative* (New York: Vintage Books, 1985).

32. M. Krelswirth, "Trusting the Tale: The Narrativist Turn in the Human Sciences," *New Literary History* 23 (1992): 629–57; D. E. Polkinghorne, *Narrative Knowing and the Human Sciences* (Albany, N.Y.: State University of New York Press, 1988).

33. W. Booth, *The Rhetoric of Fiction,* 2d ed. (Chicago: University of Chicago Press, 1983); W. Benjamin, *Illuminations,* trans. H. Zohn (New York: Schocken, 1969); P. Riceur, *Time and Narrative,* trans. K. McLaughlin and D. Pellauer (Chicago: University of Chicago Press, 1985).

34. E. Mishler, *The Discourse of Medicine: Dialectics of Medical Interviews* (Norwood, N.J.: Ablex, 1984); S. K. Toombs, "Illness and the Paradigm of Lived Body," *Theor. Med.* 9 (1988): 201–26.

35. J. M. Borkin et al., "Finding Meaning after the Fall: Injury Narratives from Elderly Hip Fracture Patients," *Soc. Sci. Med.* 33 (1991): 947–57; U. Gerhardt, "Qualitative Research on Chronic Illness: The Issues and the Story," *Soc. Sci. Med.* 30 (1990): 1149–59; M. J. Del Vecchio Good et al., "Oncology and Narrative Time," *Soc. Sci. Med.* 38 (1994): 855–62.

36. K. M. Hunter, *Doctors' Stories: The Narrative Structure of Medical Knowledge* (Princeton, N.J.: Princeton University Press, 1992).

37. S. Toulmin, "The Construal of Reality: Criticism in Modern and Postmodern Science," in *The Politics of Interpretation,* ed. W. T. Mitchell (Chicago: University of Chicago Press, 1983), 99–117.

38. K. M. Hunter, ed., Narrative and Medical Knowledge: *Literature and Medicine* 13, no. 1 (Baltimore: Johns Hopkins University Press, 1994).

39. J. S. Terry and E. L. Gogol, "Poems and Patients: The Balance of Interpretation," *Lit. Med.* 6 (1987): 43–53; J. B. Younger, "Literary Works as a Mode of Knowing," *Image: Journal of Nursing Scholarship* 22 (1990): 39–43; R. S. Downie, "Literature and Medicine," *J. Med. Ethics* 17 (1991): 93–96; K. C. Calman et al., "Literature and Medicine: A Short Course for Medical Students," *Med. Educ.* 22 (1988): 265–69; R. Charon, "The Narrative Road to Empathy," in *Empathy and the Practice of Medicine: Beyond Pills and the Scalpel,* ed. H. M. Spiro et al. (New Haven, Conn.: Yale University Press, 1993), 147–59; K. D. Clouser, "Humanities in Medical Education: Some Contributions," *J. Med. Philos.* 15 (1990): 289–301.

40. J. L. Coulehan, "Teaching the Patient's Story," *Qualitative Health Research* 2 (1992): 358–66.

41. R. Charon, "To Render the Lives of Patients," *Lit. Med.* 5 (1986): 58–74; P. A. Marshall and J. P. O'Keefe, "Medical Students' First Person Narrative of a Patient's Story of AIDS," *Soc. Sci. Med.* 40 (1994): 67–76; A. Shafer and M. P. Fish, "A Call for Narrative: The Patient's Story and Anesthesia Training," *Lit. Med.* 13 (1994): 124–42; S. C. Vaughan, "Joint Authorship in the Physician-Patient Interaction," *Pharos* 53, no. 3 (1990): 38–42.

42. R. Selzer, *Mortal Lessons* (New York: Simon & Schuster, 1987); J. R. Nashold, "Doctors Who Write: Spies in the Heart of Love," *N. C. Med. J.* 53, no. 5 (1992): 205–9; H. J. Daniel, III, "Medicine and the Biological Sciences: New Vistas for Verse," *N. C. Med. J.* 51, no. 8 (1990): 406–9.

43. M. Konner, *Medicine at the Crossroads: The Crisis in Health Care* (New York: Pantheon Books, 1993).

44. A. L. Suchman and D. A. Matthews, "What Makes the Patient-Doctor Relationship Therapeutic? Exploring the Connexional Dimension of Medical Care," *Ann. Intern. Med.* 108 (1988): 125–30.

45. Coles, *The Call of Stories: Teaching and the Moral Imagination*; S. H. Miles, "The Case: A Story Found and Lost," *Second Opinion* 15 (1990): 55–59; C. Radey, "Imagining Ethics: Literature and the Practice of Ethics," *J. Clin. Ethics* 3 (1992): 38–45.

46. D. Burrell and S. Hauerwas, "From System to Story: An Alternative Pattern for Rationality in Ethics," in *Knowledge, Value and Belief: The Foundations of Ethics and Its Relationship to Science,* vol. 2, ed. H. T. Englehardt and D. Callahan (Hastings-on-Hudson, N.Y.: Hastings Center, Institute of Society, Ethics and the Life Sciences, 1977), 111–52; W. T. Reich, "Experiential Ethics as a Foundation for Dialogue between Health Communication and Health-Care Ethics," *J. Applied Communication Research,* 16 (1988): 16–28; J. M. Gustafson, "Moral Discourse about Medicine: A Variety of Forms," *J. Med. Philos.* 15 (1990): 125–42.

47. L. R. Churchill, "The Human Experience of Dying: The Moral Primacy of Stories over Stages," *Soundings* 62 (1979): 24–37; A. H. Jones, "Literature and Medicine: Illness from the Patient's Point of View," in *Personal Choices and Public Commitments: Perspectives on the Medical Humanities,* ed. W. J. Winslade (Galveston, Tex.: Institute for the Medical Humanities, 1988), 1–15.

48. M. A. Schwartz and O. P. Wiggins, "Systems and the Structuring of Meaning: Contributions to a Biopsychosocial Medicine," *Am. J. Psychiatry* 143 (1986): 1213–21; P. R. Slavney and P. R. McHugh, "Life Stories and Meaningful Connections: Reflections on a Clinical Method in Psychiatry and Medicine," *Perspect. Biol. Med.* 27 (1984): 279–88.

49. A. Jonsen and S. Toulmin, *The Abuse of Casuistry: A History of Moral Reasoning* (Berkeley, Calif.: University of California Press, 1988); R. A. Carson, "Interpretive Bioethics: The Way of Discernment," *Theor. Med.* 11 (1990): 51–59; S. H. Miles and K. M. Hunter, eds., "Case Stories: A Series," *Second Opinion* 11 (1990): 54.

50. J. E. Connelly and S. DalleMura, "Ethical Problems in the Medical Office," *JAMA* 260 (1988): 812–15; J. L. Puma and D. L. Schiedermayer, "Outpatient Clinical Ethics," *J. Gen. Intern. Med.* 4 (1989): 413–20; J. E. Connelly and C. Campbell, "Patients Who Refuse Treatment in Medical Offices," *Arch. Intern. Med.* 147 (1987): 1829–33.

51. S. M. Radwany and B. H. Adelson, "The Use of Literary Classics in Teaching Medical Ethics to Physicians," *JAMA* 257 (1987): 1629–31; L. L. Nixon and D. Wear, "'They Will Put It Together and Take It Apart': Fiction and Informed Consent," *Law. Med. Health Care* 19 (1991): 291–95; C. Radey, "Telling Stories: Creative Literature and Ethics," *Hastings Center Report* 20, no. 11 (1990): 25.

52. A. H. Jones, "Literary Value: The Lesson of Medical Ethics," *Neohelicon* 14 (1987): 383–92.

53. W. Booth, *The Company We Keep: An Ethics of Fiction* (Berkeley, Calif.: University of California Press, 1988); J. H. Miller, *The Ethics of Reading: Kant, de Man, Eliot, Trollope, James, and Benjamin* (New York: Columbia University Press, 1987); T. Siebers, *The Ethics of Criticism* (Ithaca, N.Y.: Cornell University Press, 1988).

54. M. C. Nussbaum, *Love's Knowledge: Essays in Philosophy and Literature* (New York: Oxford University Press, 1990); I. Murdoch, *The Sovereignty of Good* (London: Ark Paperbacks, 1986).

55. R. Charon, "Narrative Contributions to Medical Ethics: Recognition, Formulation, Interpretation, and Validation in the Practice of the Ethicist," in *A Matter of Principles? Ferment in United States Bioethics,* ed. E. R. DuBose et al. (Valley Force, Penn.: Trinity Press International, 1994), 260–83.

56. P. Benner, "The Role of Experience, Narrative, and Community in Skilled Ethical Comportment," *ANS Adv. Nurs. Sci.* 14, no. 2 (1991): 1–21.

57. W. Iser, *The Act of Reading: A Theory of Aesthetic Response* (Baltimore: Johns Hopkins University Press, 1978); J. Culler, "Stories of Reading," in *On Deconstruction: Theory and Criticism after Structuralism* (Ithaca, N.Y.: Cornell University Press, 1982), 64–83; N. Holland, *The Dynamics of Literary Response* (New York: Columbia University Press, 1989); J. Tompkins, ed., *Reader Response Criticism: From Formalism to Post-Structuralism* (Baltimore: Johns Hopkins University Press, 1980).

58. R. Barthes, "Semiology and Medicine," in *The Semiotic Challenge,* trans. R. Howard (New York: Hill and Wang, 1988), 202–13; M. Foucault, *The Birth of the Clinic: An Archaeology of Medical Perception,* trans. A. M. Sheridan-Smith (New York: Pantheon, 1973).

59. P. de Man, *Blindness and Insight* (Minneapolis, Minn.: University of Minnesota Press, 1986); H. Bloom et al., *Deconstruction and Criticism* (New York : Continuum, 1985); J. Derrida, *Of Grammatology,* trans. G. C. Spivak (Baltimore: Johns Hopkins University Press, 1976); M. M. Bakhtin, *The Dialogic Imagination: Four Essays by M. M. Bakhtin,* ed. M. Holquist, trans. C. Emerson and M. Holquist (Austin, Tex.: University of Texas Press, 1976).
60. S. Poirier and D. J. Brauner, "Ethics and the Daily Language of Medical Discourse," *Hastings Cent. Rep.* 18, no. 8–9 (1988): 5–9; J. T. Banks and A. H. Hawkins, ed., The Art of the Case History: *Literature and Medicine* 11, no. 1 (Baltimore: Johns Hopkins University Press, 1992).
61. S. Poirier and D. J. Brauner, "The Voices of the Medical Record," *Theor. Med.* 11 (1990): 29–39; W. J. Donnelly, "Righting the Medical Record: Transforming Chronicle into Story," *JAMA* 260 (1988): 823–25; A. H. Hawkins, "Oliver Sacks' 'Awakenings': Reshaping Clinical Discourse," *Configurations* 2 (1993): 229–45.
62. E. S. More and M. A. Milligan, eds., *The Empathic Practitioner: Empathy, Gender, and Medicine* (New Brunswick, N.J.: Rutgers University Press, 1994).
63. S. Gilbert and S. Gubar, *The Madwoman in the Attic: The Woman Writer and the Nineteenth-Century Literary Imagination* (New Haven, Conn.: Yale University Press, 1979).
64. E. Flynn and P. Schweickart, eds., *Gender and Readings: Essays on Readers, Texts, and Contexts* (Baltimore: Johns Hopkins University Press, 1986); E. Showalter, ed., *The New Feminist Criticism: Essays on Women, Literature, and Theory* (New York: Pantheon, 1985).
65. S. Marcus, "Freud and Dora: Story, History, and Case History," in *In Dora's Case: Freud-Hysteria-Feminism,* ed. C. Bernheimer and C. Kahane (New York: Columbia University Press, 1985), 56–91; J. Hillman, "The Fiction of Case History: A Round with Freud," in *Healing Fiction* (Barrytown, N.Y.: Station Hill Press, 1983), 3–49.
66. M. W. Alcorn and M. Bracher, "Literature, Psychoanalysis, and the Re-Formation of the Self: A New Direction for Reader-Response Theory," *Proceedings of the Modern Language Association* 100 (1985): 342–54; L. Trilling, "Freud: Within and Beyond Culture," in *Beyond Culture: Essays on Literature and Learning* (New York: Harcourt Brace Jovanovich, 1965), 77–102; M. A. Skura, *The Literary Use of the Psychoanalytic Process* (New Haven, Conn.: Yale University Press, 1981).
67. Hawkins, *Reconstructing Illness: Studies in Pathography*; Frank, "The Rhetoric of Self-change: Illness Experience as Narrative."
68. Billings, "A Seminar in 'Plain Doctoring'"; Calman et al., "Literature and Medicine: A Short Course for Medical Students"; Marshall and O'Keefe, "Medical Students' First Person Narrative of a Patient's Story of AIDS"; Radwany and Adelson, "The Use of Literary Classics in Teaching Medical Ethics to Physicians"; J. Wilson and B. Blackwell, "Relating Literature to Medicine: Blending Humanism and Science in Medical Education," *Gen. Hosp. Psychiatry* 2 (1980): 127–33.
69. Connelly, "The Whole Story"; Charon, "The Narrative Road to Empathy"; Coulehan, "Teaching the Patient's Story"; T. E. Quill and R. M. Frankel, eds., "Special Stories Issue," *Medical Examiner* 11, no. 1 (1994).
70. T. M. Gill and A. R. Feinstein, "A Critical Appraisal of the Quality of Quality-of-Life Measurements," *JAMA* 272 (1994): 618–26; H. Spiro, "What Is Empathy and Can It Be Taught?" *Ann. Intern. Med.* 116 (1992): 843–46.

CHAPTER 52

Ethically Responsible Creativity—Friendship of an Understanding Heart: A Cognitively Affective Model for Bioethical Decision Making

John F. Monagle

Ethically Responsible Creativity—Friendship of an Understanding Heart is offered as a contemporary caring and helpful bioethical decision-making model. At this time in the evolution of models, theories, methods, paradigms, and matrices, old and new methodologies are either deficient (lacking an essential component), defective (the meanings of terms have been weakened by ambiguity), or too embryonic to be decisively applied to contemporary bioethical experiences.[1]

Furthermore, the increase of and advancement in medical knowledge and the rapid development of biotechnologies whose applications are anxiously awaited have led to bioethical dilemmas. Medical science is able to maintain lives for years where death would previously have come quickly. Decisions to maintain life have caused serious intellectual and emotional controversies and lawsuits—with differing bioethical and legal results.[2]

Two contrasting cases are presented below: those of Nancy Beth Cruzan and Helga Wanglie and their families.[3] These two cases demonstrate the need for the ethically responsible creativity (ERC) model.

The most important question to be answered in these two cases is: Who will be empowered to be the controlling agent in the making of the ethical decision? The answer to this question is even more important than *what* the controlling agent decides.

The need to correct our models because of such contrasting cases as Cruzan and Wanglie is recognized by most bioethical pioneers. We realize the prescriptive directions, duties, rights, and obligations embedded in principles[4] as well as cookbook recipes for doing bioethics fail when they are enclosed in the ethical heat of the oven: they prove to be deficient, defective, or embryonic when applied to similar patients in similar experiences.

Some suggest applying the virtues in conjunction with the four basic principles in an attempt to account for the text and context of the physician-patient relationship.[5] The hope is that, if the virtues are recognized, cherished, and practiced, physicians will become more sensitized to the individual appropriateness of all treatments and procedures and all medical decisions, including bioethical ones.

Others are beginning the awesome adventure of inquiry, by way of narrative ethics, into the exciting world of bioethics beyond the clinical setting—an inquiry into "what is going on around me and what response is required of me to what is going on around me?"[6] They call for an experiential, inductive paradigm that is concerned with the integration of experienced values.[7] The model or paradigm is embryonic but imaginative and innovative; the quest is praiseworthy and hopefully will yield practical results when focused on bioethical decision making (a small part of the total narrative endeavor).

However, not only are the models presently inadequate to resolve critical ethical issues, but also the meaning of terms, phrases, and principles inherent in the presentations are ambiguous, too widely connotative, and perhaps in some presentations equivocal. All health care professionals involved in ordinary and critical decision making are struggling to define precisely the terms, phrases, and principles applied presently with such generally unexamined facility. Because the terms, phrases, and principles lack precise and universally accepted meanings, they lead to intellectual and emotional disagreements among physicians, patients, and their families as well as health care institutions, the community, and society at large.

The controversial terms, phrases, and principles at the top of the list include *medical necessity*, *competency*,[8] *appropriateness*, *hopelessness*, *futility*,[9] *autonomy*, *nonmalfeasance*, *beneficence*, and *justice*. The vagueness in meaning has forced some health care professionals to coin their own phrases in the hospice movement, some of which are paradoxical, such as "hopeless hope" and "futile nonfutility."

However, how do we *fix* (denote precisely) these terms, phrases, and principles? And until the meanings are settled, how can we properly discuss and finalize bioethical decisions? Until they are fixed by strict denotation through societal, medical, ethical, and legal agreement, we must deal with the problem of ambiguity.

Nevertheless, in the Bergsonian meantime we need to make use of some model that will allow us to arrive at bioethical decisions. ERC, which combines the inputting of clinical and ethical data, the application of the four basic ethical principles, and the application of the philosophy of "friendship of an understanding heart" is one such model. Through ERC, *comfortable* bioethical decisions can be reached.[10]

DESCRIPTIVE DEFINITION OF ETHICALLY RESPONSIBLE CREATIVITY

Ethics is the pattern of values and norms that is "taken for granted" in a given culture or professional or institutional setting. The ERC model is intended to be used in situations in which responses to questions of a *societal* nature are required. It is not designed for responding to "moral" questions, that is, individual cases of conscience. (The communication media and some ethicists use the terms *ethics* and *morality* interchangeably, which brings confusion, in my opinion, to the issues in need of resolution.)

The individuals involved in the bioethical decision-making process should be willing to work with the physician, the patient, the family, the health care organization, and the community at large in implementing the bioethical decision (even though the attending physician will have to take ultimate legal responsibility).[11]

Collectively these individuals are responsible for

- the model and methodology used in the decision-making process
- the medical data and ethical considerations offered for discussion and evaluation
- the persons or advisors to be consulted in the decision-making process (e.g., the patient, the family, significant others, the attending physician, consultants, representatives appointed by the health care institution, a clergyperson and/or bioethicist, and representatives of the community at large)
- the priority and significance (weight) given to the values, preferences, wishes, desires and opinions of the patient, the family, significant others, and the attending physician
- the consequences of the decision
- the documentation of the bioethical decision

The term *creativity* is used, in the tradition of Plato, Leibniz, Bergson, and Whitehead, in the sense of "becoming" or "process." In other words, the components of the ERC model are subject to dynamic medical-ethical evolution. The dynamic process of development of the model allows for change over time. As medical and biotechnical knowledge increases, as society gains greater understanding of the use and limitations of health care discoveries, and as the community develops a consensus on fundamental issues, bioethical decisions hopefully will increasingly be similar in similar cases.

Social demands, public consensus, ethical-legal definitions, court decisions, and state and federal legislation will alter the range of allowable treatments and procedures. Not all will agree with the results of the evolutionary process. Nevertheless, expensive or experimental interventions will be examined and will be permitted or denied based on a patient's diagnosis and prognosis as well as society's willingness to pay. Personal values and preferences will sometimes be overridden by state and federal legislation.[12] Whether we as a nation adopt an egalitarian, federally funded universal health care plan or an egalitarian, competitive managed care plan made accessible and available to all, we can expect that a prioritized list of allowed and denied benefits will evolve. National restrictions, no doubt, will limit individual autonomy. "This does not imply that autonomy has been superseded by other values, but that autonomy must be understood in a larger context which includes, for example, justice, allocation of resources, futility."[13]

Thankfully, we have not reached that point when money as a value has superseded life or quality of life. ERC, therefore, remains a viable model, and hopefully it will be able to adapt to the future.

THE CASES OF NANCY BETH CRUZAN AND HELGA WANGLIE

Although bioethical decision-making models have been refined methodologically and can sometimes be used to achieve the resolution of cases of minor conflict, they are not sufficiently useful in major conflicts related to complex biotechnical situations like those of Cruzan and Wanglie. A certain degree of consternation and frustration gripped me when I studied the contrasting (seemingly contradictory) positions taken by professionals and families in each case as well as the legal judgments rendered by the courts to resolve these cases. A bioethical decision outside of the court could not be made because of the deficient, defective, or embryonic models being used.

Both women, although separated by age and locality, were basically in similar persistent vegetative states. Unless there were "justifiable" reasons for contrasting (contradictory) opinions, the ethical-legal decisions should have been similar in the two cases. Similar, more harmonious, mutually agreed decisions could have been reached through the use of an adequate decision-making model, such as the ERC model.

Nancy Beth Cruzan, age 37 at death,[14] resident of Jasper County, Missouri, and patient in a Missouri state hospital, was clinically judged to be in a persistent vegetative state (PVS) and to evince no significant cognitive function. She was maintained by artificial nutrition and hydration through a gastrostomy tube implanted surgically into her stomach through an incision in her abdominal wall.

The prognosis was that she could remain in this irreversible state for as long as 30 years and that her brain would progressively deteriorate until death. Her parents, Lester and Joyce Cruzan, requested the health care administrator and the attending physician to allow the withdrawal of the intubation, which was only artificially prolonging a life that was virtually meaningless and holding Nancy Cruzan a passive prisoner of inappropriate technology.[15] The Cruzans considered Nancy's condition to be "hopeless" relative to any meaningful recovery and viewed present and future interventions as "futile." However, the attending physician refused to withdraw the artificial nutrition and hydration. His medical reasons were not altogether clear, but from a legal perspective his motivation was quite clear: Both he and the administrator were state employees. They thought that a modicum of defensive medicine was prudent. The law in Missouri was not sufficiently developed to handle this case, so they thought. They feared that they would become subjects of criminal and civil actions. A possible bioethical decision gave way to a decision based on the legal risk of criminal homicide, malpractice (negligence), or both.[16]

Nancy Cruzan's parents had to seek a court resolution. The case went through the Circuit Court of Jasper County (which granted the request of Lester and Joyce Cruzan) to the Missouri Supreme Court (which reversed the decision) to the United States Supreme Court (which affirmed the reversal of the Missouri Supreme Court). The United States Supreme Court sent the case back to the Jasper County District Court, requiring that "clear and convincing evidence" of Nancy Cruzan's wishes would have to be brought forward before the Jasper County Court could grant the parents' request.[17] The testimony of Lester and Joyce Cruzan, loving parents and closest friends, and the testimony of Nancy's sister and an acquaintance were not accepted by the United States Supreme Court as "clear and convincing evidence." The testimony of the Cruzans, according to the dissenting Justices, was disregarded.[18]

Lester and Joyce Cruzan searched and found two additional "acquaintances" who testified that Nancy had expressed to them her desire not to be maintained by artificial means if ever she was in a condition where there was no hope of recovery or even in a condition where she would find herself helpless. The Jasper County District Court had its clear and convincing evidence. The court ruled in favor of the Cruzan's request. Again, the testimony of Nancy's parents as best and closest friends, loving and caring for her, and best suited to knowing and understanding her did not constitute clear and convincing evidence in the view of the United States Supreme Court. The United States Supreme Court, as "strangers" in the case, had spoken.

Helga Wanglie, age 86, resident of Minneapolis, also was in PVS and was maintained by respirator and artificial nutrition and hydration.[19] The health care administrator and attending physician had decided that Mrs. Wanglie, despite the fact that she was fully insured, was a burden to the institution and to the attending physician, who could make more valuable use of his time since he considered all future interventions as "inappropriate."

According to the attending physician, Helga Wanglie's situation was "hopeless," "futile," and irreversible. The attending physician, therefore, sought the consent of Oliver Wanglie, her best friend and loving husband for more than 50 years, to remove the respirator and to withdraw the intubation supplying nutrition and hydration. Oliver Wanglie refused to consent because he stated (and later testified in court) that Helga Wanglie expressly had requested that she would want to be maintained by artificial life support until God decided to take her. The hospital went to court.[20]

The Honorable Patricia L. Belois, of the Fourth District Court, Hennepin County, Minnesota, heard the case and ruled on July 1, 1992, just three days before Helga Wanglie's death, in favor of Oliver Wanglie's request to maintain his wife on artificial life support. Oliver Wanglie, by substituted judgment, could decide as best he saw fit. To Judge Belois, the question of *who* would be the decision maker was more important than *what* the decision would be.

Although the judgment seemed to be in opposition to other court opinions, because it allowed continued treatment for a patient who was in an irreversible persistent vegetative state and for whom, according to the clinical judgment of a competent physician, all interventions were futile and inappropriate, Judge Belois ruled in favor of the autonomy of an incompetent patient as rightly exercised by the substituted judgment of her husband, Oliver Wanglie.[21] Although I personally do not think that the continued treatment was medically appropriate or beneficial, nevertheless I agree with the court's decision in favor of autonomy and in favor of giving the power of substituted judgment to Helga Wanglie's husband. The decision by Judge Belois confirms my conviction that the ERC model is adequate to resolve similar cases. Her Honor stated in effect that no one was better able to know, understand, appreciate, and implement the wishes of Helga Wanglie than her best friend and loving husband of over 50 years. The judge was *amicus familiae*.

THE ERC MODEL

The ERC model (Figure 52–1) is an educational framework that I have used in my pioneering past and continue to expand creatively. Other professional ethicists and more recent settlers have developed or adopted their own diagrammatic decision-making models. All models, no doubt, have been helpful in dealing with the necessary components that are essential in reaching a bioethical decision—at least until recently.

However, the Nancy Cruzan and the Helga Wanglie cases, because of their diverse conclusions, convince me that all other models are

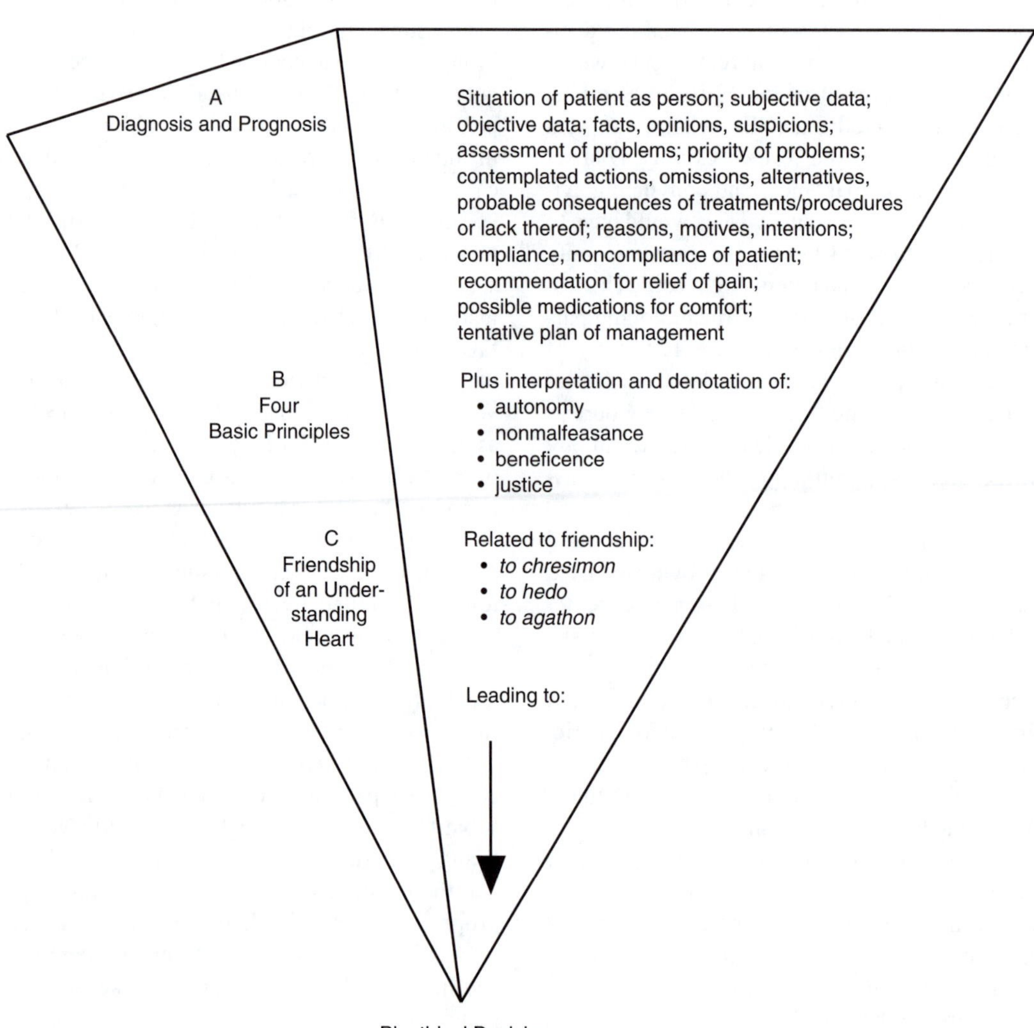

Figure 52–1 Ethically Responsible Creativity—Friendship of an Understanding Heart (a cognitively affective model for bioethical decision making).

deficient in at least one essential component and are therefore incapable of leading to acceptable bioethical decisions.

Medical-Ethical Data

In the top level of Figure 52–1 are the medical and nonprincipled ethical components that lead to a tentative, *non-infallible,* clinical diagnosis and prognosis. Each patient is recognized as unique. All subjective data that can be gleaned from the patient, the family, and significant others are included. The patient's past medical history, symptoms, and complaints are also considered. Objective data resulting from all necessary or useful treatments and technologies are scrutinized (the ruling-out process). Problems are analyzed to determine their acuity and chronicity. From an ethical perspective, all reasonable actions (omissions) are considered together with their probable consequences. Reasons, motives, and intentions are articulated and documented for review by the ethical advisory group or committee involved in making bioethical decisions.[22] Means of providing maximum comfort and relief of pain are prescribed based on the characteristics of the patient and the patient's situation. A tentative medical-ethical plan of management is outlined based on all pertinent information. The tentative plan at the same time is processed though the middle (second) level.

The Four Basic Principles

In the middle level, the four basic ethical principles of autonomy, nonmalfeasance, beneficence, and justice are applied. When their meanings are properly spelled out, these principles have a limited usefulness as tools in bioethical decision making. It is likely they were applied in both the Cruzan and Wanglie cases. However, their meanings have gone through an evolution, and, in fact, the principles are subject to diverse interpretations.

In past philosophical history and legal jurisprudence, the etymological, ethical, and legal meanings had *fixed* denotations. As language, medical knowledge, and biotechnology evolved, and as ethical-legal cases became more complex, the interpretation, priority, and "weight-value" of their meanings have become more diverse: denotations have given way to broader connotations.

Autonomy

Auto = self, one's own; *nomos* = law. Self-law is self-rule, self-determination; the meaning over time has expanded to include freedom, free choice, free decision making. Autonomy became the core of personhood, the center of moral responsibility for self in the case of both actions and consequences.

The meaning of autonomy has expanded even further to include personal values and preferences. When the patient is judged by others to be incompetent, autonomy then resides in the values, preferences, and choices of the physician (paternalistic model); in the values, preferences, and choices of the family (familial model); or in the values, preferences, and choices of the health care facility (institutional model).

Who determines the meaning of autonomy in a bioethical decision-making situation?

Nonmalfeasance

Non = not, no; *male* = bad, evil, harm; *facere* = to do. *Nonmalfeasance* means to do no harm. The principle of nonmalfeasance requires health care providers to do no harm to the patient.

The meaning of nonmalfeasance expanded from never intentionally doing harm to never unintentionally doing harm. But what is *harm*? Is there malfeasance by commission, omission, activity, or passivity? Metaethically, does malfeasance connote physical, psychological, and spiritual harm?

When the patient is competent, is nonmalfeasance or malfeasance defined by the patient's reaction or response? Does malfeasance include performing acts of "futility" in "hopeless" cases? Does malfeasance include "inappropriate" interventions?

When the patient is clinically judged to be incompetent, is malfeasance determined by the family, by the legal system, or through malpractice suits?[23] In the emergency department, does aggressive medical treatment count as nonmalfeasance? Does defensive medicine count as malfeasance?

Who determines the meaning of nonmalfeasance in a bioethical decision-making situation?

Beneficence

Bene = well; *facere* = to do. The principle of beneficence requires health care providers to act in the best interests of the patient. But what are the patient's best interests? Does the physician act in the best interests of the patient by withdrawal of treatment in futile situations? Does the physician act in the best interests of a terminally ill patient by inducing death or assisting in suicide? Is death in the best *interests* of anyone? By whom is beneficence assessed and defined—by the patient, the physician, the family, the health care facility, the community, society at large?

Who determines the meaning of beneficence in a bioethical decision-making situation?

Justice

Justitia = giving each person his or her due. But does justice mean equity? Does it require equalizing wealth by taking from the rich and giving to the poor? Is justice best served by providing everyone with exactly the same access to treatment? Or does justice merely require that all exchanges occur voluntarily, no matter what the ultimate distribution of wealth and power?

Who determines the meaning of justice in a bioethical decision-making situation?

This critique of principlism[24] is not intended to denigrate the usefulness of principles as tools, but it is intended to show that the principles do not reign supreme and that societal agreement as to which principle has priority in an individual case is lacking. The question remains: Who determines the meaning and application of ethical principles in a bioethical decision-making situation?

In the Cruzan case, the administrator and attending physician *refused to withdraw* nutrition and hydration, the court required *clear and convincing evidence*, and the family's knowledge of the patient's wishes was *not sufficient*. How were autonomy, nonmalfeasance, beneficence, and justice interpreted and by whom?

In the Wanglie case, the administrator and attending physician *insisted on the withdrawal* of life support. They went to court *against* Oliver Wanglie's wishes. The court ruled against the hospital and physician *in favor of* Oliver Wanglie and designated him as the person who should make the ultimate decision. How and by whom were the principles interpreted?

Friendship of an Understanding Heart

Aristotle describes three types of friendship: (1) friendship *to chresimon*, (2) friendship *to hedo*, and (3) friendship *to agathon* (Figure 52–2).[25] (Aristotle's terms can be translated as useful friendship, social friendship, and truly virtuous friendship.)

Before applying these types of friendships to individuals involved in bioethical decision making, we must go back in time to prepare for the future. The relationship in medicine between physician, patient, and family has historically been one of virtual strangers. In ancient Greek society, the relationship was literally between the stranger who treats and the stranger who suffers, waits, and is treated. The historical narrative of physicians as strangers is imbedded in the Hippocratic oath. Part of the oath demands that the physician keep the secrets and mysteries of medicine and pass them on only to his sons (no doubt, one of the roots of medical male chauvinism). It is only in very recent history that the relationship of stranger to stranger began to change to a still ill-defined relationship of physician to patient and family.

Perhaps early in this century, when country doctors were common providers of medical care, there was some semblance of friendship in the relationship. However, friendship was not formally encouraged and probably, when present, was overly romanticized (e.g., in the works of Norman Rockwell).

The more realistic relationship of stranger to stranger has been the prevailing one, although it hardly qualifies as a relationship at all. Aristotle states that such connections are those of

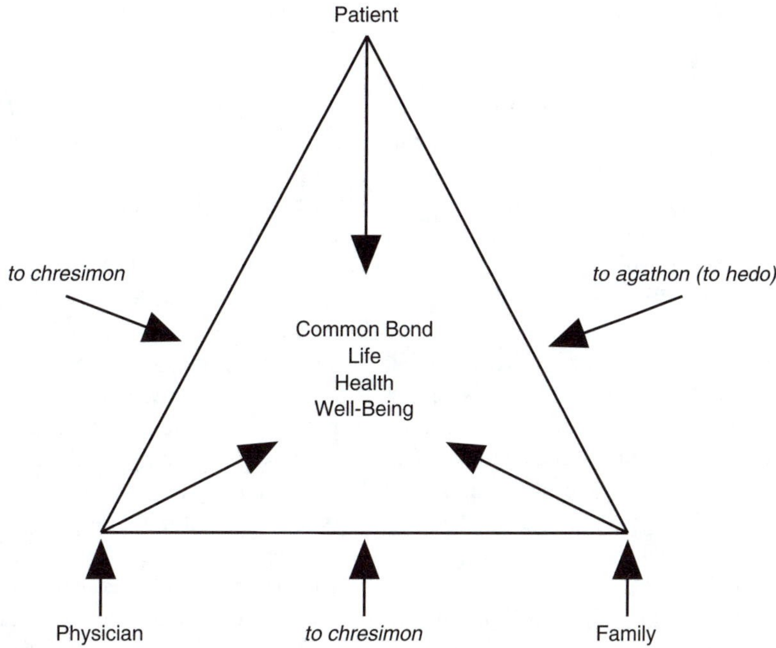

Figure 52–2 Aristotle's Three Kinds of Friendship.

"acquaintances," and he does not find a place for acquaintances in his presentation of the three kinds of friendship. He does, however, recognize that acquaintances should express themselves in language and gestures of *friendliness* to maintain a peaceful society.

It is only in the recent past, the late 1960s and early 1970s, that we began to read in the bioethical literature of the need to establish better relationships between physicians and patients and families. Paul Ramsey, in his classic work *Patient as Person*, awakened pioneering bioethicists to the need to educate physicians to treat patients as persons, not as objects or target organs.[26] The practice of treating patients as objects or target organs and their families as invaders into the private turf of medicine continued for a short time after Ramsey's book was published.

In my opinion, real progress toward better relationships occurred during the "malpractice crisis" between 1973 and 1978. The big issue became educated informed consent. Because of the overwhelming number and costs of malpractice suits, physicians in general recognized that patients could no longer be viewed as strangers, objects, or target organs. The principles of autonomy, nonmalfeasance, beneficence, and justice were accepted by physicians and other health care professionals, and presentations by bioethicists of "ethical-legal considerations regarding informed consent" were welcomed.

Nevertheless, we do not to this day have a relationship between the physician and the patient and family that is embedded in a philosophical foundation outside of medicine itself. There is such a foundation in the relationship of friend to friend. This is a caring, noncasuistic, fidelity bond. Family must be included in the bond if we are to put the proper controlling spin on uniform, comfortable bioethical decision making.

A relationship of friendship, as envisioned and practiced in Aristotle's society and down through the centuries by others, is appropriate and realistic if practiced by the physician and the patient and family and will serve as a teleological foundation for the ends of medicine.

Aristotle labels this kind of relationship friendship *to chresimon*.[27]

Friendship *to chresimon* is consistent with the philosophy expressed by Democritus and embraced by Aristotle: "Friends hold *in common* what they hold." Physicians, patients, and families hold in common the life, health, and well-being of all persons in the relationship.

Friendship *to chresimon* in contemporary practice requires the physician to do the following:

- See the patient and family at the scheduled time (without more than 15 minutes delay).
- Take the time to explain to the patient what should be explained and to answer any questions. "The issuance of a diagnosis," states E. D. Pellegrino, "and a standardized explanation may be convenient for the physician or all that his time will permit. Yet, this can be the first step in making the patient an object and not a person."[28] The patient is a person, *not* a client.
- Listen, not just hear. The physician should get to know the patient and family in a relaxed situation so as to devote full attention to what is said.
- Learn the attitudes, values, preferences, and choices of the patient and family.[29]
- Show compassion and accept the patient for who he or she is.[30] This is a component of respectful friendship.
- Give complete, honest answers to questions from the patient and family.[31] Each patient wants answers to all health questions put in the context of his or her life. Offer hope to the extent that it is realistic.
- Make house calls in necessary but non-emergency situations for patients too sick to travel rather than telling them to take a taxi or call an ambulance.
- Delete from physician bills labels such as "Pay within 10 days or this debt will be turned over to a collection agency." It would be an act of friendship to have the office staff telephone the patient or family to inquire about their ability to pay; arrange for periodic, partial payments if necessary; and eliminate any finance charge for late payments.[32]

Although friendship *to chresimon* is the lowest of Aristotle's types of friendship, nevertheless he emphasizes that it is to be cherished. This type of friendship will disappear when the benefits of the relationship are no longer needed.[33]

Aristotle describes two higher levels of friendship: friendship *to hedo* is best exemplified in relationships among family members and significant others.[34] Friendship *to hedo* also occurs among golf or tennis partners—among people who enjoy socializing with each other. This type of friendship does not usually occur between the physician and the patient and family, but it sometimes does.

Friendship to agathon is the highest type of friendship, according to Aristotle.[35] It usually requires a long time to develop. It is best exemplified by family members and friends who feel close to each other—who accept each other "as is" and for their true and virtuous worth and intrinsic goodness of character.

Aristotle expands this notion of friendship to include love that endures. Love, according to Aristotle, is a superabundance or excess of friendship *to agathon*. Loving friendship is best exemplified by the relationship between husband and wife, parents and children.

This friendship is the friendship of an *understanding heart*.[36] Whatever clinical data and ethical considerations are offered to a patient's family, for example, these will be received according to their mental capacity and ability to understand. They will be considered with an understanding heart.

The physician, on the other hand, may have a different understanding of the data because of his or her medical and biotechnical knowledge.

Confronted with ambiguous terminology and widely connotative principles, and even though the medical facts, opinions, and clinical judgment of the physician are to be respected, nevertheless, the family, relying on the known wishes of the patient (when the patient is incompetent), should make the final decisions regarding treatment based on friendship *to agathon* of an understanding heart. Even if the family's decision is considered to be clinically erroneous by the physician, it should prevail—not because it is good or bad, right or wrong, but because it is a *comfortable* decision and one based on the friendship of an understanding heart. The physician who has become a friend *to chresimon* does not relinquish professional autonomy when he or she defers to the family with regard to ultimate decisions.[37] Unless there are reasons that demonstrate that the family is unfit mentally to make such decisions, they should be allowed to decide what they think is in the best interests of their loved one (i.e., what the loved one would request if he or she were able to express his or her wishes). This is the compassionate, comfortable decision in the light (darkness) of ambiguous terminology (e.g., the meaning of "futility") and widely connotative principles (e.g., the meaning of autonomy and beneficence).

In the cases of Nancy Beth Cruzan and Helga Wanglie, if there had been friendship *to chresimon* between the physician and family, the family would have been given the right to make the final decision. There would have been no compromise of the ethical integrity of the medical profession, nor of any bioethical "norms or standards." Furthermore, there would have been no violation of proper allocation of scarce resources (since proper allocation of scarce resources is a controversial bioethical issue itself). The physician as friend *to chresimon* is not a gatekeeper responsible for implementing distributive justice.

CONCLUSION

I cannot praise the ruling of the United States Supreme Court that forced Lester and Joyce Cruzan to sacrifice the expression of their loving friendship *to agathon* for their daughter Nancy by not allowing them the right to make the final bioethical decision. They were forced to seek clear and convincing evidence of Nancy's wishes from acquaintances. The United States Supreme Court Justices in effect designated Nancy's parents as "strangers" in the case.

In the case of Helga Wanglie, I praise the decision of Judge Patricia Belois. She exercised sensitive objectivity by ruling in favor of Oliver Wanglie and by specifying him as the appropriate one to make the bioethical decision for his wife. Judge Patricia Belois put the proper control spin into effect by ruling that *who* should make the decision is more important than *what* decision should be made. She agreed that a loving husband of more than 50 years should be recognized as the one who would know best from his understanding heart what his wife would wish, and in doing so she affirmed that the rightful exercise of autonomy by substituted judgment should be exercised by the person closest (in loving friendship) to the patient. In effect, she judged in favor of the loving friendship of an understanding heart. She allowed Oliver Wanglie to make the comfortable decision.

I am convinced that Ethically Responsible Creativity—Friendship of an Understanding Heart is an adequate model for contemporary bioethical decision making. It includes the consideration of relevant medical-ethical data, the application of the four basic principles, controlled as to denotation, and the interpretation of ambiguous terminology by the appropriate decision maker.

When the patient is conscious, he or she, if competent, should be the ultimate decision maker. When the patient is unconscious or in a persistent vegetative state, the physician, as friend *to chresimon*, yields the right to the family, as friends *to agathon* to make the final bioethical decision.

The control of the interpretation of clinical-ethical data as well as the denotation of all principles together with the individualized understanding of ambiguous terminology is placed in the substituted judgment of friends *to agathon*.

This model also entails that gays and lesbians who are friends of an understanding heart should be allowed to make bioethical decisions for loved ones who are no longer able to make decisions for themselves.

Friendship of an understanding heart is the core element of ethically responsible creativity and should prevail in determining who makes what bioethical decision.

NOTES

1. T. S. Szasz and M. H. Hollender, "A Contribution to the Philosophy of Medicine: The Basic Models of the Doctor-Patient Relationship," *Archives of Internal Medicine* 97 (1956): 585–592; G. C. Graber and D. C. Thomasma, *Theory and Practice in Medical Ethics* (New York: Continuum, 1969); R. M. Veatch, "Models for Ethical Medicine in a Revolutionary Age," *Hastings Center Report* 2, no. 3 (1972): 5–7; W. T. Reich, "Narrative Bioethics: Some Comments for the SHHV Panel on Literature and Medicine" (paper delivered at the SHHV Meeting, Memphis, Tennessee, November 20, 1992); P. Benner, "Discovering Challenges to Ethical Theory in Experienced-Based Narratives of Nurses' Everyday Ethical Comportment."
2. M. N. Sheehan, "Technology, Older Persons and the Doctor-Patient Relationship."
3. *Cruzan v. Harmon, Jasper County,* State of Missouri Circuit Court Probate Division, 1989; *Cruzan v. Department of Health* et al., 760-SW 2nd 408 (1990); *Cruzan v. Director, Missouri Department of Health et al.,* 11o S Ct. 2841, 2855-56 (1990); *Cruzan v. Harmon,* final decision in favor of Cruzans (December 14, 1990); In Re *Helga Wanglie,* Fourth Judicial District Court, Probate Court Division, PX-91-283, Hennepin County, Minnesota; A. M. Capron, "In Re Helga Wanglie," *Hastings Center Report* (1991): 26–28.
4. K. D. Clouser and B. Gert, "A Critique of Principlism," *Journal of Medicine and Philosophy* 15 (1990): 219–36.
5. E. D. Pellegrino and D. C. Thomasma, *The Virtues in Medicine Practice* (New York: Oxford University Press, 1993). Perhaps in the ultimate analysis ERC is a virtue model.
6. Reich, "Narrative Bioethics."
7. In my courses for medical and nursing students, I describe values as important physical, intellectual, spiritual, moral/ethical social considerations necessary in the framework of human existence. The list of values is open-ended, and the students have offered the following: life itself; personal quality of life; environmental, social, and global quality of life; evolving self; family; friends; society; government (structure and persons); internationalism; money; sex and sexuality; professional occupation; leisure; power (authority); religion (as permeating all values and preferences); education; democracy; patriotism; human freedom; principles of autonomy, nonmalfeasance, beneficence, benevolence, justice; law and order; ethnicity; race; cultural pluralism; love.
8. B. Chell, "Competency: What It Is, What It Isn't and Why It Matters," in *Medical Ethics: A Guide for Health Professionals*, ed. J. F. Monagle and D. C. Thomasma (Gaithersburg, Md.: Aspen Publishers, Inc., 1988), 99–108.
9. S. H. Miles, "Medical Futility," Chapter 25 above (see note 8); R. Truog et al., "The Problem with Futility," Chapter 26 above (see note 8).
10. The term *comfortable* refers to those decisions that cannot be said to be good or bad, right or wrong. This is not intended to establish an emotional tenderness that leads to mayhem; rather it brings to a resolution the conflict when both sides are *right and wrong* at the same time in the same case; R. S. Loewy, "Relationships in Health Care Revisited," Chapter 40 above (see note 8).
11. J. F. Monagle, *Risk Management: A Guide For Health Care Professionals* (Gaithersburg, Md.: Aspen Publishers, Inc., 1985); A. Gruber, "Social Systems and Professional Responsibility," Chapter 16 above (see note 8). Gruber calls for more professionals and citizens to become participants in bioethical decision making.
12. For example, the Oregon Plan (disallowed by former President George Bush as discriminatory against the disabled and approved by President Bill Clinton provided that the discrimination is eliminated).
13. W. A. Atchley, "Beyond Autonomy: New International Perspectives for Bioethics," taken from the brochure announcing the Third Annual Congress, International Bioethics Institute, April 16–18, 1993, San Francisco, California.
14. Nancy Beth Cruzan was age 30 when she suffered her injuries in an automobile accident; she was married; Paul, her husband, had the marriage dissolved within the first year after the accident. She was not totally brain dead; there was limited response to painful stimuli. See *U.S. Law Week*, 26 June 1990.
15. *U.S. Law Week*, 26 June 1990.
16. Monagle, *Risk Management.*
17. *Cruzan v. Harmon.*
18. Justices Brennan, Marshall, and Blackmun dissented. In their dissenting opinion, they wrote that "the parents' interest is fundamental . . . the court failed to consider statements Nancy had made to family members and a close friend" (*U.S. Law Week*, 26 June 1990, 436).
19. L. R. Churchill, "When Patients or Families Demand Too Much," Chapter 27 above (see note 8).
20. M. Angell, "The Case of Helga Wanglie: A New Kind of Right to Die Case," *New England Journal of Medicine*, 325 (1991): 92–93.
21. In the *Cruzan* case, the United States Supreme Court questioned the right of autonomy of an incompetent patient: "This does not mean that an incompetent person should possess the same right (of autonomy) since such a person is unable to make an informed and voluntary choice to exercise that right or any other right" (*U.S. Law Week*, 26 June 1990, 419, footnote B).

22. Thomasma and Monagle, "Hospital Ethics Committees," Chapter 43 above.
23. Monagle, *Risk Management.*
24. Clouser and Gert, "A Critique of Principlism."
25. Aristotle, *Nicomachean Ethics*, trans. Martin Ostwold (New York: Bobbs-Merrill, 1962). I find an extraordinarily satisfying sense of completeness in Aristotle's treatment of the nature of friendship.

    BK VIII, 1156A, 10—*to chresimon.*

    BK VIII, 1156A, 12—*to hedo.*

    BK VIII, 1156, 6—*to agathon.*

    BK VIII, 1156, 13–17—"the other is worthy of affection because of the other's goodness in an unqualified sense"—friendship *to agathon.*

    BK IX, 1171A, 11—love is a hyperbole of friendship.

    BK VIII, 1159B, 29–32—"friends hold in common what they have (hold)."

    BK IV, 1126B, 19–20: acquaintances and friendliness.

    BK VIII, 1156A, 15–21: no longer a useful friendship.

    BK VIII, 1155A, 2–5: friendship as excellence or virtue.

    BK VIII, 1155A, 14: friendship as virtue.
26. P. Ramsey, *The Patient as Person* (New Haven, Conn.: Yale University Press, 1970).
27. Aristotle, *Nicomachean Ethics*, note 25.
28. E. D. Pellegrino, "Educating the Humanist Physician: An Ancient Ideal Reconsidered," *JAMA* 227 (1974): 1290. This article is sensitive, scholarly, and insightful. It explains the two basic components, their meanings, and their importance in medical education. One component is cognitive; the other is affective. I am emphasizing the affective component in this chapter.
29. "We now live in an era in which the ancient and long-standing image of the physician as a benign authoritarian is intolerable to most educated people. Patients have the right to make choices among alternative modes of management in keeping with the values they conceive to be most important to them. The physician must understand the basis of the patient's value choices, respect them and work within their confines much more sensitively than ever before. In a matter so personal as health, the imposition of one person's values over another's—even of the physician's over the patient's—is a moral injustice" (Pellegrino, "Educating the Humanist Physician," 1293).
30. Compassion as *philanthropia* "Compassion means co-suffering, the capacity and the willingness of the physician *somehow* to share in the pain and anguish of those who seek help from him/her . . . to see the situation as the patient does . . . to 'feel' along with the patient. When it is genuine, compassion is unmistakenly sensed by the patient and it cannot be feigned" (Pellegrino, "Educating the Humanist Physician," 1290); M. N. Sheehan, "Technology, Older Patients, and the Doctor-Patient Relationship."
31. Pellegrino, "Educating the Humanist Physician," 1290.
32. The lack of payment by the patient or family may be an expression of ethical or legal dissatisfaction with the physician's behavior, knowledge, or skill.
33. Aristotle, *Nicomachean Ethics.*
34. Aristotle, *Nicomachean Ethics*, note 25.
35. Ibid.
36. Friendship of an understanding heart—the wisdom of Solomon. In "Narrative Bioethics," Warren Reich reflects on the parable of the Good Samaritan, a religious narrative that has also had an impact on secular culture. I hope that the wisdom of Solomon might be able to influence the behavior of health care professionals. Medicine is an inexact, fallible science, and no one has all the answers: "Oh Lord, my God, you have made me your servant, king to succeed my father David: but I am a mere youth, not knowing at all how to act. I serve you in the midst of the people whom you have chosen, a people so vast that it cannot be numbered or counted. Give your servant, therefore *an understanding heart* to judge your people and to distinguish right from wrong. For who is able to govern this vast people of yours?" (1 Kings 3:7–9).
37. C. Sabatino, "Surrogate Decision-Making in Healthcare," *Real Property, Probate and Trust Law*, June 1992, 74–82; J. A. Menikoff et al., "Beyond Advance Directives: Health Care Surrogate," *New England Journal of Medicine* 327 (1992): 1165–69.

CHAPTER 53

Bioethics as Social Problem Solving

Paul T. Durbin

> Although situational or act-oriented theories recognize rules, they treat them as summary rules or rules of thumb that are expendable. Their hypothesis is that moral rules summarize the wisdom of the past by expressing better and worse ways to handle recurring problems. Such rules assist deliberation but can be set aside at any time according to the demands of the situation. . . . We have argued against this interpretation of moral rules.
>
> — Tom L. Beauchamp and James F. Childress

What I offer here are some philosophical reflections on bioethics[1] roughly in the last quarter of the twentieth century. I offer the reflections in the spirit of American pragmatism—not the recent version of Richard Rorty[2] but the older, progressive tradition of John Dewey[3] and George Herbert Mead[4] and the still older views of William James.[5]

BIOETHICS PHILOSOPHICALLY CONSTRUED

Robert Veatch quotes a representative of the American Medical Association as saying it is not up to philosophers but to the medical profession to set its moral rules:

> So long as a preponderance of the providers of medical service—particularly physicians—feel that the weight of the evidence favors the concept that the public may be better served—that the greatest good may be best accomplished—by a profession exercising its own responsibility to the state or to someone else, then the medical profession has an ethical responsibility to exert itself in making apparent the superiorities of [this] system.[6]

Veatch cites this claim in a book that places it in a broader context, within a framework of "different systems or traditions of medical ethics . . . including the Hippocratic tradition, various Western religions, ethical systems derived from secular philosophical thought, and ethics grounded in philosophical and religious systems of non-Western cultures"[7] (e.g., China and India, but also the old Soviet Union and Islamic countries). Nonetheless, Veatch takes it to be obvious that any such profession-related or parochial or denominational system of medical or health care ethics requires "critical thinking" about "how an ethic for medicine should be grounded."[8]

Far and away the most popular summation of this foundational approach is provided in Tom Beauchamp and James Childress's *Principles of Biomedical Ethics*.[9] According to Albert Jonsen, a critic of this approach, the first edition of the *Principles* filled a vacuum in the early years of the bioethics movement; it "provided the emerging field of bioethics with a methodology" that was in line with "the currently accepted approaches of moral philosophy" and thus could be readily taught and employed by practitioners.[10]

Jonsen goes on to provide a neat summary: "That method consisted of an exposition of the two major 'ethical theories,' deontology and teleology, and a treatment of four principles, autonomy, nonmaleficence, beneficence, and justice, in the light of those theories."[11] Jonsen adds that "the four principles have become the mantra of bioethics, invoked constantly in discussions of cases and analyses of issues."[12]

While Jonsen is critical of the Beauchamp-Childress approach, he recognizes that it is reflective of "currently accepted approaches in moral philosophy." As witness to this, two other popular textbooks, although broader in scope than *Principles*, can be cited.

Michael Bayles, in *Professional Ethics*,[13] provides what is probably the most widely used single-author textbook for professional ethics generally. Like Beauchamp, Bayles is a utilitarian, but his approach can be adapted easily to any other ethical theory. Bayles endorses a general rule: "When in doubt, the guide suggested here is to ask what norms reasonable persons [generally, not just in the professions] would accept for a society in which they expected to live."[14] He goes on, however, with this summary of the view he elaborates later in the book:

> There are several levels of justification. An ethical theory is used to justify social values. These values can be used to justify norms. The norms can be either universal (applying to everyone) or role related (applying only to persons in the roles). Roles are defined by norms indicating the qualifications for persons occupying them and the type of acts they may do, such as represent clients in court. Norms can then be used to justify conduct.[15]

This exactly parallels the model used by Beauchamp and Childress.[16]

Joan Callahan's *Ethical Issues in Professional Life*,[17] while perhaps not as popular as Bayles's textbook, is also widely used. It is perhaps most notable for its dependence on the notion of "wide reflective equilibrium." As her sources, Callahan cites John Rawls, Norman Daniels, and Kai Nielsen, but she could as easily have cited dozens of other philosophers espousing one version or another of what Kurt Baier calls the "moral point of view." Here is how Callahan's summary of the approach begins:

> Things are much the same in ethics [as in science]. We begin with our "moral data" (i.e., our strongest convictions of what is right or wrong in clear-cut cases) and move from here to generate principles for behavior that we can use for decision making in cases where what should be done is less clear.[18]

This lays out the top-down, theory-to-decision approach. Then Callahan says,

> But, as in science, we sometimes have to reject our initial intuitions about what is right or wrong since they violate moral principles we have come to believe are surely correct. Thus, we realize we must dismiss the initial judgment as being the product of mere prejudice or conditioning rather than a judgment that can be supported by morally acceptable principles.[19]

This is the application part, but Callahan immediately adds the other pole in the dynamic equilibrium: "On the other hand, sometimes we are so certain that a given action would be wrong (or right) that we see we must modify our moral principles to accommodate that judgment."[20]

This exactly reflects the view of Beauchamp and Childress as stated in this passage:

> Moral experience and moral theories are dialectically related: We develop theories to illuminate experience and to determine what we ought to do, but we also use experience to test, corroborate, and revise theories. If a theory yields conclusions at odds with

> our ordinary judgments—for example, if it allows human subjects to be used merely as means to the ends of scientific research—we have reason to be suspicious of the theory and to modify it or seek an alternative theory.[21]

Jonsen believes that the term *theory* here is being used very loosely,[22] but if we employ different terms and talk simply about different approaches to ethics, it is clear that some authors have opted for other approaches to bioethics that they think are more congruent with their experiences. A notable example is the team of Edmund Pellegrino and David Thomasma, who say they base their approach on Aristotle and phenomenology—but mostly on good clinical practice.[23]

In one of their books devoted to the foundations of bioethics, Pellegrino and Thomasma summarize their approach:

> Our moral choices are more difficult, more subtle, and more controversial than those of [an earlier] time. We must make them without the heritage of shared values that could unify the medical ethics of [that] era. Our task is not to abandon hope in medical ethics, but to undertake what Camus called "the most difficult task of all: to reconsider everything from the ground up, so as to shape a living society inside a dying society." That task is not the demolition of the edifice of medical morality, but its reconstruction along three lines we have delineated: (1) replacement of a monolithic with a modular structure for medical ethics, with special emphasis on the ethics of making moral choices in clinical decisions; (2) clarification of what we mean when we speak of the good of the patient, and setting some priority among the several senses in which that term may be taken; and (3) refurbishing the ideal of a profession as a true "consecration."[24]

The Pellegrino and Thomasma approach has much in common with the virtue ethic of Alasdair MacIntyre.[25] And the more recent of the two Pellegrino and Thomasma books on foundations culminates in what they call "a physician's commitment to promoting the patient's good." This updated Hippocratic-type oath has an overarching principle—devotion to the good of the patient—and 13 obligations that are said to flow from it. These range from putting the patient's good above the physician's self-interest through respecting colleagues in other health professions and accepting patients' beliefs and decisions to embodying the principles in professional life.[26] While admitting that such an oath is not likely to meet with general acceptance "given the lack of consensus on moral principles" today, Pellegrino and Thomasma end with this plea: "We invite our readers to consider this amplification of our professional commitment as a means of meriting the trust patients must place in us and as a recognition of the centrality of the patient in all clinical decisions."[27]

The Pellegrino and Thomasma reference to the current lack of a consensus on moral principles hints at a fundamental problem for bioethics. What are decision makers to do if, as seems almost inevitable, defenders of conflicting approaches to bioethics cannot reach agreement? If those attempting to justify particular ethical decisions cannot themselves reach a decision, are we unjustified in the meantime in the decisions that we do make? Beauchamp and Childress attempt to play down this issue, at least as regards utilitarian and deontological theories: "The fact that no currently available theory, whether rule utilitarian or rule deontological, adequately resolves all moral conflicts points to their incompleteness."[28] Admitting that there are many forms of consequentialism, utilitarianism, and deontology, as well as approaches that emphasize virtues or rights, they conclude by defending a *process*—which they say "is consistent with both a rule-utilitarian and a rule-deontology theory"—rather than providing an absolute theoretical justification.[29]

Not all bioethicists are satisfied with this treatment of theoretical disagreement. H. Tristram Engelhardt in particular has devoted much time and energy to arriving at a more satisfying solution.[30] He begins his daunting effort to provide a true foundation for bioethics with a framework: "Controversies regarding which lines of conduct are proper can be resolved on the basis of (1) force, (2) conversion of one party to the other's viewpoint, (3) sound argument, and (4) agreed-to procedures."[31] Engelhardt then demolishes the first three as legitimate foundations for the resolution of ethical disagreement, beginning with the easiest: "Brute force is simply brute force. A goal of ethics is to determine when force can be justified. Force by itself carries no moral authority."[32]

Engelhardt then attacks any assumed religious foundation for the resolution of moral controversy, calling "the failure of Christendom's hope" to provide such a foundation, either in the Middle Ages or after the Reformation, a major failure. He then adds, "This failure suggests that it is hopeless to suppose that a general moral consensus will develop regarding any of the major issues in bioethics."[33]

Engelhardt then turns to properly philosophical hopes: "The third possibility is that of achieving moral authority through successful rational arguments to establish a particular view of the good moral life."[34] But he adds immediately, "This Enlightenment attempt to provide a rationally justified, concrete view of the good life, and thus a secular surrogate for the moral claims of Christianity, has not succeeded."[35] The evidence for this Engelhardt supplied earlier—and it parallels the obvious disagreements among schools of thought referred to by Beauchamp and Childress.

This leaves only the fourth possibility: "The only mode of resolution is by agreement. . . . One will need to discover an inescapable procedural basis for ethics."[36] This may sound like Beauchamp and Childress's retreat to process, but Engelhardt wants to make more of it than that:

> This [procedural] basis, if it is to be found at all, will need to be disclosable in the very nature of ethics itself. . . . Such a basis appears to be available in the minimum notion of ethics. . . . If one is interested in resolving moral controversies without recourse to force as the fundamental basis of agreement, then one will have to accept peaceable negotiation among members of the controversy as the process for attaining the resolution of concrete moral controversies.[37]

This, Engelhardt says, should "be recognized as a disclosure, to borrow a Kantian metaphor, of a transcendental condition . . . of the minimum grammar involved in speaking rationally of blame and praise, and in establishing any particular set of moral commitments."[38]

The generally poor reception that Engelhardt's foundational efforts have received[39] as opposed to the wide recognition he has received for particular contributions to the discussion of concrete controversies, might suggest that there is something fundamentally wrong about the search for ultimate ethical justification in bioethics.

This suggestion leads to the final group of authors to be mentioned in these reflections on philosophical bioethics. Albert Jonsen, mentioned earlier as a critic of the Beauchamp-Childress approach, says this:

> In light of the diversity of views about the meaning and role of ethical theory in moral philosophy, we need not be surprised at the confusion in that branch of moral philosophy called "practical" or (with a bias toward one view of theory) "applied ethics." . . . Authors who begin their works with erudite expositions of teleology and deontology hardly mention them again when they plunge into a case. . . . It is this that the clinical ethicists notice and that leads some of them to answer the theory-practice question by wondering whether it is the right question and whether the connection between these classic antonyms is not just

> loose or tight, but even possible or relevant.[40]

Two of the authors Jonsen is referring to are himself and Stephen Toulmin, who, in *The Abuse of Casuistry*, argue for an approach in which bioethicists should "wrestle with cases of conscience . . . [where they will] find theory a clumsy and rather otiose obstacle in the way of the prudential resolution of cases."[41] Jonsen likens this to deconstruction in literary studies and the critical legal studies approach in philosophy of law; he is also explicit, in another place, about the rhetorical nature of the casuistic approach.[42] Without saddling these other authors with casuistry as *the* approach, Jonsen also puts his and Toulmin's critique of applied ethics within the recent movement of antitheorists headed by Richard Rorty and Bernard Williams.[43] (In a review of *The Abuse of Casuistry*, John Arras adds Stuart Hampshire and Annette Baier.)[44]

In short, recent bioethics, philosophically construed, is a confusing battleground, with contributions from absolute foundationalists to case-focused rejectors of theory and a variety of approaches in between (or all around).

BIOETHICS MORE BROADLY CONSTRUED

It should be remembered—for purposes of this chapter and more generally—that bioethics has never been exclusively or even primarily a philosopher's affair. Indeed, it could be claimed that philosophers are and ought to be outsiders to the real communities making the important bioethical decisions.[45]

One of the earliest calls for the post–World War II medical research community to police itself ethically came from a physician, Henry K. Beecher, writing in 1966 in the *Journal of the American Medical Association* and the *New England Journal of Medicine*—both regular sources of bioethics commentary right down to the present.[46]

Beecher's call for reform was followed up by sociologists (e.g., Bernard Barber et al., *Research on Human Subjects: Problems of Social Control in Medical Experimentation* [1973], and Renée Fox, *Experiment Perilous: Physicians Facing the Unknown* [1974]).[47] Historians also became interested (e.g., James Jones, *Bad Blood: The Tuskegee Syphilis Experiment* [1981]).[48]

Celebrated cases also did a great deal to coalesce the field, from Karen Quinlan and Elizabeth Bouvia to Jack Kevorkian, from Baby Doe to Baby M., from celebrated heart transplant cases to proposals for mandatory testing for the acquired immune deficiency syndrome (AIDS) virus.[49] What even the briefest reflection on these cases reminds us is how bioethics involves patients, families, hospital administrators, lawyers and judges, government officials, and even the public at large.

And public involvement reminds us, further, that significant numbers of commissions have been involved, at the local level (e.g., the New York State Task Force on Life and the Law), at the national level (e.g., the National Commission for the Protection of Human Subjects of Biomedical and Behavioral Research; the President's Commission for the Study of Ethical Problems in Medicine and Biomedical and Behavioral Research), and at the international level (e.g., the European Forum of Medical Associations).

Philosophers have, obviously, been involved in setting up prestigious bioethics institutes. But the institutes themselves are important parts of the bioethics community, with impressive numbers of nonphilosophers on their mailing lists. And physicians (e.g., Willard Gaylin at the Hastings Center, along with many others) and laypeople (the Kennedy family, who support the Kennedy Institute) have also played major roles.

For me, the proper locus of bioethics decision making is in typically small groups of physicians, nurses, administrators, lawyers, and local public officials—together with patients and their families—wrestling with specific cases and issues within their own communities. This type of group decision making is exemplified in *Moral Problems in Medicine*, one of the earliest bioethics textbooks (1976), which had six coeditors and at least another half-dozen people directly involved.[50] And it continues right down to the present, most notably in the incredible diversity of ethics committees and other groups that have sprung up in hospitals and all sorts of health care institutions since the promulgation of the Reagan Administration's Baby Doe regulations and the enactment of the Patient Self-Determination Act in 1991.[51] Philosophical bioethicists, it seems to me, do some of their best work in these groups, as they work collectively to solve local cases and issues and to formulate policies for their own institutions.

PRAGMATIC REFLECTIONS ON PHILOSOPHICAL BIOETHICS

William James, faced at the end of the nineteenth century with the same sort of disagreement about the foundations of ethics that exists 100 years later regarding the foundations of bioethics, summed up the situation this way:

> Various essences of good have thus been found and proposed as bases of the ethical system. Thus, to be a mean between two extremes; to be recognized by a special intuitive faculty; to make the agent happy for the moment; to make others as well as him happy in the long run; to add to his perfection or dignity; to harm no one; to follow from reason or universal law; to be in accordance with the will of God; to promote the survival of the human species.[52]

But, James says, none of these has satisfied everyone. So what he thinks we must do is treat them all as having some moral force and go about satisfying as many of the claims as we can while knowing we can never satisfy all of them at once. "The guiding principle for ethical philosophy," James concludes, must be "simply to satisfy at all times *as many demands as we can*."[53] And, following this rule, society has historically striven from generation to generation "to find the more and more inclusive [moral] order"—and has, James thinks, done so successfully, gradually eliminating slavery and other evils tolerated in earlier eras.[54]

In many ways this sounds like Engelhardt's condition of the possibility of ethical discourse, but James would never accept Engelhardt's characterization of the approach as Kantian-transcendental. James is simply advocating a procedural rule to be used by particular communities of ethical truthseekers attempting to find a satisfactory concrete solution for particular problems—in a process that must inevitably go on and on without end. Concrete ethical solutions are not dictated by an abstract commitment to the conditions of ethics but must be worked out arduously through the competition of different ideals.

John Dewey was as opposed to transcendental foundations as James. He would probably have been bemused—and also angry—at the persistent academic search for an ultimate foundation for our practical decisions in bioethics.[55] He would also have attempted, however, to see how the "principled" approach (e.g., of Beauchamp and Childress) is "in effect, if not in profession connected with human affairs."[56] In *Reconstruction in Philosophy*, Dewey continues his attack on ethical theory as "hypnotized by the notion that its business is to discover some . . . ultimate and supreme law"; instead, he proposed that ethics be reconstructed so that we may "advance to a belief in a plurality of changing, moving, individualized goods and ends, and to a belief that principles, criteria, laws are intellectual instruments for analyzing individual or unique situations."[57] In *A Common Faith*, Dewey adds that community efforts to solve social problems progressively can generate an attitude akin to religious faith that makes social problem solving a meaningful venture.[58] And in *Liberalism and Social Action*, Dewey tries to lead the way in applying his approach to the "confusion, uncertainty, and conflict" that marked his times,[59] just as the bioethics community is attempting to do today with respect to the confusion, uncertainty, and conflict plaguing health care today.

George Herbert Mead, an opponent of both utilitarian and Kantian approaches to ethics,[60] offers in place of those a positive formulation of what ethics should mean:

> The order of the universe that we live in *is* the moral order. It has become the moral order by becoming the self-conscious method of the members of a human society. . . . The world that comes to us from the past possesses and controls us. We possess and control the world that we discover and invent. And this is the world of the moral order.[61]

Then Mead adds, "It is a splendid adventure if we can rise to it."[62]

If we pay attention to these American pragmatists, I think what we can say about bioethics in the last quarter of the twentieth century is that philosophers contribute most when they contribute to the progressive social problem solving of particular communities (e.g., policy formulation, case resolution, etc.). Some do this, admittedly, at the national or even international level, but even in those cases they do so as members of groups that include physicians, lawyers, and other concerned citizens. And most do so at the local level—where, in Mead's words, they are only being truly ethical if they are contributing to the social problem solving of some particular group in which they represent only one voice, and a small one at that.

SOME LESSONS

Does the awareness on the part of philosophers of their limited role in bioethics suggest any lessons for us?

The most obvious lesson is humility. Philosophers can and do help to clarify issues (sometimes even provide answers), but the real moral decisions in bioethics, for the most part, are made by others.

Another lesson has to do with the urgency of the real-world problems that bioethics faces, which are, after all, what got philosophers involved in the first place. Medicine and the health care system generally—including those parts of it that operate in open or covert opposition to the entrenched power of physicians and hospitals—face enormous problems today, from rampant inflation and calls for rationing to the questioning of the very legitimacy of high-technology medicine. All the while, doctors, nurses, and other providers must continue to face life-and-death issues every day, not to mention the daunting task of treating the ordinary ills of ordinary people who, with increasing frequency, cannot pay for their medical care.

It is probably inevitable, given the structure of philosophy today as an academic institution, that philosophical bioethicists will continue narrow technical debates among themselves about ultimate justifications of bioethical decisions. But academicism and careerism in bioethics should be recognized for what they are—distractions (however necessary, for some purposes) from the *real* focus of bioethics.

Beyond these lessons for philosophers, does American pragmatism have any lessons to teach the bioethics community more generally? Probably only this: that we should all heed James's call for tolerance and openness to minority views. Bioethics has come a long way in just 25 or so years. Significant consensus has been achieved on issues from informed consent to be a research subject to the importance of asking patients what they want done, if anything, in their last weeks and days and hours. But equally significant issues remain, as they always will in a society open to change. And all of us, from the smallest local bioethics group to the international community, ought to remain open to change. As William James said,

> Every now and then . . . someone is born with the right to be original, and his revolutionary thought or action may bear prosperous fruit. He may replace old "laws of nature" by better ones; he may, by breaking old moral rules in a certain place, bring in a total condition of things more ideal than would have followed had the rules been kept.[63]

NOTES

1. A brief survey of the numerous textbooks in the field suggests that *bioethics*, although not the only label, is probably the most common one.
2. See R. Rorty, *Philosophy and the Mirror of Nature* (Princeton, N.J.: Princeton University Press, 1979); *id., Consequences of Pragmatism* (Minneapolis, Minn.: University of Minnesota Press, 1982); *id., Objectivity, Relativism, and Truth* (New York: Cambridge University Press, 1991).
3. The works in the Dewey corpus that I will refer to are *The Quest for Certainty* (New York: Putnam's, 1929); *Reconstruction in Philosophy*, 2d ed. (Boston: Beacon Press, 1948); *A Common Faith* (New Haven, Conn.: Yale University Press, 1934); and *Liberalism and Social Action* (New York: Putnam's, 1935).
4. See especially G. H. Mead, "Scientific Method and the Moral Sciences," in *Selected Writings: George Herbert Mead*, ed. A. Reck (Indianapolis, Ind.: Bobbs-Merrill, 1964), 248–66.
5. The article I refer to is W. James, "The Moral Philosopher and the Moral Life," in *The Will to Believe, and Other Essays in Popular Philosophy* (New York: Holt, 1897), reprinted in *The Writings of William James*, ed. J. McDermott (New York: Random House, 1967), 610–29.
6. R. B. Roth, "Medicine's Ethical Responsibilities," *JAMA* 215 (1971): 1956–58, reprinted in *Cross Cultural Perspectives in Medical Ethics: Readings*, ed. R. M. Veatch (Boston: Jones and Bartlett, 1989), 155.
7. Veatch, *Cross Cultural Perspectives*, 146.
8. Ibid.
9. T. L. Beauchamp and J. F. Childress, *Principles of Biomedical Ethics*, 3d ed. (New York: Oxford University Press, 1989); Also see: T. L. Beauchamp and J. F. Childress, *Principles of Biomedical Ethics,* 4th ed. (New York: Oxford University Press, 1994).
10. A. R. Jonsen, "Practice versus Theory," *Hastings Center Report* 20, no. 4 (1990): 32.
11. Ibid.
12. Ibid.
13. M. Bayles, *Professional Ethics*, 2d ed. (Belmont, Calif.: Wadsworth, 1989).
14. Ibid., 28.
15. Ibid.
16. Beauchamp and Childress, *Principles of Biomedical Ethics*.
17. J. C. Callahan, ed., *Ethical Issues in Professional Life* (New York: Oxford University Press, 1988).
18. Ibid., 10.
19. Ibid.
20. Ibid.
21. Beauchamp and Childress, *Principles of Biomedical Ethics*, 15–16.
22. Jonsen, "Practice versus Theory," 34.
23. E. D. Pellegrino and D. C. Thomasma, *A Philosophical Basis of Medical Practice* (New York: Oxford University Press, 1981), xi.
24. E. D. Pellegrino and D. C. Thomasma, *For the Patient's Good: The Restoration of Beneficence in Health Care* (New York: Oxford University Press, 1988), 134.
25. A. MacIntyre, *After Virtue* (London: Duckworth, 1981); *id., Whose Justice, Which Rationality?* (Notre Dame, Ind.: University of Notre Dame Press, 1988).
26. Pellegrino and Thomasma, *For the Patient's Good*, 205–6.
27. Ibid., 206.
28. Beauchamp and Childress, *Principles of Biomedical Ethics*, 46.
29. Ibid., 62.
30. H. T. Engelhardt, *Foundations of Bioethics* (New York: Oxford University Press, 1986); *id., Bioethics and Secular Humanism: The Search for a Common Morality* (London: SCM Press; Philadelphia: Trinity Press, 1991).
31. Engelhardt, *Foundations of Bioethics*, 30.
32. Ibid., 40.
33. Ibid.
34. Ibid.
35. Ibid.
36. Ibid., 41.
37. Ibid.
38. Ibid., 42.
39. See, for example, J. D. Moreno, "Ethics by Committee: The Moral Authority of Consensus," *Journal of Medicine and Philosophy* 13 (1988): 411–32, esp. 425ff.; K. E. Tranoy, "The Search for a Common Morality," *Medical Humanities Review* 6, no. 2 (1992): 22–25.
40. Jonsen, "Practice versus Theory," 34.
41. Ibid. The work being described is A. R. Jonsen and S. Toulmin, *The Abuse of Casuistry: A History of Moral Reasoning* (Berkeley, Calif.: University of California Press, 1988).
42. A. R. Jonsen, "Casuistry as Methodology in Clinical Ethics," *Theoretical Medicine* 12 (1991): 295–307.
43. Rorty, *Philosophy and The Mirror of Nature*; *id., Consequences of Pragmatism*; id., *Objectivity, Relativism, and Truth*; B. Williams, *Ethics and the Limits of Philosophy* (Cambridge, Mass.: Harvard University Press, 1985).

44. J. D. Arras, "Common Law Morality," *Hastings Center Report* 20, no. 4 (1990): 36; S. Hampshire, *Innocence and Experience* (Cambridge, Mass.: Harvard University Press, 1986); A. Baier, "Some Thoughts on How We Moral Philosophers Live Now," *Monist* 67 (1984): 490–97.

45. L. R. Churchill, "The Role of the Stranger: The Ethicist in Professional Education," *Hastings Center Report* 8, no. 6 (1978): 13–15.

46. H. K. Beecher, "Consent in Clinical Experimentation: Myth and Reality," *JAMA* 195 (1966): 34–35; H. K. Beecher, "Ethics and Clinical Research," *New England Journal of Medicine* 274 (1966): 1354–60.

47. B. Barber et al., *Research on Human Subjects: Problems of Social Control in Medical Experimentation* (New York: Russell Sage Foundation, 1973); R. Fox, *Experiment Perilous: Physicians Facing the Unknown* (Philadelphia: University of Pennsylvania Press, 1974).

48. J. H. Jones, *Bad Blood: The Tuskegee Syphilis Experiment,* 3d ed. (New York: The Free Press, 1993).

49. Some of the best examples are discussed in G. E. Pence, *Classic Cases in Medical Ethics,* 2nd ed. (New York: McGraw-Hill, 1995).

50. S. Gorovitz et al., *Moral Principles in Medicine* (Englewood Cliffs, N.J.: Prentice-Hall, 1976).

51. The growing literature on bioethics committees is reviewed in P. M. McCarrick, "Ethics Committees in Hospitals," *Kennedy Institute of Ethics Journal* 2 (1992): 285–305.

52. James, "Moral Philosopher and Moral Life," in *The Writings of William James*, 620.

53. Ibid., 620.

54. Ibid., 623.

55. Dewey, *The Quest for Certainty.*

56. Dewey, *Reconstruction in Philosophy*, xi.

57. Ibid., 162–63. This does not make Dewey an act utilitarian in the sense opposed by Beauchamp and Childress. Dewey, along with the other traditional pragmatists referred to here, would not have agreed with a theory/act dichotomy. Mead, for one, explicitly states that the *social praxis* of a community is the matrix within which both theories and acts emerge—and they emerge *ethically* if the social problems calling them forth are addressed in a progressive fashion (Scientific Method and the Moral Sciences).

58. Dewey, *A Common Faith*, 27.

59. Dewey, *Liberalism and Social Action*, 92.

60. See H. Joas, *G. H. Mead: A Contemporary Re-examination of His Thought* (Cambridge, Mass.: MIT Press, 1985), 124.

61. Mead, "Scientific Method and the Moral Sciences," 266.

62. Ibid.

63. James, "Moral Philosopher and Moral Life," in *The Writings of William James*, 625.

Chapter 54

Intercultural Reasoning: The Challenge for International Bioethics

Patricia A. Marshall, David C. Thomasma, and Jurrit Bergsma

The exportation of Western biomedicine throughout the world has not resulted in a systematic homogenization of scientific ideology but rather in the proliferation of many forms and practices of biomedicine. Similarly, in the last decade, bioethics has become increasingly an international enterprise. Although there may be consensus regarding the inherent value of ethical discourse as it relates to health and medical care, there are disagreements about the nature and parameters of medical morality. This lack of consensus exists because our beliefs about morality are culturally constituted, embedded in social, religious, and political ideologies that influence particular individuals and communities at specific historical moments.[1]

In a world of cultural pluralism and ethnic diversity, is it possible to achieve consensus when we talk about medical ethics and moral values? To date, little attention has been given to cross-cultural issues in bioethics. Veatch's[2] book on cross-cultural medical ethics addressed, to a certain extent, medical traditions in non-Western societies. More recently, Pellegrino and associates[3] explored problems confronting transcultural bioethics. Although sociologists such as Fox and Swazey[4] and a handful of anthropologists[5] have examined cultural factors associated with health care ethics, significant questions remain. Of particular importance are questions concerning the cultural assumptions that inform our beliefs about the significance and relevance of bioethics for the art and practice of healing.

In this chapter, we describe several examples illustrating cross-cultural dissonance regarding bioethical issues. These examples suggest that problems are associated with divergent beliefs about the meaning and perceived value of ethical concepts and medical practices. We argue that the tension among objective, rational, and analytical ethics on one hand and the complicated reality of lived experience in disparate cultural worlds on the other hand can be minimized. Intercultural bioethics discourse is enhanced when there is at least minimal agreement over the process of moral reasoning and a shared understanding about the context of particular medical practices. Finally, respect for cultural differences must be maintained without sacrificing the value placed on basic human rights.

INTERCULTURAL EXPERIENCES IN BIOETHICS REASONING

The following examples of recent experiences demonstrate difficulties in translating and transferring insights from one culture to another in bioethics. The selection of cases is somewhat arbitrary and calls attention to problems surrounding both conceptual issues and specific

Source: P. Marshall, D. C. Thomasma, and J. Bergsma, Intercultural Reasoning: The Challenge for International Bioethics, *Cambridge Quarterly of Healthcare Ethics,* Vol. 3, pp. 321–328, © 1994, Reprinted with the permission of Cambridge University Press.

applications of medical technology. We use these examples to examine some of the concepts at risk of being misunderstood and misperceived in the process of translation between disciplines and nationalities.

The Historical Importance of Autonomy

Increasingly, as bioethicists in the United States encounter their colleagues from other parts of the world, assumptions concerning both the meaning and the primacy of autonomy as an ethical concept become painfully obvious. In 1984, the Dutch Philosophy of Medicine Society held a conference to critique a new book by Pellegrino and Thomasma on the philosophy of medicine.[6] During the conference, Dutch professors criticized the authors' assumptions about individualism, individual rights, and the importance of the individual patient in the doctor-patient relationship. Exasperated, at one point, Thomasma, who was attending the meeting, made the claim that everyone would agree that the notion of individualism was the most revolutionary concept in human history because it set limits on the ability of the state and the community to govern individuals. None of the 40 professionals attending the conference in the Netherlands agreed with him. Thomasma was shocked to learn that they considered socialism to be far more revolutionary than individualism. Thomasma later returned to the United States and wrote about this difference.[7]

The Ethics of Abortion for Sexual Preference

For some time, procedures have been available for early diagnosis of genetic abnormalities in fetuses. Poor prognosis, a very poor projected quality of life, concerns about preventing psychological and social harms for the parents, and the enormous financial burden on society are just some of the reasons impelling prospective parents to choose aborting the fetus rather than carrying it to term. The use of ultrasound techniques to detect fetal abnormality is considered routine medical care by Western nations.

During a 1992 international bioethics conference in Amsterdam, however, participants were told of a study in New Delhi that found that roughly 8,300 abortions were performed in clinics employing some of the same fetal diagnostic techniques. Almost 7,900 of these aborted fetuses were female. In this case, the procedure was being used not to diagnose deformities but to identify gender. Because of cultural, social, and economic circumstances, female babies were not valued as much as male babies.

Upon hearing this, participants from the Western nations were stunned. They regarded this practice not only as a misuse of medical technology but also as an extreme form of sexual discrimination.

Pluralism without Relativism

At the same 1992 international conference, a Spanish philosopher of medicine gave one of the introductory lectures in English. During the lecture, in an almost reverent overtone, he spoke of the need to respect pluralism but immediately qualified his statement with a strong admonition against relativism.

After the speech, a Dutchman, an American, several other Spanish colleagues of the philosopher, and other Spanish-speaking bioethicists, physicians, and lawyers were conversing. The American noted how difficult it was for him to understand how the speaker could respect pluralism without at least some degree of relativism, because for the American the word *pluralism,* suggested, to a certain extent, a tolerance for relativism. The Spanish philosopher replied again that there was no room for relativism in his thinking. The Dutchman, whose country won its independence from Spain 300 years ago, launched an only slightly veiled attack on Spanish authoritarianism and Catholicism, which he understood to be the substance of the Spanish philosopher's work. This claim was vigorously denied by the philosopher. Meanwhile, his friends from Latin America started to agree with the Dutchman's perception about Spanish domination, although without forswearing their Catholic heritage. Within a matter of minutes, myriad opportunities for misunderstanding presented themselves—old political animosities, religious assumptions, Catholic rationalism versus Protestant skepticism, and New World versus Old World perceptions of reality. Although the word *relativism* was used, there were too many meanings attached to the word to provide any kind of reasonable or, as Engelhardt has called it, "peaceable" discussion of issues.[8]

The Remmelink Report

In 1992, the Dutch Remmelink Report on the nationwide status of euthanasia[9] noted that 1.8 percent of terminally ill patients in the Netherlands request euthanasia; 75 percent of these individuals want to die at home with the aid of their general practitioners. About 2,400 Dutch citizens die this way each year, 85 percent of whom are suffering from terminal cancer. Dr. Pieter Admiraal, president of the Dutch Medical Society and an early champion of euthanasia, noted that "active euthanasia can only be the last dignified act of terminal care."[10]

Following the publication of this report, there was intense criticism of a category in which cases of involuntary euthanasia were summarized. For example, a representative of the United States Bishop's pro-life secretariat claimed that the Dutch government itself had documented 1,000 cases of involuntary euthanasia, in which "physicians had killed patients without their explicit request."[11] This charge is now echoed by many health professionals, academic scholars, and the general public concerned about the Dutch experimenting with what appears to be mercy killing.

Nonetheless, the charge can be strongly disputed and has been by those skilled at caring for the hopelessly ill in clinical settings. Dr. Admiraal denied the claim that Dutch physicians are murdering unwilling and unwitting patients, noting that there has been only one such case over the past 20 years and that the physician involved was immediately and severely punished. The data on Dutch euthanasia must be read in light of clinical experience. The Dutch medical system provides medical treatment for all dying patients. The kinds of cases listed in the involuntary category in the Remmelink Report are incidents that occur frequently in medical settings worldwide. For example, a defective newborn might be denied treatment by physicians because of the severity of the problems and the grim prognosis.

Courts in the Netherlands have backed up the decision of physicians not to offer medically futile treatment and to report these cases as involuntary euthanasia. The Dutch believe that the distinction between active and passive euthanasia has no moral merit because both forms of euthanasia have the same intention—that the patient achieve relief from suffering through death.

CONCEPTS, MEANING, AND MEDICAL MORALITY IN TRANSNATIONAL CONTEXT

In the examples described, two problems emerge. First, there is confusion about the meaning and relative value of concepts such as autonomy, pluralism, and relativism. Second, clinical practices such as selective abortion and euthanasia evoke moral repugnance based on underlying normative belief systems about what is and what ought to be appropriate medical practice. Both problems call attention to the significance of cultural assumptions regarding the semantics of ethical dialects and the application of biomedical technology. At the heart of the matter is our comprehension of language and cultural context, both of which inform, maintain, and reinforce our understanding of ideal and normative moral behavior.

Pellegrino[12] observed that the challenge of transcultural biomedical ethics is "vastly complicated because medical science and technology, as well as the ethics designed to deal with its impact, currently are Western in origin." He stated that the Western values of empirical science, principle-based ethics, and democratic political philosophy "are often alien, and even antipathetic, to many non-Western world views." Yet, as we have seen, important differences also occur between individuals representing Western nationalities. The Dutch philosophers, despite their Western European identity, rejected Thomasma's claims about the overriding historical importance of autonomy. Moreover, ethnic differences in moral values related to health and illness will also occur within Western societies. Murray,[13] for example, called attention to the African-American history of dehumanization and discrimination, which results in an equal emphasis placed on values such as self-determination, truth telling, and social justice.

The preoccupation with autonomy and self-determination in Western bioethics, especially among United States bioethicists, is indicative of the extent to which cultural values influence our orientation to biomedical morality. Our beliefs about personhood and autonomy inform every aspect of medical transactions, including notions about informed consent and confidentiality in the patient-physician relationship. In the United States and other Western nations, the individual is identified as the locus of decisional capacity for informed consent. This concept is meaningless in societies that stress the overriding importance of an individual's relationship to family and community. In these contexts, decisional capacity is socially, not individually, expressed. Similarly, the notion that one's privacy and confidentiality should be respected is thought to be a shared ideal in Western cultures. However, this does not necessarily constitute a universal value. Social science research on beliefs and norms associated with the cultural construction of the self indicate significant variability concerning the relative importance of privacy.[14]

In addition to problems surrounding differences in perceptions about the meaning and value of ethical concepts, language barriers may also hinder communication among professionals attempting to discuss biomedical and ethical problems. Studies have shown, for example, that in cross-cultural clinical settings, the subtleties of dialect and the social nuances of interpersonal communication present obstacles to the consent process.[15] The linguistic framing of discourse on ethics has important implications for those seeking to bridge transcultural divides in bioethics. Does the bioethicist need to be a cultural and conversational insider to access the relevant language necessary to talk with colleagues from other countries? This question raises additional concerns about the necessity of linguistic and social convergence before understanding can be achieved. The miscommunications that occurred between the Dutch, United States, Latin American, and Spanish philosophers in their attempts to clarify relativism and pluralism demonstrate the potential for bioethical cacophony.

Knowledge of cultural context can reduce dissonance in transcultural bioethics discussion and strengthen communication. As noted earlier, the Dutch have been strongly criticized for practicing euthanasia. In particular, cases of involuntary euthanasia have elicited condemnation. Yet, there might be less criticism of involuntary euthanasia if opponents understood the meaning of the practice in social context and the specific requirements for withdrawing or withholding care. For example, although refusal of treatment for defective newborns is routinely practiced in the United States, it is characterized as a tragic but compassionate necessity, not as involuntary euthanasia. The Dutch use of the classification "involuntary euthanasia" illustrates the power of language to confound cross-cultural communication. Lack of clinical insights that elaborate contextual detail can severely impair the translation of concepts and information between cultures.

Another aspect of cultural context relates to the problem of ethical relativism. Many individuals find the practice of euthanasia and physician-assisted suicide morally reprehensible; similarly, most Westerners would agree that there is absolutely nothing socially redeeming about the practice of selective abortion on the basis of gender, which was reported to occur in New Delhi. Often, these practices evoke deep-seated reactions, reflecting the strength of our moral enculturation.

Anthropologists have engaged in prolonged debates about the theoretical and social utility of ethical relativism as it relates to cultural context.[16] A full discussion of the issues, however, is beyond the scope of this chapter. Simply stated, the problem with ethical relativism, in its broadest conceptualization, is that it seems to condone every permutation of human behavior. As Brown[17] pointed out (p. 86), "Ethical relativism is troubling because it leaves little basis for judging something to be wrong or harmful if it is to be considered only in the context in which it 'makes sense.'" Schweder[18] argued for a "qualified version of ethical relativism," noting that profound differences may exist between the moral codes of different people, but there is more than one moral code that can be rationally defended. Along different lines, Renteln[19] characterized relativism as a metaethical theory about the nature of moral perceptions and suggested that relativism is compatible with cross-cultural universals, which could indicate support for particular human rights.

CONCLUSION

The movement toward international debate regarding ethics and biomedicine will continue to grow. Consensus on issues may not always be feasible. However, several conditions for international intercultural discourse about biomedical ethics are essential for effective development of the discipline.

First, minimal agreement must be reached regarding the language, meaning, and value of ethical concepts and processes of moral reasoning. This agreement will require explicit self-critical attention to the meaning of concepts and their cultural context in ways that have not yet been present in the international dialogue.

Second, there must be a commitment to discerning cultural context. Bioethicists can be the beneficiaries of the richness that characterizes cultural diversity if opportunities are created to experience the challenge of transcultural dialogue. Yet, this challenge will require a new and perhaps uneasy acceptance (for some) of pluralism. As Marshall pointed out (p. 62),

> One person's truth is another's conundrum. . . . This perhaps is the key to understanding the subjective phenomenology and cultural diversity in questions of medical ethics. Whose judgment is correct? Where does the ownership of legitimacy reside? At the individual level, the answers to these questions are easier: the "right" morality is an expression of the heart as much as it is the head, and here we can all claim authority. But in matters of public policy, both nationally and internationally, the answers become distressingly clouded and ambiguous. Individuals may experience an abandonment of their particular "truth," and the struggle for ethical dominance and control over medical discourse and technology becomes voluble.[20]

Third, more serious philosophical work must be done on transcultural structures in human behavior and existence. One such structure may be that of human rights.

The first conference on human rights in 25 years was sponsored by the United Nations in 1993 in Vienna. Some countries, such as China, argued that nations with a different, more communal tradition should be exempt from now-standard international expectations about respecting human rights. China argued, for example, that human rights should be secondary to the needs of the state, such as law and order. This objection was roundly rejected by the majority of countries in the world.[21] In fact, the conference ended with a proposal that the U.N. establish an office of high commissioner to protect and promote human rights around the world. The conference reaffirmed the universality of human rights against a concerted effort to subordinate them to the state or to cultural considerations.[22] The same conference recognized that "women's rights are an inalienable, integral, and indivisible part of universal human rights."[23]

Such widespread theoretical acceptance of fundamental human rights around the world demonstrates that, to a large degree, our international expectations regarding individual rights help shape progress in developing our conceptions about how these rights are to be implemented. Bioethicists need to examine whether there is a basis in the structures of human existence for such rights. Just as the Roman Empire developed the Stoic theory of natural rights into a system of law, so too must we develop a newer and more sophisticated theory of natural law for the modern era. Another example of this kind of transcultural work can be found in Erich Loewy's efforts to ground ethics in the physiological capacity to suffer.

Fourth, as a consequence of the above conditions, discourse about biomedical ethics must have some a priori commitments present on the table. Among candidates for such commitments might be the goal of assisting individuals to enhance their autonomy, their moral personhood, in decisions to be made or possibly the rights of all women in the world to control their own reproductive potential. Still other candidates might include those that emerge from our collective experience in reaching a consensus about actions to be taken through ethics committee deliberations or national policy committees.

NOTES

1. W. Effelsberg and F. J. Illhardt, "Kultur und Medizin," *Curare: Zeitschrift fuer Ethnomedizin und transkulturelle Psychiatrie* 15, no. 3 (1992): 161–64.
2. R. M. Veatch, *Cross Cultural Perspectives in Medical Ethics: Readings* (Boston: Jones and Bartlett, 1989).
3. E. D. Pellegrino et al., *Transcultural Dimensions in Medical Ethics* (Frederick, Md.: University Publishing Group, 1992).
4. R. C. Fox and J. P. Swazey, "Medical Morality Is Not Bioethics: Medical Ethics in China and the United States," *Perspectives in Biology and Medicine* 27 (1984): 336–60.
5. P. M. Marshall, "Anthropology and Bioethics," *Medical Anthropology Quarterly* 6, no. 1 (1992): 49–73; P. Kunstadter, "Medical Ethics in Cross-cultural and Multi-cultural Perspective," *Social Science and Medicine* 14B (1980): 289–96; H. Fabrega, "An Ethnomedical Perspective of Medical Ethics," *Journal of Medicine and Philosophy* 15 (1990): 593–625; R. Lieban, "Medical Anthropology and the Comparative Study of Medical Ethics," in *Social Science Perspectives on Medical Ethics,* ed. G. Weisz (Philadelphia: University of Pennsylvania Press, 1990), 221–40.
6. E. D. Pellegrino and D. C. Thomasma, *A Philosophical Basis of Medical Practice* (New York: Oxford University Press, 1981).
7. D. C. Thomasma, "Limitations of the Autonomy Model for the Doctor-Patient Relationship," *The Pharos* 46 (1983): 2–5; *id.,* "Philosophy of Medicine in Europe: Challenges for the Future," *Theoretical Medicine* 6 (1985): 115–23; D. C. Thomasma and E. D. Pellegrino, "Challenges for a Philosophy of Medicine of the Future: A Response to Fellow Philosophers in the Netherlands," *Theoretical Medicine* 8 (1987): 187–204.
8. H. T. Englehardt Jr., *Bioethics and Secular Humanism: The Search for a Common Morality* (Philadelphia: Trinity Press International, 1991).
9. van de Rapport Commissie Onderzoek Medische Praktijk inzake Euthanasia, *Medische beslissingen roud het levenseinde* ('s-Gravenhage: Sdu Uitgeverij Plantijnstraat, 1991).
10. D. Scott, "Euthanasia: America's Next Challenge to Life," *The Evangelist* (Diocese of Albany, New York) 67, no. 4 (1992): 4.
11. Ibid.
12. E. D. Pellegrino, "Intersections of Western Biomedical Ethics and World Culture: Problematic and Possibility," *Cambridge Quarterly of Healthcare Ethics* 1 (1992): 191–96.
13. R. F. Murray Jr., "Minority Perspectives on Biomedical Ethics," in *Transcultural Dimensions in Medical Ethics,* ed. E. D. Pellegrino et al. (Frederick, Md.: University Publishing Group, 1992), 35–42.
14. K. Gergen, "Social Understanding and Conceptions of Self," in *Cultural Psychology,* ed. J. W. Stigler et al. (Cambridge, England: Cambridge University Press, 1990), 596–606.
15. J. M. Kaufert and J. D. O'Neil, "Biomedical Rituals and Informed Consent: Native Canadians and the Negotiation of the Clinical Trust," in *Social Science Perspectives on Medical Ethics,* ed. G. Weisz (Philadelphia: University of Pennsylvania Press, 1990), 41–64.
16. R. G. D'Andrade, "Cultural Meaning Systems," in *Cultural Theory: Essays on Mind, Emotion, Self,* ed. R. A. Shweder and R. Levine (Cambridge, England: Cambridge University Press, 1984), 88–119; E. Hatch, *Culture and Morality: The Relativity of Values in Anthropology* (New York: Columbia University Press, 1983);

H. Fabrega, "Cultural Relativism and Psychiatric Illness," *Journal of Nervous and Mental Disease* 177 (1989): 415–24; M. E. Spiro, "Cultural Relativism and the Future of Anthropology," *Cultural Anthropology* 1 (1986): 259–86; M. Douglas, "Morality and Culture," *Ethics* 93 (1983): 786–91; C. Geertz, "Anti-relativism," *American Anthropologist* 86 (1984): 263–78.

17. K. Brown, "Death and Access: Ethics in Cross-cultural Health Care," in *Choices and Conflict,* ed. E. Friedman (Chicago: American Hospital Association, 1992), 85–93.
18. R. A. Shweder, "Ethics Relativism: Is There a Defensible Version?" *Ethos* 18, no. 2 (1990): 219–23.
19. A. D. Renteln, "Relativism and the Search for Human Rights," *American Anthropologist* 90 (1988): 56–72.
20. P. A. Marshall, "Anthropology and Bioethics," *Medical Anthropology Quarterly* 6, no. 1 (1992): 49–73.
21. "Conference Resolves Dispute over Rights," *Chicago Tribune,* 20 June 1993, sec. 1, 14.
22. *Washington Post* News Service, "U.N. Parley Backs Human Rights Office," *The Sacramento Bee Final,* 26 June 1993, sec. A, 10.
23. Ibid.

Index

A

Abortion, 60–66
amniocentesis and, 16–20, 30–31
vs. costs of caring for disabled child, 33
distribution of interests regarding, 529
elements of middle ground on, 61–66
abortion for mere convenience is morally wrong, 62
abortion is frequently a subtly coerced decision, 64–65
abortion is killing act, 61–62
abortion is not a purely private affair, 63
abortion is tragic experience to be avoided if at all possible, 63
abortion to save life of mother is morally acceptable, 62
absolutely prohibitive law on abortion is not enforceable, 63–64
availability of contraception does not reduce number of abortions, 65
conditions leading to abortion should be abolished insofar as possible, 62–63
"consistent ethic of life" should be taken seriously, 66
hospitals need to have a policy on abortion, 65
judgment about morality of abortion is not simply a matter of a woman's determination and choice, 62
permissive laws forfeit notion of "sanctity of life" for unborn, 65
presumption against taking human life, 61
Roe v. Wade offends many people, 63
there should be alternatives to abortion, 63
there should be public policy restrictions on abortion, 64
unenforceable laws are bad laws, 63
when discussion becomes heated, it should cease, 66
witness is the most effective leaven and the most persuasive educator about abortion, 64
financial access to, 36, 41
frequency of, 62
hospital policy on, 464
moral status of, 31
pro-choice and pro-life positions on, 60
rights of surrogate mother to, 13
for sex selection, 31, 588
state funding for, 36
state restrictions on, 31, 36
wrongful-birth and wrongful-life torts and, 31–33
Absolute duties, 521–522
Abuse
of children, 11, 48, 51
domestic violence, 128–134
intergenerational transmission of, 130
Access to care, 299
abortion, 36, 41
intergenerational justice and, 353–364
for long-term care of elderly, 177–187
medical gatekeeping and, 413–420
national self-interest and, 402
new drugs, 251, 253 (*See also* Clinical trials)
preimplantation genetic diagnosis, 58
prioritizing of, 372
professional social obligations and, 385–386
rationing of health care and, 371–377 (*See also* Rationing of health care)
Securing Access to Health Care, 469
strict equality of treatment, 404
universal, 364

Acquired immunodeficiency syndrome. *See* Human immunodeficiency virus infection
Activities of daily living (ADLs), 178
Adoption, 6, 11–12, 48, 50, 51
Advance directives, 92–113, 289, 422
  case law challenges to, 110–112
  conscientious objection to, 99, 109
  cultural influences and, 423–425
  definition of, 93
  efficacy of, 94
  for emergency admissions, 99–100, 108
  filing of, 97, 102
  forms for, 102
  helping patients to complete, 102–103
  honoring of, 102, 110
    consequences of failing to honor, 111
  implementation of, 94
  information to be provided to patients about, 92, 107
  instructional, 93
  Joint Commission standard on, 106, 109–110
  nondiscrimination related to completion of, 99–100
  number of persons dying without, 291, 293
  Patient Self-Determination Act and, 94
  for persons with dementia, 189–191
  pregnancy and, 72–73
  prehospital, 141–142
  process for invoking, 96
  proxy, 93–94
  for psychiatric admissions, 101, 108
  public education about, 103–105, 108–109
  recognition between states, 96
  staff education about, 102–103
  updating of, 96
  variations in state laws about, 94
Advocacy
  for elderly persons' access to long-term care, 183–184
  equalizing, 401–402
AID. *See* Artificial insemination by donor
AIDS. *See* Human immunodeficiency virus infection
Alcohol consumption during pregnancy, 70
Alliance for the Mentally Ill, 165, 245, 246
Alpha$_1$-antitrypsin deficiency, 224
Alpha-fetoprotein testing, 25, 30, 40, 70–71
Alzheimer's Association, 183
Alzheimer's disease, 183, 189–198. *See also* Dementia
American Association for Retired Persons, 183
American Coalition of Citizens with Disabilities, 185
American Fertility Society (American Society of Reproductive Medicine), 5, 12
Americans with Disabilities Act, 39, 186
Amniocentesis, 15–22, 29–30, 57. *See also* Prenatal diagnosis
  procedure for, 15, 29
  purpose of, 18–20
  for reproductive counseling, 20–22
  risks, benefits, and eligibility criteria for, 16
    maternal age over 35, 17
    willingness to undergo abortion, 16–17
  selective abortion and therapeutic imperative, 18–20
  timing of, 29–30
  ultrasound guidance for, 30
Anencephalic infants, 334–335
  organ procurement from, 337–338
Angiotensin-converting enzyme, 224
Animal rights, 10–11
Applied ethics model, 541
  Belmont Report and, 230, 231, 241, 246, 522–523, 544
  casuistry as alternative to, 541, 542, 546 (*See also* Casuistry)
  role of principles in, 543–544
Aristotle's three types of friendship, 572–575
"Art of medicine," 554
Artificial insemination by donor (AID), 46, 48
Assisted-living facilities, 182
Autonomy, 156, 523, 571
  actual, 203, 205
  concept of negative freedom, 200
  cultural differences in importance of, 588, 590
  definition of, 201, 392, 393, 571
  dementia and, 190–191
  doctor-patient relationship and, 392–393
  in emergency department, 144
  family role in medical decision making and, 81–90
  identity and, 203–204
  liberty and, 168
  mental illness and, 165–169
  Patient Self-Determination Act, 92–113 (*See also* Advance directives; Patient Self-Determination Act)
  of persons in nursing homes, 195–196, 200–210
  professional responsibility and, 392–393
  realizing oneself, 203
  related to practicing and teaching on the newly dead, 142–143
  requests for physician-assisted death and, 303

responsibility and, 203–204
vs. safety in nursing homes, 205–207
social work perspective on, 393–395

B

Baby Doe case, 323, 460, 471, 583
Battered women. *See* Domestic violence
Behavior management for persons with dementia, 196–198
Belmont Report, 230, 231, 241, 246, 522–523, 544
Beneficence, 156, 165, 414, 522, 572
Bernardin, Cardinal Joseph, 61, 66
Bias in clinical trials, 260–261
Birth-control pills, 8
Blood transfusion
history of, 343
religious refusal of, 120–123
Bouvia case, 465, 485–486
Brain death, 330–339, 529
cardiac arrest and, 332–333
as condition for withdrawal of life support, 336
criterion for, 330
diagnosis of, 338–339
electroencephalographic activity and, 330
Harvard Criteria for diagnosis of, 335–336
higher-brain formulation of, 334–335
hypothermia and, 330
loss of homeostatic equilibrium and, 332–333
maintaining somatic existence of brain-dead pregnant woman until fetus reaches viable gestation, 333
organ procurement and, 333, 336–338
resource allocation and, 336
vs. returning to traditional cardiorespiratory standard for determining death, 335–339
tests for, 331–332
whole-brain standard for, 330, 331
alternatives to, 334–339
critique of, 331–334
inconsistencies between tests and criterion, 331–332

C

Caesarian-section births, 71
Cancer
childhood, related to prenatal exposure to X-rays, 69
cultural influences on decisions about end-of-life care for, 422–429
Capital punishment, 61, 66
Capitation, 445–446
Caregiving
devaluation of, 193–194
by family members, 181–182, 194–195
gender differences in, 194
for persons with dementia, 193–196
Caring, 437, 510–511
Case management
for chronic schizophrenics, 175
for medically fragile, technology-dependent children, 153
Casuistry, 13, 541–552, 582
as alternative to applied ethics model, 541, 542
as case-driven method, 542–543
definition of, 541, 542
history of, 541
practical problem-solving emphasis of, 541
problems with casuistical method, 546–551
conventionalism and critique, 549–550
determining whether it is really theory free, 547–548
identification of cases, 546–547
indeterminacy and consensus, 548–549
reinforcing individualism of bioethics, 550–551
revival of, 541–542
role of principles in, 543–546
derivation and meaning of principles, 543
open texture of principles, 544
priority of practice, 543–544
teaching and learning, 544–546
CDR. *See* Clinical Dementia Rating
Certification of bioethicists, 467–468
Character theories, 524, 533–535
application of, 533–535
Childrearing, 48–52
Children
abuse of, 11, 48, 51
advances in neonatology, critical care, and rehabilitation medicine for, 149–150
genetic testing of, 217
"vulnerable child syndrome," 217
impoverished or neglected, 74
medically fragile, technology-dependent, 146–162 (*See also* High-technology home care)
bringing public attention to, 151
in critical care era, 149–151
education of, 155
future of, 155–161
in polio era, 148–149
psychosocial/developmental needs of, 154–155

public policy responses to meet needs of, 151–152
reimbursement for care of, 147, 152–154, 160
service delivery to, 152, 154–155
prenatal X-ray exposure and cancer in, 69
Choice in Dying, 93, 97
Chorionic villi sampling (CVS), 15, 20, 30, 57. *See also* Prenatal diagnosis
advantages of, 30
to detect treatable defects, 23–25
procedure for, 15, 30
risks and cost of, 30
timing of, 30
Cimetidine, 235
Clinical Dementia Rating (CDR), 191
Clinical research. *See* Research on human subjects
Clinical trials, 251–257
access to new drugs and, 251, 253
attacks on traditional methods of, 252–255
beginning of, 259
bias in, 260–261
as cooperative ventures, 255, 261–262
critics of, 256–257
paternalism, 256
therapeutic obligation, 256
defenders of, 255–256
ending of, 261
experimental design of, 267–268
hard vs. soft endpoints in, 254
inclusion of representative populations in, 253–254, 260–261
moral and value judgments in, 259–261
number of participants in, 267
Phases I to IV studies, 253
protectionism and, 251–252
randomization in, 258, 260
selecting subjects for, 259–260, 268–269
understanding vs. control in, 257–258
use of placebos in, 259, 267
Cloning, 3–7
of frogs, 3
history of, 3
human, 3–7
Clonaid offer for, 3, 4
denied federal funding for, 4
possible uses for, 4–5
to prevent disease, 5
to replace a loved one, 7
to solve reproductive problems, 5–6
to supply tissues or organs for transplantation, 6–7
mammalian, 3–4
obstacles to, 4
reasons for pursuing, 3
sheep, 3, 4
scientific enthusiasm for, 3
Cognitively affective model for ethical decision making, 566–575. *See also* Ethically responsible creativity decision-making model
Commercialization of health care, 508–512
"Common-law morality," 543, 545
Communitarian position on family role in decision making, 81–88
Competency, 117–125
comprehension and, 245–247
conclusions about determination of, 123–124
definition of, 118–119, 125
essence of, 119–120
ethical decision making and, 535–536
family role in medical decision making for competent patients, 82–84
to give informed consent for human experimentation, 233–236, 245–247
importance of, 124–125
rationality and, 119–120
religious refusal of treatment, 120–123
tests of, 118–119
what it is and is not, 117–118
Confidentiality
doctor-patient relationship and, 74–75
fetal, 31
of genetic testing, 216–217
Consequentialism, 518, 531. *See also* Teleological theories
Consultation. *See* Health care ethics consultation
Continuing care retirement communities, 182
Contraception
education in schools about, 45
number of abortions related to availability of, 65
sterilization of persons with mental illness, 239–240
Cost containment, 153, 371, 416, 443–445. *See also* Managed care organizations
Costs. *See also* Funding; Reimbursement for services
of abortion vs. caring for child with disability, 33
of chorionic villi sampling, 30
of health care, 371, 419, 452, 505
of HIV drug therapy, 251
for long-term care, 180–181
of in vitro fertilization, 57
Counseling, reproductive, 20–22

- Critically ill and dying patients. *See also* Death
  - advance directives for, 92–113
  - concept of brain death, 330–339
  - family decision making for, 288–293
  - futile treatment of, 323–328
  - human cloning to replace a loved one, 7
  - improving quality of care for, 308–309
  - international perspectives on euthanasia, 311–322
    - cultural differences, 318–322
    - Germany, 315–317
    - Netherlands, 312–315, 317, 589
    - United States, 311–312, 318
  - multiculturalism, bioethics, and end-of-life care, 421–429
    - case examples, 425–428
    - disclosure of diagnosis of terminal illness, 422–423
    - use of advance directives, 423–425
  - physician-assisted death and, 302–309
    - suicide, 295–300
  - tissue waste, communities, and presumed consent, 342–349
  - use of consistent process in end-of-life ethics case consultations, 479–480
  - withdrawal of fluids and nutrition from, 198, 279–286
- Cruzan case, 94, 95, 289, 327, 471, 566, 568–569, 572, 575
- Cultural influences, 587–592. *See also* Racial-ethnic issues
  - on bioethics reasoning, 587–589
    - abortion for sexual preference, 588
    - historical importance of autonomy, 588
    - pluralism without relativism, 588–589
    - Remmelink Report, 313, 589
  - concepts, meaning, and medical morality in transnational context, 589–591
  - cultural diversity of United States, 421
  - on dealing with dying, 318–322
  - on decisions about end-of-life care, 421–429
    - case examples, 425–428
    - disclosure of diagnosis of terminal illness, 422–423
    - use of advance directives, 423–425
  - disability and, 39–41
  - high-technology home care and, 147
  - language barriers and, 590
- Cultural Pluralism and Ethical Decision-Making Project, 425
- CVS. *See* Chorionic villi sampling
- Cystic fibrosis, 57, 58
  - before-birth vs. after-birth information about, 38
  - prenatal diagnosis of, 29, 36

D

- Death, 311–322. *See also* Critically ill and dying patients
  - concept of brain death, 330–339, 529
  - criterion for, 330
  - definition of, 330
  - diagnosis of, 338–339
  - disposition of remains after, 342
  - dying in intimacy, 290–293
  - physician-assisted, 302–309
    - euthanasia, 311–322
    - suicide, 295–300
  - practicing and teaching on the newly dead, 142–143
  - returning to traditional cardiorespiratory standard for determination of, 335–339
  - "right to die," 95
  - romanticizing of, 290
  - tests for, 330–331
  - tissue waste and, 342–349
- Decision making. *See* Health care decision making
- Declaration of Helsinki, 230, 232, 240, 244
- Deinstitutionalization of schizophrenics, 164–175. *See also* Schizophrenics
- Dementia, 189–198
  - advance directives for persons with, 189–191
  - behavior control for persons with, 196–198
    - environmental modifications, 197
    - family interventions, 197
    - pharmacotherapy, 197–198
    - supportive therapy, 197
  - disclosing diagnosis of, 189–190
  - euthanasia of persons with, 198
  - hospice care for persons with, 192
  - long-term care for persons with, 183, 193–196
  - patient autonomy and, 190–191
  - quality of life and just treatment limitations for, 191–193
  - rating scale for, 191
  - research on mentally disabled persons, 239–248 (*See also* Research on human subjects)
  - viewed as terminal disease, 191, 195
  - withholding or withdrawing food and fluids from persons with, 198
- Deontological theories, 521–524, 531–533
  - absolute duties, 521–522
  - application of, 532–533

definition and description of, 517–518
Kant, 521
prima facie duties, 522
prima facie principles in medical ethics, 522–523
Depression in elderly persons, 196
Determinism, 221–222
Deutsche Gesellschaft für Humanes Sterben, 315–317
Diagnosis-related groups (DRGs), 160, 415–418
Dideoxyinosine, 254
Diethylstilbestrol (DES), 46, 70
Disability, 37–40
abortion vs. costs of caring for child with, 33
access to long-term care for elderly persons with, 177–187
Americans with Disabilities Act, 39, 186
before-birth vs. after-birth information about, 38
culture and, 39–41
disability-rights activists, 37–39
home care for medically fragile, technology-dependent children, 146–162 (*See also* High-technology home care)
prenatal diagnosis, abortion, and, 37–40
religions' views of, 39
social response to, 38
Disclosing diagnosis of terminal illness, 422–423
Discrimination
gender, 130
sex selection, 22–23, 31, 38, 218, 588
genetic, 219–220
nondiscrimination provision of Patient Self-Determination Act, 99-100
Disrespect, 10–11
DNA databanks, 219
DNA testing. *See* Genetic testing
Do not resuscitate (DNR) orders, 324, 325
without consent of patient or family, 323, 324
hospital policy on, 464
prehospital, 100, 141–142
Doctor-patient relationship, 385, 401–402
Aristotle's three types of friendship applied to, 572–575
compared with researcher-subject relationship, 229–230
confidentiality and, 74–75
contractual model of, 393
as fiduciary relationship, 229, 230, 401
informed consent and, 401–402
patient autonomy and, 392–393
physician-assisted suicide and, 297, 298
during pregnancy, 68, 72, 74–75
redressing inequality in, 401–402
related to technology and caring for elderly, 433–440
Domestic violence, 128–134
abuse of HIV-positive women, 130
asking women about, 133
impact of theory on clinical practice related to, 130–132
changing theory and incorporating context, 131–132
inadvertent retraumatization, 131
limitations of mental health models, 131
medicalization of social problems, 130
implications for training and practice, 133–134
interdisciplinary response to, 133
mandatory reporting of, 133
personal and social barriers to effective response to, 129
as social problem, 128–129
standards of care for, 128
structural constraints on response to, 132–133
systemic barriers to effective response to, 129–130
impact of medical training, 128, 129
professional socialization and intergenerational transmission of abuse, 130
Double effect principle, 312
Down's syndrome
before-birth vs. after-birth information about, 38
fluorescent in situ hybridization diagnosis of, 57
maternal age and incidence of, 17
prenatal diagnosis of, 17, 29
DRGs. *See* Diagnosis-related groups
Drug testing. *See* Clinical trials
Durable power of attorney for health care, 72, 93–94, 422. *See also* Advance directives
Duties
absolute, 521–522
prima facie, 522

E

Easter Seals, 154
Economic issues. *See* Funding; Health care as business; Reimbursement for services
Education of public. *See also* Training, professional
about advance directives, 103–105, 108–109
about medically fragile, technology-dependent children, 155
contraceptive education in schools, 45
genetic literacy, 220
Elbaum v. Grace Plaza of Great Neck, Inc., 111

Elderly persons
  access to long-term care for, 177–187 (*See also* Long-term care)
  advocates for, 183–184
  assisted-living facilities for, 182
  avoiding polypharmacy in, 197
  cared for by family members, 177, 181–182, 194–195
  continuing care retirement communities for, 182
  dementia in, 189–198 (*See also* Dementia)
  dependence of, 201
  depression in, 196
  growing numbers of, 177, 179–180, 353, 432
  health insurance for, 367–368
  income of, 181
  intergenerational justice and, 353–364
  life care at home for, 182
  respecting autonomy of persons in nursing homes, 195–196, 200–210 (*See also* Nursing homes)
  social isolation of, 196
  use of high technology for, 432–440
    relationships and caring, 437–440
Elizabeth Bouvia v. Superior Court of the State of California of the County of Los Angeles (Glenchur), 465, 485–486
Embryos. *See also* Fetus; Pregnancy
  donors of, 52–53
  human cloning, 3–7
  microsurgery on, 56
  moral status of, 11–13
  preimplantation genetic diagnosis of, 15, 16, 20, 56–58
  transplantation of, 48
Emergency medicine issues, 138–144
  advance directives in emergency situations, 100–101
  assisted suicides and emergency department resuscitations, 140–141
  determining futility of care, 140
  determining patient's decision-making capacity, 144
  emergency department as health safety net, 138–139, 402
  emergency departments that refuse care, 139
  ethical dilemmas, 138
  managed care, 139–140
  overriding patient autonomy, 144
  pain management, 144
  paternalism, 140
  practicing and teaching on the newly dead, 142–143
  prehospital advance directives or prehospital do not resuscitate orders, 141–142
  provider safety and security, 142
  research under unusual circumstances, 143–144
Entitlement theory of rights, 507
Equality and inequality in health care, 381, 399–408. *See also* Justice
  building equality, 400–404
    advocacy, 401–402
    matters of fact, 400–401
    national self-interest, 402–404
  gender-related inequalities in health insurance, 368–369
  justice, prudence, and equality, 404–408
    equality and community, 407–408
    justice and social contract, 404–405
    playing, paying, and national health insurance, 406–407
    strict equality of treatment, 404
    supernatural lottery, 405–406
  related to race and socioeconomic status, 399–400
ERC. *See* Ethically responsible creativity decision-making model
Estriol, unconjugated, 30
Ethical Issues in Professional Life, 579
Ethical relativism, 588–591
Ethically responsible creativity (ERC) decision-making model, 566–575. *See also* Health care decision making
  basic principles and, 571–572
    autonomy, 571
    beneficence, 572
    justice, 572
    nonmalfeasance, 571–572
  descriptive definition of, 567–568
  dynamic process of development of, 568
  friendship of an understanding heart, 572–575
    Aristotle's three types of friendship, 572–575
    doctor-patient relationship, 573–575
  medical-ethical data in, 571
Ethics, defined, 567
Ethics advisory groups, 464–465. *See also* Health care ethics consultation
Ethics committees, 460–469
  difficulties and needs of ethicists and, 467–469
  educational and training standards for, 491
  legal cases involving, 465, 485–486
  membership of, 465, 475–476, 477
  reporting structure of, 476, 477
  roles of, 460–465, 476–477

consultation, 464–465 (*See also* Health care ethics consultation)
institutional commitment, 463
multidisciplinary discussion, 461–462
policy formulation, 463–464
resource allocation, 462–463
staff education, 461
structural models of, 466–467
administration model, 467
governing-board model, 467
medical staff organizational model, 467
Ethnicity. *See* Cultural influences; Racial-ethnic issues
Eugenics, 36–37, 39
definition of, 239
genetic testing and, 223
Nazi racial hygienists, 239–240
prenatal diagnosis and, 36–37, 39
sterilization of persons with mental illness, 239–240
Euthanasia. *See also* Physician-assisted death
international perspectives on, 311–322
cultural differences, 318–322
Germany, 315–317
Netherlands, 312–315, 317, 589
objections to models of dying, 316–318
United States, 311–312
passive, 312
of persons with dementia, 198
vs. physician-assisted suicide, 296
selective abortion as, 18–20
U.S. laws regarding, 296
voluntary active, 302, 313
Experimental design, 267–268
open-label extension study, 267–268
randomized, double-blind, placebo-controlled clinical study, 267–268
Extracorporeal membrane oxygenation, 324, 325

F

Familial breast-ovarian cancer syndrome, 57, 58
Families U.S.A. Foundation, 183
Family
breakdown of, 48
caregiving by, 181–182, 194–195
definitions of, 49
extended, 49
genetic testing and, 212–225
new reproductive technologies and, 49–52
nuclear, 49
Family role in medical decision making, 81–90
about physician-assisted suicide, 298
communitarian defense of, 81–82, 84–86
for competent patients, 82–84
for critically ill or dying patient, 288–293
demonizing of family, 289–290
failure of communitarian challenge regarding, 86–88
family involvement, 88–90
futile treatment, 323–328
for incompetent patients, 247
system of proxies for, 293
Family systems approach to battered women, 131
Family Voices, 155
Fee-for-service model, 443–445
Fetus. *See also* Embryos; Pregnancy
abortion and rights of, 60–66
biopsy of, 15
emerging relationship between state and, 72–75
exposure to alcohol, 70
exposure to X-rays, 68–69
maternal-fetal conflicts, 69
teratogenic drugs affecting, 46, 70
visualization of, 69
Fidelity, 522, 523
Fluids, withholding of. *See* Withholding or withdrawal of life-sustaining treatment
Fluorescent in situ hybridization (FISH), 57, 217
Fragile X syndrome, 224
Friendship, 572–575
of an understanding heart, 574–575
Aristotle's three types of, 572–575
doctor-patient relationship and, 573–575
Funding. *See also* Health care as business; Reimbursement for services
for abortion, 36
for care of medically fragile, technology-dependent children, 147, 152–154, 160
for human cloning, 4
for long-term care, 179, 181–184
through voluntary/community agencies, 154
for work of hospital ethics committees, 467, 468
Futile treatment, 323–328, 460. *See also* Withholding or withdrawal of life-sustaining treatment
Baby Doe case, 323, 460, 471, 583
case law on, 323–324, 327
for chronic schizophrenia, 170
concept of physiologic futility, 325
for dementia, 191–193
do not resuscitate orders and, 324, 325
in emergency medicine, 140

extracorporeal membrane oxygenation and, 324, 325
Helga Wanglie case, 566, 569–570, 572, 575
judgments about what is in the patient's best interest, 326–327
for persons in persistent vegetative state, 323–324, 328
professional ideals and, 327
resource allocation and, 326
social consensus on, 327
statistical uncertainty and, 325–326
values and, 324–325

G

Gametes, moral status of, 11–13
Gatekeeping, medical, 453
by managed care organizations, 139–140, 153–154, 445
by physicians, 413–420
beneficence and, 414
de facto conflict of interest and, 413–414
morally obligatory, 413–415
negative, 413, 415–417
positive, 413, 415–418
Gender issues. *See also* Women
discrimination, 130
health insurance, 366–369
maintaining relationships as a value, 520–521
prenatal diagnosis and, 34–35
sex selection, 22–23, 38, 218, 588
women as caregivers, 194
Gene mapping, 213
Gene therapy, 58
Genetic counseling, 20–22, 26
Genetic diseases, 399
human cloning for prevention of, 5
preimplantation genetic diagnosis of, 56–58
prenatal diagnosis of, 15–26, 29–41
Genetic testing, 212–225
challenges in, 213–218
individual and familial, 214
professional, 215–218
confidentiality, 216–217
indications for testing, 217
informed consent, 216
limitations of testing, 217–218
quality control, 216
when to disclose information, 215–216
of children, 217
diagnostic, 223
genetic profiling, 223
ideologic archeology of clinical genetics, 221–223
professional ethos of medical genetics, 222–223
prognostic uncertainty and therapeutic impotence, 223
respect for reproductive autonomy, 223
shadow of eugenics, 223
social power of genetic information, 221–222
determinism, 221–222
familial implications, 222
reductionism, 222
new lexicon for, 223–225
policy issues related to, 218–220
genetic discrimination, 219–220
genetic literacy, 220
genetic services and public health, 218
private control of genetic information, 218–219
predictive, 223
prenatal, 15–26, 29–41, 217–218 (*See also* Prenatal diagnosis)
probabilistic, 223
prognostic, 223
prophylactic, 223
weather watching, fortunetelling, and, 213
Germany, 315–317
Gilgunn v. Massachusetts General Hospital, 111
Golden rule tradition, 380–381
Gratitude, 522

H

HCEC. *See* Health care ethics consultation
HCG. *See* Human chorionic gonadotropin
Health care as business, 505–512
caring model of health care, 510–511
commercialization of medicine, 508–512
economic egoism, 505, 507
entitlement theory of rights, 507
ideal political economy, 510
justice, 511–512
market model of health care, 505–507
moral psychology, 508–509
overlapping spheres of concern in health care, 507
professionalism, 511
technology model of health care, 507, 510
Health care costs, 371, 419, 452, 505
Health care decision making, 471, 515, 527–537. *See also* Autonomy
advance directives and, 92–113
competency for, 117–125

cultural influences on decisions about end-of-life care, 421–429
in emergency department, 144
ethically responsible creativity model for, 566–575 (*See also* Ethically responsible creativity decision-making model)
family's role in, 81–90
in home care vs. medical model, 147–148
inadequacies of present models for, 566–567
Cruzan and Wanglie cases, 568–570
information required for patients "on admission," 97–98, 107–108
informed consent for (*See* Informed consent)
key concepts and their bearing on dilemmas, 527–531
interests, 528–529
patient's moral status, 529–530
social ties, 530–531
welfare, 528
method for, 527, 535–537
in medical dilemmas, 535–536
competent patients, 535
incompetent patients, 535–536
newborns, 536
nondilemmatic, 536–537
moral decisions, 515
moral theories and, 517–524, 531–535 (*See also* Theories in medical ethics)
character theories, 524, 533–535
consequentialism (teleological theories), 518–521, 531
deontological theories, 521–524, 531–533
Patient Self-Determination Act and, 92–113
related to genetic testing, 220
religious refusals of treatment, 120–123 (*See also* Refusal of treatment)
statement of state law on, 93, 96–97
truth telling required for, 422
vagueness of terminology for, 567
Health Care Decision Making Surveys, 468
Health care ethics consultation (HCEC), 471–481, 484–494
access to, 475
accountability in, 485–486
approaches for, 474–475
certifying or accrediting programs for, 493
characteristics of, 489
combined Integrated Model for, 472
demographics of ethics consultants, 473, 478–479
description of process for, 477–478
educational and training standards for, 484–494
credentialing, certifying, or licensing and, 493
ethics committee subgroup or independent consultation team, 491–492
full ethics committee, 491
identification of, 490–491
implementation of, 492–493
individual consultants, 492
recommendations for, 492–493
as veiled power play, 487
goals of, 488
institutional settings for, 473, 474
justifiability in our society, 486–487
legal cases related to, 465, 485–486
limitations in managed care organizations, 468
limitations of study of, 480–481
maintaining disciplinary diversity in, 487
methodology for study of, 471–472
proper scope of, 489
role of ethics committees, 464–465, 476–477 (*See also* Ethics committees)
skills, knowledge, and character traits required for, 487–488
Society for Bioethics Consultation, 468, 472, 478
survey questionnaire on, 472–473
reliability and validity of, 472–473
use of consistent process in end-of-life cases, 479–480
Health Care Financing Administration, 95, 107
Health care institutional ethics, 497–504. *See also* Ethics committees
changing trends in, 497
clinical concerns, 498
human resources, 498–499
work and, 499–500
organizational identity and strategic direction, 500–502
public nature of corporation, 502–504
Health care practitioners
membership on hospital ethics committees, 465
moral universe of professions, 396
physicians and managed care organizations, 443–445
financial incentives, 443–445
utilization review and practice guidelines, 445
physicians as medical gatekeepers, 413–420 (*See also* Gatekeeping)
professional challenges in genetic testing, 215–218
professional ideals and futile treatment, 327
relationship with clients, 385 (*See also* Doctor-patient relationship)
social obligations of, 378, 383–390

social systems and professional responsibility of, 392–397
training of (*See* Training, professional)
Health care proxy, 72, 93–94
Health care reform, 452
national self-interest and, 402–404
play-or-pay approach to, 406–407
Health insurance coverage. *See also* Managed care organizations; Reimbursement for services
gender and, 366–369
elderly adults, 367–368
inequalities, 368–369
Medicaid, 368
nonelderly adults and private insurance, 366–367
reform proposals, 369
for long-term care, 182
Medicaid, 368
for medically fragile, technology-dependent children, 152–154
Medicare, 367–368
Medigap policies, 367–368
national health care insurance, 452
play-or-pay approach to, 406–407
national self-interest and, 402
for victims of domestic violence, 132–133
Health maintenance organizations (HMOs), 415, 443–445, 452. *See also* Managed care organizations
care for medically fragile, technology-dependent children, 153
characteristics of ethical HMO, 447–448
group model, 444
staff model, 444–445
Hedonism, 519
Helga Wanglie case, 566, 569–570, 572, 575
High-technology home care (HTHC), 146–162
background of, 146–147
culture and, 147
definition of home care, 147
distinction from medical model, 147–148
future of, 155–161
applying ethical principles to adult case examples, 156–158
assessing values with agreed-upon criteria, 155
considering human values in complex life situation, 155
ongoing ethical issues, 158–159
organizational planning approaches, 161
organizational strategies, 160–161
reimbursement, 160
resolving value conflicts, 155–156
reimbursement for, 147, 152–154
scope of home care practice, 147
services provided for medically fragile, technology-dependent children, 152, 154–155
educational, 155
health care, 154
psychosocial/developmental, 154–155
understanding past of, 148–152
critical care era, 149–151
advances in neonatology, critical care, and rehabilitation medicine, 149–150
initial home care experiences, 150–151
initial hospital-based solutions, 150
polio era, 148–149
community-based solutions, 149
organizational advances, 149
technological advances, 148–149
recent past, 151–152
private reimbursement practices, 152
public attention to technology-dependent children, 151
public policy to meet needs of technology-dependent children, 151–152
service delivery, 152
Hippocratic Oath, 317, 453
Hitler, Adolf, 239–240
HIV. *See* Human immunodeficiency virus infection
Home care
for elderly, 181–182
life care at home, 182
high-technology home care for medically fragile, technology-dependent children, 146–162
Homelessness and mental illness, 168–173
Honesty, 523
Hospice care, 100, 192
Hospital ethics committees. *See* Ethics committees
HTHC. *See* High-technology home care
Human chorionic gonadotropin (HCG), 30
Human cloning. *See* Cloning
Human experimentation. *See* Research on human subjects
Human genome project, 58
Human immunodeficiency virus (HIV) infection
abuse of women with, 130
access to new drugs for, 251–254
AIDS activists and their legacy for research policy, 251–262 (*See also* Clinical trials; Research policy)
AIDS dementia, 189 (*See also* Dementia)
cost of drug therapy for, 251
pregnancy and
mandatory testing, 74–75
zidovudine therapy, 74–75, 251–252

Human Life Statute, 64
Human resources issues, 498–500
Human rights tradition, 382–383
Humility, 584
Huntington's disease, 57, 224

I

IADLs. *See* Instrumental activities of daily living
Identity
  autonomy and, 203–204
  and sense of home in nursing home, 207–209
Immunization against polio, 149
In vitro fertilization (IVF), 57–58. *See also* Reproductive technologies
  cost of, 57
  efficiency of, 57–58
  preimplantation genetic diagnosis after, 57–58
Incest, 51
Incompetency. *See* Competency
Independent practice associations (IPAs), 160, 415, 443–445. *See also* Managed care organizations
Indigent persons, 399–400
  children, 74
  emergency department as health safety net for, 138–139, 402
Indignity, 10–11
Inequality. *See* Equality and inequality
Infertility. *See also* Reproductive technologies
  human cloning and, 5–6
  new reproductive technologies for, 45–54
Informed consent
  doctor-patient relationship and, 401–402
  for genetic testing, 216
  for human experimentation, 228–237, 270–275
    coercion and minimal requirements for, 235–236
    competency and, 233–236, 245–247
    content of consent forms for, 229
    cornerstones of, 244
    Declaration of Helsinki, 230, 232, 240, 244
    definitional problem of, 228–232
    ethical justification for, 236–237
    information required for, 233
    institutional review boards and, 229, 236, 241–242, 270–275
    International Covenant on Civil and Political Rights, 244
    legal requirements for, 228
    on mentally disabled persons, 244–245, 274–275
      in emergency situations, 274–275
    Nuremberg Code, 228–229, 240, 244
    risk-benefit considerations for, 233–234, 265
    Tuskegee syphilis study, 37, 240–241
    on vulnerable subjects, 234, 241–242
  language of document for, 271
  for practicing and teaching on the newly dead, 142–143
  required elements of, 270–271
  for sickle cell anemia screening, 37
  for therapy, 229
  time and place of, 271–272
  for withdrawal of fluids and nutrition, 281, 282
Institutional review boards (IRBs), 143, 229, 236, 241–242, 265–276
  meeting spirit of regulations, 266
  overview of past 25 years of, 266–267
  procedural correctness of, 266
  quality control of decisions of, 266
  review of clinical research protocol, 266–270
    commitment to research, 269
    dynamic nature of approval process, 270
    experimental design, 267–268
    method of analysis, 267
    participant number, 267
    qualifications of investigator, 269
    selection of participants, 268–269
    worth of research, 269–270
  review of informed consent for clinical research, 270–275
    consent and cognitively impaired, 274–275
    consent language, 271
    required elements of consent, 270–271
    specific consent issues, 272–274
    time and place of consent, 271–272
Instrumental activities of daily living (IADLs), 178
Insurance. *See* Health insurance coverage; Reimbursement for services
Integrated delivery systems, 160
Intensive care unit, pediatric, 149–150
Interests, 528–529
International Covenant on Civil and Political Rights, 244
International issues. *See* Cultural influences
IPAs. *See* Independent practice associations
IRBs. *See* Institutional review boards
IVF. *See* In vitro fertilization

J

Jehovah's Witnesses, 120–122, 123
Joint Commission on Accreditation of Healthcare Organizations, 106, 109–110, 485, 498

Judgments, 515–517
  character, 516, 524
  evaluative, 515–516, 524
  moral obligation, 516, 524
Justice, 156, 509, 522, 523, 572
  consensus about, 355–356
  definition of, 353–355, 572
  distributive, 354, 404
  equality and inequality in health care, 399–408
  intergenerational, 353–364
    Catholic perspective on, 356–364
    public policy and, 364
  mercy and, 363
  mutual obligation and, 354
  policy based on, 511–512
  as a principle and as a virtue, 353–354
  social contract and, 404–405

K

Kaiser Permanente, 443. *See also* Managed care organizations
Kant, Immanuel, 521
Karen Quinlan case, 283, 312, 327, 471, 544, 545
Klinefelter's syndrome, 57
Koop, C. Everett, 149, 151

L

Labor law, 500
Language barriers, 590
Least restrictive environment concept, 169
Lesch-Nyhan syndrome, 57
Libertarianism, 378–380
Liberty, 167–169
  reproductive rights, 5–6
  rights of elders in nursing homes, 202
Life care at home, 182
Life expectancy, 194
Life-sustaining treatment, 100, 471
  futile, 323–328
    Wanglie case, 566, 569–570, 572, 575
  withholding or withdrawal of, 303, 311–312
    brain death as condition for, 336
    fluids and nutrition, 279–286
    frequency of, 312
    Karen Quinlan case, 283, 312, 327, 471, 544, 545
    Nancy Cruzan case, 94, 95, 289, 327, 458–459, 471, 566, 568–569, 572, 575
    number of deaths related to, 312
Li-Fraumeni syndrome, 213–214, 221, 224
Literature and medicine studies, 554–561
  contributions to achievement in human dimensions of medicine, 555
  to gain narrative knowledge, 557–559
  goals of, 554, 561
  literary theory and, 560–561
  in medical schools, 555
  narrative ethics and, 559–560
  outcome research on, 561
  of patient's life, 555–556
  of physician's work, 556–557
Living will, 72, 92, 93, 190, 289, 422. *See also* Advance directives
Long-term care, 177–187
  access to, 180–187
    advocacy for, 183–184
    caregiving role of families, 181–182
    costs of care, 180–181
    forces for improving, 183–184
    prospects for improving, 184–187
    role of Medicaid, 182–184
    role of private insurance, 182
  alternatives for, 182
    assisted-living facilities, 182
    continuing care retirement communities, 182
    life care at home, 182
  constituencies perceiving importance of, 177
  financing of, 179, 181–184, 195
  growing need for, 178–180, 194
  for persons with dementia, 183, 193–196
  range of services needed in, 178
  respecting autonomy of persons in nursing homes, 195–196, 200–210 (*See also* Nursing homes)
Lying, 515, 517

M

Managed care organizations (MCOs), 442–448, 446–447, 452. *See also* Health insurance coverage; Reimbursement for services
  capitation in, 445–446
  characteristics of ethical health maintenance organization, 447–448
  consequences of financial incentives of, 446–447
  cost containment by, 153, 443–445
  emergency medicine and, 139–140
  vs. fee-for-service model, 443–445
  for-profit vs. nonprofit, 442–443
  funding for care of medically fragile, technology-dependent children, 153–154

gatekeepers for, 139–140, 153–154, 445
limitations on ethics consultation by, 468
physicians and, 443–445
financial incentives, 443–445
utilization review and practice guidelines, 445
professional social obligations and, 386–388
response to domestic violence, 132–133
variations among, 442
March of Dimes, 149
Market model of health care, 505–507
Maternal age
eligibility for amniocentesis based on, 17
incidence of Down's syndrome related to, 17
Maternal serum screening, 15, 25, 30, 40, 70–71
Maternal-infant bonding, 34, 35
MCOs. *See* Managed care organizations
Medicaid, 368, 406
asset sheltering and eligibility for, 183
gender and, 368
for long-term care for elderly, 182–184
for medically fragile, technology-dependent children, 152–153
Medical charts, 560
Medicare, 367–368, 452
Medicare Catastrophic Coverage Act of 1988, 185
Medigap insurance, 367–368
Mental illness
in defense of providing new type of asylum for, 173
deinstitutionalization of chronic schizophrenics, 164–175
historical perspective on, 166–168
history of medical abuse of persons with, 239–241
homelessness and, 168–173
hospitalization for, 165
imprisonment and, 171–173
noncompliance with treatment for, 165
patient autonomy and, 165–169
providing advance directive information for psychiatric admissions, 101
reform of mental health care system, 164
research on mentally disabled persons, 239–248 (*See also* Research on human subjects)
societal attention to, 165
sterilization of persons with, 239–240
Mitochondrial diseases, 5
Moral decisions, 515
Moral obligation theories, 517–524. *See also* Theories in medical ethics
Moral psychology, 508–509
Moral reference group, 8–10, 518
Moral status of patient, 529–530
Muscular dystrophy, 29
Muscular Dystrophy Association, 154

N

Nancy Cruzan case, 94, 95, 289, 327, 471, 566, 568–569, 572, 575
Narrative ethics, 559–560, 566–567
National Commission for the Protection of Human Subjects, 242, 544, 582
National Foundation for Infantile Paralysis, 149
National Institutes of Health Human Embryo Research Panel, 4
National Research Act of 1974, 241
Nazism, 239–240, 315, 517
Neonatology, 149–150
Netherlands, 312–315, 317, 588, 589
Neural tube defects, 29–30
Newborns, 536. *See also* Prenatal diagnosis
anencephalic, 334–335
organ procurement from, 337–338
NIH Revitalization Act, 254, 260, 261
Nonmalfeasance, 522, 571–572
Nuremberg Code, 228–229, 240, 244
Nursing homes, respecting autonomy of persons in, 195–196, 200–210
actual autonomy and identity, 202–204
decision to enter nursing home, 200
identity and sense of home, 207–209
access to private and communal spaces, 208–209
personal items, 207
visitors, 208
independence, rights, and paradox of autonomous life in nursing home, 200–202
institutional nature of nursing homes, 201, 204–205
misconceptions about elders in nursing homes, 209
safety vs. autonomy, 205–207
social contacts, 210
therapeutic potential of physical environment, 206
Nutrition, withholding of. *See* Withholding or withdrawal of life-sustaining treatment

O

OBRA. *See* Omnibus Budget Reconciliation Act
Office for Protection from Research Risk guidebook, 241–242

Older Americans Act, 182, 183
Omnibus Budget Reconciliation Act (OBRA), 92, 95, 106
Open-label extension study, 267–268
Opioids, high-dose, 303
Organ procurement. *See* Transplantation
Organizational identity and strategic direction, 500–502
Outcomes research, 452–458
  conflict of interest related to profits from, 457
  definition of, 453
  to generate report cards on patient care, 456–457
  on intensive care units, 455
  on literature and medicine studies, 561
  postoperative outcome, 454
  potential for depersonalization of treatment and, 457–458
  predictive accuracy of, 455–456
  severity of illness and, 454–456
  software for, 456
  steps in, 453
  subjectivity in defining outcome, 453–454
  treatment standardization based on, 454–455

P

p53 gene, 213–214, 221, 224
Pain management in emergency department, 144
Parenthood determination, 8, 9, 50
Paternalism, 392, 531
  in emergency medicine, 140
  therapeutic obligation and, 256
Paternity testing, 216
Patient Self-Determination Act (PSDA), 92–113, 498. *See also* Advance directives; Autonomy
  advance directives, 93–94
  applied to emergency admissions, 100–101, 108
  applied to psychiatric admissions, 101, 108
  background of, 93–96
  conscientious objection and, 99, 109
  ensuring compliance with, 98, 109
  five-year implementation update on, 105–113
    case law challenges to advance directives, 110–112
    Final Rule (1995), 106–109
    Interim Final Rule (1992), 106
    Joint Commission standards, 109–110
  information required for patients "on admission," 97–98, 107–108
  information to be provided to patients under, 92, 107
  nondiscrimination requirement of, 99–100
  public education about, 103–105, 108–109
  staff education about, 102–103
  statement of state law, 93, 96–97
Patients' experience of illness, 555–556
Patients' moral status, 529–530
PCR. *See* Polymerase chain reaction
Pediatric intensive care unit, 149–150
Persistent vegetative state
  futile treatment and, 323–324, 328
  guidelines for diagnosis of, 334
  higher-brain death and, 334–335
  Karen Quinlan case, 283, 312, 327, 471, 544, 545
Personnel issues, 498–499
  work and, 499–500
PGD. *See* Preimplantation genetic diagnosis
Phenylketonuria (PKU), 24–25, 219, 224
Philosophical bioethics, 578–582, 583–584
  vs. bioethics more broadly construed, 582–583
  lessons from, 584
  pragmatic reflections on, 583–584
Phronesis, 546
Physician hospital organizations (PHOs), 160
Physician-assisted death, 302–309
  clinical management of requests for, 306–308
    assure adequate comfort care, 307–308
    assure voluntariness and reasonableness of request, 308
    listen openly and evaluate underlying issues, 306–307
    share personal stance with patient, 307
  as compassionate response to suffering, 304
  definitions related to, 302
  euthanasia, 311–322 (*See also* Euthanasia)
  in Germany, 315–317
  in Netherlands, 312–315, 317, 589
  patient integrity and autonomy and, 303
  placing debate in context, 308–309
  professional integrity and, 305
  safeguards and slippery slope argument regarding, 304–305
  substituted judgment principle and, 305
  in United States, 312
  what it is not, 303
Physician-assisted suicide, 295–300
  balancing risks and benefits of, 299–300
  definition of, 296, 302
  doctor-patient relationship and, 297, 298
  documentation for, 298
  emergency department resuscitations and, 140–141
  vs. euthanasia, 296
  family and, 298

frequency of, 296, 312
method of, 298–299
policy proposal for, 296–297
proposed clinical criteria for, 297–298
public support for, 296
U.S. laws regarding, 296, 312
Physicians. *See* Doctor-patient relationship; Health care practitioners
PKU. *See* Phenylketonuria
Placebos, 259, 267
Planned Parenthood, 60
Pluralism, 425, 519–520, 588–589, 591
Point of service plans, 452
Policy issues
ethical policy subcommittees, 463–464
genetic testing, 218–220
medically fragile, technology-dependent children, 151–152
physician-assisted suicide, 296–297
policy based on precepts of justice, 511–512
rationing of health care, 376–377
research policy, 251–262 (*See also* Research policy)
Polio pandemic, 148–149
Politics, 407–408
Polymerase chain reaction (PCR), 56–57, 217, 219
Polypharmacy, 197
Poverty. *See* Indigent persons; Socioeconomic status
Preembryos, 12–13
Preferred provider organizations (PPOs), 443–445, 452. *See also* Managed care organizations
Pregnancy, 67–76. *See also* Reproductive issues
alcohol consumption during, 70
Caesarian-section births, 71
emerging relationship between state and fetus, 72–75
impact on doctor-patient relationship, 72, 74–75
implications for doctors and pregnant women, 74–75
state's expanding role in treatment of pregnant women, 72–74
widespread use of unproved technologies, 72
ethical dilemmas about treatment of, 67–68
"good" vs. "bad" pregnant women, 70–71, 76
high technology and emergence of fetus as "patient," 68–71
maternal-doctor conflicts, 69–71
visualizing fetus, 69
X-ray exposure, 68–69
HIV infection and
mandatory testing for, 74–75
zidovudine for, 74–75, 251–252
maintaining somatic existence of brain-dead pregnant woman until fetus reaches viable gestation, 333
maternal-doctor relationship, 68
Preimplantation genetic diagnosis (PGD), 15, 16, 20, 56–58
access to, 58
for carriers of genetic diseases, 58
ethics of, 57–58
technology for, 56–57
creation of zona pellucida, 56
fluorescent in situ hybridization, 57
polymerase chain reaction, 56–57
timing of, 56
Prenatal diagnosis, 15–26, 29–41, 217–218
criticisms of, 33–41
diversity and reductionism, 35, 39–41
gender issues, 34–35
meaning and experience of disability, 37–39
racial-ethnic and class issues, 35–37, 41
to detect treatable defects, 23–25
fetal confidentiality and, 31
fetus as patient in, 18
financial access to, 36
maternal-infant bonding and, 34, 35
opponents of, 33–34
parental responsibility and, 31–33
public health uses of, 25–26
purpose of, 18–20
religions' views of, 39
risks, benefits, and eligibility criteria for, 16–18
selective abortion and therapeutic imperative, 18–20, 30–31
for sex selection, 22–23, 38, 218
support for, 31–33
techniques for, 15, 29–31, 57 (*See also* specific techniques)
amniocentesis, 15–22, 29–30
chorionic villi sampling, 15, 30
maternal serum screening, 15, 30
ultrasound, 30
uncertainty and ethics of reproductive counseling, 20–22
women's responses to offer of screening, 70–71
wrongful-birth and wrongful-life torts and, 31–33
Prenatal treatment, 19
President's Commission for the Study of Ethical Problems in Medicine and Biomedical and Behavioral Research, 485, 582
President's Commission on Mental Health, 169
Prevention of disease, human cloning for, 5
Prima facie duties, 522

Prima facie principles in medical ethics, 522–523
Primary care networks, 415
Principles of Biomedical Ethics, 578–579
Principlism, 515, 571–572. *See also* Theories in medical ethics
Prison population and mental illness, 171–173
Privacy, 543
Pro-choice and pro-life positions, 60–66. *See also* Abortion
Professional Ethics, 579
Prospective payment systems, 415–417
PSDA. *See* Patient Self-Determination Act

Q

Quality control in genetic testing, 216
Quality of life, 419–420
  and just treatment limitations for dementia, 191–193
  withdrawal of fluids and nutrition and, 285–286
Quinlan case, 283, 312, 327, 471, 544, 545

R

Racial-ethnic issues. *See also* Cultural influences
  eugenic practices, 36–37
  prenatal diagnosis and, 35–37, 41
  racism, 399–400
Randomized, double-blind, placebo-controlled clinical study, 267–268
Randomized clinical trials, 258, 260
Rationing of health care, 371–377
  definition of, 371–373
  due to inability to pay, 372
  equitable application of policies for, 375
  ethics of, 373–374
  ethics of medical gatekeeping, 413–420 (*See also* Gatekeeping)
  ideal conditions for, 374
  inevitability of, 419–420
  justifying in real world, 374–375
  self-imposed limits for, 375
  social-ethical concomitants of, 418–419
  who makes decisions about, 375–377
Reductionism, 35, 39–41, 222
Refusal of treatment, 422
  based on religious beliefs, 120–123
  competency and, 117–125
  by emergency departments, 139
  Karen Quinlan case, 283, 312, 327, 471, 544, 545
  Nancy Cruzan case, 94, 95, 289, 327, 471, 566, 568–569, 572, 575
  withdrawal of fluids and nutrition, 198, 279–286
Reimbursement for services, 462–463. *See also* Health insurance coverage; Managed care organizations
  in future, 160
  in managed care organizations, 443–446
  for medically fragile, technology-dependent children, 147, 152–154, 160
  for victims of domestic violence, 132–133
Relativism, ethical, 588–591
Religious beliefs
  about prenatal diagnosis and disability, 39
  casuistic ethics and, 541–542
  Catholic perspective on intergenerational justice, 353–364
  court judgments about, 121
  differentiating from religious delusions, 122
  refusal of treatment based on, 120–123
Remmelink Report, 313, 589
Reparation, 522
Reproductive issues
  abortion, 60–66
  determination of parenthood, 8, 50
  diversity and reductionism, 35, 39–41
  eugenic practices, 36–37
  human cloning, 3–7
  moral status of gametes and embryos, 8–13
  parental responsibility and right to reproduce, 31–33
  pregnancy and medical ethics in 21st century, 67–76
  preimplantation genetic diagnosis and embryo selection, 56–58
  prenatal diagnosis, 15–26, 29–41
  reproductive counseling, 20–22
  reproductive technologies, 45–54
  sterilization of persons with mental illness, 239–240
  ways to create a baby, 9
Reproductive rights, 5–6
  liberty rights, 5–6
  welfare rights, 6
Reproductive technologies, 45–54
  availability to single persons or homosexual couples, 51
  basis for developing ethical position on, 46–47
  determination of parenthood related to, 8, 9
  family and, 49–52
    child, 51–52
    parents and spouses, 50–51
  human cloning, 5–6
  inadequate approaches to ethical assessment of, 45–46

moral status of gametes and embryos, 11–13
proposed ethical standard for, 47–48
social systems and, 48
surrogate mothers, 13, 48, 53
using third-party donors, 48, 50–53
cultural ethos and, 52–53
Research on human subjects, 228–237
in acute care, 143–144
categories of, 232
clinical research protocol for, 266–270
commitment to research, 269
experimental design, 267–268
method of analysis, 267
participant number, 267
qualifications of investigator, 269
selection of participants, 268–269
worth of research, 269–270
cloning, 3–7
"Common Rule" on, 241
definition of experimentation, 231
informed consent for, 228–237, 270–275 (*See also* Informed consent)
innovations and nonvalidated practices, 231
institutional review boards and, 229, 236, 241–242, 265–276 (*See also* Institutional review boards)
mentally disabled persons, 239–248
abuses, 242–244
federal laws on, 241–242
guidelines for future, 245–247
legal competence, 245–247
morally justified experiments, 247
therapeutic vs. nontherapeutic research, 245
history of medical abuse, 239–241
informed consent for, 244–245, 274–275
in emergency situations, 274–275
morally justified experiments, 247
National Commission for the Protection of Human Subjects, 242
Office for Protection from Research Risk guidebook on, 241–242
outcomes research, 452–458
radiation experiments, 247
requirements for, 240
researcher-subject relationship, 229–230
risk-benefit considerations for, 233–234, 265
therapeutic vs. nontherapeutic, 230–232, 245
Tuskegee syphilis study, 37, 240–241
Universal Moral Principles for, 247
vulnerable subjects, 234, 241–242
Research policy, 251–262
case for research as cooperative venture, 261–262
concept of understanding vs. control, 257–258
critics of research as cooperative venture, 255–257
critics of traditional clinical trials, 256–257
defenders of traditional clinical trials, 255–256
influence of AIDS activists on, 251–252
moral and value judgments, 259–261
beginning trials, 259
bias, 260–261
ending trials, 261
randomization, 258, 260
selecting subjects, 259–260
using placebos, 259, 267
traditional methods under attack, 252–255
Resource allocation
brain death and, 336
futility and, 326
hospital ethics committees' role in, 462–463
intergenerational justice and, 353–364
under managed care, 386
professional social obligations and distribution of care, 385–386
vs. rationing of health care, 372–373
scarce resources and organ donations, 343, 345–346
universal access to health care, 364
Resource-based relative value scale, 160
Respect, 10–11
for autonomy of persons in nursing homes, 195–196, 200–210
for life, 523
for persons, 523
for reproductive autonomy, 223
Resuscitation, 288
assisted suicide and, 140–141
do not resuscitate (DNR) orders
futility and, 324, 325
prehospital, 100, 141–142
"Right to die," 95
Risk assessment, genetic. *See* Genetic testing
Roe v. Wade, 61–64. *See also* Abortion

S

Safety
vs. autonomy in nursing homes, 205–207
domestic violence, 128–134
in emergency department, 142
"Sanctity of life" for unborn, 65. *See also* Abortion
Scapegoating within family, 51
Schizophrenics
deinstitutionalization of, 164–175
background of, 164–168
concept of least restrictive environment, 169

in defense of providing new type of asylum, 173
factors contributing to impetus for, 164–165
futility of treatment and, 170
homelessness and, 168–173
prison populations and, 171–173
related to right to life, liberty, and pursuit of happiness, 168–169
socioethical dilemmas in treatment, 169–170
statistical data on, 170–173
informed consent for research on, 245
washout/relapse experiments on, 243
Screening, prenatal. *See* Prenatal diagnosis
Securing Access to Health Care, 469
Self-improvement, 522
Senility. *See* Dementia
Sex selection, 22–23, 38, 218
abortion for, 31, 588
Sexual harassment, 130
Sickle cell disease, 29, 37
Social obligations, 378–390
conflict of, 388–390
golden rule tradition, 380–381
of health care practitioners, 378, 383–386
central values, 385
distribution of care, 385–386
expertise, 384
impact on central values, 385
individual and collective control, 384–385
managed care and, 386–388
relationship to clients, 385
sacrifice and limits of professional obligation, 386
human rights tradition, 382–383
libertarianism, 378–380
utilitarianism, 382
Social problems
abortion, 60–66
bioethics as social problem solving, 578–584
deinstitutionalized chronic schizophrenics, 164–175
disability, 37–40
domestic violence, 128–134
genetic services, 218
intergenerational justice, 353–364
medicalization of, 130, 139
prenatal diagnosis, 25–26
rationing of health care, 371–377
Social Services Block Grants, 182, 183
Social systems and professional responsibility, 392–397
moral universe of professions, 396
social work perspective, 396–397
new bioethics and, 395–396
new model of autonomy and, 392–393
social work perspective, 393–395
Social ties, 530–531
Society for Bioethics Consultation, 468, 472, 478
Society for Health and Human Values, 555
Socioeconomic status, 399–400. *See also* Indigent persons
prenatal diagnosis and, 35–37, 41
Spouse abuse. *See* Domestic violence
Stavudine, 255
Stepfamilies, 51
Substance abuse among women, 130
Substituted judgment, 305, 569
Suicide
assisted, in Germany, 315–317
physician-assisted, 295–300, 302 (*See also* Physician-assisted suicide)
prehospital advance directives and prehospital do not resuscitate orders, 141–142
protection of suicidal persons, 141
Surrogate mothers, 13, 48, 53

T

Tay-Sachs disease, 57
Technology, 460, 471
futile treatment, 323–328, 460
home care for medically fragile, technology-dependent children, 146–162 (*See also* High-technology home care)
human relationships and, 433–437
reproductive, 45–54 (*See also* Reproductive technologies)
technology model of health care, 507, 510
use for elderly persons, 432–440
relationships and caring, 437–440
withholding or withdrawal of life-sustaining treatment, 303, 311–312
Teleological theories, 518–521, 531
act vs. rule approach, 521
application of, 531
definition and description of, 517
moral reference group, 8–10, 518
principle of teleologism, 518
theories of value, 518–521
hedonism, 519
maintaining relationships as a value, 520–521
pluralism, 519–520

subjective preference, 519
values in medicine, 520
Teratogenic drugs, 46, 70, 72
Terminally ill patients. *See* Critically ill and dying patients; Death
Thalidomide, 46, 70, 72
Theories in medical ethics, 515–525
ethical judgments, 515–517
moral decisions, 515
narrative approaches, 524–525
theories of character, 524, 533–535
theories of moral obligation, 517–524
definitions and descriptions of, 517–518
deontological theories, 521–524, 531–533
absolute duties, 521–522
Kant, 521
prima facie duties, 522
prima facie principles in medical ethics, 522–523
utilitarianism and other teleological theories, 518–521, 531
act vs. rule approach, 521
moral reference group, 8–10, 518
theories of value, 517–521
Tissue waste, 342–349
Training, professional
about advance directives, 102–103
about domestic violence, 128, 129, 133–134
for ethics consultation, 484–494
hospital ethics committees' role in, 461
practicing and teaching on the newly dead, 142–143
Transplantation
allowing donation of organs for, 343–344
casuist approach to funding for heart transplantation, 550–551
community, justice, and mutual obligation related to, 344–345
history of, 342–343
human cloning to supply tissues or organs for, 6–7
objections to customary tissue salvage for, 346–347
fears of violating symbols, 347–348
possible resolution, 347–349
procuring organs for, 337–338
from anencephalic infants, 337–338
brain death and, 333, 336–338
justified killing for, 338, 339
presumed consent for, 344, 348–349
scarce resources and organ donations for, 343, 345–346
just distribution of, 372, 374
tissue waste and, 342–349
Trisomies, prenatal diagnosis of, 17, 29, 57
Turner's syndrome, 57
Tuskegee syphilis study, 37, 240–241

U

Ultrasound, prenatal, 30, 69
Unconjugated estriol, 30
Unconsciousness, death and, 334–335
Uniform Determination of Death Act, 330
United Cerebral Palsy, 154
United Way, 154
Universality, 380
Utilitarianism, 382, 518, 531. *See also* Teleological theories
Utilization review, 445. *See also* Gatekeeping

V

Values
assessing with agreed-upon criteria, 155
in complex life situations, 155
futile treatment and, 324–325
interests, 528–529
professional social obligations and, 385
resolving conflicts about, 155–156
theories of value, 518–521
hedonism, 519
maintaining relationships as a value, 520–521
pluralism, 519–520
subjective preference, 519
values in medicine, 520
Ventilator-dependent children. *See* Children, medically fragile, technology-dependent
Violence
child abuse, 11, 48, 51
domestic, 128–134
in emergency department, 142
Virtues, 524

W

Wanglie case, 566, 569–570, 572, 575
Washington University Clinical Dementia Rating (CDR), 191
Webster v. Reproductive Health Services, 36
Welfare concept, 528
Welfare dependency, 403
Wilmut, Ian, 3, 4

Withholding or withdrawal of life-sustaining treatment, 303, 311–312, 460. *See also* Futile treatment
brain death as condition for, 336
fluids and nutrition, 198, 279–286
benefit vs. burden of treatment, 283–284, 286
bodily integrity of patient and, 281–282
distinction between food and drink and nutrition and hydration, 280–281
doctor-patient relationship and, 284
easing discomfort of terminal illness, 284–285
ethical justification for, 279
Helga Wanglie case, 566, 569–570, 572, 575
informed consent for, 281, 282
as issue of cure vs. care, 280
Karen Quinlan case, 283, 312, 327, 471, 544, 545
Nancy Cruzan case, 94, 95, 289, 327, 471, 566, 568–569, 572, 575
purpose of artificial feeding, 280
quality of life and, 285–286
frequency of, 312
impact on staff, 462
in the Netherlands, 312
number of deaths related to, 312
in United States, 311–312
Women. *See also* Gender issues
abuse of, 128–134 (*See also* Domestic violence)
application of feminist literary methods to physician-patient interactions, 560–561
as caregivers, 194
health insurance for, 366–369
elderly adults, 367–368
inequalities, 368–369
Medicaid, 368
nonelderly adults and private insurance, 366–367
reform proposals, 369
HIV-infected, 130
inclusion in clinical trials, 253–254
moral issues of feminists, 546
substance abuse among, 130
Work and human resources, 499–500
Wrongful-birth torts, 31–32
Wrongful-life torts, 6, 31–33

X

X-rays during pregnancy, 68–69

Z

Zidovudine
clinical trials of, 258, 261
given during pregnancy, 74–75, 251–252